Communities in Action
Pathways to Health Equity

Committee on Community-Based Solutions to Promote
Health Equity in the United States

James N. Weinstein, Amy Geller, Yamrot Negussie,
and Alina Baciu, *Editors*

Board on Population Health and Public Health Practice

Health and Medicine Division

A Report of

The National Academies of
SCIENCES • ENGINEERING • MEDICINE

THE NATIONAL ACADEMIES PRESS
Washington, DC
www.nap.edu

THE NATIONAL ACADEMIES PRESS   500 Fifth Street, NW   Washington, DC 20001

This activity was supported by the Robert Wood Johnson Foundation under contract number 72444. Any opinions, findings, conclusions, or recommendations expressed in this publication do not necessarily reflect the views of any organization or agency that provided support for the project.

Library of Congress Cataloging-in-Publication Data

Names: Weinstein, James N., editor. | Geller, Amy (Amy B.), editor. |
  Negussie, Yamrot, editor. | Baciu, Alina, editor. | National Academies of
  Sciences, Engineering, and Medicine (U.S.). Committee on Community-Based
  Solutions to Promote Health Equity in the United States, issuing body.
Title: Communities in action : pathways to health equity / James N.
  Weinstein, Amy Geller, Yamrot Negussie, and Alina Baciu, editors.
Description: Washington, DC : National Academies Press, 2017. | Includes
  bibliographical references.
Identifiers: LCCN 2017005055 | ISBN 9780309452960 (paperback) | ISBN
  0309452961 (paperback) | ISBN 9780309452977 (pdf)
Subjects: | MESH: Health Equity | Healthcare Disparities | Community Health
  Planning | Health Promotion | Socioeconomic Factors | United States
Classification: LCC RA418 | NLM W 76 AA1 | DDC 362.1—dc23 LC record available at https://lccn.loc.gov/2017005055

Digital Object Identifier: 10.17226/24624

Additional copies of this publication are available for sale from the National Academies Press, 500 Fifth Street, NW, Keck 360, Washington, DC 20001; (800) 624-6242 or (202) 334-3313; http://www.nap.edu.

Copyright 2017 by the National Academy of Sciences. All rights reserved.

Printed in the United States of America

Suggested citation: National Academies of Sciences, Engineering, and Medicine. 2017. *Communities in action: Pathways to health equity*. Washington, DC: The National Academies Press. doi: 10.17226/24624.

The National Academies of
SCIENCES • ENGINEERING • MEDICINE

The **National Academy of Sciences** was established in 1863 by an Act of Congress, signed by President Lincoln, as a private, nongovernmental institution to advise the nation on issues related to science and technology. Members are elected by their peers for outstanding contributions to research. Dr. Marcia McNutt is president.

The **National Academy of Engineering** was established in 1964 under the charter of the National Academy of Sciences to bring the practices of engineering to advising the nation. Members are elected by their peers for extraordinary contributions to engineering. Dr. C. D. Mote, Jr., is president.

The **National Academy of Medicine** (formerly the Institute of Medicine) was established in 1970 under the charter of the National Academy of Sciences to advise the nation on medical and health issues. Members are elected by their peers for distinguished contributions to medicine and health. Dr. Victor J. Dzau is president.

The three Academies work together as the **National Academies of Sciences, Engineering, and Medicine** to provide independent, objective analysis and advice to the nation and conduct other activities to solve complex problems and inform public policy decisions. The National Academies also encourage education and research, recognize outstanding contributions to knowledge, and increase public understanding in matters of science, engineering, and medicine.

Learn more about the National Academies of Sciences, Engineering, and Medicine at **www.national-academies.org**.

The National Academies of
SCIENCES · ENGINEERING · MEDICINE

Reports document the evidence-based consensus of an authoring committee of experts. Reports typically include findings, conclusions, and recommendations based on information gathered by the committee and committee deliberations. Reports are peer reviewed and are approved by the National Academies of Sciences, Engineering, and Medicine.

Proceedings chronicle the presentations and discussions at a workshop, symposium, or other convening event. The statements and opinions contained in proceedings are those of the participants and are not necessarily endorsed by other participants, the planning committee, or the National Academies of Sciences, Engineering, and Medicine.

For information about other products and activities of the National Academies, please visit nationalacademies.org/whatwedo.

COMMITTEE ON COMMUNITY-BASED SOLUTIONS TO PROMOTE HEALTH EQUITY IN THE UNITED STATES

JAMES N. WEINSTEIN (*Chair*), Dartmouth-Hitchcock Health System
HORTENSIA DE LOS ANGELES AMARO, University of Southern California School of Social Work and Keck School of Medicine
ELIZABETH BACA, California Governor's Office of Planning and Research
B. NED CALONGE, University of Colorado and The Colorado Trust
BECHARA CHOUCAIR, Kaiser Permanente (*formerly Trinity Health until November 2016*)
ALISON EVANS CUELLAR, George Mason University
ROBERT H. DUGGER, ReadyNation and Hanover Provident Capital, LLC
CHANDRA FORD, University of California, Los Angeles, Fielding School of Public Health
ROBERT GARCÍA, The City Project and Charles Drew University of Medicine and Science
HELENE D. GAYLE, McKinsey Social Initiative
ANDREW GRANT-THOMAS, EmbraceRace
SISTER CAROL KEEHAN, Catholic Health Association of the United States
CHRISTOPHER J. LYONS, University of New Mexico
KENT McGUIRE, Southern Education Foundation
JULIE MORITA, Chicago Department of Public Health
TIA POWELL, Montefiore Health System
LISBETH SCHORR, Center for the Study of Social Policy
NICK TILSEN, Thunder Valley Community Development Corporation
WILLIAM W. WYMAN, Wyman Consulting Associates, Inc.

Study Staff

AMY GELLER, Study Director
YAMROT NEGUSSIE, Research Associate
SOPHIE YANG, Research Assistant (*from June 2016*)
ANNA MARTIN, Senior Program Assistant
ALINA BACIU, Senior Program Officer (*from October 2016*)
MICAELA HALL, Intern (*from June 2016 to August 2016*)
HOPE HARE, Administrative Assistant
ROSE MARIE MARTINEZ, Senior Board Director
DORIS ROMERO, Financial Associate

National Academy of Medicine/American Academy of Nursing/American Nurses Association/American Nurses Foundation Distinguished Nurse Scholar-in-Residence
SUZANNE BAKKEN, Columbia University School of Nursing

James C. Puffer, M.D./American Board of Family Medicine Fellowship
KENDALL M. CAMPBELL, East Carolina University, Brody School of Medicine

Consultants
ARIEL COLLINS, The City Project
DEBORAH KIMBELL, The Dartmouth Institute for Health Policy and Clinical Practice
NANCY NEGRETE, The City Project
RON SUSKIND, Harvard Law School
MAKANI THEMBA, Higher Ground Change Strategies
CESAR DE LA VEGA, The City Project
SUNMOO YOON, Columbia University

Reviewers

This report has been reviewed in draft form by individuals chosen for their diverse perspectives and technical expertise. The purpose of this independent review is to provide candid and critical comments that will assist the institution in making its published report as sound as possible and to ensure that the report meets institutional standards for objectivity, evidence, and responsiveness to the study charge. The review comments and draft manuscript remain confidential to protect the integrity of the deliberative process. We wish to thank the following individuals for their review of this report:

DOLORES ACEVEDO-GARCIA, Brandeis University
MARION DANIS, National Institutes of Health Clinical Center
JOSÉ J. ESCARCE, University of California, Los Angeles
RAUL GUPTA, West Virginia Bureau for Public Health
MEGAN HABERLE, Poverty and Race Research Action Council (PRRAC)
ROBERT A. HAHN, U.S. Centers for Disease Control and Prevention, Community Guide Branch
VALARIE BLUE BIRD JERNIGAN, University of Oklahoma Health Sciences Center
HOWARD KOH, Harvard T.H. Chan School of Public Health
MARGARET LEVI, Stanford University
MAHASIN S. MUJAHID, University of California, Berkeley
ADEWALE TROUTMAN, University of South Florida

WILLIAM A. VEGA, University of Southern California School of Social Work
CHRISTOPHER WILDEMAN, Cornell University
EARNESTINE WILLIS, Medical College of Wisconsin

Although the reviewers listed above have provided many constructive comments and suggestions, they were not asked to endorse the conclusions or recommendations nor did they see the final draft of the report before its release. The review of this report was overseen by **JACK EBELER** and **SARA ROSENBAUM,** the George Washington University Milken Institute School of Public Health. They were responsible for making certain that an independent examination of this report was carried out in accordance with institutional procedures and that all review comments were carefully considered. Responsibility for the final content of this report rests entirely with the authoring committee and the institution.

Preface

Our nation's founders wrote that all people are created equal with the right to "life, liberty, and the pursuit of happiness." Therefore, the principles of equality and equal opportunity are deeply rooted in our national values, and in the notion that everyone has a fair shot to succeed with hard work. However, our nation's social and economic well-being depends in part on the well-being of its communities, and many are facing great and evolving challenges. Across the country there are communities with insufficient access to jobs, adequate transit, safe and affordable housing, parks and open space, healthy food options, or quality education—the necessary conditions and opportunities to fully thrive. This lack of opportunity is particularly evident in the disparities that exist in health status and health outcomes between different zip codes or census tracts.

Other wealthy developed countries outperform the United States in health status, despite our high level of spending on health care. For example, not only does the nation's life expectancy when compared to peer nations lag behind,[1] but life expectancy in the United States also varies dramatically—by roughly 15 years for men and 10 years for women—depending on income level, education, and where a person lives. In the poorest parts of the country, rates of obesity, heart disease, cancer, diabetes, stroke, and kidney disease are substantially higher than in more affluent regions. Tragically, infant mortality—the number of deaths under

---

[1] National Research Council and Institute of Medicine. 2013. *U.S. health in international perspective: Shorter lives, poorer health.* Washington, DC: The National Academies Press.

1 year of age per 1,000 live births—is much higher in certain populations. In 2013, among non-Hispanic whites, 5.06 infants of every 1,000 live births died before their first birthday; among African Americans, that rate was double, at 11.1 per 1,000.[2] Rates were also higher for Native American (7.61 per 1,000) and Puerto Rican (5.93 per 1,000) infants, as well as for low-income white infants in the Appalachian region, where in 2012, 7.6 infants died for every 1,000 live births.[3] Research has shown that access to health care is important, but it is not sufficient to improve health outcomes (see, for example, Hood et al., 2016[4]). To change the current state will require addressing the underlying social, economic, and environmental factors that contribute to health inequities. This report has examined the evidence on the current status of health disparities as well as the research examining the underlying conditions that lead to poor health and health inequities.

It will take local, state, and national leadership in the public and private sectors to improve the underlying conditions of inequity, and that will take time. However, there is great promise in communities that are taking action against health inequities across the United States. Moreover, advancements in the use of large disparate, population-based data with sophisticated analytic tools allow us to be more focused on possible solutions that tackle the multiple factors that shape health in communities. New partners in education, transportation, housing, planning, public health, business, and beyond are joining forces with community members to promote health equity. In this report the committee examines and shares examples of solutions implemented in several communities in the hope that other communities might adapt relevant elements and lessons learned to foster community-based approaches in their own unique environments. The report presents thorough evidence that health equity adds an important perspective in trying to improve community well-being, economic vitality, and social vibrancy.

During the committee's time together, while reviewing the large body of scientific evidence and hearing from expert researchers on the social, economic, and environmental factors that affect health, several public health crises surfaced, including lead-contaminated water poisoning of children and other residents in Flint, Michigan, and the worsening opioid

---

[2] Mathews, T. J., M. F. MacDorman, and M. E. Thoma. 2015. *Infant mortality statistics from the 2013 period linked birth/infant death data set.* Hyattsville, MD: National Center for Health Statistics.

[3] Children's Defense Fund. 2016. *Ohio's Appalachian children at a crossroads: A roadmap for action.* Columbus, OH: Children's Defense Fund-Ohio.

[4] Hood, C. M., K. P. Gennuso, G. R. Swain, and B. B. Catlin. 2016. County health rankings: Relationships between determinant factors and health outcomes. *American Journal of Preventive Medicine* 50(2):129–135.

drug epidemic primarily affecting low-income people in rural communities across the country. These events are not the first of their kind, but they underscore the potential to galvanize public attention on health inequity at the community level.

In preparing this report, the committee took seriously its charge to review the state of health disparities and explore the underlying conditions and root causes that contribute to health inequity in order to inform much-needed efforts to reverse such inequities. The committee urges looking at disparities through the lens of health equity, as well as from other perspectives, to inform the changes necessary to improve the well-being of communities and our nation. The committee's recommendations are offered with a focus on health equity as an essential component of health and well-being, but also with an awareness of the work at many levels necessary to address the myriad of challenges facing those most in need.

Health inequities are a problem for us all: the burden of disparities in health adversely affects our nation's children, our business efficiency and competitiveness, our economic strength, national security, our standing in the world, and our national character and commitment to justice and fairness of opportunity.

This committee is grateful to the Robert Wood Johnson Foundation for the opportunity to delve deeply into the nature and causes of health inequity, to understand the critical need for solutions, and to examine the inspirational work that is being done in many communities to improve their well-being for themselves and for generations to come. It is the committee's hope that this report will inform, educate, and ultimately inspire others to join in efforts across the nation so that members of all communities can enjoy life, liberty, and the pursuit of happiness undeterred by poor health.

James N. Weinstein, *Chair*
Committee on Community-Based Solutions to
Promote Health Equity in the United States

Acknowledgments

The committee wishes to acknowledge and thank the many individuals and organizations that contributed to the study process and the development of *Communities in Action: Pathways to Health Equity*. Their contributions significantly enriched the committee's information gathering and enhanced the quality of this report.

To begin, the committee would like to thank the sponsor of this study. Support for the committee's work was provided by the Robert Wood Johnson Foundation.

The committee found the perspectives of multiple individuals and groups immensely helpful in informing its deliberations through presentations and discussions that took place at the committee's public meetings. The speakers whose presentations informed the committee's work include, in order of appearance, Steven H. Woolf, Camara Jones, Rachel Davis, Richard Hofrichter, Edward Ehlinger, Martha Halko, Gregory Brown, Anna Ricklin, Sam Zimbabwe, Robert Bullard, Marianne Engelman Lado, Thomas LaVeist, David Zuckerman, Michelle Chuk Zamperetti, Katie Loovis, Doran Schrantz, Nina Wallerstein, Manal Aboelata, Beatriz Solís, and David Erickson. The public meeting agendas are provided in Appendix C.

The committee also greatly appreciated the input of the Association of State and Territorial Health Officials, National Association of County and City Health Officials, Mildred Thompson at PolicyLink, Prevention Institute, Liz Welch at Thunder Valley Community Development Corporation, and Richard Wood at the University of New Mexico.

The committee extends its utmost gratitude to the individuals who served as consultants to the committee by sharing their time and expertise during the writing of this report. They were instrumental to the study process as the committee explored the complex issues of health inequity and the role of community-based solutions in advancing equity. These individuals include Ariel Collins, Deborah Kimbell, Nancy Negrete, Ron Suskind, Makani Themba, Julie Troccio, Cesar De La Vega, William Weeks, and Sunmoo Yoon.

The committee is especially grateful to the nine inspiring communities highlighted in this report for generously sharing their experiences, challenges, and achievements. Specifically, the committee would like to thank Sasha Cotton and Gretchen Musicant (Minneapolis Blueprint for Action to Prevent Youth Violence); John Fairman and Neuaviska Stidhum (Delta Health Center); Juan Leyton, Andrew Seeder, and Harry Smith (Dudley Street Neighborhood Initiative); Mary Ellen Burns, Henrietta Muñoz, Sebastian Schreiner, and Jeniffer Richardson (Eastside Promise Neighborhood); Shoshanna Spector (Indianapolis Congregation Action Network); Patricia Bowie, Ron Brown, and Lila Guirguis (Magnolia Community Initiative); Trisha Chakrabarti and Dana Harvey (Mandela MarketPlace); Clarke Gocker, Ahmad Nieves, and Julia White (People United for Sustainable Housing, Buffalo); and Peggy Shepard (WE ACT for Environmental Justice).

The committee thanks the National Academies of Sciences, Engineering, and Medicine staff who contributed to the production of this report, including study staff Amy Geller, Yamrot Negussie, Sophie Yang, Anna Martin, Alina Baciu, Micaela Hall, Hope Hare, and Rose Marie Martinez. The committee thanks the National Academies communications and report production staff, including Greta Gorman, Nicole Joy, Sarah Kelley, and Tina Ritter. Thanks also to other staff of the Board on Population Health and Public Health Practice who provided occasional support. The committee was also fortunate to have support from Suzanne Bakken and Kendall Campbell, who contributed their time and expertise throughout the report development. This project received valuable assistance from Daniel Bearss and Ellen Kimmel (National Academies Research Center); Dana Korsen and Jennifer Walsh (Office of News and Public Information); Doris Romero (Office of Financial Administration); and Clyde Behney, Chelsea Frakes, Lauren Shern, and colleagues (Health and Medicine Division Executive Office and Office of Review and Communications).

Finally, the National Academies staff offers additional thanks to the executive assistants of committee members, without whom scheduling the multiple committee meetings and conference calls would have been nearly impossible: Sandra Aponte, Tiffany Eckert, Robbie Fox-Dunigan, Maria Gallegos, Chandra Halstead, Faith Johnston, Ruth Ann Keister, Lorena Maldonado, Cheryl Mance, Justin Nguyen, and Lauren Pell.

Contents

ACRONYMS AND ABBREVIATIONS	xix
KEY TERMS	xxiii
SUMMARY	1
1 THE NEED TO PROMOTE HEALTH EQUITY	**31**

Introduction, 31
Defining Health Equity, 32
Disparities in Health Outcomes, 33
Social Determinants of Health, 38
Impacts of Health Inequity in the United States, 38
Changing Social and Environmental Context, 41
Why Communities?, 43
Momentum for Achieving Health Equity, 43
About This Report, 44
Concluding Observations, 52
References, 52

2 THE STATE OF HEALTH DISPARITIES IN THE UNITED STATES	**57**

Health Disparities, 57
Addressing Health Inequity in Unique Populations, 64
Place Matters, 79

Evidence Gaps, 85
References, 88

3 THE ROOT CAUSES OF HEALTH INEQUITY   **99**
How Structural Inequities, Social Determinants of Health, and Health Equity Connect, 100
Structural Inequities, 102
Social Determinants of Health, 116
Concluding Observations, 161
References, 164

4 THE ROLE OF COMMUNITIES IN PROMOTING HEALTH EQUITY   **185**
Community Action: Vitally Necessary, 189
The Evidence on Community-Based Efforts, 191
Elements of Successful Community Efforts, 196
Building Evidence to Support Community Action, 202
References, 207

5 EXAMPLES OF COMMUNITIES TACKLING HEALTH INEQUITY   **211**
Process of Selection, 211
Community Examples, 213
Summary of Challenges, 315
Summary of Key Elements, Levers, Policies, and Stakeholders, 315
Conclusion, 320
Annex, 323
   Selection Process for Community Examples, 323
References, 327

6 POLICIES TO SUPPORT COMMUNITY SOLUTIONS   **335**
Taxation and Income Inequality, 337
Housing and Urban Planning Policies, 341
Education Policies, 347
Civil Rights Law and Policy, 351
Health Policy, 362
Criminal Justice Policy, 368
Concluding Observations, 372
References, 372

7 PARTNERS IN PROMOTING HEALTH EQUITY IN COMMUNITIES 383
Finance, 384
Anchor Institutions, 392
Other Community-Based Partners, 411
Role of Government, 414
Cross-Sector Collaboration—Health in All Policies, 427
Concluding Observations, 437
References, 438

8 COMMUNITY TOOLS TO PROMOTE HEALTH EQUITY 447
Tools for Community Success, 447
Crosscutting Tools and Processes, 448
Making Health Equity a Shared Vision and Value, 479
Increasing Community Capacity to Shape Health Outcomes, 481
Fostering Multi-Sector Collaboration, 488
Community Tool Kits, 492
Conclusion, 495
References, 495

9 CONCLUSION 503
References, 506

APPENDIXES

A	Native American Health: Historical and Legal Context	507
B	Community-Level Indicators and Interactive Tools for Health Equity	519
C	Public Meeting Agendas	539
D	Committee Biographical Sketches	545

Acronyms and Abbreviations

AA	associate of arts
ACA	Patient Protection and Affordable Care Act
ACLU	American Civil Liberties Union
ACS	American Community Survey
AHA	American Hospital Association
AHRQ	Agency for Healthcare Research and Quality
AIDS	acquired immune deficiency syndrome
APA	American Planning Association
APHA	American Public Health Association
API	academic performance index
ASPPH	Association of Schools and Programs of Public Health
BPA	bisphenol A
CBA	community benefits agreement
CBO	Congressional Budget Office
CBPR	community-based participatory research
CCCEH	Columbia Center for Children's Environmental Health
CCP	Community College Pathways
CCPH	Community–Campus Partnerships for Health
CDA	child development associate
CDC	U.S. Centers for Disease Control and Prevention
CDC	community development corporation
CDE	common data element

CEHNM	Center for Environmental Health in Northern Manhattan
CHNA	community health needs assessment
CI:Now	Community Information Now
CLT	community land trust
CMS	Centers for Medicare & Medicaid Services
COPC	community-oriented primary care
COR	Council of Representative
CPED	Community Planning and Economic Development
CPLC	Chicanos Por La Causa, Inc.
CTSA	Clinical and Translational Science Award
DEP	New York City Department of Environmental Protection
DHC	Delta Health Center, Inc.
DOT	U.S. Department of Transportation
DSNI	Dudley Street Neighborhood Initiative
EBALDC	East Bay Asian Local Development Corporation
ED	U.S. Department of Education
EHJLT	Environmental Health and Justice Leadership Training
EITC	earned income tax credit
EJI	Environmental Justice Institute
EPA	U.S. Environmental Protection Agency
EPN	Eastside Promise Neighborhood
ESSA	Every Student Succeeds Act
FIHET	Federal Interagency Health Equity Team
FQHC	federally qualified health center
GDP	gross domestic product
GED	General Education Development
GPRA	Government Performance Results Act
HEZ	health enterprise zone
HHS	U.S. Department of Health and Human Services
HIAP	Health In All Policies
HIV	human immunodeficiency virus
HRSA	Health Resources and Services Administration
HUD	U.S. Department of Housing and Urban Development
IHI	Institute for Healthcare Improvement
IHS	Indian Health Service
IndyCAN	Indianapolis Congregation Action Network

ACRONYMS AND ABBREVIATIONS xxi

IOM	Institute of Medicine
IVE	Integrated Voter Engagement

KCHD	Kansas City Health Department

LACDPH	Los Angeles County Department of Public Health
LEED	Leadership in Energy and Environmental Design
LGBT	lesbian, gay, bisexual, and transgender
LIHTC	Low Income Housing Tax Credit
LOC	local organizing committee

MCI	Magnolia Community Initiative
MST	military sexual trauma
MTA	Metropolitan Transit Authority
MTS	marine transfer station

NAACP	National Association for the Advancement of Colored People
NACCHO	National Association of County and City Health Officials
NAMI	National Alliance on Mental Illness
NASEM	National Academies of Sciences, Engineering, and Medicine
NCHS	National Center for Health Statistics
NIEHS	National Institute of Environmental Health Sciences
NIH	National Institutes of Health
NPA	National Partnership for Action to End Health Disparities
NPA	National People's Action
NPS	National Park Service
NRC	National Research Council
NRDC	Natural Resources Defense Council
NSDUH	National Survey on Drug Use and Health
NTFAI	National Task Force on Anchor Institutions
NVSS	National Vital Statistics Survey
NYPIRG	New York Public Interest Research Group
NYSDOH	New York State Department of Health
NYSTEA	New York State Transportation Equity Alliance

OEO	Office of Economic Opportunity

PACE	Program of All-inclusive Care for the Elderly
PaCT	Promise and Choice Together
PACT	Partnership of Academicians and Communities for Translation
PAD	Parks after Dark
PICO	People Improving Communities through Organizing

PRAPARE   Protocol for Responding to and Assessing Patients' Assets, Risks, and Experiences
PTSD   posttraumatic stress disorder
PUSH   People United for Sustainable Housing

QCDO   Quitman County Development Organization

RBA   results-based accountability
RHEC   regional health equity council
RWJF   Robert Wood Johnson Foundation

SAISD   San Antonio Independent School District
SAMHSA   Substance Abuse and Mental Health Services Administration
SES   socioeconomic status
SKCHD   Seattle & King County Health Department
SNAP   Supplemental Nutrition Assistance Program
SPARCC   Strong, Prosperous, and Resilient Communities Challenge
SQUIRE   Standards for Quality Improvement Reporting Excellence
SSI   Supplemental Security Income
STD   sexually transmitted disease
STEM   science, technology, engineering, and mathematics

TCEP   tris(2-carboxyethyl)phosphine hydrochloride [flame retardant]
TCI   Transforming Communities Initiative
TRAC   Transit Riders Action Committee

UDS   Uniform Data System
USDA   U.S. Department of Agriculture
UWPHI   University of Wisconsin Population Health Institute

VA   U.S. Department of Veterans Affairs
VHA   Veterans Health Administration
VSAT   Veterans Sustainable Agriculture Training Program

WHO   World Health Organization

YMCA   Young Men's Christian Association

Key Terms

community	Any configuration of individuals, families, and groups whose values, characteristics, interests, geography, and/or social relations unite them in some way.
community-based solution	An action, policy, program, or law driven by the community that impacts community-level factors and promotes health equity.
health	A state of complete physical, mental, and social well-being and not merely the absence of disease.
health disparities	Differences that exist among specific population groups in the United States in the attainment of full health potential that can be measured by differences in incidence, prevalence, mortality, burden of disease, and other adverse health conditions.

health equity	The state in which everyone has the opportunity to attain full health potential and no one is disadvantaged from achieving this potential because of social position or any other socially defined circumstance.
public policy	A law, regulation, procedure, administrative action, incentive, or voluntary practice of governments and other institutions that affects a whole population.
social determinants of health	The conditions in the environments in which people live, learn, work, play, worship, and age that affect a wide range of health, functioning, and quality-of-life outcomes and risks. For the purposes of this report, the social determinants of health are education; employment; health systems and services; housing; income and wealth; the physical environment; public safety; the social environment; and transportation.

Summary

Health equity is the state in which everyone has the opportunity to attain full health potential and no one is disadvantaged from achieving this potential because of social position or any other socially defined circumstance. Health equity and opportunity are inextricably linked. Currently in the United States, the burdens of disease and poor health and the benefits of well-being and good health are inequitably distributed. This inequitable distribution is caused by social, environmental, economic, and structural factors that shape health and are themselves distributed unequally, with pronounced differences in opportunities for health.

Community is any configuration of individuals, families, and groups whose values, characteristics, interests, geography, or social relations unite them in some way (adapted from Dreher, 2016[1]). However, the word is used to denote both the people living in a place and the place itself. In this report the committee generally focuses on shared geography—in other words, community is defined as the people living in a place such as a neighborhood. Therefore, a community-based solution is an action, policy, program, or law that is driven by community members, affects local factors that can influence health, and has the potential to advance health equity.

---

[1] Draft manuscript from Melanie C. Dreher, Rush University Medical Center, provided to staff on February 19, 2016, for the Committee on Community-Based Solutions to Promote Health Equity in the United States. Available by request from the National Academies of Sciences, Engineering, and Medicine's Public Access Records Office. For more information, email PARO@nas.edu.

The potential of community-based solutions to advance health equity is a focus because the Robert Wood Johnson Foundation (RWJF) asked the Committee on Community-Based Solutions to Promote Health Equity in the United States to consider solutions that could be identified, developed, and implemented at the local or community level. However, the report focus should not be interpreted to suggest that community-based solutions represent the primary or sole strategy or the best opportunity to promote health equity (see Box S-1 for an outline of the report in brief). Communities exist in a milieu of national-, state-, and local-level policies, forces, and programs that enable and support or interfere with and impede the ability of community residents and their partners to address the conditions that lead to health inequity. Therefore, the power of community actors is a necessary and essential, but not a sufficient, ingredient in promoting health equity.

In addition to the support of high-level policies, such as those that address structural inequities (e.g., residential segregation), community-based solutions described in this report also rely on multi-sectoral and multilevel collaborations and approaches: for example, engaging businesses, the faith community, and other nontraditional partners. It is a strength of multi-sectoral collaboration and efforts that are not primarily health-focused that they, by definition, ensure diverse approaches to

---

BOX S-1
Report in Brief

A. **Health equity is crucial for the well-being and vibrancy of communities.** The United States pays the high price of health inequity in lost lives, potential, and resources. (Chapters 1 and 2)
B. **Health is a product of multiple determinants.** Social, economic, environmental, and structural factors and their unequal distribution matter more than health care in shaping health disparities. (Chapter 3)
C. **Health inequities are in large part a result of poverty, structural racism, and discrimination.** (Chapter 3)
D. **Communities have agency to promote health equity.** However, community-based solutions are necessary but not sufficient. (Chapters 4 and 5)
E. **Supportive public and private policies at all levels and programs facilitate community action** (infrastructure of policies, funding, political will, etc.). (Chapter 6)
F. **The collaboration and engagement of new and diverse (multi-sector) partners is essential to promoting health equity.** (Chapter 7)
G. **Tools and other resources exist to translate knowledge into action to promote health equity.** (Chapter 8)
H. **Conclusion** (Chapter 9)

improving community health and well-being. Such diverse approaches also are a manifestation of the fact that not all communities start out observing the differences in life expectancy between one side of town and another and seek to address those inequities. Some communities aim to improve high school graduation, expand affordable housing, or create jobs. This report is for communities that believe improving health among their residents is important, but it is also for communities that believe better transit, more affordable housing, safer streets, and more small businesses are important. Whether health is the end or the means to an end, communities can benefit by understanding how health is connected to other goals important to them, and that improving education, housing, safety, employment, or the environment can also help improve health and mitigate health inequity.

HEALTH EQUITY IS CRUCIAL

Health equity is fundamental to the idea of living a good life and building a vibrant society because of its practical, economic, and civic implications. Shifts in economic mobility, income inequality, and persisting legacies of social problems such as structural racism are hampering the attainment of health equity, causing economic loss, and, most overwhelmingly, the loss of human lives and potential.

Although moral arguments to promote health equity exist,[2] promoting health equity could afford considerable economic, national security, and other benefits. The premise that there is social mobility, the opportunity to succeed with hard work, and the opportunity to achieve prosperity is fundamental to the "American Dream" (Carr and Wiemers, 2016). However, recent research demonstrates that worsening social, economic, and environmental factors are affecting the public's health in serious ways that compromise opportunity for all (Chetty et al., 2016; Rudolph et al., 2015; Woolf et al., 2015).

Health inequity is costly. For example, a 2009 analysis by LaVeist and colleagues found that "eliminating health disparities for minorities would have reduced direct medical care expenditures by $229.4 billion for the years 2003–2006" (LaVeist et al., 2009, p. 4). In 2009 the Urban Institute

---

[2] For example, Jones and colleagues cite valuing all people equally as foundational to the concept of equity, noting that the equal worth of all people is at the core of the human rights principle that all human beings equally possess certain rights (Jones, 2009). Braveman and colleagues point out that health differences adversely affecting socially disadvantaged groups are particularly unacceptable because ill health can be an obstacle to overcoming social disadvantage. They further note that this "consideration resonates with common sense notions of fairness, as well as with ethical concepts of justice" (Braveman et al., 2011, p. S150).

projected that from 2009 to 2018, racial disparities in health would cost U.S. health insurers approximately $337 billion total (Waidmann, 2009). Disparities in access to and in the quality of care (e.g., delayed care, inadequate coverage) account for a portion of these costs.

Beyond adding to health care costs, health inequity has consequences for the U.S. economy, national security, business viability, and public finances. In the domain of national security, diminished health means a diminished capacity to participate in military service—a concern shared by hundreds of senior military leaders. More than 75 percent of 17- to 24-year-olds—more than 26 million young adults—in the United States cannot qualify to serve in the armed forces because they experience persistent health problems—often untreated, ranging from obesity to dependencies on prescription and nonprescription drugs—are poorly educated, or have been convicted of a felony (Christeson et al., 2009). Nearly one-third (32 percent) of all young people experience health problems—other than their weight—that will keep them from serving. Many are disqualified from serving for asthma, eyesight or hearing problems, mental health issues, or recent treatment for attention deficit hyperactivity disorder. Navy Rear Admiral Robert Besal (ret.) has asserted that young people who are physically unfit for "productive employment or military service represent a staggering loss of individual potential and collective strength for the nation as well" (Council for a Strong America, 2016).

Just as a healthy military is viewed as a necessity for national security, a healthy, productive workforce is a prerequisite for a thriving economy (HERO, 2015; IOM, 2015a). The impact of poor health on private businesses is significant. Research from the Urban Institute shows that those young adults with health problems who cannot find jobs in the mainstream economy are less productive and generate higher health care costs for businesses (Woolf et al., 2015).

Three indicators provide summary information about the overall health of a population or subpopulation: infant mortality, age-adjusted death rates, and life expectancy. In international rankings, the United States ranks lower than other wealthy nations on each of these indicators; data on U.S. states show that racial and ethnic disparities are found in each of these indicators (NRC and IOM, 2013; OECD, 2015). In addition to sharp and persistent racial and ethnic disparities, other significant trends have surfaced: a slight decline in life expectancy of white women in the past several years (Arias, 2016), income inequality, drug use, suicide, and the relative deprivations of rural life have all emerged as key themes.

Report Conceptual Model

As part of its statement of task, the committee was asked to review the state of health disparities in the United States and to explore the underlying conditions and root causes contributing to health inequities and the interdependent nature of the factors that create them. The committee drew on existing literature and comprehensive reviews to examine the state of health disparities by race and ethnicity, gender, sexual orientation, and disability status, highlighting those populations that are disproportionately affected by inequity. Health disparities stem from systematic differences—those that are preventable and unjust—among groups and communities occupying unequal positions in society (Graham, 2004).

Figure S-1 is a conceptual model that grounds the report of the Committee on Community-Based Solutions to Promote Health Equity in the

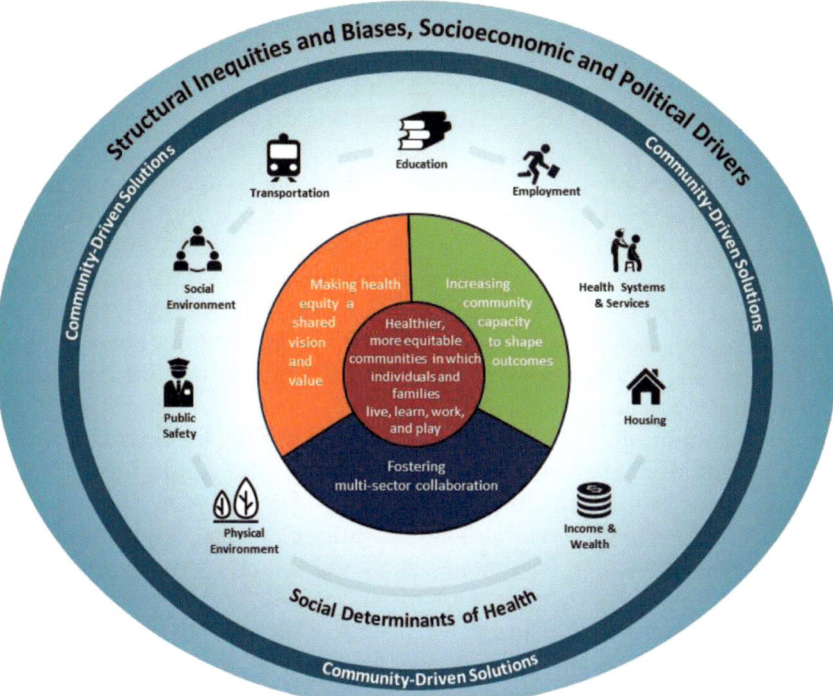

FIGURE S-1 A conceptual model for community-based solutions to promote health equity.
NOTES: Multi-sector collaboration can include partners from agriculture, banking/finance, business/industry, economic development, education, health care, housing, human/social services, justice, labor, land use and management, media, public health, transportation, and workforce development, among other sectors.
SOURCES: Informed by the Robert Wood Johnson Foundation (RWJF) Culture of Health Action Framework and the Prevention Institute's *Systems Framework to Achieve an Equitable Culture of Health.*

United States. The model adapts elements of the RWJF Culture of Health Action Framework and the Prevention Institute's *Systems Framework to Achieve an Equitable Culture of Health*. The figure applies the culture of health lens to the committee's understanding of the underlying causes and conditions of health inequity in addition to the community-based solutions that promote health equity.

Unlike a logic model, which is linear and progresses neatly from inputs to outputs and outcomes, the model in Figure S-1 is circular to reflect the topic's complexity, with inputs shown in the outer circle and background—depicting the context of structural inequities, socioeconomic and political drivers, and determinants of health in which health inequities and community-driven solutions exist. Community-driven solutions that target the nine determinants of health listed in the model (e.g., education, housing) likely share three key elements the committee identified at the beginning of its work. The committee adapted two action areas of the Culture of Health Action Framework"Making health equity a shared vision and value" and "Fostering multi-sector collaboration"as two elements of community-based solutions to promote health equity. Based on the committee's information-gathering sessions, relevant literature, and committee deliberations, the committee also articulated a third element: "Increasing community capacity to shape outcomes." These elements of community-based efforts are discussed in Chapter 4. The RWJF action area "Creating healthier, more equitable communities" has been incorporated into the model at the center of the diagram as the outcome of the community-driven solutions.

The community examples featured in this report (see Chapter 5) highlight solutions that have been implemented at the community level to target one or more of the nine determinants of health using the three elements identified in the model. These solutions, which hold health equity (or its determinants) as a shared vision and value, increase community capacity to shape outcomes, and foster multi-sector collaboration, can help create equal opportunity for health, which is the foundation for health equity.

MANY FACTORS SHAPE HEALTH AND HEALTH EQUITY

The committee took a multifactor view of health status and health inequities, in recognition that only some aspects of a person's health status depend on individual behaviors and choice. Community-wide problems such as poverty, unemployment, low educational attainment, inadequate housing, lack of public transportation, exposure to violence, and neighborhood deterioration (social or physical) shape health and contribute to health inequities. The historic and ongoing interplay of structures, policies, norms, and demographic and geographic patterns shapes the life of every individual across the country, and its effects persist over multiple generations (Braveman and Gottlieb, 2014; Krieger, 2014; Marmot et al., 2010; Williams and Collins, 2001). These factors are not intractable, and such inequities[3] can be mitigated by policies and community action in powerful ways (see Chapter 3 for a discussion of these factors).

It is becoming clearer that health insurance coverage alone will not address health disparities, including those across race, ethnicity, socioeconomic status (SES), and geography (Kenney and Huntress, 2012; Ubri and Artiga, 2016). Signed into law in 2010, the Patient Protection and Affordable Care Act (ACA) has accelerated progress toward health equity by expanding health insurance coverage to about 20 million Americans (Uberoi et al., 2016). However, challenges remain to fully addressing health care equity, including policy hurdles affecting access and utilization among subgroups of the population.[4]

Health inequity arises from root causes that could be organized in two clusters:

1. Intrapersonal, interpersonal, institutional, and systemic mechanisms (also referred to as structural inequities) that organize the distribution of power and resources differentially across lines of race, gender, class, sexual orientation, gender expression, and other dimensions of individual and group identity.
2. The unequal allocation of power and resources—including goods, services, and societal attention—which manifests itself in unequal social, economic, and environmental conditions, also called the determinants of health.

Interventions targeting those factors hold the greatest promise for promoting health equity. The root causes of inequity are diverse, complex, evolving, and interdependent in nature (Williams and Collins, 2001), and while society has made substantial progress toward equity, disparities in health outcomes and opportunities for health persist. Poverty, race, and ethnicity continue to be associated with poorer health and poorer

---

[3] That is, differences that exist among specific population groups in the United States in the attainment of full health potential and in the incidence, prevalence, mortality, and burden of disease and other adverse health conditions (NIH, 2014).

[4] For example, a lack of coverage for some immigrants and asylum seekers or those subject to deferred action for childhood arrivals; a limited system capacity or competence to care for some populations, such as lesbian, gay, bisexual, or transsexual (LGBT) persons (e.g., newly covered partners of insured LGBT individuals); and the lack of health data to monitor the health needs of some populations (e.g., for American Indians, of whom approximately 20 percent live on rural reservations) (Kruse et al., 2016).

conditions for health. For example, evidence indicates that the conditions that exist in low-income communities, such as concentrated poverty, low housing values, and low high school graduation rates, foster violence and increase the risk of homicide (Prevention Institute, 2011). Those conditions themselves are shaped by interconnected structures, policies, and norms that affect people differently along lines of class, race, and ethnicity. Taking low high school graduation rates, for example, research indicates that race and class differences in adverse childhood experiences, chronic stress and trauma, and lead exposure in the environment affect children's ability to learn (Aizer et al., 2015; Bethell et al., 2014; Jimenez et al., 2016; Levy et al., 2016). Moreover, a growing body of research indicates that minority students are disproportionately affected by school discipline policies that lead students to drop out of school (Howard, 2010; Losen et al., 2015; Reardon et al., 2012; Skiba et al., 2011; Smith and Harper, 2015). Chapters 3 and 6 describe more of the evidence on how inequitable structures, policies, and norms influence the determinants—from housing to education to employment—that make it considerably harder for people who are poor and for people of color to achieve good health.

Conclusion 3-2: Based on its review of evidence, the committee concludes that health inequities are the result of more than individual choice or random occurrence. They are the result of the historic and ongoing interplay of inequitable structures, policies, and norms that shape lives.

These structures, policies, and norms—such as segregation, redlining and foreclosure, and implicit bias—play out on the terrain of the social, economic, environmental, and cultural determinants of health.

COMMUNITY AGENCY TO PROMOTE HEALTH EQUITY

A community is the place where one lives, works, and plays. It serves as the bedrock of health that shapes lives and behaviors. Indeed, as detailed in Chapters 2 and 3, research consistently indicates that where one lives is a greater predictor of one's health than individual characteristics or behaviors. Communities encompass multiple spheres of interaction, from the individual to the organizational level to the physical setting, and each level of interaction affects health outcomes. Communities also are unique in the nature and extent of health inequities, and so are the means to address those issues, such as the locus of power and community values.

Communities across the United States are developing and putting into action strategies to reduce health inequities. Often these community efforts go unseen in the media, while stories of blight, crime, or community unrest are more visible. Community assets can be built, leveraged, and modified and can create a context in which to foster health equity. The committee was asked to identify and examine six or more examples of community-based solutions that address health inequities, drawing from deliberate and indirect interventions or activities that promote equal opportunity for health. The nine examples in Chapter 5 span health and non-health sectors and take into account the range of factors that contribute to health inequity in the United States, such as systems of employment, public safety, housing, transportation, education, and others. See Table S-1 for a list and brief description of each community example. The committee used a set of core inclusion criteria to select the examples for this report. According to these core criteria, the community examples must

- address at least one (or preferably more) of the nine social determinants of health identified by the committee—education, employment, health systems and services, housing, income and wealth, physical environment, public safety, social environment, and transportation—and be:
  o community-driven;
  o multi-sectoral; and
  o evidence-informed.

The committee also strove to capture examples of communities that were able to engage nontraditional partners, work in an interdisciplinary and multilevel manner, and document plans to achieve their outcomes and sustain its efforts. These communities represent a diversity of geography, environments, challenges, and resources. Chapter 5 provides a summary of each example to demonstrate the innovative work conducted by communities and the challenges they face. In Chapter 5 the committee comments on a number of crosscutting essential elements that show promise for promoting health equity in communities. These elements include, but are not limited to, creating a shared vision and building trust in the community, leadership development, building a diverse network of partners through relationship building and mutual accountability, governing processes that have a grassroots component, fostering creativity, leveraging resources, and training and commissioning technical expertise where necessary.

To succeed, communities need evidence (from research); a broader context of policy, resources, and political will that nurtures local efforts; and tools.

TABLE S-1 Overview of Community Examples to Promote Health Equity

Name *Location*	Brief Description	Primary Social Determinant(s) of Health Targeted
Blueprint for Action *Minneapolis, MN*	A strategic plan that employs the public health approach to youth violence prevention that arose from a community-driven, grassroots response to the issue.	Public safety
Delta Health Center *Mound Bayou, MS*	The first rural federally qualified health center, employing a community-oriented primary care model.	Health systems and services
Dudley Street Neighborhood Initiative *Boston, MA*	A nonprofit, community-driven organization that empowers residents to drive economic development and neighborhood revitalization.	Physical environment Employment
Eastside Promise Neighborhood *San Antonio, TX*	An implementation site of the Promise Neighborhood grant program, developing collaborative solutions to address barriers to education.	Education
Indianapolis Congregation Action Network *Indianapolis, IN*	A multi-faith, nonpartisan organization that catalyzes marginalized people and faith communities to organize for racial and economic equity.	Employment Public safety
Magnolia Community Initiative *Los Angeles, CA*	An initiative that seeks to increase social connectedness, community mobilization, and access to vital supports and services to improve outcomes for children.	Social environment
Mandela MarketPlace *Oakland, CA*	A nonprofit organization that addresses issues of food insecurity and economic divestment through the creation of sustainable food systems.	Physical environment
People United for Sustainable Housing *Buffalo, NY*	A nonprofit organization that mobilizes residents to secure quality, affordable housing and advance economic justice.	Housing
WE ACT for Environmental Justice *Harlem, NY*	A nonprofit organization that engages in community organizing, community-based participatory research, and advocacy to confront environmental injustice.	Physical environment

DISPARITIES AND THEIR ROOTS

Health disparity research has evolved from describing associations (e.g., between SES and health) to describing the mechanisms linking SES and health, to more recent work on the interactions among factors (Adler and Stewart, 2010). More epidemiological studies employing a combination of research strategies (i.e., mixed-methods qualitative and quantitative research) in addressing health disparities are needed to provide guidance for community interventions in this complex arena (Diez Roux and Mair, 2010).

Conclusion 2-1: To enable researchers to fully document and understand health inequities, to provide the foundation for solution development, and to measure solution outcomes longitudinally, the following are needed:
- *An expansion of current health disparity indicators and indices to include other groups beyond African Americans and whites, such as Hispanics and their major subgroups, Native Americans, Asian Americans, Pacific Islanders, and mixed race, in addition to LGBT individuals, people with disabilities, and military veterans.*
  - *Including consideration of methods to generate stable estimates of disparities through oversampling certain populations where necessary.*
- *An expansion of metrics and indicators capturing the broader definition of health, including health equity and the social determinants of health.*
- *Longer-term studies, as many health outcomes take years (or decades) to see quantifiable changes in health outcomes related to the social determinants of health.*
- *Studies examining the ways in which a single structural factor may influence multiple health outcomes.*
- *Increased funding opportunities dedicated to developing and testing relevant theories, measures, and scientific methods, with the goal of enhancing the rigor with which investigators examine structural inequities such as structural racism and health disparities.*

Unequal treatment in the health care delivery system has been well documented elsewhere (IOM, 2003), as has implicit bias and the need for cultural competence (IOM, 2003; Sabin et al., 2009). Greater diversity in the health sector workforce could help improve cultural competence and offer additional benefits (Cooper et al., 2003). Also, additional research could inform health care organizations, academic health centers, and others about the effects of and effective strategies to address the health-related harms of structural racism and implicit and explicit bias across categories of race, ethnicity, gender, disability status, age, sexual orientation, gender identity, and other marginalized statuses. For example, the literature does not clearly elucidate the relationship between health care workforce pipeline programs (e.g., to grow the numbers of minority providers) and their impact on the social determinants of health for poor and underserved communities.

> **Recommendation 3-1: The committee recommends that research funders[5] support research on (a) health disparities that examines the multiple effects of structural racism (e.g., segregation) and implicit and explicit bias across different categories of marginalized status on health and health care delivery; and (b) effective strategies to reduce and mitigate the effects of explicit and implicit bias.**

There have been promising developments in the search for interventions to address implicit bias, but more research is needed, and engaging community members in this and other aspects of research on health disparities is important for ethical and practical reasons (Minkler et al., 2010; Mosavel et al., 2011; Salway et al., 2015). In the context of implicit bias in workplaces and business settings, including individuals with relevant expertise in informing and conducting the research could also be helpful. Therefore, research teams could be composed of such nontraditional participants as community members and local business leaders, in addition to academic researchers.

> **Recommendation 3-2: The committee recommends that research funders support and academic institutions convene multidisciplinary research teams that include nonacademics to (a) understand the cognitive and affective processes of implicit bias and (b) test interventions that disrupt and change these processes toward sustainable solutions.**

As communities pursue broader change in the conditions for health, they find a dearth of systematic, organized information and guidance to help them: set common goals and measures of success; select multifaceted and mutually reinforcing strategies, grounded in strong theory; align implementation efforts; and make the necessary system and community-level changes to adapt and continuously improve. A centralized resource for communities is needed, and several partially relevant models exist,

---

[5] Funders include government agencies, private foundations, and other sources such as academic centers of higher education.

some of which could potentially be modified to operate in an expanded capacity. These include the County Health Rankings (CHR) What Works for Health database, the U.S. Centers for Disease Control and Prevention's (CDC's) Community Health Improvement (CHI) Navigator, and also, perhaps, the Agency for Healthcare Research and Quality's Measures Clearinghouse and the National Library of Medicine (which serves as a knowledge curation resource through its special queries). The CHR What Works for Health database provides information for community health improvement organized by expected beneficial outcomes, potential beneficial outcomes, evidence of effectiveness, impact on disparities, implementation examples, implementation resources, and citations. The CHI Navigator is intended for individuals and groups who lead or participate in CHI work "within hospitals and health systems, public health agencies, and other community organizations. It is a one-stop shop that offers community stakeholders expert-vetted tools and resources for: depicting visually the who, what, where, and how of improving community health; making the case for collaborative approaches to community health improvement; establishing and maintaining effective collaborations; and finding interventions that work for the greatest impact on health and well-being for all" (CDC, 2015). The Urban Institute Metropolitan Housing and Communities Policy Center's What Works Collaborative[6] is another evidence database that conducts research to support evidence-based housing and urban policy. Another resource is the Guide to Community Preventive Services,[7] whose health equity focus includes systematic reviews examining the influence of educational interventions on long-term health.

Recommendation 4-1: A public–private consortium[8] should create a publicly available repository of evidence to inform and guide efforts to promote health equity at the community level. The consortium should also offer support to communities, including technical assistance.

---

[6] For more information, see http://www.urban.org/policy-centers/metropolitan-housing-and-communities-policy-center/projects/what-works-collaborative (accessed October 28, 2016).

[7] For more information, see https://www.thecommunityguide.org/topic/health-equity (accessed October 28, 2016).

[8] This could be done through such mechanisms as a collaboration among CDC (home of the Community Health Improvement Navigator initiative), university-based centers (see the example of the University of Wisconsin Population Health Institute that operates the County Health Rankings [CHR] What Works for Health database), and one or more philanthropic organizations.

The repository would include databases that provide information at the national, state, and metropolitan levels as well as for smaller local geographies such as census tracts; information on effective interventions and approaches; and the knowledge necessary to strengthen the capacity of communities to act on topics such as education, income, employment, transportation, nutrition, civil rights, housing, and other determinants of health by race, ethnicity, gender, disability status, age, sexual identity/ orientation, and other demographic characteristics.

POLICY CONTEXT AND PARTNERS

Adding to the complexity of developing and implementing community interventions to promote health equity are significant changes in the sociocultural, demographic, economic, and political landscape affecting health disparities and the social determinants of health. These changes include an increase in income inequality (e.g., incomes in the top 10 percent average 9 times the income of the bottom 90 percent, and incomes in the top 0.1 percent are more than 184 times those of the bottom 90 percent); the demographic shift to a larger proportion of people of color in the U.S. population (e.g., by 2040, the number of U.S. counties in which the majority of the population is people of color is expected to more than double), with implications for expanding health inequity; and increasing disparities. Recent events involving race and law enforcement relations have offered a disturbing illustration of systematically unequal treatment that is causing fear, mistrust, anger, and divisiveness. Moreover, there is a growing bipartisan recognition that mass incarceration, which affects individuals of color disproportionately, plays a major role in damaging families and communities, constitutes an unsustainable use of taxpayer dollars, and, in connection with the larger policy milieu in both the private and the public sector, leads to poor employment prospects and voting disenfranchisement (Clear, 2008; NRC, 2014). These current realities serve as reminders that the vision of a truly inclusive and equitable society is not yet within reach. However, community-driven solutions, such as those that his report highlights, can help move the nation in that direction. For example, Multnomah County, Oregon, applies an "equity and empowerment lens" to local policy (Multnomah County, 2014a,b, n.d.), and Seattle–King County implemented an "equity in all policies" approach to all decision making and annually reports on what it terms "the determinants of equity" in the county (Beatty and Foster, 2015).

In a 2011 Institute of Medicine (IOM) report, the authoring committee recommended that "states and the federal government develop and employ a Health In All Policies (HIAP) approach to consider the health effects—both positive and negative—of major legislation, regulations, and other policies that could potentially have a meaningful impact on the public's health" (IOM, 2011, p. 9). The committee further recommended that "state and federal governments evaluate the health effects and costs of major legislation, regulations, and policies that could have a meaningful impact on health. This evaluation should occur before and after enactment" (p. 11). The recommendation below is made with acknowledgment of the ongoing work in many jurisdictions around the country and of the previous IOM recommendations.

> **Recommendation 6-1:** All government agencies that support or conduct planning related to land use, housing, transportation, and other areas that affect populations at high risk of health inequity should:
> - Add specific requirements to outreach processes to ensure robust and authentic community participation in policy development.
> - Collaborate with public health agencies and others to ensure a broad consideration of unintended consequences for health and well-being, including whether the benefits and burdens will be equitably distributed.[9]
> - Highlight the co-benefits of—or shared "wins" that could be achieved by—considering health equity in the development of comprehensive plans[10] (e.g., improving public transit in transit-poor areas supports physical activity, promotes health equity, and creates more sustainable communities).
> - Prioritize affordable housing, implement strategies to mitigate and avoid displacement (and its serious health effects), and document outcomes.

An additional way to think about promoting community-based strategies for reducing education and health disparities is to consider the existing infrastructure of policies and programs within the education sector with an eye for how this infrastructure might be strengthened, modified, and expanded in the interest of improving health outcomes. The committee considered the role of the education sector in shaping health and health equity, given the strong relationship between educational achievement and health outcomes. Recently updated requirements for school

---

[9] See Recommendation 7 in *For the Public's Health: Revitalizing Law and Policy to Meet New Challenges* (IOM, 2011).
[10] See, for example, ChangeLab Solutions' "Model Comprehensive Plan Language on Complete Streets" (ChangeLab Solutions, 2016).

assessment of student health needs also appear to align well with needs assessments required in the health sector, for both public health agencies and tax-exempt hospitals and health systems (IRS, 2016; PHAB, 2011).

> **Recommendation 6-2:** State departments of education should provide guidance to schools on how to conduct assessments of student health needs and of the school health and wellness environment. This guidance should outline a process by which schools can identify model needs assessments, including those with a focus on student health and wellness.

> **Recommendation 6-3:** To support schools in collecting data on student and community health, tax-exempt hospitals and health systems and state and local public health agencies should:
> - Make schools aware of existing health needs assessments to help them leverage current data collection and analyses.[11]
> - Assist schools and school districts in identifying and accessing data on key health indicators that should inform school needs assessments and any related school improvement plans.

Hospitals are demonstrating greater interest in community-wide health investments and underlying factors that affect population health, rather than maintaining a more narrow focus on health care services and funding offsets. In *Can Hospitals Heal America's Communities,* Norris and Howard (2015) write that "addressing these social determinants of health through their business and non-clinical practices (for example, through purchasing, hiring, and investments), hospitals and health systems can produce increased measurably beneficial impacts on population and community health" (pp. 1–2). Examples of efforts to build, hire, and invest locally include Kaiser Permanente in California and elsewhere and ProMedica in Cleveland (NASEM, 2016d).

> **Recommendation 6-4:** Through multi-sectoral partnerships, hospitals and health care systems should focus their community benefit dollars to pursue long-term strategies (including changes in law, policies, and systems) to build healthier neighborhoods, expand access to housing, drive economic development, and advance other upstream initiatives aimed at eradicating the root causes of poor health, especially in low-income

---

[11] See, for example, the Healthy Students, Promising Futures tool kit from the U.S. Departments of Education and Health and Human Services (ED, 2016a).

communities. Hospital and health systems should also advocate for the expansion of efficient and effective services responding to health-related social needs[12] for vulnerable populations and people living in poverty.

Because health care payment reform (among other public policies) may have unintended consequences such as reproducing health disparities, efforts to mitigate negative consequences are needed. However, mitigating efforts can be addressed only by including the perspectives of populations most affected by such programs.

Recommendation 6-5: Government and nongovernment payers and providers should expand policies aiming to improve the quality of care, improve population health, and control health care costs[13] to include a specific focus on improving population health for the most vulnerable and underserved. As one strategy to support a focus on health disparities, the Centers for Medicare & Medicaid Services could undertake research on payment reforms that could spur accounting for social risk factors in the value-based payment programs it oversees.

The National Academies' Committee on Accounting for Socioeconomic Status in Medicare Payment Programs has shown in its reports (NASEM, 2016a,b,c,e) that value-based payment systems that do not account for social risk factors can have unintended adverse consequences, including providers and health plans avoiding low-income patients and underpayment to providers disproportionately serving socially at-risk populations (such as safety-net providers). These unintended consequences could in turn lead to deterioration in the quality of health care for socially at-risk populations and widening health disparities. That committee has stated that reducing disparities in access, quality, and outcomes is one of four policy goals in accounting for social risk factors (NASEM, 2016a,b,c,e), and its reports suggest that reforms to value-based payment programs that compensate providers fairly and increase fairness and

---

[12] Alley et al. (2016) describe services addressing health-related social needs, including transportation and housing. Others define services addressing such needs as "wraparound services," referring to linkages or services health care providers can offer to ensure, for example, that patients have transportation to routine health care appointments, have adequate food in their homes, and obtain legal (e.g., for tenant-landlord disputes about environmental exposure to asthma triggers) or social service assistance. See, for example, (Bell and Cohen, 2009).

[13] Better care, better population health, and lower cost are often described as the Triple Aim (Berwick et al., 2008).

accuracy in public reporting can help achieve goals to reduce disparities and improve quality and efficiency of care for all patients.

Civil rights, health, and environmental justice laws and policies provide a framework that promotes equal access to publicly funded resources and prohibit discrimination based on race, color, national origin, income, gender, disability, and other factors. This is a crosscutting framework that applies across different areas such as health, park access, education, housing, transportation, and others. Using the framework to support community-driven solutions draws on lessons from the civil rights movement and related movements, such as the women's movement. Specific actions by several federal agencies illustrate how civil rights can be promoted to advance health equity through the planning framework.

Conclusion 6-1: In the committee's judgment, civil rights approaches have helped mitigate the negative impacts of many forms of social and health discrimination. Continuing this work is needed to overcome discrimination and the structural barriers that affect health.

Conclusion 6-2: The committee concludes that using civil rights approaches in devising and implementing community solutions to promote health equity can guard against unjustified and unnecessary discriminatory impacts, as well as against intentional discrimination in programs that affect health. For example, those implementing community solutions can employ methods and data in ways that include full and fair participation by diverse communities.

The philanthropy sector has a number of tools available to support communities as they design, implement, and evaluate interventions to promote health equity. In broad categories, these tools include convening, leadership and capacity development, model testing, topic studies and reports, project and program funding, advocacy support, and social movement building. Advocacy funding may present challenges for certain foundations for which funding issue-specific advocacy strategies, such as lobbying, is prohibited by federal tax law. Nevertheless, such foundations can support advocacy groups with general operating funds (as distinguished from program-specific funds) that can be used to lobby, as long as the foundation is not involved with decision making about what issues the advocacy group chooses to take on. Foundations can also support social movement building by providing support for organizations that use community organizing to address important social issues.

Recommendation 7-1: Foundations and other funders should support community interventions to promote health equity by:

- Supporting community organizing around important social determinants of health;
- Supporting community capacity building;
- Supporting education, compliance, and enforcement related to civil rights laws; and
- Prioritizing health equity and equity in the social determinants of health through investments in low-income and minority communities.

Past IOM reports have reflected on the limitations of randomized controlled trials for public health and related research and on the need for a broader array of research tools to inform community health improvement efforts (IOM, 2012; IOM and NRC, 2013). To inform community-based efforts to promote health equity, novel research is needed, but to make that possible, changes to the dominant research paradigm are needed.

While social epidemiology has made highly important contributions to our understanding of the social determinants of health and population health, it "does not have the breadth, or imply all of the multiple interactions and pathways" involved in population health (Kindig and Stoddart, 2003, p. 382). Thus, models for the training of population and place-based scientists and practitioners are needed in order to develop the research required to guide upstream approaches, including place-based interventions, which address contextual factors that shape major public health problems such as obesity, interpersonal violence, infant and maternal health problems, cardiovascular diseases, infectious diseases, substance use disorders, and mental health disorders. Therefore, based on the committee's expertise and its examination of the available evidence, the committee recommends the following:

Recommendation 7-2: A number of actions to improve the knowledge base for informing and guiding communities should be taken, including
- Public and private research funders should support communities and their academic partners in the collection, analysis, and application of evidence from the experience of practitioners, from leaders of community-based organizations, and from traditionally underrepresented participants who are typically left out of such partnerships.
- Universities, policy centers, and academic publications should modify current incentive[14] structures to encourage and reward more research on the social distribu-

---

[14] Such incentives may include funding, publication standards, and rules governing tenure.

tion of risks and resources and the systematic generation and dissemination of the evidence needed to guide the complex, multi-faceted interventions that are most likely to reduce inequities in health outcomes.[15]
- Academic programs should promote the development of and dialogue on theory, methods, and the training of students to create a more useful knowledge base in the next generation of researchers on how to design, implement, and evaluate place-based initiatives to improve community health.

Anchor institutions—a wide range of local institutions that include hospitals and universities, local government, sports venues, and museums—are "firmly rooted in their locales" and constitute "sticky capital" (i.e., capital that is resistant to change). Such institutions: (1) are affected by their local environment and, as such, have a stake in the health of surrounding communities; (2) have a moral and an ethical responsibility to contribute to the well-being of surrounding communities because they can make a difference; and (3) when involved in solving real-world local problems, are more likely to advance learning, research, teaching, and service (Harkavy et al., 2014).

Rubin and Rose (2015) and others (Martin et al., 2005; Miller and Rivera, n.d.; O'Mara, 2012) have highlighted the complex, sometimes contentious relationships and history between anchor institutions and their communities (e.g., community perception that they receive no benefit and may even be harmed by the local anchor institution). However, the potential of anchor institutions to engage with communities to improve well-being has also been explored and numerous examples provided (Dubb et al., 2013; Norris and Howard, 2015; NTFAI, 2010). Anchor institution motivations to engage with community partners vary and may include one or more of the following: "an economic self-interest in helping ensure that the communities in which they are based are safe, vibrant, and healthy" (Serang et al., 2013, p. 4); an interest in contributing to economic development; a sense of social responsibility; and a desire to pursue public–private partnerships to address mutually relevant challenges. The

---

[15] SQUIRE (Standards for Quality Improvement Reporting Excellence) is an example of concerted efforts by leaders in one sector—health care—to change powerful incentives. SQUIRE guidelines provide an explicit framework for reporting new knowledge about system-level work to improve the quality, safety, and value of health care in the hope of shifting the emphasis and rewards from a near-exclusive emphasis on experimental findings to examining interventions closely, carefully, and in detail; generating important new knowledge about systems of care; and learning about how best to change those systems (Davidoff and Batalden, 2005).

anchor institution approach of an articulated mission, strategies, and metrics to improve community conditions has gained increasing attention and buy-in in a number of major metropolitan areas (e.g., Cleveland, Ohio; Detroit, Michigan; Philadelphia, Pennsylvania; Phoenix, Arizona). Such anchors have made significant investments, usually with a number of other anchor partners including city government and, often, private investors. Data on how such efforts have improved the living conditions of long-term and low-income residents are not yet available.

> **Recommendation 7-3:** The committee recommends that anchor institutions (such as universities, hospitals, and businesses) make expanding opportunities to promote health equity in their community a strategic priority. This should be done by:
> - Deploying specific strategies to address the multiple determinants of health on which anchors can have a direct impact or through multi-sector collaboration; and
> - Assessing the negative and positive impacts of anchor institutions in their communities and how negative impacts may be mitigated.[16]

Policy makers include a wide variety of actors (e.g., city council members, mayors, school board members, state legislators, etc.) whose work spans the spectrum from very local policy development, such as zoning, to national policy development, such as the Fair Housing Act. Furthermore, policy shapes the social determinants of health and the conditions of communities (IOM, 2011). Historically, policy has arguably been a driver of health inequity (e.g., redlining and urban renewal policies) (Williams and Collins, 2001). Thus, policy makers can play a significant leadership role in advancing progress in communities toward health equity.

> **Recommendation 7-4:** The committee recommends that local policy makers assess policies, programs, initiatives, and funding allocations for their potential to create or increase health inequities in their communities.

Public health agencies can bring data, epidemiologic expertise, partnerships, and community engagement capacity in addition to commitments to achieving health equity. Because of previously established relationships, public health agencies are also natural conveners of certain health equity stakeholders, including health care systems, community organizations, and insurance companies. In addition, because

---

[16] See, for example, McNeely and Norris (2015).

nontraditional partnerships are needed to successfully address the social, economic, and environmental factors influencing health equity, public health agencies can become conveners of community development organizations, faith-based organizations, businesses, and governmental agencies (e.g., transportation, housing, education). Furthermore, public health agencies have some of the data needed to link nontraditional partners' work and interests to health and can serve as a source of evidence-based approaches that nontraditional partners can implement or support. The capacity of public health agencies as data repositories could be enhanced if more data were available and stratified by neighborhood levels for specific populations and health-related indicators, and if agencies could obtain data from a range of public- and private-sector sources, analyze it, and share it with partners and users in the community in a timely manner (RESOLVE, 2014).

In early 2016 the Governance Institute convened the first in a series of intensive trainings as part of Alignment of Governance & Leadership in Healthcare: Building Momentum for Transformation. The training, which will recur, was designed to orient health care delivery system executives to the potential of interfacing and partnering with the community development sector. Moreover, the Build Healthy Places Network, the Center on Social Disparities in Health, and RWJF have together put forward *Making the Case for Linking: Community Development and Health*, a brief highlighting multiple models and examples of health and development sector partnerships from around the country (Edmonds et al., 2015). The growing recognition that health is powerfully shaped by place calls on health sector practitioners, researchers, and decision makers to strengthen their relationships with the community development sector, from community development corporations that work to expand opportunity in communities to community development financial institutions and others.

> **Recommendation 7-5: The committee recommends that public health agencies and other health sector organizations build internal capacity to effectively engage community development partners and to coordinate activities that address the social and economic determinants of health. They should also play a convening or supporting role with local community coalitions to advance health equity.**

New federal education legislation, the Every Student Succeeds Act,[17] is a new mandate that requires school-level needs assessments, although

---

[17] S.1177—Every Student Succeeds Act. Public Law 114-95 (December 10, 2015), 114th Cong.

access to quality data may persist as a barrier. For example, not all schools have good data on chronic absenteeism (ED, 2016b). Nor is information on school climate and neighborhood and on the community factors that affect learning widely available. See Chapter 6 for a recommendation (Recommendation 6-2) on state department guidance for student health needs assessments.

> Recommendation 7-6: Given the strong effects of educational attainment on health outcomes and their own focus on equity (ED, 2016c), the U.S. Department of Education Institute for Educational Science and other divisions in the department should support states, localities, and their community partners with evidence and technical assistance on the impact of quality early childhood education programs, on interventions that reduce disparities in learning outcomes, and on the keys to success in school transitions (i.e., pre-K and K–12 or K–12 postsecondary).

Given the crucial importance of health equity to the nation's economic and growth prospects and to communities' well-being and vibrancy, high-level attention and coordination are needed to ensure that efforts to rein in inequity succeed. The current state of health disparities has severe consequences for the nation, and it is a call to action to stem the high human and economic cost of health inequity. Clearly, considerable support for addressing health equity has been established in the U.S. Department of Health and Human Services and across the executive branch through the Federal Interagency Health Equity Taskforce. In November 2016, the President signed an executive order establishing a community solutions council charged with fostering "collaboration across agencies, policy councils, and offices to coordinate actions, identify working solutions to share broadly, and develop and implement policy recommendations that put the community-driven, locally led vision at the center of policymaking" (The White House, 2016). Sustaining and elevating cross-government effort is important to help galvanize a national effort toward promoting health equity and to encourage ongoing multi-sectoral community-based efforts around the country.

> Recommendation 7-7: The committee recommends that key federal government efforts, such as the Community Solutions Council, that are intended to support communities in addressing major challenges, consider integrating health equity as a focus.

A health equity focus could mean undertaking such approaches as:
(a) Determining how government decisions in health and non-health sectors could affect low-income and minority populations.
(b) Convening key stakeholders to explore financing structures through which companies, philanthropy, and government can together fund key health equity initiatives, including efforts to generate better, timelier, and more locally relevant data.

The importance of considering the unintended consequences of government policies is evident. For example, Chapter 3 describes examples of historical government policies that shaped government investment, land use, transportation, planning, and other features of communities with disproportionately negative effects on access to housing, safety, social cohesion, family stability, and health outcomes in low-income and minority populations (Freeman and Braconi, 2002; Fullilove and Wallace, 2011; IOM, 2003; Levy et al., 2006; Prevention Institute, 2011; Vélez, 2001; Zuk et al., 2015). Weighing the consequences on health outcomes, however, will require access to more varied and meaningful sources of data and may demand resources for analysis and assessment. The unique circumstances and context of each community (defined by census tract or zip code) may make it difficult to undertake such an assessment of potential consequences in a way that considers their full scope.

Public–private partnerships offer opportunities for innovation and alignment of resources that can achieve greater efficiency and effectiveness. Examples include pay-for-success financing models to support early childhood development and other programs, the Sustainable Communities federal partnership that brought together public- and private-sector actors to align their efforts, and clean energy financing arrangements (IOM, 2015b; PolicyLink, n.d.; Probst, 2014).

TOOLS

In its gathering of community examples and review of the literature, the committee identified a number of guiding principles for community consideration. They are provided in Box S-2, along with the three key elements found in all nine examples of community-based solutions to promote health equity highlighted in Chapter 5.

Chapter 8 provides a range of tools for facilitating multi-sector collaboration, making health equity a shared vision and value, and building capacity to shape outcomes in the community. Depending on a specific community's needs and current available resources, some tools may be more applicable for them than others. The tools outlined in this chapter include making the case for health equity; meeting data information

> **BOX S-2**
> **Some Guiding Principles for Community Consideration**
>
> As described above, community-based efforts to promote health equity require the following three key elements: (1) making health equity a shared vision and value, (2) increasing community capacity to shape outcomes, and (3) fostering multi-sector collaboration. Although no recipe for successful collaboration to promote health equity exists, some additional characteristics emerging from the literature and community-based practices are:
>
> **Process**
>
> - Leverage existing efforts whenever possible.
> - Adopt explicit strategies for authentic community engagement, ownership, involvement, and input throughout all stages of such efforts.
> - Nurture the next generation of leadership.
> - Foster flexibility, creativity, and resilience where possible.
> - Seriously consider potential community partners, including nontraditional ones.
> - Commit to results, systematic learning, cross-boundary collaboration, capacity building, and sustainability.
> - Partner with public health agencies whenever possible, no matter the focus of the effort.
>
> SOURCES: Community Tool Box, 2016; FSG, 2011, 2013; Prybil et al., 2014; Verbitsky-Savitz et al., 2016.

needs, with available data sources and interactive tools outlined; adopting theories of change; using civil rights law; medical–legal partnerships; health impact assessments; funding mechanisms; public will building; capacity building for multiple purposes; and a list of community tool kits.

CONCLUDING OBSERVATIONS

There are systemic root causes of health inequities in this country that can seem overwhelming to local communities working to tackle unemployment, concentrated poverty, and school dropout rates. It will take considerable time to address these root causes, and it will require system-level changes to reduce poverty, eliminate structural racism, improve income equality, increase educational opportunity, and fix the laws and policies that perpetuate structural inequities. All actors in the community—businesses, state and local governments, anchor institutions, and other community residents—have the power to change the narrative and help promote health equity. Although the report focuses on community-based solutions, where possible, promising strategies to address these hard-to-tackle root causes at higher levels are provided, including the policy context and the supportive actions of partners.

REFERENCES

Adler, N. E., and J. Stewart. 2010. Health disparities across the lifespan: Meaning, methods, and mechanisms. *Annals of the New York Academy of Sciences* 1186:5–23.
Aizer, A., J. Currie, P. Simon, and P. Vivier. 2015. Inequality in lead exposure and the black-white test score gap. *Institute for Public Policy and Social Research.* https://www.ippsr.msu.edu/research/inequality-lead-exposure-and-black-white-test-score-gap (accessed December 9, 2016).
Alley, D. E., C. N. Asomugha, P. H. Conway, and D. M. Sanghavi. 2016. Accountable Health Communities—Addressing Social Needs through Medicare and Medicaid. *The New England Journal of Medicine* 374(1):8.
Arias, E. 2016. *Changes in life expectancy by race and Hispanic origin in the United States, 2013–2014.* Hyattsville, MD: National Center for Health Statistics.
Beatty, A., and D. Foster. 2015. *The determinants of equity: Identifying indicators to establish a baseline of equity in King County.* King County, WA: King County Office of Performance, Strategy, and Budget.
Bell, J., and L. Cohen. 2009. *The Transportation Prescription: Bold new ideas for healthy, equitable transportation reform in America, 2009. Commissioned by the Convergence Partnership.* https://www.preventioninstitute.org/sites/default/files/publications/The%20Transportation%20Prescription_0.pdf (accessed December 14, 2016).
Berwick, D. M., T. W. Nolan, and J. Whittington. 2008. The triple aim: Care, health, and cost. *Health Affairs* 27(3):759–769.
Bethell, C. D., P. Newacheck, E. Hawes, and N. Halfon. 2014. Adverse childhood experiences: Assessing the impact on health and school engagement and the mitigating role of resilience. *Health Affairs* 33(12):2106–2115.
Braveman, P., and L. Gottlieb. 2014. The social determinants of health: It's time to consider the causes of the causes. *Public Health Reports* 129(Suppl 2):19–31.
Braveman, P. A., S. Kumanyika, J. Fielding, T. LaVeist, L. N. Borrell, R. Manderscheid, and A. Troutman. 2011. Health disparities and health equity: The issue is justice. *American Journal of Public Health* 101(Suppl 1):S149–S155.
Carr, M. D., and E. Wiemers. 2016. *The decline in lifetime earnings mobility in the U.S.: Evidence from survey-linked administrative data.* Washington, DC: Washington Center for Equitable Growth.
CDC (U.S. Centers for Disease Control and Prevention). 2015. *CDC community health improvement navigator.* http://www.cdc.gov/chinav/ (accessed October 28, 2016).
ChangeLab Solutions. 2016. *Model Comprehensive Plan Language on Complete Streets: A framework to embrace complete streets principle.* http://www.changelabsolutions.org/publications/comp-plan-language-cs (accessed October 24, 2016).
Chetty, R., M. Stepner, S. Abraham, S. Lin, B. Scuderi, N. Turner, A. Bergeron, and D. Cutler. 2016. The association between income and life expectancy in the United States, 2001–2014. *JAMA* 315(16):1750–1766.
Christeson, W., A. D. Taggart, and S. Messner-Zidell. 2009. *Ready, willing, and unable to serve: 75 percent of young adults cannot join the military. Early education across America is needed to ensure national security.* Washington, DC: Mission: Readiness.
Clear, T. R. 2008. The effects of high imprisonment rates on communities. *Crime and Justice* 37(1):97–132.

Community Tool Box. 2016. Chapter 1. Section 7. *Working together for healthier communities: A framework for collaboration among community partnership, support organizations, and funders.* http://ctb.ku.edu/en/table-of-contents/overview/model-for-community-change-and-improvement/framework-for-collaboration/main (accessed October 18, 2016).

Cooper, L. A., D. L. Roter, R. L. Johnson, D. E. Ford, D. M. Steinwachs, and N. R. Powe. 2003. Patient-centered communication, ratings of care, and concordance of patient and physician race. *Annals of Internal Medicine* 139(11):907–915.

Council for a Strong America. 2016. New 50-state index from Council for a Strong America shows most young adults not "citizen-ready": Crime and inability to join military or workforce present national crisis. *Marketwired*, September 13.

Davidoff, F., and P. Batalden. 2005. Toward stronger evidence on quality improvement. Draft publication guidelines: The beginning of a consensus project. *Quality & Safety in Health Care* 14(5):319–325.

Diez Roux, A. V., and C. Mair. 2010. Neighborhoods and health. *Annals of the New York Academy of Sciences* 1186(1):125–145.

Dubb, S., S. McKinley, and T. Howard. 2013. *Achieving the anchor promise: Improving outcomes for low-income children, families and communities.* Takoma Park, MD: Democracy Collaborative.

ED (U.S. Department of Education). 2016a. Healthy students, promising futures: State and local action steps and practices to improve school-based health toolkit. https://www2.ed.gov/admins/lead/safety/healthy-students/toolkit.pdf (accessed October 17, 2016).

ED. 2016b. Chronic absenteeism in the nation's schools: An unprecedented look at a hidden educational crisis. https://www2.ed.gov/datastory/chronicabsenteeism.html (accessed October 28, 2016).

ED. 2016c. The fiscal year 2017 budget: Promoting greater use of evidence and data as a lever for advancing equity. In Homeroom: The Official Blog of the U.S. Department of Education. http://www2.ed.gov/admins/lead/safety/healthy-students/index.html (accessed October 24, 2016).

Edmonds, A., P. Braveman, E. Arkin, and D. Jutte. 2015. *Making the case for linking community development and health: A resource for those working to improve low-income communities and the lives of the people living in them.* UCSF Center on Social Disparities in Health, Robert Wood Johnson Foundation, and the Build Healthy Places Network.

Freeman, L., and F. Braconi. 2002. Gentrification and displacement. *The Urban Prospect* 8(1).

FSG (Foundation Strategy Group). 2011. *Collective impact.* http://www.fsg.org/ideas-in-action/collective-impact (accessed October 18, 2016).

FSG. 2013. *Using collective impact in a public health context: Introduction.* http://www.fsg.org/blog/using-collective-impact-public-health-context-introduction (accessed October 18, 2016).

Fullilove, M. T., and R. Wallace. 2011. Serial forced displacement in American cities, 1916–2010. *Journal of Urban Health* 88(3):381–389.

Graham, H. 2004. Social determinants and their unequal distribution: Clarifying policy understandings. *Milbank Q* 82(1):101–124.

Harkavy, I., M. Hartley, R. A. Hodges, A. Sorrentino, and J. Weeks. 2014. Effective governance of a university as an anchor institution: University of Pennsylvania as a case study. *Leadership and Governance in Higher Education* 2:98–116.

HERO (Health Enhancement Research Organization). 2015. Exploring the value proposition for workforce health: Business leader attitudes about the role of health as a driver of productivity and performance. http://hero-health.org/wp-content/uploads/2015/02/HPP-Business-Leader-Survey-Full-Report_FINAL.pdf (accessed October 24, 2016).

Howard, T. C. 2010. *Why race and culture matter in schools: Closing the achievement gap in America's classrooms.* New York: Teachers College Press.

IOM (Institute of Medicine). 2003. *Unequal treatment: Confronting racial and ethnic disparities in health care.* Washington, DC: The National Academies Press.
IOM. 2011. *For the public's health: Revitalizing law and policy to meet new challenges.* Washington, DC: The National Academies Press.
IOM. 2012. *For the public's health: Investing in a healthier future.* Washington, DC: The National Academies Press.
IOM. 2015a. *Business engagement in building healthy communities: Workshop summary.* Washington, DC: The National Academies Press.
IOM. 2015b. *Financing population health improvement.* Washington, DC: The National Academies Press.
IOM and NRC (Institute of Medicine and National Research Council). 2013. *Priorities for research to reduce the thread of firearm-related violence.* Washington, DC: The National Academies Press.
IRS (Internal Revenue Service). 2016. Statistics for tax returns with EITC. https://www.eitc.irs.gov/ EITC-Central/eitcstats?_ga=1.80629535.982617637.1477348670 (accessed December 19, 2016).
Jimenez, M. E., N. E. Reichman, R. Wade, Y. Lin, and L. M. Morrow. 2016. Adverse experiences in early childhood and kindergarten outcomes. *Pediatrics* 137(2).
Jones, H. 2009. *Equity in development: Why it is important and how to achieve it.* London, UK: Overseas Development Institute.
Kenney, G. M., and M. Huntress. 2012. *The Affordable Care Act: Coverage implications and issues for immigrant families.* https://aspe.hhs.gov/basic-report/affordable-care-act-coverage-implications-and-issues-immigrant-families (accessed October 24, 2016).
Kindig, D., and G. Stoddart. 2003. What is population health? *American Journal of Public Health* 93(3):380–383.
Krieger, N. 2014. Discrimination and Health Inequities. *International Journal of Health Services* 44(4):643–710.
Kruse, C. S., S. Bouffard, M. Dougherty, and J. S. Parro. 2016. Telemedicine use in rural Native American communities in the era of the ACA: A systematic literature review. *Journal of Medical Systems* 40(6):145.
LaVeist, T. A., D. J. Gaskin, and P. Richard. 2009. *The economic burden of health inequalities in the United States.* Washington, DC: Joint Center for Political and Economic Studies.
Levy, D. J., J. A. Heissel, J. A. Richeson, and E. K. Adam. 2016. Psychological and biological responses to race-based social stress as pathways to disparities in educational outcomes. *American Psychologist* 71(6):455–473.
Levy, D. K., J. Comey, and S. Padilla. 2006. *In the face of gentrification: Case studies of local efforts to mitigate displacement.* Washington, DC: Urban Institute.
Losen, D., C. Hodson, M. A. Keith II, K. Morrison, and S. Belway. 2015. *Are we closing the school discipline gap?* Los Angeles: University of California.
Marmot, M., J. Allen, P. Goldblatt, T. Boyce, D. McNeish, M. Grady, and I. Geddes. 2010. *Fair society, healthy lives: Strategic review of health inequalities in England post-2010.* London: The Marmot Review.
Martin, L. L., H. Smith, and W. Phillips. 2005. Bridging 'town & gown' through innovative university-community partnerships. *The Innovation Journal: The Public Sector Innovation Journal* 10(2). http://www.innovation.cc/volumes-issues/martin-u-partner4final.pdf (accessed October 20, 2016).
McNeely, E., and G. Norris. 2015. *SHINE summit 2015: Innovating for NetPositive impact: Summary report.* Boston, MA: Sustainability and Healthy Initiative for NetPositive Enterprise.
Miller, D. S., and J. D. Rivera. n.d. Town and gown: Understanding the past to improve the future. *International Journal of the Humanities* 3(8):215–224.

Minkler, M., A. P. Garcia, J. Williams, T. Lopresti, and J. Lilly. 2010. Si se puede: Using participatory research to promote environmental justice in a Latino community in San Diego, California. *Journal of Urban Health* 87(5):796–812.

Mosavel, M., R. Ahmed, D. Daniels, and C. Simon. 2011. Community researchers conducting health disparities research: Ethical and other insights from fieldwork journaling. *Social Science & Medicine* 73(1):145–152.

Multnomah County. 2014a. *Foundational assumptions of the equity and empowerment lens logic model.* https://multco.us/file/31824/download (accessed October 28, 2016).

Multnomah County. 2014b. *Multnomah County Office of Diversity and Equity: Equity and empowerment lens.* https://multco.us/diversity-equity/equity-and-empowerment-lens (accessed October 24, 2016).

Multnomah County. n.d. *What is the equity and empowerment lens?* https://multco.us/diversity-equity/equity-and-empowerment-lens (accessed October 28, 2016).

NASEM (National Academies of Sciences, Engineering, and Medicine). 2016a. *Accounting for social risk factors in Medicare payment: Identifying social risk factors.* Washington, DC: The National Academies Press.

NASEM. 2016b. *Accounting for social risk factors in Medicare payment: Criteria, factors, and methods.* Washington, DC: The National Academies Press.

NASEM. 2016c. *Accounting for social risk factors in Medicare payment: Data.* Washington, DC: The National Academies Press.

NASEM. 2016d. *The role of business in multisector obesity solutions: Working together for positive change: Workshop in brief.* Washington, DC: The National Academies Press.

NASEM. 2016e. *Systems practices for the care of socially at-risk populations.* Washington, DC: The National Academies Press.

NIH (National Institutes of Health). 2014. *Health disparities.* http://www.nhlbi.nih.gov/health/educational/healthdisp/ (accessed November 2, 2016).

Norris, T., and T. Howard. 2015. *Can Hospitals Heal America's Communities?*

NRC (National Research Council). 2014. *The growth of incarceration in the United States: Exploring causes and consequences.* Washington, DC: The National Academies Press.

NRC and IOM. 2013. *U.S. health in international perspective: Shorter lives, poorer health.* Washington, DC: The National Academies Press.

NTFAI (National Task Force on Anchor Institutions). 2010. *Anchor institutions task force.* http://www.margainc.com/files_images/general/anchor_task_force_statement.pdf (accessed October 20, 2016).

OECD (Organisation for Economic Co-operation and Development). 2015. *Health at a glance: OECD indicators.* Paris: OECD Publishing.

O'Mara, M. P. 2012. Beyond town and gown: University economic engagement and the legacy of the urban crisis. *Journal of Technology Transfer* 37(2):234–250.

PHAB (Public Health Accreditation Board). 2011. *Public Health Accreditation Board standards & measures, version 1.0.* http://www.phaboard.org/wp-content/uploads/PHAB-Standards-and-Measures-Version-1.01.pdf (accessed December 2, 2016).

PolicyLink. n.d. *Center for Infrastructure Equity: Sustainable communities.* http://www.policylink.org/focus-areas/infrastructure-equity/sustainable-communities (accessed December 1, 2016).

Prevention Institute. 2011. *Fact Sheet: Links between violence and health equity.* Oakland, CA: Prevention Institute.

Probst, C. S. 2014. *Private sector financing and public-private partnerships for financing clean energy.* Research Program on Sustainability Policy and Management, Earth Institute, Columbia University.

Prybil, L., F. D. Scutchfield, R. Killian, A. Kelly, G. Mays, A. Carman, S. Levey, A. McGeorge, and D. W. Fardo. 2014. Improving community health through hospital–public health collaboration: Insights and lessons learned from successful partnerships. In *Health*

Management and Policy Faculty Book Gallery: Book 2. Lexington, KY: Commonwealth Center for Governance Studies, Inc.

Reardon, S. F., R. A. Valentino, and K. A. Shores. 2012. Patterns of literacy among U.S. students. *Future of Children* 22(2):17–37.

RESOLVE. 2014. *The high achieving governmental health department in 2020 as the community chief health strategist.* Washington, DC: RESOLVE.

Rubin, V., and K. Rose. 2015. *Strategies for strengthening anchor institutions' community impact.* Oakland, CA: PolicyLink.

Rudolph, L., S. Gould, and J. Berko. 2015. Climate change, health, and equity: Opportunities for action. https://www.phi.org/uploads/application/files/h7fjouo1i38v3t-u427p9s9kcmhs3oxsi7tsg1fovh3yesd5hxu.pdf (accessed October 24, 2016).

Sabin, J., B. A. Nosek, A. Greenwald, and F. P. Rivara. 2009. Physicians' implicit and explicit attitudes about race by MD race, ethnicity, and gender. *Journal of Health Care for the Poor and Underserved* 20(3):896–913.

Salway, S., P. Chowbey, E. Such, and B. Ferguson. 2015. Researching health inequalities with community researchers: Practical, methodological and ethical challenges of an "inclusive" research approach. *Research Involvement and Engagement* 1(1).

Serang, F., J. P. Thompson, and T. Howard. 2013. *The anchor mission: Leveraging the power of anchor institutions to build community wealth.* Takoma Park, MD: The Democracy Collaborative.

Skiba, R. J., R. H. Horner, C.-G. Chung, M. K. Rausch, S. L. May, and T. Tobin. 2011. Race is not neutral: A national investigation of African American and Latino disproportionality in school discipline. *School Psychology Review* 40(1):85–107.

Smith, E. J., and S. R. Harper. 2015. *Disproportionate impact of K-12 school suspension and explusion on black students in southern states.* Philadelphia, PA: Penn Graduate School of Education Center for the Study of Race and Equity in Education.

The White House. 2016. *Executive Order—Establishing a Community Solutions Council.* https://www.whitehouse.gov/the-press-office/2016/11/16/executive-order-establishing-community-solutions-council (accessed December 1, 2016).

Uberoi, N., K. Finegold, and E. Gee. 2016. *Health insurance coverage and the Affordable Care Act, 2010-2016.* Office of the Assistant Secretary for Planning and Evaluation, U.S. Department of Health and Human Services.

Ubri, P., and S. Artiga. 2016. *Disparities in health and health care: Five key questions and answers.* http://files.kff.org/attachment/Issue-Brief-Disparities-in-Health-and-Health-Care-Five-Key-Questions-and-Answers (accessed October 24, 2016).

Vélez, M. B. 2001. Role of public social control in urban neighborhoods: A multi-level analysis of victimization risk. *Criminology* 39(4):837-864.

Verbitsky-Savitz, N., M. B. Hargreaves, S. Penoyer, N. Morales, B. Coffee-Borden, and E. Whitesell. 2016. *Preventing and mitigating the effects of ACEs by building community capacity and resilience: APPI cross-site evaluation findings.* Washington, DC: Mathematica Policy Research.

Waidmann, T. 2009. *Estimating the cost of racial and ethnic health disparities.* Washington, DC: Urban Institute.

Williams, D. R., and C. Collins. 2001. Racial residential segregation: A fundamental cause of racial disparities in health. *Public Health Reports* 116(5):404–416.

Woolf, S. H., L. Aron, L. Dubay, S. M. Simon, E. Zimmerman, and K. X. Luk. 2015. *How are income and wealth linked to health and longevity?* Washington, DC: Urban Institute and Virginia Commonwealth University.

Zuk, M., A. H. Bierbaum, K. Chapple, K. Gorska, A. Loukaitou-Sideris, P. Ong, and T. Thomas. 2015 (unpublished). *Gentrification, displacement, and role of public investment: A literature review.* Federal Reserve Bank of San Francisco.

1

The Need to Promote Health Equity

INTRODUCTION

In the United States, health equity and equal opportunity are inextricably linked, and the burdens of disease and poor health and the benefits of wellness and good health are inequitably distributed among groups of people.

Although biology, genetics, and individual behaviors play a role in these differences, many health outcomes are more substantially affected by social, economic, and environmental factors. Understanding the social determinants of health requires a shift toward a more "upstream" perspective—that is, the conditions that constitute the context in which an individual's behaviors are shaped. To put this more simply, Keyes and Galea (2016) describe the relationship between an individual and the conditions in which one lives using the metaphor of a fishbowl. If the bowl in which a fish lives is dirty, or the glass is cracked and the water is leaking, the fish will never reach its full health potential, despite any individual effort. Although the life of a person is clearly more complex than that of a fish, this metaphor illustrates the futility of only addressing individual behaviors without considering the context. People inhabit environments shaped by policies, forces, and actions that influence their individual choices and behaviors over a lifetime and over generations. Community-wide and national problems like poverty, unemployment, poor education, inadequate housing, poor public transportation, exposure to violence, and neighborhood deterioration (social or physical) are among the factors that shape people's health, and they do so in unequal ways, thus contributing to health inequities. The historic and ongoing interplay of structures, policies, norms, and demographic/geographic patterns shapes the life of every individual across the country. These factors are not intractable, and inequities in these factors can be mitigated by policies and community action in powerful ways (see Chapter 3 for a discussion of the evidence). Community assets can be built, leveraged, and modified to create a context to achieve health equity.

People are heavily influenced by the communities they work and live in, and the diverse actors that make up the community ecosystem can be powerful producers of health and well-being. Therefore, this report focuses on the promise of communities to create opportunities for their members to achieve their full health potential. By showcasing many creative, forward-looking, and bold community-led solutions for achieving health equity, this report aims to provide a new narrative about health in the United States. In addition to actors in communities, the report examines other elements that address the structures, policies, and norms needed to promote health equity.

DEFINING HEALTH EQUITY

This report makes frequent reference to a number of terms with meanings that vary depending on the context and the community of users. Such terms include "disparities," "inequities," "equity," "racism," and "bias," and they are defined in the glossary of key terms and when first introduced in the report.

It is difficult to fully separate the concepts of equity and equality because they are intertwined. Different fields have used varying terminology in legal, public health, government, and other contexts. This report uses the term "health equity" by applying the term equity to the field of public health. *Health equity* is the state in which everyone has the opportunity to attain full health potential and no one is disadvantaged from achieving this potential because of social position or any other socially defined circumstance. In this report promoting health equity means creating the conditions where individuals and communities have what they need to enjoy full, healthy lives. Health equity requires focused and sustained societal efforts to confront historical and contemporary injustices and eliminate health disparities (Brennan Ramirez et al., 2008; HHS, n.d.). *Health disparities* are differences that exist among specific population groups in the attainment of full health potential and in incidence, prevalence, mortality, and burden of disease and other adverse health conditions (NIH, 2010), and they stem from systematic differences—that are preventable and unjust—among groups and communities occupying unequal positions in society (Graham, 2004).

As discussed later in this chapter, studies of health inequities have focused largely on health disparities across racial and ethnic populations. Although such studies have uncovered patterns of discrimination and inequitable health outcomes, enlarging this work to assess the effects of poverty, unemployment, toxic stress, and the many secondary unintended consequences (e.g., drug use and violence) for minority and other disproportionately impacted populations is needed. It is well documented that low socioeconomic status (SES) hampers an individual's ability to achieve optimal health by limiting access to health-preserving resources (Williams and Purdie-Vaughns, 2015; Woolf and Braveman, 2011). However, SES does not fully explain health disparities based on race and ethnicity, sexual orientation and gender identity (Williams and Purdie-Vaughns, 2015).

In the following sections, the nature and implications of disparities on three key health indicators and for health care are discussed. This discussion is followed by a brief introduction to the social determinants of health and the impacts of health inequities on society. Next, the changing social and environmental context and the role of communities in addressing health inequity are described. Finally, this chapter highlights the ongoing support for accelerating the progress to achieve health equity before providing an overview of the rest of the report.

DISPARITIES IN HEALTH OUTCOMES

The existence of racial and ethnic disparities in morbidity, mortality, and many indicators of health for African Americans, Native Americans, Hispanics,[1] and Asians/Pacific Islanders was first acknowledged by the federal government in the 1985 *Report of the Secretary's Task Force on Black and Minority Health* (Heckler, 1985). Since then, research has sought to identify additional disparities and explain the mechanisms by which these disparities occur.

Three indicators provide summary information about the overall health of a population or subpopulation: *infant mortality, age-adjusted death rates*, and *life expectancy*. The United States ranks lower than most peer nations on these indicators; moreover, racial and ethnic disparities exist in quality and length of life among U.S. residents. The failure to address growing income inequality, along with health inequities by race

---

[1] Hispanic/Latino identification with country of origin: Four decades after the U.S. government mandated the use of Hispanic or Latino for data collection (e.g., in the decennial census), most Americans with roots in Spanish-speaking countries prefer to be identified by their country (51 percent versus 24 percent who prefer a pan-ethnic term). Also, 69 percent respond that they believe there are multiple cultures, not one monolithic "Hispanic" or "Latino" culture (Taylor et al., 2012).

and ethnicity, contributes to the United States' low health ranking among peer nations (Davis et al., 2014).

Infant mortality rates reflect the number of infants in a population who die before their first birthday per 1,000 live births. U.S. infant mortality rates have decreased since 2005 for the overall population and within each racial and ethnic group; however, sharp racial and ethnic disparities persist. In 2013, as in previous years, the infant mortality rate among African Americans (11.1 per 1,000 live births) was double the rate among whites (5.06 per 1,000 live births) (Mathews et al., 2015). American Indians/Alaska Natives and Puerto Ricans also experienced higher infant mortality rates (of 7.61 and 5.93 per 1,000 live births, respectively) than whites (Mathews et al., 2015). Infant mortality rates among Asians/Pacific Islanders and non-Puerto Rican Hispanics were lower than those of whites. If white America and black America were two separate nations, white America's infant mortality rate would rank 49th in the world, while black America's would be ranked 95th out of 224 nations listed by the U.S. Central Intelligence Agency's World Factbook, following Botswana, Sri Lanka, the United Arab Emirates, and Turks and Caicos Islands (WHO, 2015).

Life expectancy, the average number of years a person is expected to live based on current mortality rates (typically reported as life expectancy at birth or average number of years a newborn would be expected to live), captures the degree to which all of the individual-level socioeconomic, environmental, and health care–related resources in a society enable members of that society to achieve a long and healthy life. Better living conditions and better access to health care–related resources throughout the lifespan extend longevity. From 1980 to 2014, U.S. life expectancy (at birth) increased by approximately 6 years for males, reaching 76.4 years, and increased 3 years for females, reaching 81.2 years. Racial and ethnic disparities decreased, but they were not eliminated. In 2014, the life expectancy for African American males was 72.0 years, while that for white males was 76.5 years and that for Latino males was 79.2 years. In the same year, life expectancy was 78.1 years for African American females, 81.1 years for white females, and 84.0 years for Latina females (Arias, 2016). Childhood obesity, which disproportionately affects Hispanic and African American youth (Asieba, 2016; Taveras et al., 2013), has been projected to reduce the steady increase in overall life expectancy in this century (Olshansky et al., 2005).

Age-adjusted mortality rates capture population deaths due to all causes, and especially those not due to old age. High death rates suggest that a population not only faces serious threats to health but also lacks the resources needed to address them. The 2012 to 2014 U.S. age-adjusted rates ranged considerably. By race and ethnicity, they ranged from 399.8

per 100,000 people among Asian/Pacific Islanders to 858.1 among African Americans. From 2007 to 2009, the rate was even higher (943.0 per 100,000) among American Indian/Alaska Natives (IHS, 2016). Although the overall death rate among whites (729.1 per 100,000) was substantially lower than the rate among African Americans, it exceeded that of Asian/Pacific Islanders and American Indian/Alaska Natives (NCHS, 2014) for causes including liver disease, suicide, and unintentional injury (Kochanek et al., 2016). Looking at more distal causes, research indicates that age-adjusted death rates among whites are higher for those who live in rural settings (Caldwell et al., 2016) and have lower incomes (HRSA, 2015).

The patterns of health disparities among immigrants and their children that emerge from available data are not straightforward. More than half of U.S. citizens of Asian/Pacific Islander and Hispanic background come from families that emigrated to the United States since 1965. Considerable socioeconomic and cultural heterogeneity exists within these groups, and some subpopulations (e.g., the Hmong population of Asian descent) experience particularly severe health disparities (Cho and Hummer, 2001; de Souza and Anand, 2014; Vang et al., 2015). However, recent immigrant status has also shown positive health impact in some populations (Hummer et al., 2007; Lee et al., 2013; Markides and Coreil, 1986).

Along with race and ethnicity, sexual orientation and gender identity have emerged as important factors in the study of health disparities. Recent epidemiologic surveys have attempted to comprehensively assess the physical and mental health of lesbian, gay, bisexual, and transgender (LGBT) persons (Hsieh and Ruther, 2016; IOM, 2011). The available evidence shows that the LGBT population does experience health disparities and that the disparities are exacerbated for those who hold multiple minority statuses: this "intersectional" perspective describes the recognition that when multiple identities intersect, they represent overlapping inequalities or types of disadvantage (IOM, 2011). Thus, LGBT persons who are also racial/ethnic minorities have worse outcomes than do white LGBT individuals (Hsieh and Ruther, 2016).

Health Care

It is becoming clearer that health insurance coverage alone will not address health disparities associated with race, ethnicity, SES, and geography (Kenney and Huntress, 2012; Ubri and Artiga, 2016). The Patient Protection and Affordable Care Act (ACA), passed in 2010, has accelerated progress toward improved health equity by expanding health insurance coverage to about 20 million Americans (Uberoi et al., 2016). However, challenges remain in fully addressing health care inequity, including policy hurdles affecting subgroups of the population (e.g., lack of coverage for some immigrants and asylum seekers, or those subject to Deferred Action for Childhood Arrivals) (HealthCare.gov, n.d.); limited system capacity or competence to care for some populations, such as LGBT persons (e.g., newly covered partners of insured LGBT individuals); and the lack of health data to monitor the health needs of some populations (e.g., for American Indians, of whom approximately 20 percent live on rural reservations) (Kruse et al., 2016).

Merely increasing the availability of health care services does not necessarily reduce health care disparities. Consider how the availability of effective antiretroviral therapies has not reduced the rate of acquired immune deficiency syndrome (AIDS) equally across groups. In the U.S. context, the progression to AIDS may signal a failure to access treatment in a timely and appropriate manner as indicated by racial and ethnic trends that have been followed since the beginning of the epidemic, as shown in Figure 1-1.

Though AIDS diagnoses have decreased over time for all groups since the introduction of antiretroviral therapy, the proportion of diagnoses among whites has decreased substantially, while the percentage has increased for other groups, and most substantially for African Americans. Another striking example is found in the domain of clinical research,

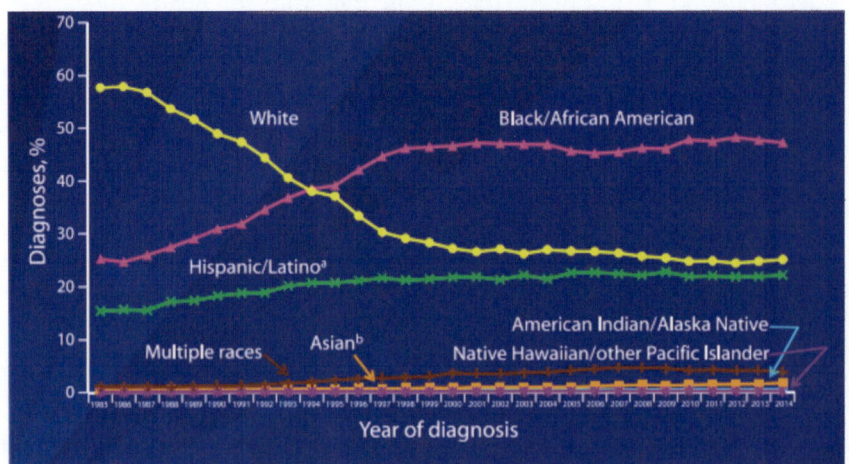

FIGURE 1-1 AIDS classifications among individuals with diagnosed HIV infection by race and ethnicity and year of diagnosis.
NOTE: All displayed data have been statistically adjusted to account for reporting delays, but not for incomplete reporting.
[a] Hispanics/Latinos can be of any race.
[b] Includes Asian/Pacific Islander legacy cases.
SOURCE: CDC, 2014.

where clinical trials of drugs and devices are not always carried out in diverse populations; therefore, the outcomes of trials may be biased toward the populations studied and fail to account for cultural or other factors that may influence effectiveness (George et al., 2014).

From a policy standpoint, the ACA has achieved its primary goal: the proportion of people who lack health insurance is lower than it has ever been. In the 29 states that have to date elected to participate in the ACA, Medicaid expansion has resulted in more than 10 million low-income individuals now being insured; furthermore, the associated reduction of cost-shifting for uncompensated care has benefited hospital budgets, particularly for disproportionate share hospitals (CMS, 2016; Cunningham et al., 2015). However, the costs of care for these patients are often greater than expected, and Medicaid's reimbursement rates are a small fraction of the reimbursement rates from commercial payers; therefore, cost-shifting persists. The ACA has increased the availability of outpatient care for low-income persons through increased funding for the operation, expansion, and construction of community health centers.

Challenges remain, however. As noted above, access to insurance does not directly translate into health equity. The traditional fee-for-service system persists and influences utilization patterns more heavily than patient need or evidence-based practice guidelines (The National Commission on Physician Payment Reform, 2013; Page, 2013; Robinson, 2001). Patients need only to receive the care they want and need. Also, there is still a subset of people without adequate insurance, and some commercial payers are leaving the exchanges, premiums are on the rise again, and pharmaceuticals and specialty drugs are increasing in complexity and pricing, untouched by the ACA.

A significant group of workers earn too much to qualify for Medicaid, but too little to afford health insurance. Also, the law does not address the needs of undocumented residents who are among the poorest people in the United States. Nearly one-third of all noncitizen immigrants lack insurance (Barry-Jester and Casselman, 2015). Underutilization of health care services among subpopulations of Hispanic and Asian immigrants has been documented (Alegria et al., 2006). The reasons for underutilization are complex and include an inability to speak the language, differences in the circumstances of immigration (e.g., refugees versus recruited professionals), and the fear of inadvertently outing family members who are in the country without documentation (Ortega et al., 2015).

Because the law is still relatively new, researchers are investigating its outcomes, but there are concerns that some lower-income working class individuals remain underinsured but have had more cost of health care shifted to them (Saloner et al., 2014), and the variations in use and cost persist.

SOCIAL DETERMINANTS OF HEALTH

Although most of the research being conducted at the time of the *Heckler Report* sought to explain how behavioral and other individual-level factors contribute to health and health care disparities, the evidence accrued since 1985 has led the field toward examining the social, environmental, economic, and cultural determinants of health. These determinants are the conditions in which one lives, learns, works, plays, worships, and ages, and these conditions are shaped by historical and contemporary policies, law, governance, investments, culture, and norms. Addressing the root causes of health inequities, such as the social determinants of health, is important in part to help enable sustainable interventions by engaging multiple sectors and addressing multiple health outcomes simultaneously. The solutions highlighted in this report recognize that national and state leadership are important to effect change in these determinants, but the report specifically addresses these interrelated determinants at the community level (see Chapter 3 for a detailed discussion of the root causes of health disparities, including the social determinants of health).

IMPACTS OF HEALTH INEQUITY IN THE UNITED STATES

Although moral arguments to promote health equity exist[2] advancing progress toward health equity could produce economic, national security, and other benefits for the nation. The premise that social mobility, opportunity to succeed with hard work, and opportunity to achieve prosperity exist is fundamental to the American Dream (Carr and Wiemers, 2016). However, recent literature demonstrates that worsening social, economic, and environmental factors are affecting health in serious ways that compromise opportunity for all (Chetty et al., 2016; Rudolph et al., 2015; Woolf et al., 2015). Health is more than life expectancy, infant health, and fitness and nutrition—it is the ability to lead a full and productive life. Additionally, an opportunity to achieve good health is crucial to U.S. democracy, national security, and economic vitality, as described below. The burden

---

[2] For example, Jones and colleagues cite valuing all people equally as foundational to the concept of equity, noting that the equal worth of all people is at the core of the human rights principle that all human beings equally possess certain rights (Jones, 2009). Braveman and colleagues point out that health differences adversely affecting socially disadvantaged groups are particularly unacceptable because ill health can be an obstacle to overcoming social disadvantage. They further note that this "consideration resonates with common sense notions of fairness, as well as with ethical concepts of justice" (Braveman et al., 2011). Daniels argues for the moral importance of health by exploring the necessities for justice as it relates to health care and the social determinants of health (Daniels, 2008).

of disparities lowers the nation's overall health status and its ranking relative to other nations.

Political and Economic Impacts of Health Disparities

In addition to the dollar cost of health care, because health inequities contribute to overall poor health for the nation, health inequity has consequences for the U.S. economy, national security, business workforce, and public finances.

Consequences for the Next Generation

American children rank behind their peers in most Organisation for Economic Co-operation and Development (OECD) nations in health status and on key determinants of health, and they experience growing disparities on multiple measures of child well-being (OECD, 2009; Seith and Isakson, 2011). Poverty, food insecurity, lack of stable housing, and lack of access to high-quality and developmentally optimal early childhood education are among the childhood factors that contribute to "chronic adult illnesses and to the intergenerational perpetuation of poverty and ill health found in many communities (e.g., obesity, diabetes, cardiovascular disease, poor educational outcomes, unemployment, poverty, early death)" (AAP, 2010, p. 839). Young children are most likely to live in poverty, and children from low-income and minority communities are most vulnerable (Burd-Sharps and Lewis, 2015). The nation's growing racial and ethnic diversity, coupled with the conditions that lead to serious early life disadvantage, have serious implications for health and health disparities in later life, leading to squandering human lives and their potential (OECD, 2009).

Consequences for the Economy

The economic effects of health inequity are the result of both unsustainable and wasteful health care spending and diminished productivity in the business sector. Health care spending accounted for 17.5 percent of gross domestic product (GDP) in 2014, and health disparities contribute to a significant amount of financial waste in the health care system.

LaVeist and colleagues (2009) calculated that eliminating health disparities for minorities would have reduced indirect costs associated with illness and premature death by more than $1 trillion between 2003 and 2006. In 2009, the Urban Institute projected that from 2009 to 2018, racial disparities in health will cost U.S. health insurers approximately $337 billion in total (Waidmann, 2009). Disparities in access to health care and in the quality of care can be costly to individuals, health care providers, health insurers, and taxpayers. Obtaining care late in the course of disease (i.e., delayed care) and inadequate health care coverage may increase the cost of care exponentially due to the exacerbation of complications, the need for more expensive care (e.g., emergency department services), and the need for more extensive care; furthermore, such treatment can increase longer-term reliance on the health care system for the management of unintended consequences on one hand and preventable chronic diseases on the other (IOM, 2009).

Consequences for National Security

For a nation that prizes military readiness, the effects of poor health status on entrance to military service and the readiness of the force matter. Military leaders reported that more than 75 percent of 17- to 24-year-olds—more than 26 million young adults—in the United States cannot qualify to serve in the armed forces because they have health problems ranging from obesity to dependencies on prescription and nonprescription drugs, are poorly educated, or are involved in crime (Christeson et al., 2009). According to more than 500 retired admirals, generals, and other senior military leaders, the health of our nation's youth represents a serious national security concern (Christeson et al., 2009, 2010). Individuals who are not healthy enough to participate in the workforce will not be afforded the same employment opportunities as their healthy counterparts. Rear Admiral Robert Besal (ret.) has asserted that young people who are physically unfit for "productive employment or military service represent a staggering loss of individual potential and collective strength for the nation as well" (Council for a Strong America, 2016).

Consequences for Business

A healthy, productive workforce is a prerequisite to a thriving economy (HERO, 2015; IOM, 2015). The impact of poor health on private businesses is significant. Research from the Urban Institute shows that those young adults with health problems who can find jobs in the mainstream economy are less productive and generate higher health care costs for businesses than those without health problems (Woolf et al., 2015).

Consequences for Income Inequality

Research finds that people in counties with an inequitable distribution of opportunities for good health are more likely to die before the age of 75 than people in counties with more equitable opportunities for health (health status), even if the average incomes are the same (University of Wisconsin Population Health Institute, 2015). Political scientists at Princeton and Georgetown University are finding that crippling political polarization and gridlock are linked to income and wealth inequality (Ferejohn, 2009; Voorheis et al., 2015). But income and wealth are not what worries Americans. Instead, it is what can be obtained with income and wealth that worries them most, and, of these, Gallup reports that health care is at the top of the list (Swift, 2015). Health problems often reduce personal income in ways that worsen inequity, which in turn may lead to further inequity. For states, it is well understood that as health care spending through state Medicaid increases, the funds available to support state universities decrease (Orszag and Kane, 2003).

CHANGING SOCIAL AND ENVIRONMENTAL CONTEXT

There are significant changes in the sociocultural (including demographic, economic, and political) and environmental landscapes affecting health disparities and the determinants of health.

The changing economic context is characterized by growing income inequality. According to an analysis performed by the Institute for Policy Studies, the income gap between higher- and lower-income individuals has increased substantially over the past 30 years, to the point that those with incomes in the top 10 percent average nine times the income of those in the bottom 90 percent, and those with incomes in the top 0.1 percent have incomes that are more than 184 times that of the bottom 90 percent (Asante-Muhammad et al., 2016). This income inequality has a remarkable impact on individual health, as higher-income earners have longer life expectancies than lower-income earners in every region of the United States. There are significant economic changes that affect other social determinants as well. For instance, urban centers across the country are dealing with shifting demographics that can result in the displacement of long-term residents. The economic advantages of changing land value due to these shifts largely benefit those who are already in higher-income brackets. In contrast, dislocated low-income households face overwhelming challenges in efforts to find new housing with access to high-quality schools, jobs, and other essential social services that are vital to optimal health. The lasting effects of the 2008 recession and the resulting displacement of vulnerable populations exacerbated the impact on both their health and their economic well-being—resulting in greater income inequality and wealth inequality (Smeeding, 2012).

Recent changes in U.S. demographics underscore the urgency of finding ways to attain health equity. For example, from 2000 to 2010 the African American population increased by 11 percent (Rastogi et al., 2010), and the Hispanic population increased by 43 percent (Ennis et al., 2011), while the white population increased by only 1.2 percent (Hixson et al., 2011). By 2040 the number of U.S. counties in which the majority of the population is comprised of people of color is expected to more than double; those counties will then represent about one-third of the United States (Frey, 2015). Without significant and fundamental policy changes, these changes in the racial and ethnic composition of U.S. communities can be expected to further widen health inequities associated with race and class. Disparities in health, income, and education have also all been increasing over time (see Chapters 2 and 3 for more information).

Climate change will increasingly affect health. In 2015, at the United Nations Climate Change Conference—also known as COP 21—multiple nations, including the United States, came together to create an agreement to combat climate change and attempt to prevent the global temperature from rising more than 2 degrees Celsius. Health representatives played an integral role in the conference, as health is and will continue to be significantly affected by climate change. Climate change is happening in all areas, but its impacts are not distributed equally. It exacerbates vulnerabilities in communities that are already disproportionately affected by preexisting social, economic, and environmental factors. Extreme weather events are one of the many examples of the ways in which climate change will impact health. Hurricane Katrina was not necessarily the direct result of climate change. However, it offers many important lessons on mitigating risk and increasing resiliency in making plans to help the entire population, especially the most vulnerable. Although there is a risk that climate change could worsen health inequities, there is also great opportunity to integrate efforts to promote health into mitigation and adaptation efforts to support more resilient, healthy, and equitable communities (Rudolph et al., 2015).

Finally, recent events involving race and law enforcement relations have elucidated systematically unequal treatment in the criminal justice system (The President's Task Force on 21st Century Policing, 2015). Moreover, there is a growing and bipartisan recognition that mass incarceration, which affects individuals of color disproportionately, plays a major role in the breakdown of families and communities, constitutes an unsustainable use of taxpayer dollars, and leads, in connection with the larger policy milieu in both the private and the public sector, to poor employment prospects and voter disenfranchisement (Clear, 2008; NRC, 2014). These current realities serve as reminders that the vision of an equitable society will be challenging to reach, but community-driven solutions, such as those this report highlights, can help move in that direction on a local scale.

WHY COMMUNITIES?

Individuals and families are part of communities, and the role of communities is crucial to promoting health equity for several reasons. First, as discussed earlier, medical interventions are insufficient to address health equity, and behavioral health promotion continues to show little success in reducing disparities (Baum and Fisher, 2014). Community-based and -driven efforts are needed to alter environmental, socioeconomic, and cultural conditions in ways that promote health equity. Community health refers to the overall well-being of a community at all levels (including the individuals within the community and the physical setting), which may involve multi-sector and multidisciplinary collaborative approaches to optimizing the health and quality of life of all persons who live, work, or are otherwise active in a defined community (Goodman et al., 2014). A healthy community is the foundation for achieving all other goals, as it is essential for a productive society. (For example, a community with a healthy workforce has a good base upon which to build its economy, and healthier students are more equipped to learn and be successful academically.) Furthermore, communities differ in the local quality and availability of health care providers, the affordability and quality of housing, employment opportunities, transportation systems, the availability of parks, green space, and other aspects of the physical environment. Communities are uniquely positioned to drive solutions tailored to their needs that target the multiple determinants of health.

MOMENTUM FOR ACHIEVING HEALTH EQUITY

There is a clear urgency for the nation to fully address health inequity. An analysis of current trends provides evidence of persistent health inequity, but there are reasons for optimism. Turning the tide is not only possible, it is imperative; many organizations in the public and private sectors have recognized this, making health equity an explicit or implicit priority. These organizations span the sectors of finance, philanthropy, public health, community development, academia, and beyond. Local, regional, and state governments have also taken on issues essential to achieving health equity. For example, the Federal Reserve Bank and community development financial institutions are engaging in improving community development, employment, and housing—which drive health improvement—and they are making investments that expand access to healthy and affordable foods and neighborhoods with open space to promote physical activity and community safety (Andrews and Erickson, 2012). Health equity is a guiding priority for the American Public Health Association in its initiative to make the United States the healthiest nation in a generation, with 2030 as a goalpost (APHA, n.d.). In

2016 the Association of State and Territorial Health Officials' President's Challenge is to "Advance health equity and optimal health for all," and "Cultivating a culture of health equity" was the theme for the National Association of County and City Health Officials' annual meeting. Numerous states, including California, Colorado, Massachusetts, Pennsylvania, and Wyoming, have created statewide offices of health equity that work in collaboration with other agencies and departments to inform policies that promote health equity. Health equity has become central to the goals of some of the nation's largest philanthropic organizations, including The California Endowment, Ford Foundation, Kresge, and Kellogg. Advancing health equity is at the core of the Robert Wood Johnson Foundation's (RWJF's) new push for a culture of health (RWJF, 2015). The federal government is investing heavily in health equity as well, and it recently established a National Institutes of Health research program to address health disparities in chronic disease as well as the National Partnership for Action to End Health Disparities. These investments seek to "transform lives and places for disinvested people" (The Housing Fund, 2015), and at their core they are investments to create opportunity for all to achieve optimal health.

> *Conclusion 1-1: The persistent state of health disparities and health inequity in the United States has profound implications for the country's overall health standing, economic vitality, and national security. Thus, addressing health inequities is a critical need that requires this issue to be among our nation's foremost priorities.*

ABOUT THIS REPORT

RWJF, as part of its Culture of Health Initiative,[3] asked the Health and Medicine Division of the National Academies of Sciences, Engineering, and Medicine to help delineate the causes of and the solutions to health inequities in the United States. The charge to the committee is provided below (see Box 1-1 for the full statement of task). To respond to the charge, the Committee on Community-Based Solutions to Promote Health Equity in the United States was formed.

The focus of this report is on what communities can do to promote health equity and on the broader policy context and contributions of stakeholders that can support communities. In addition to the root causes and structural barriers that need to be overcome, the committee also examined levers and policies to support change, some of which span

---

[3] For more information, see http://www.rwjf.org/en/culture-of-health.html (accessed October 28, 2016).

> **BOX 1-1**
> **Statement of Task**
> **Committee on Community-Based Solutions to**
> **Promote Health Equity in the United States**
>
> The Robert Wood Johnson Foundation, as part of its Culture of Health initiative, has asked the Health and Medicine Division of the National Academies of Sciences, Engineering, and Medicine to assist in delineating causes of and solutions to health inequities in the United States. A consensus committee will be formed to examine the evidence on solutions to promote health equity.
>
> As part of its work a committee convened for this purpose will:
>
> - Review the state of health disparities in the United States and explore the underlying conditions and root causes contributing to health inequity and the interdependent nature of the factors that create them (such as systems of employment, public safety, housing, transportation, education, and others).
> - Where appropriate, the committee will draw from existing literature and syntheses on health disparities and health inequity.
> - Identify and examine a minimum of six examples of community-based solutions that address health inequities, drawing both from deliberate and indirect interventions or activities that promote equal opportunity for health. The examples should span health and non-health sectors and should take into account the range of factors that contribute to health inequity in the United States (such as systems of employment, public safety, housing, transportation, education, and others).
>   - The committee may review appropriate frameworks for assessing policies and actions to address health inequalities and use these to examine the examples of community-based solutions.
>   - The committee will review the identified community-based solutions through the lens of the culture of health action areas, drivers, and measures.
> - Identify the major elements of effective or promising solutions and their key levers, policies, stakeholders, and other elements that are needed to be successful.
> - Recommend elements of short- or long-term strategies and solutions that communities may consider to expand opportunities to advance health equity.
> - Recommend key research needs to help identify and strengthen evidence-based solutions and other recommendations as viewed appropriate by the committee to reduce health disparities and promote health equity.

national, state, regional, and other contexts for the work of communities. To address its charge, the committee reviewed examples of community efforts across the country and was inspired by how these communities are rising to the challenge to address the difficult challenges and barriers to health and well-being.

Culture of Health Lens

RWJF defines a culture of health broadly "as one in which good health and well-being flourish across geographic, demographic, and social sectors; fostering healthy equitable communities guides public and private decision making; and everyone has the opportunity to make choices that lead to healthy lifestyles" (RWJF, n.d.). RWJF also says that "the exact definition of a culture of health can look very different to different people. A national culture of health must embrace a wide variety of beliefs, customs and values. Ultimately it will be as diverse and multifaceted as the population it serves" (RWJF, n.d.). The culture of health framework was developed by the foundation in collaboration with RAND Corporation through a combination of literature review and structured discussions with stakeholders (Chandra et al., 2016). The framework includes four action areas that are interdependent—none can be achieved alone (Plough and Chandra, 2016). The four action areas are

1. Making health a shared value
2. Fostering cross-sector collaboration to improve well-being
3. Creating healthier, more equitable communities
4. Strengthening the integration of health systems and services

The committee used the framework as a guide for this report and adapted it to apply specifically to its statement of task and at the community level.

The committee also referred to the ecological model illustrated in the 2003 Institute of Medicine (IOM)[4] report *The Future of the Public's Health in the 21st Century*. This figure shows the multiple determinants of health, beginning with an individual's biology (and the biology of diseases) at the center, followed by individual behavior, and in the outermost layer, the highest level of social, economic, cultural, health, and environmental conditions and policy (IOM, 2003). The committee was charged with examining community-based solutions, and it developed a simple model to show what it concluded are three important elements of community-based efforts to promote health equity. The community-based level of intervention is situated in the second and third outermost circles of Figure 1-2 (i.e., social, family, and community networks; living and working conditions). As Figure 1-2 clearly indicates, community effort is necessary, but it is not a sufficient contributor to population health and, by extension, health equity. The outermost ring—the broad milieu of social,

---

[4] As of March 15, 2016, the Health and Medicine Division (HMD) carries out the work previously undertaken by the IOM.

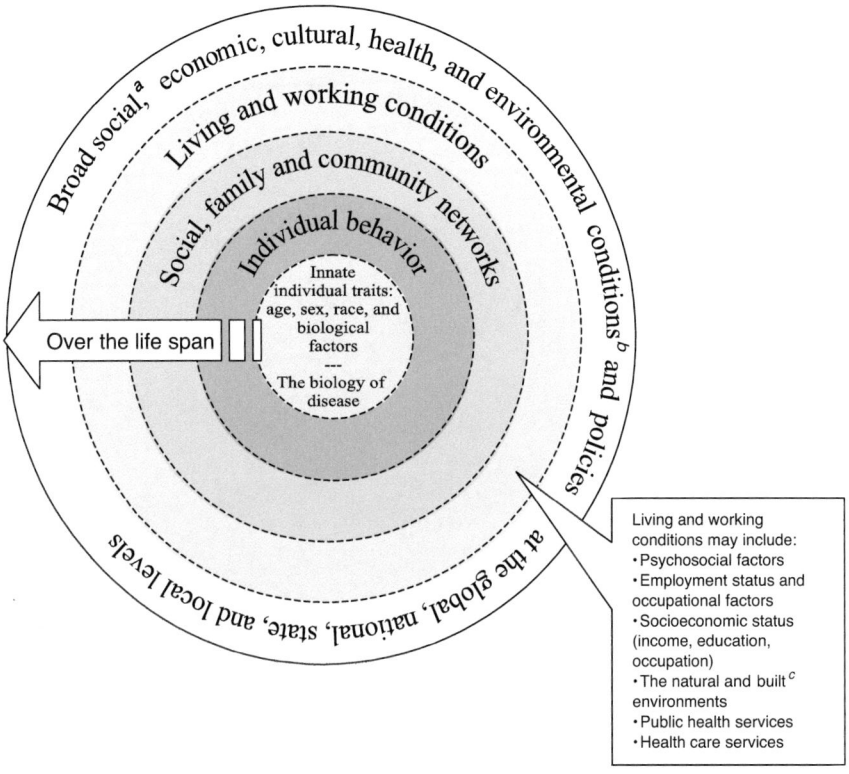

FIGURE 1-2 A guide to thinking about the determinants of population health.

[a] Social conditions include, but are not limited to economic inequality, urbanization, mobility, cultural values, attitudes and policies related to discrimination and intolerance on the basis of race, gender, and other differences.

[b] Other conditions at the national level might include major sociopolitical shifts, such as recession, war, and governmental collapse.

[c] The built environment includes transportation, water and sanitation, housing, and other dimensions of urban planning.
SOURCE: IOM, 2003.

economic, and environmental conditions and policies—is crucial to support community-level efforts.

Report Conceptual Model

Figure 1-3 is a conceptual model that grounds the committee's report. The model adapts elements of the Culture of Health Action Framework

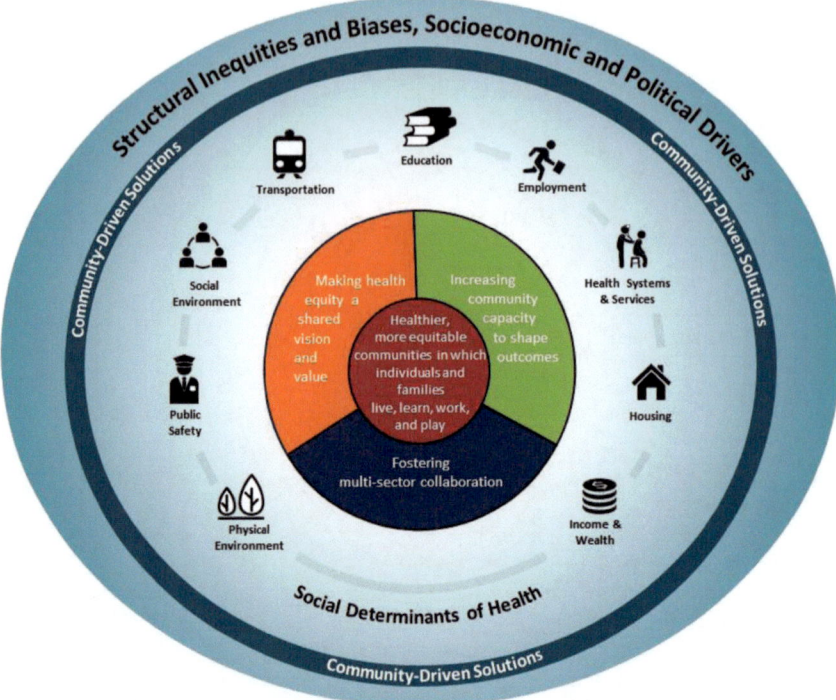

FIGURE 1-3 Report conceptual model for community solutions to promote health equity.
NOTES: Multi-sector collaboration includes partners from agriculture, banking/finance, business/industry, economic development, education, health care, housing, human/social services, justice, labor, land use and management, media, public health, transportation, and workforce development, among other sectors.
SOURCES: Informed by the Robert Wood Johnson Foundation (2015) Culture of Health Action Framework and the Prevention Institute's (2016) *Systems Framework to Achieve an Equitable Culture of Health.*

(RWJF, 2015) and the Prevention Institute's *Systems Framework to Achieve an Equitable Culture of Health* (Prevention Institute, 2016). The model applies the culture of health lens to the committee's understanding of the underlying causes and conditions of health inequity in addition to the community-based solutions that promote health equity.

The model begins with the outer circle and background as the context in which health inequities and community-driven[5] solutions exist.

---

[5] The committee chose the term "community-driven solutions" because the community will be the driving force behind the solutions in this report.

The "socioeconomic and political context" was adapted from the World Health Organization Conceptual Framework for Action on the Social Determinants of Health (WHO, 2010) and encompasses policies, law, governance, and culture. In the report conceptual model, this socioeconomic and political context includes structural inequities and biases that are produced along the axes of race, gender, class, sexual orientation, and other social domains. These inequities are manifested in systematic disadvantages that lead to inequitable access to or experience of the determinants of health. The committee adapted the determinants of health identified by the Achieving Health Equity Team at the RWJF, separating the social and physical environments, and adding transportation. Although the framework incorporates transportation as part of the "physical and social environment," transportation is vital to many areas of health (e.g., the ability to travel to health care facilities, community events, accessing jobs) and, alternatively, can have detrimental impacts on health (e.g., air pollution, unintentional injuries), and thus it has been highlighted in the model. (See Chapter 3 for a more detailed description of each determinant of health and the ways in which they affect health and well-being.)

The committee adapted two of the Culture of Health Action Framework Action Areas for community-level solutions: "Making health equity a shared vision and value" and "Fostering multi-sector collaboration." Based on the committee's information-gathering sessions, relevant literature, and committee deliberations, the committee also identified a third action area of importance for the framework when proposing solutions at the community level: "Increasing community capacity to shape outcomes." This is a process that has emerged as essential for communities to have the power to address inequities and to sustain their efforts. (These three elements are discussed in more detail in Chapter 4.) To align with its statement of task, the committee incorporated equity at the community level in its conceptual model. The Culture of Health action area "Creating healthier, more equitable communities" has been incorporated into the conceptual model as the outcome of the community-driven solutions in the center of the diagram.

The community examples featured in this report will highlight solutions that have been implemented at the community level to target one or more of the nine determinants of health using the processes identified in the conceptual model (see Chapter 5). By making health equity a shared vision and value, increasing community capacity to shape outcomes, and fostering multi-sector collaboration, these solutions foster equal opportunity for health, which is the foundation for a vibrant, healthy community.

Community Health

This report does not focus on interventions that target a single health condition, but on community-level changes and impacts on health through a holistic lens. The development of a community-based solution is a community-driven process that includes fair participation by the community in the decision-making process, in which all people have access to the information necessary to understand the matter and the process and which produces outcomes that the people accept as fair, equitable, and nondiscriminatory in the context of addressing health disparities. Therefore, the terms "community-driven solutions" and "community-based solutions" will be used interchangeably for the remainder of this report (see Box 1-2 for definitions). The importance of communities and their role and potential to promote health equity is discussed in Chapter 4.

Overview of the Study Process

To address its charge, the committee gathered information through a variety of means. It held three information-gathering meetings that were open to the public and webcast live. The first, held in January 2016, focused on obtaining information on health disparities and their root causes, including an overview from the report sponsor. The second, held in March 2016, focused on many of the social determinants of health and

---

BOX 1-2
Definitions

Community is any configuration of individuals, families, and groups whose values, characteristics, interests, geography, or social relations unite them in some way (adapted from Dreher, 2016).[a] However, the word is used to denote both the people living in a place, and the place itself. In this report the committee focuses on shared geography, i.e., place, as a key component of community—in other words, community is defined as the people living in a place, such as a neighborhood. Therefore a *community-based solution* to promote health equity is an action, policy, program, or law that is driven by the community (members), and that affects local factors that can influence health and has the potential to advance progress toward health equity.

[a] Draft manuscript from Melanie C. Dreher, Rush University Medical Center, provided to staff on February 19, 2016, for the Committee on Community-Based Solutions to Promote Health Equity in the United States. Available by request from the National Academies of Sciences, Engineering, and Medicine's Public Access Records Office. For more information, email PARO@nas.edu.

included presentations on how transportation, planning, environmental justice, and civil rights law affect health. The third meeting was held in April 2016, and presentation topics included faith-based community organizing, community-based participatory research, place-based factors and policy at the community level, and the economics of community development (meeting agendas are in Appendix C). The committee met in executive sessions for deliberative discussion throughout the study process. The committee received public submissions of materials for its consideration at the meetings and by e-mail throughout the course of the study.[6] A website was created to provide information to the public about the committee's work and to facilitate communication between the public and the committee.[7] The process used to identify the community examples highlighted is outlined in the Chapter 5 Annex.

Overview of Report

Chapter 2 begins with a description of the state of health disparities in the United States by geography, income, race and ethnicity, and other categories. Chapter 3 discusses how structural and institutional inequities have led to disparate health outcomes and highlights historical issues that continue to affect health outcomes today, as well as the ways in which current and emerging issues ultimately affect communities. This is followed by a discussion on the multiple determinants of health and how they affect health equity. Chapter 4 discusses the role and capacity of communities to promote health equity and explains the larger context in which communities are situated, as well as the types of evidence needed to support communities. Chapter 5 provides nine examples of communities that are tackling health inequity and the lessons learned from these efforts. Chapter 6 addresses the policies that ultimately affect communities and that could either hinder or promote solutions at the level of individual communities. Chapter 7 discusses the roles of various stakeholders and the actions that these actors could undertake in their communities, with an emphasis on multi-sector collaboration. Chapter 8 is geared toward communities and provides an array of strategies, tools, and activities available to communities to help them promote health equity. Chapter 9 provides brief summarizing thoughts.

---

[6] Public access materials can be requested from http://www8.nationalacademies.org/cp/projectview.aspx?key=IOM-BPH-15-15 (accessed December 23, 2016).
[7] See http://www.nationalacademies.org/hmd/Activities/PublicHealth/Culture-of-Health.aspx (accessed December 23, 2016).

CONCLUDING OBSERVATIONS

There are systemic root causes of health inequities in this country that can be overwhelming and that will take considerable time to address. It will require system-level changes to eliminate structural racism, reduce poverty, improve income equality, increase educational opportunity, and fix the laws and policies that perpetuate structural inequities. Until these root causes are addressed nationally, health equity will not be fully realized. However, actors at the community level—policy makers, businesses, state and local governments, anchor institutions, and community residents—are agents of local change who have the power to change the narrative and take action that will promote health equity. The latter is what this report will focus on, although, where possible, it will provide promising strategies to address these hard-to-tackle root causes at higher levels.

REFERENCES

AAP (American Academy of Pediatrics). 2010. Health equity and children's rights. *Pediatrics* 125(4):838–849.

Alegria, M., Z. Cao, T. G. McGuire, V. D. Ojeda, B. Sribney, M. Woo, and D. Takeuchi. 2006. Health insurance coverage for vulnerable populations: Contrasting Asian Americans and Latinos in the United States. *Inquiry* 43(3):231–254.

Andrews, N. O., and D. J. Erickson. 2012. *Investing in what works for America's communities: Essays on people, place & purpose.* Federal Reserve Bank of San Francisco and Low Income Investment Fund.

APHA (American Public Health Association). n.d. *Health equity.* https://www.apha.org/topics-and-issues/health-equity (accessed October 24, 2016).

Arias, E. 2016. Changes in life expectancy by race and Hispanic origin in the United States, 2013-2014. *National Center for Health Statistics* NCHS data brief no. 244.

Asante-Muhammad, D., C. Collins, J. Hoxie, and E. Nieves. 2016. *The ever-growing gap: Without change, African-American and Latino families won't match white wealth for centuries.* Washington, DC: Institute for Policy Studies and CFED.

Asieba, I. O. 2016. Racial/ethnic trends in childhood obesity in the United States. *Journal of Childhood Obesity* 1(1):1–6.

Barry-Jester, A. M., and B. Casselman. 2015. 33 million Americans still don't have health insurance. *FiveThirtyEight*, September 28. http://fivethirtyeight.com/features/33-million-americans-still-dont-have-health-insurance (accessed January 9, 2017).

Baum, F., and M. Fisher. 2014. Why behavioural health promotion endures despite its failure to reduce health inequities. *Sociology of Health and Illness* 36(2):213–225.

Braveman, P. A., S. Kumanyika, J. Fielding, T. LaVeist, L. N. Borrell, R. Manderscheid, and A. Troutman. 2011. Health disparities and health equity: The issue is justice. *American Journal of Public Health* 101(Suppl 1):S149–S155.

Brennan Ramirez, L. K., E. A. Baker, and M. Metzler. 2008. *Promoting health equity: A resource to help communities address social determinants of health.* Atlanta: U.S. Department of Health and Human Services, U.S. Centers for Disease Control and Prevention.

Burd-Sharps, S., and K. Lewis. 2015. *Geographies of opportunity: Ranking well-being by congressional district.* New York: Social Science Research Council.

Caldwell, J. T., C. L. Ford, S. P. Wallace, M. C. Wang, and L. M. Takahashi. 2016. Intersection of living in a rural versus urban area and race/ethnicity in explaining access to health care in the United States. *American Journal of Public Health* 106(8):1463–1469.
Carr, M. D., and E. E. Wiemers. 2016. *The decline in lifetime earnings mobility in the U.S.: Evidence from survey-linked administrative data*. Washington, DC: Washington Center for Equitable Growth.
CDC (U.S. Centers for Disease Control and Prevention). 2014. *Epidemiology of HIV infection through 2014*. https://www.cdc.gov/hiv/pdf/library/slidesets/cdc-hiv-surveillance-genepi.pdf (accessed October 24, 2016).
Chandra, A., J. Acosta, K. G. Carman, T. Dubowitz, L. Leviton, L. T. Martin, C. Miller, C. Nelson, T. Orleans, M. Tait, M. Trujillo, V. Towe, D. Yeung, and A. L. Plough. 2016. *Building a national culture of health: Background, action framework, measures, and next steps*. Santa Monica, CA: RAND Corporation.
Chetty, R., M. Stepner, S. Abraham, S. Lin, B. Scuderi, N. Turner, A. Bergeron, and D. Cutler. 2016. The association between income and life expectancy in the United States, 2001–2014. *JAMA* 315(16):1750–1766.
Cho, Y., and R. A. Hummer. 2001. Disability status differentials across fifteen Asian and Pacific Islander groups and the effect of nativity and duration of residence in the U.S. *Social Biology* 48(3–4):171–195.
Christeson, W., A. D. Taggart, and S. Messner-Zidell. 2009. *Ready, willing, and unable to serve: 75 percent of young adults cannot join the military; early education across America is needed to ensure national security*. Washington, DC: Mission: Readiness.
Christeson, W., A. D. Taggart, and S. Messner-Zidell. 2010. *Too fat to fight: Retired military leaders want junk food out of America's schools*. Washington, DC: Mission: Readiness.
Clear, T. R. 2008. The effects of high imprisonment rates of communities. *Crime and Justice* 37(1):97–132.
CMS (Centers for Medicare & Medicaid Services). 2016. *Disproportionate share hospital (DSH)*. https://www.cms.gov/medicare/medicare-fee-for-service-payment/acutein patientpps/dsh.html (accessed October 24, 2016).
Council for a Strong America. 2016. New 50-state index from Council for a Strong America shows most young adults not "citizen-ready." http://www.marketwired.com/press-release/new-50-state-index-from-council-strong-america-shows-most-young-adults-not-citizen-ready-2157947.htm (accessed October 24, 2016).
Cunningham, P. J., R. Garfield, and R. Rudowitz. 2015. How are hospitals faring under the Affordable Care Act? Early experiences from Ascension Health. The Kaiser Commission on Medicaid and the Uninsured. http://kff.org/health-reform/issue-brief/how-are-hospitals-faring-under-the-affordable-care-act-early-experiences-from-ascension-health/ (accessed October 24, 2016).
Daniels, N. 2008. *Just health: Meeting health needs fairly*. New York: Cambridge University Press.
Davis, K., K. Stremikis, D. Squires, and C. Schoen. 2014. *Mirror, mirror on the wall, 2014 update: How the U.S. health care system compares internationally*. The Commonwealth Fund.
de Souza, R. J., and S. S. Anand. 2014. Cardiovascular disease in Asian Americans: Unmasking heterogeneity. *Journal of the American College of Cardiology* 64(23):2495–2497.
Ennis, S. R., M. Rios-Vargas, and N. G. Albert. 2011. *The Hispanic population: 2010*. U.S. Census Bureau.
Ferejohn, J. 2009. Is inequality a threat to democracy? In *The unsustainable American state*, edited by L. R. Jacobs and D. S. King. New York: Oxford University Press. Pp. 34–60.
Frey, W. H. 2015. A pivotal period for race in America. In *Diversity explosion: How new racial demographics are remaking America*. Washington, DC: Brookings Institution Press.

George, S., N. Duran, and K. Norris. 2014. A systematic review of barriers and facilitators to minority research participation among African Americans, Latinos, Asian Americans, and Pacific Islanders. *American Journal of Public Health* 104(2):16–31.

Goodman, R. A., R. Bunnell, and S. F. Posner. 2014. What is "community health"? Examining the meaning of an evolving field in public health. *Preventive Medicine* 67(Suppl 1):S58–S61.

Graham, H. 2004. Social determinants and their unequal distribution: Clarifying policy understandings. *Milbank Q* 82(1):101–124.

HealthCare.gov. n.d. *Immigration status and the marketplace.* https://www.healthcare.gov/immigrants/immigration-status (accessed October 24, 2016).

Heckler, M. M. 1985. *Report of the Secretary's Task Force on Black & Minority Health.* Washington, DC: U.S. Department of Health and Human Services.

HERO (Health Enhancement Research Organization). 2015. Exploring the value proposition for workforce health: Business leader attitudes about the role of health as a driver of productivity and performance. http://hero-health.org/wp-content/uploads/2015/02/HPP-Business-Leader-Survey-Full-Report_FINAL.pdf (accessed October 24, 2016).

HHS (U.S. Department of Health and Human Services). n.d. *Disparities.* https://www.healthypeople.gov/2020/about/foundation-health-measures/Disparities (accessed October 24, 2016).

Hixson, L., B. B. Hepler, and M. O. Kim. 2011. *The white population: 2010.* U.S. Census Bureau.

HRSA (Health Resources and Service Administration). 2015. *Mortality and life expectancy in rural America: Connecting the health and human service safety nets to improve health outcomes over the life course.* National Advisory Committee on Rural Health and Human Services.

Hsieh, N., and M. Ruther. 2016. Sexual minority health and health risk factors: Intersection effects of gender, race, and sexual identity. *American Journal of Preventive Medicine* 50(6):746–755.

Hummer, R. A., D. A. Powers, S. G. Pullum, G. L. Gossman, and W. P. Frisbie. 2007. Paradox found (again): Infant mortality among the Mexican-origin population in the United States. *Demography* 44(3):441–457.

IHS (Indian Health Service). 2016. *Disparities.* https://www.ihs.gov/newsroom/factsheets/disparities (accessed October 24, 2016).

IOM (Institute of Medicine). 2003. *The future of the public's health in the 21st century.* Washington, DC: The National Academies Press.

IOM. 2009. *America's uninsured crisis: Consequences for health and health care.* Washington, DC: The National Academies Press.

IOM. 2011. *The health of lesbian, gay, bisexual, and transgender people: Building a foundation for better understanding.* Washington, DC: The National Academies Press.

IOM. 2015. *Business engagement in building healthy communities: Workshop summary.* Washington, DC: The National Academies Press.

Jones, H. 2009. *Equity in development: Why it is important and how to achieve it.* London: Overseas Development Institute.

Kenney, G. M., and M. Huntress. 2012. *The Affordable Care Act: Coverage implications and issues for immigrant families.* https://aspe.hhs.gov/basic-report/affordable-care-act-coverage-implications-and-issues-immigrant-families (accessed October 24, 2016).

Keyes, K. M., and S. Galea. 2016. *Population health science.* New York: Oxford University Press.

Kochanek, K. D., E. Arias, and B. A. Bastian. 2016. The effect of changes in selected age-specific causes of death on non-Hispanic white life expectancy between 2000 and 2014. *National Center for Health Statistics* NCHS data brief no. 250.

Kruse, C. S., S. Bouffard, M. Dougherty, and J. S. Parro. 2016. Telemedicine use in rural Native American communities in the era of the ACA: A systematic literature review. *Journal of Medical Systems* 40(6):145.

LaVeist, T. A., D. J. Gaskin, and P. Richard. 2009. *The economic burden of health inequalities in the United States*. Washington, DC: Joint Center for Political and Economic Studies.

Lee, S., A. H. O'Neill, E. S. Ihara, and D. H. Chae. 2013. Change in self-reported health status among immigrants in the United States: Associations with measures of acculturation. *PLOS One* 8(10):e76494.

Markides, K. S., and J. Coreil. 1986. The health of Hispanics in the southwestern United States: An epidemiologic paradox. *Public Health Reports* 101(3):253–265.

Mathews, T. J., M. F. MacDorman, and M. E. Thoma. 2015. Infant mortality statistics from the 2013 period linked birth/infant death data set. *National Vital Statistics Reports* 64(9):1–28.

NCHS (National Center for Health Statistics). 2014. *Health, United States, 2014: With special feature on adults aged 55–64*. Hyattsville, MD: U.S. Centers for Disease Control and Prevention.

NIH (National Institutes of Health). 2010. *NIH announces Institute on Minority Health and Health Disparities*. https://www.nih.gov/news-events/news-releases/nih-announces-institute-minority-health-health-disparities (accessed October 24, 2016).

NRC (National Research Council). 2014. *The growth of incarceration in the United States: Exploring causes and consequences*. Washington, DC: The National Academies Press.

OECD (Organisation for Economic Co-operation and Development). 2009. United States country highlights: Doing better for children. https://www.oecd.org/unitedstates/43590390.pdf (accessed December 15, 2016).

Olshansky, S. J., D. J. Passaro, R. C. Hershow, J. Layden, B. A. Carnes, J. Brody, L. Hayflick, R. N. Butler, D. B. Allison, and D. S. Ludwig. 2005. A potential decline in life expectancy in the United States in the 21st century. *New England Journal of Medicine* 352(11):1138–1145.

Orszag, P. R., and T. J. Kane. 2003. *Higher education spending: The role of Medicaid and the business cycle*. https://www.brookings.edu/research/higher-education-spending-the-role-of-medicaid-and-the-business-cycle (accessed October 24, 2016).

Ortega, A. N., H. P. Rodriguez, and A. Vargas Bustamante. 2015. Policy dilemmas in Latino health care and implementation of the Affordable Care Act. *Annual Review of Public Health* 36:525–544.

Page, L. 2013. Will fee-for-service really disappear? *Medscape*. http://www.medscape.com/viewarticle/812672 (accessed November 17, 2016).

Plough, A., and A. Chandra. 2016. *From vision to action: A framework and measures to mobilize a culture of health*. Robert Wood Johnson Foundation. http://www.rwjf.org/content/dam/COH/RWJ000_COH-Update_CoH_Report_1b.pdf (accessed December 23, 2016).

Prevention Institute. 2016. *Countering the production of health inequities: An emerging systems framework to achieve an equitable culture of health*. Oakland, CA: The Prevention Institute.

Rastogi, S., T. D. Johnson, E. M. Hoeffe, and M. P. Drewery. 2010. *The black population: 2010*. U.S. Census Bureau.

Robinson, J. C. 2001. Theory and practice in the design of physician payment incentives. *Milbank Quarterly* 79(2):149–177.

Rudolph, L., S. Gould, and J. Berko. 2015. *Climate change, health, and equity: Opportunities for action*. Oakland, CA: Public Health Institute.

RWJF (Robert Wood Johnson Foundation). 2015. *From vision to action: A framework and measures to mobilize a culture of health*.

RWJF. n.d. *What is a culture of health?* http://www.evidenceforaction.org/what-culture-health (accessed October 24, 2016).

Saloner, B., L. Sabik, and B. D. Sommers. 2014. Pinching the poor? Medicaid cost sharing under the ACA. *New England Journal of Medicine* 370(13):1177–1180.

Seith, D., and E. Isakson. 2011. *Who are America's children: Examining health disparities among children in the U.S.* New York: National Center for Children in Poverty.

Smeeding, T. 2012. *Income, wealth, and debt and the Great Recession.* Stanford, CA: Stanford Center on Poverty and Inequality.

Swift, A. 2015. *Americans see healthcare, low wages as top financial problems.* http://www.gallup.com/poll/181217/americans-healthcare-low-wages-top-financial-problems.aspx (accessed October 24, 2016).

Taveras, E. M., M. W. Gillman, K. P. Kleinman, J. W. Rich-Edwards, and S. L. Rifas-Shiman. 2013. Reducing racial/ethnic disparities in childhood obesity. *JAMA Pediatrics* 167(8):731–738.

Taylor, P., M. H. Lopez, J. Martinez, and G. Velasco. 2012. *When labels don't fit: Hispanics and their values of identity.* Pew Hispanic Center. http://www.pewhispanic.org/2012/04/04/when-labels-dont-fit-hispanics-and-their-views-of-identity (accessed October 25, 2016).

The Housing Fund. 2015. *The Housing Fund, Inc. wins $100,000 Wells Fargo next award for innovative strategy to improve consumer finance.* http://thehousingfund.org/next-award (accessed October 24, 2016).

The National Commission on Physician Payment Reform. 2013. *Report of the National Commission on Physician Payment Reform.* Society of General Internal Medicine.

The President's Task Force on 21st Century Policing. 2015. *Final report of the President's Task Force on 21st Century Policing.* http://cops.usdoj.gov/pdf/taskforce/TaskForce_FinalReport.pdf (accessed October 18, 2016).

Uberoi, N., K. Finegold, and E. Gee. 2016. *Health insurance coverage and the Affordable Care Act, 2010–2016.* Office of the Assistant Secretary for Planning and Evaluation, U.S. Department of Health and Human Services.

Ubri, P., and S. Artiga. 2016. *Disparities in health and health care: Five key questions and answers.* http://files.kff.org/attachment/Issue-Brief-Disparities-in-Health-and-Health-Care-Five-Key-Questions-and-Answers (accessed October 24, 2016).

University of Wisconsin Population Health Institute. 2015. *2015 county health rankings: Key findings report.* Madison: University of Wisconsin Population Health Institute.

Vang, Z. M., I. T. Elo, and M. Nagano. 2015. Preterm birth among the Hmong, other Asian subgroups and non-Hispanic whites in California. *BMC Pregnancy and Childbirth* 15:184.

Voorheis, J., N. McMaety, and B. Shor. 2015. *Unequal incomes, ideology and gridlock: How rising inequality increases political polarization.* https://papers.ssrn.com/sol3/papers.cfm?abstract_id=2649215 (accessed October 24, 2016).

Waidmann, T. A. 2009. *Estimating the cost of racial and ethnic health disparities.* Washington, DC: Urban Institute.

WHO (World Health Organization). 2010. *A conceptual framework for action on the social determinants of health.* Geneva: World Health Organization.

WHO. 2015. *World health statistics 2015.* Geneva, Switzerland: World Health Organization.

Williams, D. R., and V. Purdie-Vaughns. 2015. Social and behavioral interventions to improve health and reduce disparities in health. In *Population health: Behavioral and social science insights.* Rockville, MD: Agency for Healthcare Research and Quality and Office of Behavioral and Social Science Research.

Woolf, S. H., and P. Braveman. 2011. Where health disparities begin: The role of social and economic determinants—and why current policies may make matters worse. *Health Affairs* 30(10):1852–1859.

Woolf, S. H., L. Aron, L. Dubay, S. M. Simon, E. Zimmerman, and K. X. Luk. 2015. *How are income and wealth linked to health and longevity?* Washington, DC: Urban Institute and Virginia Commonwealth University.

2

The State of Health Disparities in the United States

As part of its statement of task, the committee was asked to review the state of health disparities in the United States and to explore the underlying conditions and root causes contributing to health inequities and the interdependent nature of the factors that create them (drawing from existing literature and syntheses on health disparities and health inequities). In this chapter the committee reviews the state of health disparities in the United States by race and ethnicity, gender, sexual orientation and gender identity, and disability status, highlighting populations that are disproportionately impacted by inequity. In addition, this chapter summarizes data related to military veterans as well as rural versus urban-area differences. The committee drew on existing literature, comprehensive reviews (AHRQ, 2016; NCHS, 2016), and recent studies. In Chapters 2 and 3, the report features examples of communities that are taking action to address the root causes of health inequity. These brief examples are meant to be illustrative of the work being undertaken by communities throughout the country. In Chapter 5 the report takes a more in-depth look into nine examples of community-driven solutions to promote health equity.

HEALTH DISPARITIES

For the purposes of this report, *health disparities* are differences that exist among specific population groups in the United States in the attainment of full health potential that can be measured by differences in incidence, prevalence, mortality, burden of disease, and other adverse health conditions (NIH, 2014). While the term disparities is often used or interpreted to reflect differences between racial or ethnic groups, disparities can exist across many other dimensions as well, such as gender, sexual orientation, age, disability status, socioeconomic status, and geographic location. According to Healthy People 2020, all of these factors, in addition to race and ethnicity, shape an individual's ability to achieve optimal health (Healthy People 2020, 2016). Indeed, the existing evidence on health disparities does reveal differential health outcomes across and within all of the aforementioned identity groups. Health disparities can stem from health inequities—systematic differences in the health of groups and communities occupying unequal positions in society that are avoidable and unjust (Graham, 2004). These are the type of disparities that are reflected in the committee's charge and that will be addressed for the remainder of this report. In this section, we describe health disparities affecting populations across multiple dimensions.

Racial and Ethnic Disparities

Race and ethnicity are socially constructed categories that have tangible effects on the lives of individuals who are defined by how one perceives one's self and how one is perceived by others. It is important to acknowledge the social construction (i.e., created from prevailing social perceptions, historical policies, and practices) of the concepts of race and ethnicity because it has implications for how measures of race have been used and changed over time. Furthermore, the concept of race is complex, with a rich history of scientific and philosophical debate as to the nature of race (James, 2016). Racial and ethnic disparities are arguably the most obstinate inequities in health over time, despite the many strides that have been made to improve health in the United States. Moreover, race and ethnicity are extremely salient factors when examining health inequity (Bell and Lee, 2011; Smedley et al., 2008; Williams et al., 2010). Therefore, solutions for health equity need to take into account the social, political, and historical context of race and ethnicity in this country.

The criteria people use to classify themselves and others racially and ethnically and the attitudes that people hold about race and ethnicity have been changing significantly in the early 21st century. According to the U.S. Census Bureau, 37.9 percent of the population was identified to be racial or ethnic minorities in 2014 (NCHS, 2016). "Minority" populations, which already constitute majorities in some cities and states (e.g., California), will become the majority nationwide within 30 years. By the year 2044, they will account for more than half of the total U.S. population, and by 2060, nearly one in five of the nation's total population will be foreign born (Colby and Ortman, 2014).

For racial and ethnic minorities in the United States, health disparities take on many forms, including higher rates of chronic disease and premature death compared to the rates among whites. It is important to note that this pattern is not universal. Some minority groups—most notably, Hispanic immigrants—have better health outcomes than whites (Lara et al., 2005). This "immigrant paradox" appears to diminish with time spent in the United States, however (Lara et al., 2005). For other indicators, disparities have shrunk, not because of improvements among minorities but because of declines in the health of majority groups. For example, white females have experienced increased death rates due to suicide and alcohol-related diseases. Research suggests that the recent drug overdose epidemic, along with the rise of suicide and alcohol-related diseases, has contributed to the first increase in the national death rate in decades and to the unusual recent decline in life expectancy for white females (Arias, 2016; Case and Deaton, 2015; NCHS, 2016).[1]

Although significant progress has been made in narrowing the gap in health outcomes (NCHS, 2016), the elimination of disparities in health has yet to be achieved. Furthermore, this narrowing of health gaps does not hold true for a number of outcomes. Rather, despite overall improvements in health over time, some health disparities persist. This is true with many human immunodeficiency virus (HIV)-related outcomes. For instance, the magnitude of the African American–white disparity in acquired immunodeficiency syndrome (AIDS) diagnoses and mortality has actually grown substantially over time (Levine et al., 2001, 2007).

Infant gestational age, which is an important predictor of morbidity and infant mortality, differs among racial and ethnic groups. The National Center for Health Statistics (NCHS) reports that among the five racial and ethnic groups[2] measured in the National Vital Statistics Survey (NVSS) in 2014, African American women had the highest percentage of preterm singleton births at 11.1 percent, while Asian or Pacific Islander women had the lowest at 6.8 percent (NCHS, 2016). Within the Hispanic ethnic group, there is considerable variation in health outcomes based on country of origin. For example, the 2014 NVSS findings revealed that Puerto Rican mothers had the highest percentage of preterm singleton births at 9.1 percent, and Cuban mothers the lowest at 7.2 percent (NCHS, 2016).

---

[1] At the time this report was being finalized in December 2016, the U.S. Centers for Disease Control and Prevention's National Center for Health Statistics published a new data brief on 2015 data from the National Vital Statistics System, indicating that U.S. life expectancy decreased 0.1 year between 2014 (78.9 years) and 2015 (78.8 years), and that "the age-adjusted death rate increased 1.2 percent from 724.6 deaths per 100,000 standard population in 2014 to 733.1 in 2015" (Xu et al., 2016, p. 1).

[2] These groups include African American; American Indian or Alaska Native; Hispanic; white; and Asian or Pacific Islander.

While national infant mortality rates decreased overall by 14 percent from 2004 to 2014, disparities among racial and ethnic groups persisted (NCHS, 2016). For indigenous populations, infant mortality rates are staggering. Native Americans and Alaska Natives have an infant mortality rate that is 60 percent higher than the rate for their white counterparts (HHS, 2014). In 2013, infants born to African American mothers experienced the highest rates of infant mortality (11.11 infant deaths per 1,000 births), and infants born to Asian or Pacific Islander mothers experienced the lowest rates (3.90 infant deaths per 1,000 births) (NCHS, 2016). In 2015 the percentage of low-birthweight infants rose for the first time in 7 years. For white infants, the rate of low-birthweight infants was essentially unchanged, but for African American and Hispanic infants, the rate increased (Hamilton et al., 2016).

Obesity, a condition which has many associated chronic diseases and debilitating conditions, affects racial and ethnic minorities disproportionately as well. This has major implications for the quality of life and well-being for these population groups and their families. From 2011 to 2014, Hispanic children and adolescents ages 2 to 19 had the highest prevalence of obesity in the United States (21.9 percent), and Asians had the lowest (8.6 percent) (NCHS, 2016). Again, there is variation among Hispanics; Mexican Americans suffer disproportionately from diabetes (HHS, 2015).

Heart disease and cancer are the leading causes of death across race, ethnicity, and gender (see Table 2-1). African Americans were 30 percent more likely than whites to die prematurely from heart disease in 2010, and African American men are twice as likely as whites to die prematurely from stroke (HHS, 2016b,d). The U.S. Centers for Disease Control and Prevention (CDC) reports that nearly 44 percent of African American men and 48 percent of African American women have some form of cardiovascular disease (CDC, 2014a). Moreover, African American and American Indian/Alaska Native females have higher rates of stroke-related death than Hispanic and white women (Blackwell et al., 2014).

Homicide-related deaths, another instance of health disparities, are highest for African American men (4.5 percent) and are at least 2 percent for American Indian/Alaska Native and Hispanic men. The rate of suicide is highest for male American Indians/Alaska Natives, who are also more likely than other racial and ethnic groups to die by unintentional injury (12.6 percent of all deaths) (CDC, 2013d).

It is important to be cautious with data on disparities in poverty, obesity, and diabetes for several reasons. First, surveillance and other data are adequate at capturing black–white disparities in part because of their large sample sizes. Other groups, however, are not studied in as much detail because their sample sizes can be small. Moreover, heterogeneous groups may be folded together—for example, Native Americans

TABLE 2-1 Leading Causes of Death by Race, Ethnicity, and Gender, 2013

Rank	Gender	All	African American	American Indian/Alaska Native	Asian/Pacific Islander	Hispanic	White
1	Female	Heart disease 22.4%	Heart disease 23.6%	Cancer 18.9%	Cancer 26.4%	Cancer 22.6%	Heart disease 22.4%
	Male	Heart disease 24.6%	Heart disease 24.0%	Heart disease 19.8%	Cancer 26.1%	Heart disease 20.7%	Heart disease 24.8%
2	Female	Cancer 21.5%	Cancer 22.5%	Heart disease 16.8%	Heart disease 20.8%	Heart disease 20.0%	Cancer 21.2%
	Male	Cancer 23.5%	Cancer 22.4%	Cancer 17.74%	Heart disease 23.6%	Cancer 20.7%	Cancer 23.7%
3	Female	Chronic lower respiratory diseases 6.1%	Stroke 6.0%	Unintentional injuries 8.5%	Stroke 8.0%	Stroke 5.8%	Chronic lower respiratory diseases 6.6%
	Male	Unintentional injuries 6.3%	Unintentional injuries 5.8%	Unintentional injuries 12.6%	Stroke 6.1%	Unintentional injuries 9.9%	Unintentional injuries 6.3%
4	Female	Stroke 5.8%	Diabetes 4.7%	Diabetes 6.1%	Diabetes 3.7%	Diabetes 5.0%	Stroke 5.8%
	Male	Chronic lower respiratory diseases 5.4%	Stroke 4.7%	Chronic liver disease 5.5%	Unintentional injuries 5.0%	Diabetes 4.4%	Chronic lower respiratory diseases 5.7%

continued

TABLE 2-1 Continued

Rank	Gender	All	African American	American Indian/Alaska Native	Asian/Pacific Islander	Hispanic	White
5	Female	Alzheimer's disease 4.6%	Chronic lower respiratory diseases 3.3%	Chronic liver disease 5.6%	Influenza and pneumonia 3.5%	Unintentional injuries 4.4%	Alzheimer's disease 4.9%
	Male	Stroke 4.1%	Homicide 4.5%	Diabetes 5.3%	Diabetes 4.0%	Stroke 4.3%	Stroke 4.0%
6	Female	Unintentional injuries 3.8%	Kidney disease 3.0%	Chronic lower respiratory diseases 5.0%	Alzheimer's disease 3.4%	Alzheimer's disease 3.8%	Unintentional injuries 3.9%
	Male	Diabetes 3.1%	Diabetes 4.1%	Suicide 4.3%	Chronic lower respiratory diseases 3.6%	Chronic liver disease 4.0%	Diabetes 2.9%
7	Female	Diabetes 2.8%	Unintentional injuries 3.0%	Stroke 4.4%	Unintentional injuries 3.3%	Chronic lower respiratory diseases 3.1%	Diabetes 2.5%
	Male	Suicide 2.5%	Chronic lower respiratory diseases 3.3%	Chronic lower respiratory diseases 4.0%	Influenza and pneumonia 3.3%	Chronic lower respiratory diseases 2.9%	Suicide 2.6%

8	Female	Influenza and pneumonia 2.3%	Alzheimer's disease 2.7%	Influenza and pneumonia 2.4%	Chronic lower respiratory diseases 2.5%	Influenza and pneumonia 2.4%	Influenza and pneumonia 2.4%
	Male	Influenza and pneumonia 2.1%	Kidney disease 2.6%	Stroke 2.7%	Suicide 2.6%	Suicide 2.6%	Alzheimer's disease 2.1%
9	Female	Kidney disease 1.8%	Septicemia 2.3%	Alzheimer's disease 2.1%	Kidney disease 2.0%	Chronic liver disease 2.1%	Kidney disease 1.7%
	Male	Alzheimer's disease 2.0%	Septicemia 1.9%	Influenza and pneumonia 2.0%	Kidney disease 1.9%	Homicide 2.4%	Influenza and pneumonia 2.1%
10	Female	Septicemia 1.6%	Hypertension 2.0%	Kidney disease 2.1%	Hypertension 1.9%	Kidney disease 2.0%	Septicemia 1.5%
	Male	Chronic liver disease 1.8%	Influenza and pneumonia 1.7%	Homicide 2.0%	Alzheimer's disease 1.4%	Influenza and pneumonia 2.0%	Chronic liver disease 1.9%

SOURCES: CDC, 2013b,c.

across tribes, rural and urban areas, or Pacific Islanders and Asians as one group—which may mask differences in poverty, obesity, and diabetes (Bauer and Plescia, 2014; Holland and Palaniappan, 2012). For Hispanics, an ethnic group among which there is substantial heterogeneity by country of origin, many data sources report health outcomes for the entire population, despite evidence for within-group variation on important outcomes such as HIV (Garcia et al., 2015). Relative to black–white disparities, the literature examining disparities across other racial and ethnic populations is extremely limited. Considering the significant growth of minority populations in the United States, the insufficient knowledge base to date about the health conditions of a number of these groups presents a serious challenge to understanding and addressing health disparities among specific populations.

ADDRESSING HEALTH INEQUITY IN UNIQUE POPULATIONS

In the sections that follow, the committee discusses in some detail health disparities that affect several populations unique for various reasons ranging from data challenges (e.g., one group is severely underrepresented in public health data collection) to mental health considerations (e.g., one group experiences posttraumatic stress disorder (PTSD) at a rate much higher than the average). Community-based solutions for these population groups—Native Americans; female gender; lesbian, gay, bisexual, transgender (LGBT) individuals; individuals with disabilities; and veterans—will require attention to unique needs and assets identified by members of those communities. For example, communities that are focusing on addressing health disparities among people with disabilities, could include such approaches as universal design (accessible to all) and maximizing the opportunities offered by technologic innovations, such as telemedicine.

Native American Health

Why Are Native Americans a Unique Population for Health Equity?

Native Americans, or American Indians and Alaska Natives, are a significant population for health equity considerations, especially at the community level. An extremely heterogeneous population, the 5.4 million Native Americans make up about 2 percent of the total population living in the United States, with 44 percent identifying as at least one other race (Norris et al., 2012). There are 567 federally recognized Native American tribes in the United States (GPO, 2016a) and many more that are not recognized by the government. U.S. Census estimates reveal that the majority of people who identify as Native American (78 percent) live outside of regions that are considered traditional Native American areas[3] (Norris et al., 2012).

Native Americans have a unique historical and legal background in the United States (see Appendix A for more detail on the historical and legal context), which provides the basis for the federal government's trust obligation to Native American tribes. Unlike other racial and ethnic minority groups in this country, Native Americans possess legal rights to federal health care services. Despite these legal rights, the current state of health among this population is starkly worse than its counterparts in large part due to historical and legal contexts and the subsequent conditions of Native American communities. Furthermore, the body of literature on Native Americans has not been sufficient for a number of reasons, including small sample sizes, the heterogeneity of the population, and racial misclassification on disease registries and death certificates (Jim et al., 2014).

Health Disparities Among Native Americans

Although the creation of the Indian Health Service (IHS) and a trend toward self-determination have contributed to improvement of Native American health across many areas, including infectious disease prevention and sanitation (Rhoades and Rhoades, 2014), racial and ethnic health disparities have persisted for this population. The National Interview Health Survey revealed that 13.2 percent of Native Americans report being in fair or poor health, compared to only 9.8 percent of the total population (Adams and Benson, 2015).

Mortality Overall, mortality rates for Native Americans are almost 50 percent higher than that of their white counterparts (Bauer and Plescia, 2014). Additionally, Native Americans have an infant mortality rate that is 1.5 times the rate of whites (Mathews et al., 2015). While research shows that whites experienced a significant decline in all-cause mortality rates from 1990 to 2009, Native Americans did not (Espey et al., 2014).

Burden of diseases The health and overall well-being of Native Americans reflect a higher risk and higher rates of chronic diseases when compared to other racial and ethnic groups. For example, Native Americans are twice as likely to have diabetes as whites (HHS, 2016c). This is especially

---

[3] This includes federal American Indian reservations and off-reservation trust lands, Oklahoma tribal statistical areas, tribal designated statistical areas, state American Indian reservations, and state-designated American Indian statistical areas.

true for specific subgroups of Native Americans, such as the Pima Indians, who have historically been identified as having the world's highest recorded prevalence and incidence of type 2 diabetes (HHS, 2016c; Schulz et al., 2006). While overall population rates of diabetes as an underlying cause of death have been decreasing over time, the rates of diabetes as an underlying cause of death and a multiple cause of death have remained 2.5 to 3.5 times higher for Native Americans than for whites of all ages 20 and older, for every IHS region except Alaska (Cho et al., 2014).

A 10-year analysis revealed that Native Americans were 1.21 times as likely to die from heart disease as an underlying cause of death than were whites (Veazie et al., 2014). In 2012 the tuberculosis rate for Native Americans was 6.3 percent, as compared with 0.8 percent for the white population (HHS, 2016c). This disparity is especially striking when examined against the backdrop of successful infectious disease prevention efforts that have almost eliminated the burden of tuberculosis in other racial and ethnic populations.

While overall rates of cancer are lower for Native Americans than for other racial and ethnic groups, there are specific cancers for which this population is at high risk. These include stomach, liver, cervix, kidney, gallbladder, and colorectal cancer (Espey et al., 2014; White et al., 2014). Research suggests that the burden of disease from these types of cancer is in large part attributable to the high rates of alcohol consumption among Native Americans (Landen et al., 2014). From 1990 to 2009, overall cancer death rates increased significantly for Native Americans, whereas these rates declined for white men during the entire period, and for white women during most of the 19-year period (White et al., 2014).

Mental health Native Americans have had a complex and tumultuous history in the United States. The resulting historical trauma is an important context for the discourse on mental health issues that are faced by Native American communities today. Although research on mental health is limited because of the size and heterogeneity of this population, there is literature that suggests that Native Americans disproportionately suffer from mental health disorders and related conditions. These include, but are not limited to, increased prevalence and risk factors for depression, suicide, drug and alcohol abuse, and PTSD (Berman, 2014; Herne et al., 2014; HHS, 2016c; Landen et al., 2014). When compared to the general U.S. population, Native Americans experience PTSD more than twice as often and experience psychological distress 1.5 times more often (APA, 2010). These experiences have major implications for suicide rates in Native American communities. A 10-year analysis of death certificate data linked with IHS health data found that death rates from suicide were approximately 50 percent higher among Native Americans than among whites (Herne et al., 2014). Recently, suicide has replaced homicide as the second leading cause of death among U.S. teenagers, and the highest rates are among Native American youth (VanOrman and Jarosz, 2016).

A Shift in the Narrative

Despite the barriers to achieving health and well-being that Native Americans face, there have been positive advancements by communities and community partners toward improving the health of this population. For example, the emergence of tribal health research infrastructures has been supported by National Institutes of Health funding of the Native American Research Centers for Health, which started in 2001 (Jernigan et al., 2015; Kelley et al., 2013). Furthermore, resilient Native American communities have followed the trend toward self-governance and have taken the initiative to create community-driven solutions to address the severe health conditions discussed in this section. Box 2-1 briefly introduces one of these communities and its path to health (see Chapter 4 for a more in-depth discussion of another Native American community that is taking action on health inequity).

BOX 2-1
Menominee Nation's Path to Health

The Menominee Nation in Menominee County, Wisconsin, faced increasing rates of substance abuse, domestic violence, poverty, and low graduation rates when the tribe decided to confront its historical oppression and associated trauma. An RWJF Culture of Health prize-winning community, the Menominee Nation is applying a trauma-informed care model to provide social and behavioral health services to its residents.

Some of the policy and systemic changes in Menominee County include

- A new grocery store close to the high school
- Greenhouses, gardens, and orchards at schools
- Enhancing physical education programs
- Workplace wellness culture shifts
- Community-led group activities centered around cultural practices
- Installing sidewalks and streetlights

SOURCE: RWJF, 2015.

Gender Disparities

When discussing health disparities across gender groups, it is important to acknowledge that while the basis of some disparities is biological (e.g., rates of ovarian and prostate cancers), the majority of the disparities discussed in this section are not based in biological mechanisms unless otherwise stated. Nonbiological health disparities stem from socioeconomic conditions that can shape gender differences in health outcomes such as mortality rates, alcohol and substance abuse, mental health disorders, and violence victimization.

In 2014 life expectancy at birth was 81.2 years for women and 76.4 years for men (NCHS, 2016). From 2004 to 2014, the gap in life expectancy between men and women decreased from 5.1 years to 4.8 years (NCHS, 2016). While the narrowing of the life expectancy gap could be considered a positive trend, it is in fact a troubling trend because it stems from a rise in mortality rates among women over the past two decades in many areas (Arias, 2016). Kindig and Cheng found that from 1992 to 2006, as mortality decreased in most U.S. counties, female mortality rates increased in 42.8 percent of counties. During this same period, only 3.4 percent of counties saw an increase in male mortality rates (Kindig and Cheng, 2013).

More specifically, recent evidence reveals an unprecedented increase in the death rates among white women and a decline in life expectancy, changes that white men did not experience (Arias, 2016). Findings on the causes of death among white women point to accidental poisoning (related to the rise in prescription opioid use), suicide, obesity, and smoking-related diseases (Astone et al., 2015). Figure 2-1 shows that across multiple racial groups, women—particularly white women—have been more affected than men by the increasing rates of drug poisonings (NASEM, 2016a).

In terms of alcohol and illicit drug use, men ages 12 and older report higher usage rates than women (SAMHSA, 2015a,b). While women have lower rates of alcohol and substance use, they are more likely to have a serious mental illness than men (SAMHSA, 2015a). Research shows that women are more likely to be diagnosed with anxiety or depression (including post-partum depression) and men are more likely to have substance abuse or antisocial disorders (Eaton, 2012). In fact, depression is the number one cause of women's disability in the United States (NASEM, 2016a).

Gender disparities are present across all social determinants of health, with some more prominent than others. In education, the historical gender gap has narrowed over the past 50 years, with the percentage of men and women older than 25 years with bachelor's degrees roughly equal now (32 percent and 33 percent, respectively), and the percentage of women

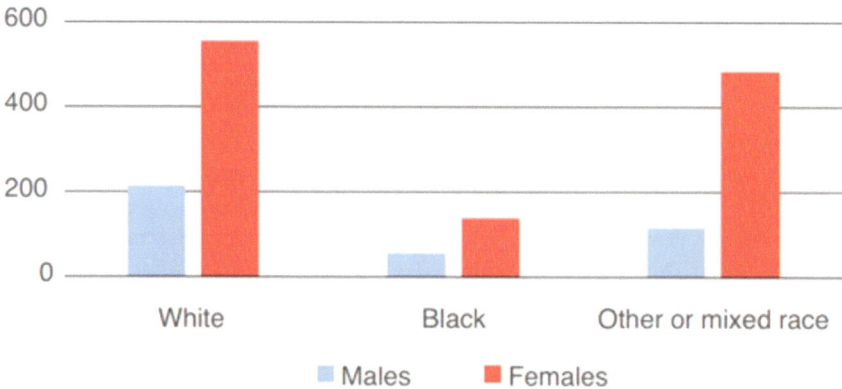

FIGURE 2-1 Percentage increase in drug poisonings between 1994 and 2010.
SOURCE: NASEM, 2016a.

ages 25–29 with a bachelor's degree exceeds that of men. However, men still outnumber women in the attainment of degrees beyond a bachelor's degree (Ryan and Bauman, 2016). The gender pay gap, a widely reported disparity in income, has implications for health inequities because income is closely tied to health. A report by the National Academies of Sciences, Engineering, and Medicine examined gains in life expectancy across different income groups over time and found that while men in the top 60 percent of the income distribution were making gains in life expectancy at age 50, women were experiencing losses in expected life expectancy at age 50 in the bottom two income quintiles and no progress in the third or fourth quintiles (NASEM, 2015).

Access to routine, quality health care is essential for both men and women. The uninsured rate is higher for men, even after the passage of the Patient Protection and Affordable Care Act (ACA), in part because men have not historically qualified for Medicaid (NASEM, 2016a). Reproductive and sexual health services are an especially important consideration for women because of their ability to bear children. Unintended pregnancy can have an impact on the overall health and well-being of women. From 2007 to 2010 teenage pregnancy rates in the United States declined 17 percent (Hamilton and Ventura, 2012).

For women, experiencing violence is a strong predictor of health, and violence against women is primarily in the form of intimate partner violence (IOM, 2010; Tjaden and Thoennes, 2000). Living in low-income neighborhoods is associated with an increased risk of intimate partner violence for African American and white women (Cunradi et al., 2000). Women are more likely than men to sustain injuries from an assault

(Tjaden and Thoennes, 2000). In addition to injury, research suggests that women's health can be greatly affected over time after experiencing violence. For example, women who experience violence are at increased risk of arthritis, asthma, heart disease, gynecological problems, and risk factors for HIV or sexually transmitted diseases (STDs) than those who do not experience violence (Campbell and Boyd, 2000; IOM, 2010). For men, community violence is likely to affect their health, and this is particularly true for men of color, who experience disproportionate amounts of violence (Prevention Institute, 2011). Men are also much more likely to commit suicide than women, regardless of age, race, or ethnicity, with overall rates at almost four times those of women (CDC, 2013a).

Lesbian, Gay, Bisexual, and Transgender Health Disparities

Who Are LGBT Persons?

LGBT persons are considered sexual minorities because of their non-heterosexual sexual orientation (i.e., lesbian, gay, or bisexual) or their gender identity (i.e., transgender).[4] Sexual orientation and gender identity minorities are often referred to using the acronym LGBT (i.e., lesbian, gay, bisexual, and transgender persons) as an umbrella term even though the forms of sexual and gender expression that exist within this population are greater than the acronym suggests. For instance, intersex persons who have both male and female sex characteristics are also considered under this rubric (Makadon et al., 2008). Until recently, LGBT populations were excluded from many of the rights and social advantages of our society and were routinely targeted for hate crimes. A 2011 Institute of Medicine (IOM) report assessed the state of the evidence and determined it was lacking with respect to demography research, evidence on social influences for LGBT people, inequities in health care, intervention research, and transgender-specific health needs. The report defined LGBT populations and outlined needs for advancing a research agenda on LGBT health disparities (IOM, 2011).

Both sex and gender are relevant to sexual orientation and gender identity. "Sex" is a biological construct that has at least two categories, male and female. Gender is a social construct reflecting one's social sense of self. It exists on a continuum ranging from masculine to feminine and has at least two categories, man and woman. Gender identity combines the biological construct of sex and the social construct of gender. It

---

[4] For a more detailed discussion of LGBT populations and how to define them, see the IOM report *The Health of Lesbian, Gay, Bisexual, and Transgender People: Building a Foundation for Better Understanding* (IOM, 2011).

has two categories, cis gendered and trans gendered. As implied by the *Diagnostic and Statistical Manual of Mental Disorders* (DSM-5) definition of gender dysphoria, transgender persons are those for whom the sex (male versus female) and gender (masculine versus feminine) categories do not align, leading a person of one gender to feel trapped in the body of the opposite sex. The LGBT population is a microcosm of the broader society and, therefore, reflects its demographic and social diversity as well as its socioeconomic and racial and ethnic inequities.

Challenges to achieving LGBT health equity stem primarily from the "invisibility" of LGBT individuals and communities, the forms of stigma and social and legal discrimination to which they are susceptible, and the paucity of data on the factors influencing LGBT health (HHS, 2011). Recent civil rights gains have helped to increase LGBT visibility, reduce stigma, and facilitate access to health insurance and health care; however, standardized competencies on LGBT health for health professionals and health care organizations are not yet required nationally. Therefore, the care that LGBT persons receive may not yet reflect an awareness of LGBT-specific concerns.

Health Disparities

Overall LGBT population The LGBT population experiences all of the same diseases and conditions that are prevalent in the broader society (e.g., cardiovascular disease) as well as other conditions such as HIV/AIDS that affect the LGBT population disproportionately. The social determinants of health are particularly influential drivers of LGBT health disparities. High rates of unemployment or underemployment, limited access to appropriate health care, and social discrimination affect the behaviors in which LGBT people engage and the strategies needed to improve the health of this population.

LGBT health disparities occur across the life course. LGBT youth are more likely than their non-LGBT peers to be bullied, commit suicide, engage in sexual risk behaviors, and run away or be forced to leave home (Robinson and Espelage, 2013). The social challenges that accompany their high rates of homelessness include mental health issues, violence, HIV and other STDs, poverty, substance abuse, and food insecurity (Garofalo and Bush, 2008). LGBT seniors are more likely than non-LGBT seniors to live alone. They are also less likely to have children, which can limit their access to sources of social support for assistance with the activities of daily living and with chronic or acute medical needs (Henning-Smith et al., 2015; Wallace et al., 2011).

Social discrimination and inadequate legal protections directly affect health behaviors (e.g., substance use) and access to health care; the data on mental health disparities are mixed. Violence, including bias crimes, remains a major public health issue for LGBT persons, although the levels and types of violence differ across LGBT subpopulations. In a rare national study, an estimated 39 percent of gay men, 15 percent of lesbians, 20 percent of bisexual men, and 15 percent of bisexual women reported having ever experienced physical violence, property crime, or attempted crime due to anti-LGBT bias (Herek, 2009). LGBT youth and transgender women are particularly susceptible to physical assault, sexual assault, and murder (Grant et al., 2011; Office for Victims of Crime, n.d.). Though sexual forms of victimization are poorly documented, the available data suggest that the lifetime prevalence is higher among lesbian and bisexual women (43.4 percent) than among gay and bisexual men, and that bias-related victimization, including murder, is higher among transgender women than among any other group (Grant et al., 2011; Rothman et al., 2011). Stark racial and ethnic disparities exist; transgender women of color experience higher levels of such violence than members of any other group (Grant et al., 2011).

Lesbian women Timely and appropriate health screenings for preventable diseases can prevent many of the health issues affecting lesbians. Lesbians have higher rates of alcohol, tobacco, and other drug use, which are associated with cardiovascular disease and obesity (O'Hanlan and Isler, 2007). On average, lesbians have greater body mass index than heterosexual women, and they are less responsive to social pressures to lose weight (Roberts et al., 2010). Lesbians also have an elevated risk for some cancers because of a combination of lifestyle factors and other risk factors. They experience disparities in breast, colon, and lung cancers due to obesity and tobacco and alcohol use. They have an elevated risk for gynecological cancers, such as ovarian and breast cancer, because of such risk factors as a lower likelihood of ever being pregnant and delayed or inadequate gynecological screenings (O'Hanlan and Isler, 2007).

Gay men Among gay men, HIV and AIDS remain major threats to health. In 2013, 81 percent of all new diagnoses of HIV (30,689 new cases) infection in the United States occurred among gay and bisexual men, with African American men having the highest rates (AHRQ, 2015). The high prevalence of HIV in this population means that any member of this population who engages in HIV-risk behaviors has an elevated risk of acquiring it. Based on 2008 surveillance data among gay and bisexual men screened for HIV infection, the CDC estimates that HIV prevalence among gay and bisexual men to be 19 percent (CDC, 2010a). An emerging set of concerns pertain to negative body image, eating disorders such as anorexia, and related mental health disorders, especially among white men; however, large population-based studies have yet to confirm this (Burns et al., 2015; Ruble and Forstein, 2008).

Bisexual persons Except for the disproportionate burden of HIV/AIDS among bisexual men, health disparities uniquely affecting bisexual men and women are poorly understood, as studies often add bisexual persons to the homosexual category. One issue that appears to affect bisexual men and women disproportionately is intimate partner violence (Brown and Herman, 2015). Estimates from the National Intimate Partner and Sexual Violence Survey document that in 2010, 61 percent of bisexual women, as compared with 44 percent of lesbians and 35 percent of heterosexual women, experienced intimate partner violence–related physical violence, stalking, or rape; 37 percent of bisexual men, as compared with 29 percent of heterosexuals and 26 percent of gay men, experienced these outcomes (Walters et al., 2013).

Transgender persons Transgendered persons, especially transgendered women, experience particularly dire disparities, which are driven primarily by the social determinants of health. The inability to secure employment as an openly transgendered person or to maintain employment while transitioning from one sex to the other helps to explain why the occurrence of annual household incomes of $10,000 or less is nearly four times higher in this population than in the overall U.S. population (Grant et al., 2011). Poverty leads many transgender women to engage in sex work, which places them at risk for incarceration, violence, substance abuse, and HIV as well as other sexually transmitted infections. African American and Hispanic transgender women are disproportionately impacted (Reisner et al., 2014). Other health disparities affecting this subpopulation include depression, self-harm, suicide, and complications due to the use of cross-sex hormones, some of which may be obtained illegally or of poor quality (Kaufman, 2008; Lawrence, 2007).

Some of the disparities that LGBT persons experience reflect the ways that LGBT status may intersect with other minority statuses. For instance, among transgender women, racial and ethnic minorities report disproportionately higher levels of incarceration than their nonminority peers, and qualitative findings suggest that concerns about racism may be at least as salient as those of sexual orientation and gender identity (Sausa et al., 2007).

Health Care Disparities

Sexual minorities face several barriers to care, including their exclusion from a partner's health insurance, provider-related discrimination, psychosocial barriers (e.g., fear of disclosing sexual orientation and gender identity or illegal behaviors), and poor matches between the needs of LGBT people and the kinds of services that are available (HHS, 2011).

Poor matches typically occur if the available services are intentionally (e.g., obstetric/gynecologic) or unintentionally (e.g., intimate partner violence) developed and provided with a particular gender in mind. For instance, both providers and transgender persons may fail to pursue the standard screening for breast cancer for transgender men, even though they may continue to be at risk. With respect to intimate partner violence, while some of the challenges faced by survivors are universal to all survivors (e.g., physical and emotional pain, the need for shelter), other issues (e.g., distinguishing perpetrators and victims in same-sex couples) affect the LGBT population specifically. Most intimate partner violence–related services are typically designed to assist heterosexual women battered by male partners (Ford et al., 2013), so providers and social service agencies may not know how to address the issues uniquely affecting LGBT survivors, though trainings are available to address this.

Perhaps the greatest challenges faced by transgendered persons and their providers involve the need for multiple surgeries and the long-term administration of sex hormones. Both require substantial reliance on the health care system, and some insurers may not reimburse the expenses fully. The need for these services is compounded by the particularly low levels of income and health insurance in this population (Center for American Progress and Movement Advancement Project, 2015; dickey et al., 2016).

Disability Status and Health Disparities

Disabilities,[5] whether present or acquired at birth or developed later in the life course, can manifest as physical, cognitive, or mental health-related impairments, which can affect health outcomes. People with disabilities represent about 18.7 percent of the U.S. population (Brault, 2012). Although there is ample evidence to suggest that people with disabilities are at increased relative risk for poor well-being (see Figure 2-2), until recently this population has been overlooked in population health data collection, analyses, and reports (Krahn et al., 2015). One of the major

---

[5] The WHO *International Classification of Functioning, Disability, and Health* (ICF) defines disability as an umbrella term for impairments, activity limitations, and participation restrictions (WHO, 2001).

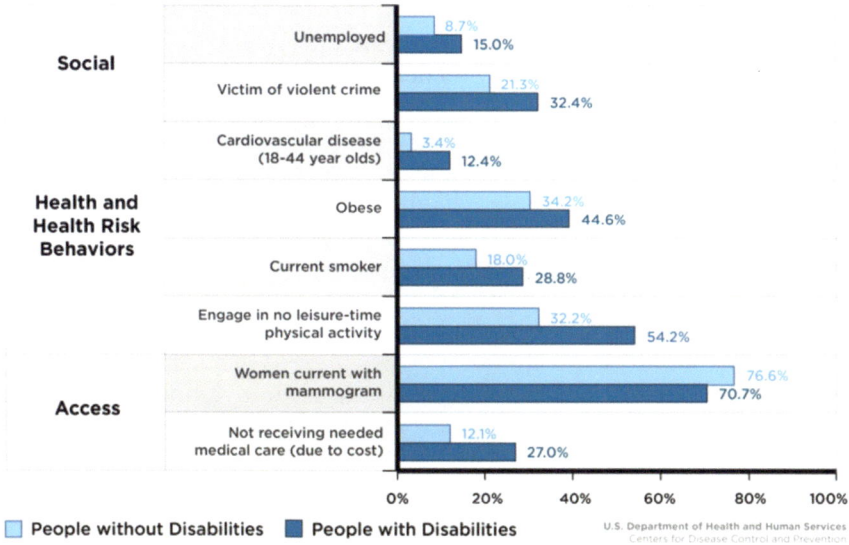

FIGURE 2-2 Factors affecting the health of people with disabilities and without disabilities.
SOURCE: CDC, 2015.

challenges in data collection has been the lack of consensus on a clear and specific definition of disability (Oreskovich and Zimmerman, 2012). There has been an emerging effort to document and address health disparities among people with disabilities (CDC, 2013a; HHS, 2016a; NASEM, 2016b), in addition to the ACA requirement to improve data collection and reporting on disability, among other factors.

Adults with disabilities are four times as likely as adults with no disabilities to report having fair or poor health (40.3 percent versus 9.9 percent) (Krahn et al., 2015). People with disabilities also report higher rates of obesity, lack of physical activity, smoking, and three to four times the rate of cardiovascular disease versus people without disabilities (CDC, 2014b, 2016c; Reichard and Stolzle, 2011; Reichard et al., 2011). For specific subgroups of this population, factors such as race and ethnicity, age, language, sex or gender, poverty, and low education can compound the effects of having a disability (Krahn et al., 2015). Furthermore, living with a disability shapes one's experiences of the social, economic, and environmental determinants of health. For instance, having a disability is associated with an increased likelihood of not having a high school education, less likelihood of employment, less access to the Internet, an increased likelihood of having an annual income less than $15,000, and inadequate access to transportation (Krahn et al., 2015).

Living with a disability can present barriers to accessing health care services and navigating the health care system (WHO, 2016). People with disabilities, including those with health insurance and those without, were more than twice as likely as people without disabilities to not receive medical care because of cost in 2009 (CDC, 2010b). While they experience higher rates of chronic disease than the general population, people with disabilities are significantly less likely to receive preventive care (Krahn et al., 2015). Additional barriers include common misconceptions, stigma, and attitudes among providers (CDC, 2016b).

Disability types vary in prevalence and in how they are associated with health disparities. In the United States, disabilities in mobility and cognition are the most commonly reported types (Courtney-Long et al., 2015). People with cognitive limitations are up to five times more likely to have diabetes than the general population (Reichard and Stolzle, 2011). Disability severity also has implications for the economic factors that shape health. According to U.S. Census data, in 2010 approximately 28.6 percent of people ages 15 to 64 with severe disabilities were in poverty, compared with 17.9 percent of adults with non-severe disabilities and only 14.3 percent of adults with no disability (Brault, 2012).

Veterans Health

As a vulnerable and growing population, military veterans are an important focus of many ongoing efforts to promote health equity. Many veterans experience lasting trauma from their military service as well as socioeconomic disadvantages post-deployment that can significantly influence their physical and mental well-being. These conditions have resulted in health and health care disparities both relative to the general population and among certain veteran subpopulations. For the purposes of this report, veterans are defined as those "who served in the active military, naval, or air service, and who [were] discharged or released therefrom under conditions other than dishonorable,"[6] who receive health care from the Veterans Health Administration (VHA) as well as those who are not enrolled.

Many conditions and factors contribute to premature mortality among veterans, including higher rates of suicide risk, homelessness, and mental health issues. The risk of suicide in the veteran population is higher than in the general population and has become an increasingly serious problem among younger veterans. A study of 1.3 million veterans who served in Iraq and Afghanistan between 2001 and 2007 found that non-deployed and deployed veterans had 61 and 41 percent higher

---

[6] 38 U.S. Code § 101.

risks of suicide, respectively, than members of the general population (Kang et al., 2015). The U.S. Department of Veterans Affairs (VA) recently examined suicide rates among VA-enrolled veterans from all states and found that in 2014, VA-enrolled veterans accounted for 17.9 percent of suicide deaths among U.S. adults and had a 21 percent higher risk of suicide relative to the general adult population (VA, 2016). The higher risk of suicide among younger veterans has also drawn significant attention. Specifically, between 2006 and 2011, the suicide rate among young California veterans (a yearly average of 27 suicides per 100,000 veterans) was 57 percent higher than the rate among active duty military personnel (Zarembo, 2013).

Mental illness and related psychopathological problems, including PTSD, depression, substance abuse, and sexual trauma, are significantly more prevalent among the veteran population. Despite the high burden, calculated prevalence rates have varied significantly because of substantial variations in many components of study design. The prevalence of these disorders among veterans who receive care from the VA and among those who do not can be even more difficult to discern. The prevalence of PTSD in veterans who were deployed to Afghanistan and Iraq is two to three times greater than in the overall population, with many studies estimating that the prevalence among this veteran cohort ranges from 13 to 20 percent (IOM, 2012). PTSD is closely linked to military sexual trauma (MST), which federal law defines as "psychological trauma, which in the judgment of a mental health professional employed by the VA, resulted from a physical assault of a sexual nature, battery of a sexual nature, or sexual harassment which occurred while the veteran was serving on active duty, active duty for training, or inactive duty training."[7] Sexual trauma is far more prevalent among veterans and military personnel than in the general population and is likely to be considerably underreported. Recently, data from the National Health and Resilience in Veterans Study collected in 2013 revealed a prevalence rate of 7.6 percent, with 32.4 percent of female veterans and 4.8 percent of male veterans reporting MST (Klingensmith et al., 2014). MST disproportionately affects female veterans but is also a pervasive problem among male veterans, and it detrimentally affects both mental and physical health. It has been linked to suicidal ideation, substance abuse, PTSD, depression, anxiety, eating disorders, and impaired mental and cognitive functioning (Klingensmith et al., 2014; Mondragon et al., 2015; O'Brien and Sher, 2013). It has also been linked to greater symptoms of physical pain (Mondragon et al., 2015; O'Brien and Sher, 2013). Sexual trauma suffered during military service may also affect the social well-being of veterans after they are deployed,

---

[7] 38 U.S. Code § 1720D. Counseling and treatment for sexual trauma.

as MST has been negatively correlated with emotional and social support post-deployment (Mondragon et al., 2015).

Disparities related to access to and use of health care as well as higher prevalence of certain chronic diseases are also present in the veteran population. A review of studies examining racial and ethnic health care disparities in the VA found that relative to white veterans, African American veterans experience lower levels of arthritis and cardiovascular disease management, lower levels of participation in surgery related to cancer and cardiovascular disease, and a lower quality of diabetes care (Saha et al., 2007). Prevalence rates for certain chronic diseases are also disproportionately high in the veteran population. Among African American male veterans born between 1945 and 1965, the prevalence of hepatitis C virus was 17.7 percent, a fivefold greater rate than the 3.5 percent prevalence found in the same birth cohort of the general population between 2001 and 2010 (Backus et al., 2014).

Veteran homelessness is one of the most staggering and urgent issues affecting veteran health; although the number of homeless veterans has decreased in recent years, veterans remain at significantly higher risk than members of the general population for becoming homeless (Tsai and Rosenheck, 2015). Point-in-time counts by the U.S. Department of Housing and Urban Development across all states estimated 47,725 homeless veterans in 2015 and 39,471 homeless veterans in 2016, a decrease of 17.3 percent between the 2 years[8] (HUD, 2016). Studies with more geographically focused sampling also illustrate the continuing pervasiveness of veteran homelessness. In a study of homeless veterans 65 years and older in Los Angeles between 2003 and 2005, 56 percent were found to be chronically homeless, with African American veterans accounting for 42 percent of this number (van den Berk-Clark and McGuire, 2013). Additionally, female veterans are at higher risk of homelessness than both male veterans and females in the civilian population and account for an increasing proportion of homeless veterans, as the number of female veterans increases (Balshem et al., 2011; Byrne et al., 2013). Box 2-2 briefly describes a community-based program that was designed to address a few of the barriers that veterans face.

---

[8] Note: Comparison of prevalence estimates over time is flawed due to differences in counting and estimation methods.

> **BOX 2-2**
> **Veterans Sustainable Agricultural Training Program**
>
> Former Marine Sergeant Colin Archipley and his wife, Karen, bought a small 200-tree avocado farm which they named "Archi's Acres." Their search for more sustainable farming methods, coupled with a desire to stay connected in a meaningful way to the Marine Corps, led to development of the Veterans Sustainable Agriculture Training Program (VSAT). Offered in collaboration with California State Polytechnic University, VSAT's aim is to help others achieve meaningful employment in sustainable agriculture. This collaboration and the structure of the 6-week "agricultural entrepreneurial incubator" program for which students can receive 17 quarter units of academic credit are key to its success. In addition:
>
> - The partnership with the university provides the foundation for nationally recognized accreditation.
> - The program meets the U.S. Department of Agriculture's (USDA's) experience requirements—completing VSAT is equivalent to 1 year of farm management experience or a 4-year degree in soil science—so consequently, graduates qualify for a USDA-guaranteed farm loan.
> - Veterans and active duty service members can use their existing educational benefits (e.g., GI Bill, VA Vocational Rehabilitation, or tuition assistance) to cover the program's $4,500 tuition. Other veteran-serving nonprofits also provide tuition grants for qualifying veterans (Stand for the Troops Inc., 2016).
>
> To facilitate the success of its graduates, VSAT complements technical content with the business aspects of sustainable farming: sustainable farming production methods, agricultural irrigation planning and techniques, organic hydroponic techniques, greenhouse design considerations, farm ownership and management, business development and implementation, business plan development, hands-on training approach, introduction to farm service agency loan programs training, and introduction to the agricultural marketplace and network (Archi's Acres Inc., 2016).
> More than 80 VSAT students are veterans and many are struggling with health issues such as "invisible" wounds (e.g., PTSD) and other service-connected disabilities (Stand for the Troops Inc., 2016). Thus, VSAT and the subsequent employment in sustainable agriculture have the potential to also influence the health of veterans. As of 2012, VSAT had helped more than 100 military veterans transition to the civilian workforce.

PLACE MATTERS

In the following section, the committee discusses the relationship between people and place and implications for health disparities. One of the most consistent findings in the health disparities literature is that place matters. Research shows that there are systematic disparities in morbidity, mortality, and other measures of well-being across different areas of the country, even across small areas that lie relatively close together. At a larger level of analysis, life expectancy varies between states by up to 7.0 years for males and 6.7 years for females (NRC and IOM, 2013). Historically, many analyses compared health and life expectancy rates across wide areas, such as regions or states. Thus, it can be stated that obesity—a condition associated with chronic disease, mortality, and decreased overall well-being—is concentrated in the South and Midwest (Levi et al., 2015b). Likewise, people living in the South are more likely to be diagnosed with HIV over the course of their lifetime than other Americans, with the highest risk in Washington, DC (1 in 13), Maryland (1 in 49), Georgia (1 in 51), Florida (1 in 54), and Louisiana (1 in 56) (CDC, 2016d).

However, the availability of more granular data has allowed for the observation of even larger disparities across smaller geographic regions such as zip codes, counties, and census tracts (see Figures 2-3 and 2-4) (Kulkarni et al., 2011; UWPHI, 2016; Zimmerman and Woolf, 2014). In some cities, for example, life expectancy can differ by as much as 25 years

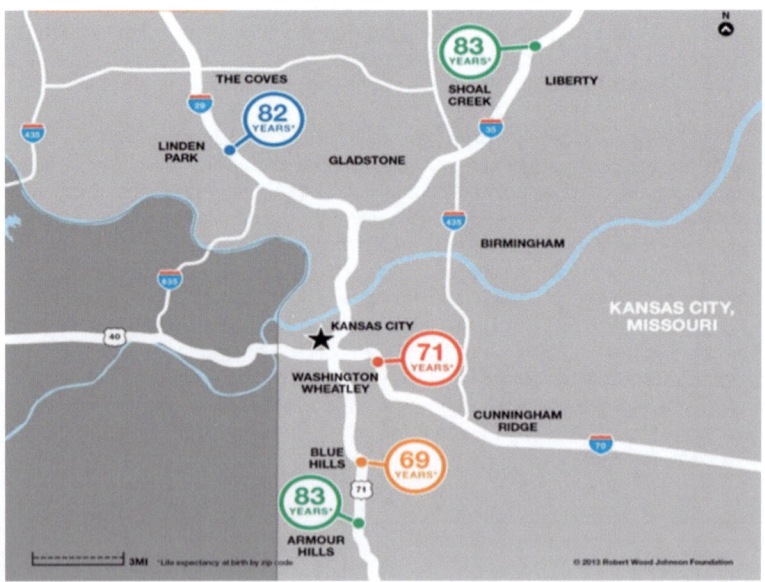

FIGURE 2-3 Map of life expectancy disparities in Kansas City, Missouri.
NOTE: The average life expectancy gap for babies born to mothers in Kansas City can reach up to 14 years.
SOURCE: RWJF, 2013a. Used with permission from the Robert Wood Johnson Foundation.

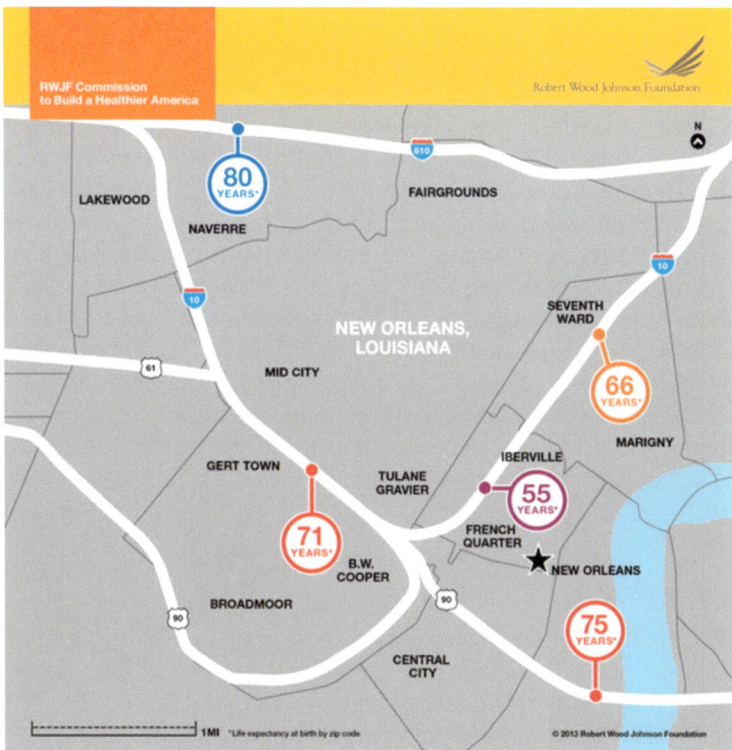

FIGURE 2-4 Map of life expectancy disparities in New Orleans, Louisiana.
NOTE: The average life expectancy gap for babies born to mothers in New Orleans can reach up to 25 years.
SOURCE: RWJF, 2013b. Used with permission from the Robert Wood Johnson Foundation.

from one neighborhood to the next (Figure 2-4 illustrates this disparity between New Orleans neighborhoods) (Evans et al., 2012; Zimmerman and Woolf, 2014). Life expectancy is but one measure of these disparities. Similar gaps in health-related outcomes across geographic areas can be found for infant mortality, obesity, violence, and chronic diseases (UWPHI, 2016). There is also research suggesting that African Americans and whites living in similar neighborhood conditions do not experience the racial disparities in health that national data reflect (LaVeist et al., 2011).

Health Disparities in Rural Places

Health equity for rural communities brings considerations that may not be as prevalent in urban and suburban communities. Singh and Siahpush found that rural areas have not made the same strides in improving life expectancy as urban areas have, with the gap between rural and urban areas widening from 0.4 years in 1969–1971 to 2.0 years in 2005–2009 (Singh and Siahpush, 2014). Rural counties[9] have always had the highest premature death rates among the various types of counties. However, the County Health Rankings Report revealed that after a period of steady decline over decades, rural counties are experiencing an increase in the number of premature deaths (UWPHI, 2016). The evidence also shows that, compared with their urban counterparts, rural communities have higher rates of preventable conditions (such as obesity, diabetes, cancer, and injury), and higher rates of related high-risk health behaviors (such as smoking, physical inactivity, poor diet, and limited use of seatbelts) (Crosby et al., 2012).

Appalachian Health

In Appalachia[10] the proportion of the population living in rural communities is double that of the population in the nation living in rural areas (42 percent and 20 percent, respectively) (CREC and WVU, 2015). Mortality measures show that in Appalachia, mortality rates have increased, particularly in central and southern Appalachian counties, while they have been decreasing in the country overall (CREC and WVU, 2015). Yao et al. (2012) analyzed spatial disparities in white infant mortality rates over time and found that disparities in infant mortality rates between Appalachian counties and non-Appalachian counties have persisted since the 1970s. High infant mortality in Appalachia is associated with high poverty rates, residence in more rural areas, and lower physician density (Yao et al., 2012). Health perception has also been shown to be worse among residents who live in communities in Appalachian counties when compared to other residents living in the same state, but in non-Appalachian counties (McGarvey et al., 2011). This association persisted even among those with health insurance.

This region has historically been affected by poverty and lack of opportunities for achieving optimal health, including factors such as

---

[9] Rural classification here is adapted from the National Center for Health Statistics' urban–rural classification based on Metropolitan Statistical Area designations.

[10] The Appalachian region includes the entire state of West Virginia and parts of the following states: Alabama, Georgia, Kentucky, Maryland, Mississippi, New York, North Carolina, Ohio, Pennsylvania, South Carolina, Tennessee, and Virginia (CREC and WVU, 2015).

employment, education, housing, and access to transportation. From 2010–2014, in the region's most rural counties, 15 percent of residents were not covered by health insurance, compared to 14 percent in the nation (Pollard and Jacobsen, 2016). Unemployment rates among the population in Appalachia suggest that this population has not rebounded from the economic downturn in 2007–2009. The labor force participation rate was almost a full percentage point lower in 2010–2014 than its rate in 2005–2009 (Pollard and Jacobsen, 2016).

Limited timely access to a health care provider, poor management of chronic disease, and limited subspecialty availability are very real concerns for rural communities (Wong and Regan, 2009). Health systems in rural communities are often under-resourced, understaffed, and of small scale, and in recent years many rural hospitals have closed. The small scale may make it easier for health care providers to discriminate, as a single provider may be able to dictate the treatment, cost, and quality of service (Bull et al., 2001) and there may be little recourse for the rural resident. Transportation challenges also pose a problem for rural health care delivery systems.

Despite these challenges, rural communities may not suffer disadvantages in all areas of health when compared to urban and suburban communities. Both rural and urban areas tend to have higher rates of adverse health outcomes than suburban areas (Eberhardt and Pamuk, 2004).

The nature of racial and ethnic disparities in rural areas is rather complex and intersectional. It appears to vary depending in part on the region of the country and the racial and ethnic groups being considered (e.g., rural Native American reservations; Hispanic farm workers; African Americans residing in rural parts of the South, which may include historically African American municipalities as well as those in which African Americans constitute a minority of the population; and rural communities with large immigrant or Hispanic populations). For migrant and seasonal farmworkers, 78 percent of whom are foreign born, there are many unique health concerns that stem from occupational hazards, poverty, substandard living conditions, language and cultural barriers, and inadequate preventive care (Hansen and Donohoe, 2003; NCFH, 2009).

The health issues facing U.S. rural communities are not necessarily due to rurality per se. In part these place-based health disparities are driven by

- demographic shifts in which rural areas are losing population as young people migrate to cities for work, school, etc.;
- inefficiency associated with providing health care services, which leads to, for instance, hospital closures in rural areas;

- a primary focus on and allocation of resources for interventions to address issues facing urban populations;
- a lack of the necessary technological infrastructure (e.g., a lack of reliable Internet service), which limits the possible alternative strategies for health promotion; and
- place-specific exposures such as those associated with mining and farming (pesticide exposures, etc.).

Health Disparities in Urban Places

There are unique features of urban regions as well as unique population characteristics and barriers to health that shape urban disparities. The food environment is a widely examined feature of urban areas that shapes health outcomes. When examining the 10 counties with the highest number of food-insecure individuals in the country, all of the 10 counties spanned over large urban cities (e.g., Chicago, Illinois; Houston, Texas; Los Angeles, California; New York, New York; Phoenix, Arizona) (Gundersen, 2015). In addition to the nutritional impact of urban food deserts, there is a social dynamic process that affects health disparities in these urban environments. The processes involved in the growth, purchase, preparation, consumption, and sharing—or absence—of food within communities can shape how residents in urban food deserts interact with food (Cannuscio et al., 2010).

Violence, in addition to the resulting injuries and trauma, affects urban regions at higher rates than in other regions. Approximately two-thirds of all U.S. firearm homicides occur in large urban areas, with inner cities as the most affected by firearm homicide (Prevention Institute, 2011). Youth violence is highest in cities (469 per 100,000) and less in metropolitan counties (259 per 100,000) and suburban areas (252 per 100,000) (Levi et al., 2015a). One of the downstream effects of violence is the chronic stress that is associated with living in an unsafe community. In urban areas where violence is pervasive, community-level trauma can manifest in which residents experience psychological trauma, with some exhibiting signs of PTSD (Pinderhughes et al., 2015). According to the Prevention Institute, 35 percent of urban youth exposed to community violence develop PTSD, a rate higher than that among soldiers deployed to combat (Prevention Institute, 2011). Unsafe neighborhoods can also lead to anxiety, depression, and stress, all of which are in turn associated with preterm births and low birth weight (Egerter et al., 2011).

Urban communities have been characterized by a high burden of asthma for decades. For children, specifically, the data reveal higher rates of morbidity due to asthma for those living in crowded, urban neighborhoods (Gern, 2010). This association has been attributed to the presence of environmental hazards such as pollution, pest allergens, and exposure to indoor and outdoor smoke (Kozyrskyj et al., 2004). However, findings suggest that other factors, such as race, ethnicity, and income, may have more important roles in shaping risk of asthma in children than their physical environment (Keet et al., 2015).

EVIDENCE GAPS

Since the publication of Heckler's 1985 *Report of the Secretary's Task Force on Black & Minority Health* (the *Heckler Report*) and even the IOM's 2003 *Unequal Treatment: Confronting Racial and Ethnic Disparities in Health Care* report, significant progress has been made in the science of health inequities. Scientific progress is evident in the development of conceptual models of the multilevel factors that shape health inequities, a greater standardization and collection of data on race and ethnicity, more sophisticated data analytic tools and methods, and the exponential growth of published studies on health inequities. Adler and colleagues provided a review of progress to date in the field of health inequities and note in detail the scientific advances, challenges, and future directions for research (Adler and Stewart, 2010).

Yet, compared to other fields of health research, health inequities is still a relatively new field. It faces significant research and practical application challenges that need to be addressed in order to offer knowledge that can strategically and accurately inform interventions aimed at reducing or eliminating health inequities.

First, the collection and use of data on race, ethnicity, and language are key parts of the process of identifying health and health care needs and eliminating disparities. Yet, work remains to be done in ensuring that our current data systems capture the appropriate categories and that these are consistently collected across studies and data systems. Toward this aim, in 2009, the IOM report *Race, Ethnicity, and Language Data: Standardization for Health Care Quality Improvement* proposed templates of granular ethnicity and language categories for national adoption so that entities wishing to collect detailed data can do so in systematic, uniform ways. The Office of Management and Budget (OMB) is currently undertaking a review of the current classifications for race and ethnicity and has issued a call for comments, including on the salience of the terminology used for race and ethnicity classifications and other language in the standard (GPO, 2016b).

Beyond the collection of data on race and ethnicity, a significant challenge has been the lack of sufficiently large samples of some racial and ethnic groups and their subgroups in population-level epidemiological studies such as the National Health and Nutrition Examination Survey and the National Survey on Drug Use and Health. Insufficiently large samples of some groups (e.g., Native Americans/American Indians, Hispanics and subgroups, and Asian and Pacific Islanders and subgroups) result in unreliable estimates of health indicators and resulting limitations on studies to investigate the factors that contribute to disparities within and across groups. Oversampling of these groups in national epidemiological studies is needed to yield appropriate estimates of health conditions.

Reliable estimates of health indicators can sometimes be derived by collapsing data across years, but this also poses some limitations on tracking health changes over time and providing up-to-date estimates. For smaller and geographically concentrated racial and ethnic groups (which are not well represented in national studies), specialized ongoing periodic studies are needed to track health conditions and the progress in reducing health inequities. For example, the National Latino and Asian American Study, while limited to one administration, provided previously unavailable but highly valuable data on Hispanic and Asian populations (Burnham and Flanigan, 2016).

Beyond race and ethnicity, the 2011 IOM report, *The Health of Lesbian, Gay, Bisexual, and Transgender People: Building a Foundation for Better Understanding* made recommendations regarding data collection about sexual orientation and gender identity in federal surveys and in electronic health records; implementation of the recommendations will provide essential data to document and monitor progress on LGBT health. For example, questions on sexual orientation and gender identity are included in recent versions of the Behavioral Risk Factor Surveillance Survey (CDC, 2016a).

Second, one of the important areas of knowledge advancement in health disparities research has been the integration of neighborhood-level factors that contribute to or are associated with health inequities. For example, measures of neighborhood-level segregation (e.g., the Diversity Index [National Equity Atlas, 2016], public school segregation [JSRI, 2016], and community diversity and distances between communities with different racial or ethnic profiles [VDH, 2016]); income inequality (National Equity Atlas, 2016; RWJF, 2016a; United Health Foundation, 2016), health equity (e.g., National Equity Atlas: Economic Vitality, Readiness, Connectedness, Economic Growth [National Equity Atlas, 2016]), social cohesion and social capital (e.g., group membership, volunteerism [Opportunity Index, 2016], linguistic isolation [Brandeis University, 2016]), gentrification (e.g., change in median income [United Health Foundation, 2016]), and housing affordability (Brandeis University, 2016) have been developed and used to document the associations and effects of these features of neighborhoods on health and health equity. The integration of these and other neighborhood-level features, if added to existing epidemiological health studies, could facilitate researchers' use of these measures in studies of health equity.

An additional challenge is that most studies of the features of the neighborhood environment and their impacts on health and health equity have been cross-sectional and are thus limited in establishing causal relationships (Diez Roux and Mair, 2010). As noted by Diez-Roux and Mair, the field needs longitudinal studies of neighborhood features and their relationships to health outcomes that use statistical controls for baseline differences and longitudinal analyses relating changes in outcomes to changes in predictors. While such studies are still observational, they can employ a number of statistical approaches that are preferable to cross-sectional analyses as they build a case for experimental studies and for rigorous intervention evaluations. Similarly, longitudinal studies of life-course processes on the impacts of neighborhood level factors on health and health equity are needed. For example, in considering residential mobility, Diez Roux and Mair note the limited work on characterizing neighborhood environments across the life course and the need to develop strategies to link cohort data to historical neighborhood data (Diez Roux and Mair, 2010).

Third, health disparity research has developed from a description of associations (e.g., socioeconomic status and health) to mechanisms linking socioeconomic status and health and multilevel influences to more recent work on the interactions among factors (Adler and Stewart, 2010). Yet, epidemiological studies on the factors that contribute to health and health inequities have not yet consistently provided clear answers regarding the most powerful and promising candidate levers to be targeted in community interventions. Although we cannot wait for the science to develop to the point of being able to provide exact answers, pilot interventions need to be based on the best available evidence and to be carefully evaluated with the most rigorous methods possible. However, in order to have a more definitive scientific basis for intervention approaches in this complex arena—with the myriad factors and ways that neighborhood and other factors affect health—a combination of research strategies, including rigorous observation studies, natural experiences or feasible experiments, and simulation studies, is needed (Diez Roux and Mair, 2010). Based on the data presented in this chapter and the current gaps in the evidence, the committee concludes the following:

Conclusion 2-1: To enable researchers to fully document and understand health inequities, to provide the foundation for solution development, and to measure solution outcomes longitudinally, the following are needed:

- *An expansion of current health disparity indicators and indices to include other groups beyond African Americans and whites, such as Hispanics and their major subgroups, Native Americans, Asians, Pacific Islanders, and mixed race, in addition to LGBT individuals, people with disabilities, and military veterans.*
  - Including consideration of methods to generate stable estimates of disparities through oversampling certain populations where necessary.
- *An expansion of metrics and indicators capturing the broader definition of health, including health equity and the social determinants of health.*
- *Longer-term studies, as many health outcomes take years (or decades) to see quantifiable changes in health outcomes related to the social determinants of health.*
- *Studies examining the ways in which a single structural factor may influence multiple health outcomes.*
- *Increased funding opportunities dedicated to developing and testing relevant theory, measures, and scientific methods, with the goal of enhancing the rigor with which investigators examine structural inequities such as structural racism and health disparities.*

REFERENCES

Adams, P., and V. Benson. 2015. Tables of summary health statistics for the U.S. population: 2014 National Health Interview Survey: U.S. Centers for Disease Control and Prevention.

Adler, N. E., and J. Stewart. 2010. Health disparities across the lifespan: Meaning, methods, and mechanisms. *Annals of the New York Academy of Sciences* 1186:5–23.

AHRQ (Agency for Healthcare Research and Quality). 2015. HIV and AIDS: Chartbook on effective treatment. http://www.ahrq.gov/research/findings/nhqrdr/2014chartbooks/effectivetx/eff-hiv.html (accessed October 24, 2016).

AHRQ. 2016. 2015 *National Healthcare Quality and Disparities Report and 5th Anniversary Update on the National Quality Strategy*. Rockville, MD: Agency for Healthcare Research and Quality. April 2016. AHRQ Pub. No. 16-0015.

American Psychological Association (APA). 2010. APA fact sheet: Mental health disparities: American Indians and Alaska Natives. http://www.integration.samhsa.gov/workforce/mental_health_disparities_american_indian_and_alaskan_natives.pdf (accessed October 21, 2016).

Archi's Acres Inc. 2016. Cal Poly's sustainable agriculture training at Archi's Acres. http://archisacres.com/page/sat-program (accessed October 21, 2016).

Arias, E. 2016. *Changes in life expectancy by race and Hispanic origin in the United States, 2013-2014*. Hyattsville, MD: National Center for Health Statistics.

Astone, N. M., S. Martin, and L. Aron. 2015. Death rates for U.S. women ages 15–54. Washington, DC: Urban Institute.

Backus, L. I., P. S. Belperio, T. P. Loomis, and L. A. Mole. 2014. Impact of race/ethnicity and gender on HCV screening and prevalence among US veterans in Department of Veterans Affairs care. *American Journal of Public Health* 104(S4):S555–S561.

Balshem, H., V. Christensen, A. Tuepker, and D. Kansagara. 2011. VA evidence-based synthesis program reports. In *A critical review of the literature regarding homelessness among veterans*. Washington, DC: U.S. Department of Veterans Affairs. VA-ESP Project #05-225.

Bauer, U. E., and M. Plescia. 2014. Addressing disparities in the health of American Indian and Alaska Native people: The importance of improved public health data. *American Journal of Public Health* 104(Suppl 3):S255–S257.

Bell, J., and M. M. Lee. 2011. *Why place and race matter: Impacting health through a focus on race and place*. Oakland, CA: PolicyLink.

Berman, M. 2014. Suicide among young Alaska Native men: Community risk factors and alcohol control. *American Journal of Public Health* 104(S3):S329–S335.

Blackwell, D. L., J. W. Lucas, and T. C. Clarke. 2014. Summary health statistics for U.S. adults: National Health Interview Survey, 2012. *Vital and Health Statistics* 10(260). February 2014. National Center for Health Statistics.

Brandeis University. 2016. Diversitydatakids.org. http://www.diversitydatakids.org (accessed October 21, 2016).

Brault, M. W. 2012. Americans with disabilities: 2010. Current Population Reports. July 2012. http://www.census.gov/prod/2012pubs/p70-131.pdf (accessed October 21, 2016).

Brown, T. N. T., and J. L. Herman. 2015. *Intimate partner violence and sexual abuse among LGBT people: A review of existing research*. Los Angeles, CA: The Williams Institute.

Bull, C. N., J. A. Krout, E. Rathbone-McCuan, and M. J. Shreffler. 2001. Access and issues of equity in remote/rural areas. *Journal of Rural Health* 17(4):356–359.

Burnham, W. D., and W. Flanigan. 2016. State-level presidential election data for the United States, 1824-1972 (icpsr 0019). http://www.icpsr.umich.edu/icpsrweb/ICPSR/studies/0019 (accessed October 21, 2016).

Burns, M. N., D. T. Ryan, R. Garofalo, M. E. Newcomb, and B. Mustanski. 2015. Mental health disorders in young urban sexual minority men. *Journal of Adolescent Health* 56(1):52–58.

Byrne, T., A. E. Montgomery, and M. E. Dichter. 2013. Homelessness among female veterans: A systematic review of the literature. *Women & Health* 53(6):572–596.

Campbell, J. C., and D. Boyd. 2000. Violence against women: Synthesis of research for health care professionals. NCJ 199761. December 2000. Washington, DC: National Institute of Justice.

Cannuscio, C. C., E. E. Weiss, and D. A. Asch. 2010. The contribution of urban foodways to health disparities. *Journal of Urban Health* 87(3):381–393.

Case, A., and A. Deaton. 2015. Rising morbidity and mortality in midlife among white non-Hispanic Americans in the 21st century. *Proceedings of the National Academy of Sciences of the United States of America* 112(49):15078–15083.

CDC (U.S. Centers for Disease Control and Prevention). 2010a. Prevalence and awareness of HIV infection among men who have sex with men—21 cities, United States, 2008. *Morbidity and Mortality Weekly Report* 59(37):1201–1207.

CDC. 2010b. Quickstats: Delayed or forgone medical care because of cost concerns among adults aged 18–64 years, by disability and health insurance coverage status—National Health Interview Survey, United States, 2009. *Morbidity and Mortality Weekly Report* 59(44). http://www.cdc.gov/mmwr/preview/mmwrhtml/mm5944a7.htm (accessed December 7, 2016).

CDC. 2013a. CDC health disparities and inequalities report: United States, 2013. *Morbidity and Mortality Weekly Report* 62(Suppl 3).

CDC. 2013b. Leading causes of death by age group, race/ethnicity males, United States, 2013. http://www.cdc.gov/men/lcod/2013/Race_ethnicityMen2013.pdf (accessed October 21, 2016).

CDC. 2013c. Leading causes of death by race/ethnicity, all females, United States, 2013. https://www.cdc.gov/women/lcod/2013/womenrace_2013.pdf (accessed October 21, 2016).

CDC. 2013d. Leading causes of death by race/ethnicity, all males, United States, 2013. http://www.cdc.gov/men/lcod/2013/Race_ethnicityMen2013.pdf (accessed November 2, 2016).

CDC. 2014a. African Americans heart disease and stroke fact sheet. http://www.cdc.gov/dhdsp/data_statistics/fact_sheets/fs_aa.htm (accessed December 7, 2016).

CDC. 2014b. Cigarette smoking among adults with disabilities. http://www.cdc.gov/ncbddd/disabilityandhealth/smoking-in-adults.html (accessed December 7, 2016).

CDC. 2015. Common barriers to participation experienced by people with disabilities. http://www.cdc.gov/ncbddd/disabilityandhealth/disability-barriers.html (accessed October 21, 2016).

CDC. 2016a. BRFSS questionnaires. http://www.cdc.gov/brfss/questionnaires (accessed October 21, 2016).

CDC. 2016b. Common barriers to participation experienced by people with disabilities. http://www.cdc.gov/ncbddd/disabilityandhealth/disability-barriers.html (accessed December 7, 2016).

CDC. 2016c. Disability and obesity. http://www.cdc.gov/ncbddd/disabilityandhealth/obesity.html (accessed December 7, 2016).

CDC. 2016d. Half of black gay men and a quarter of Latino gay men projected to be diagnosed within their lifetime. http://www.cdc.gov/nchhstp/newsroom/2016/croi-press-release-risk.html (accessed October 21, 2016).

Center for American Progress and Movement Advancement Project. 2015. *Paying an unfair price: The financial penalty for being transgender in America*. Washington, DC: Center for American Progress; Denver, CO: Movement Advancement Project.

Cho, P., L. S. Geiss, N. Rios Burrows, D. L. Roberts, A. K. Bullock, and M. E. Toedt. 2014. Diabetes-related mortality among American Indians and Alaska Natives, 1990–2009. *American Journal of Public Health* 104(S3):S496–S503.

Colby, S. L., and J. M. Ortman. 2014. Projections of the size and composition of the U.S. population: 2014 to 2060. Washington, DC: U.S. Census Bureau.

Courtney-Long, E. A., D. D. Carroll, Q. C. Zhang, A. C. Stevens, S. Griffin-Blake, B. S. Armour, and V. A. Campbell. 2015. Prevalence of disability and disability type among adults—United States, 2013. *Morbidity and Mortality Weekly Report* 64(29):777–783.

CREC and WVU (Center for Regional Economic Competitiveness and West Virginia University). 2015. Appalachia then and now: Examining changes to the Appalachian region since 1965. Appalachian Regional Commission.

Crosby, R. A., M. L. Wendel, R. C. Vanderpool, and B. R. Casey. 2012. Rural populations and health: Determinants, disparities, and solutions. San Francisco, CA: Jossey-Bass.

Cunradi, C. B., R. Caetano, C. Clark, and J. Schafer. 2000. Neighborhood poverty as a predictor of intimate partner violence among white, black, and Hispanic couples in the United States: A multilevel analysis. *Annals of Epidemiology* 10(5):297–308.

dickey, l. m., S. L. Budge, S. L. Katz-Wise, and M. V. Garza. 2016. Health disparities in the transgender community: Exploring differences in insurance coverage. *Psychology of Sexual Orientation and Gender Diversity* 3(3):275–282.

Diez Roux, A. V., and C. Mair. 2010. Neighborhoods and health. *Annals of the New York Academy of Sciences* 1186(1):125–145.

Eaton, N. R. 2012. Testing gender and ethnicity invariance of the comorbidity structure of common mental disorders. PhD diss. University of Minnesota, Minneapolis. http://conservancy.umn.edu/bitstream/handle/11299/136815/Eaton_umn_0130E_12995.pdf?sequence=1 (accessed October 21, 2016).

Eberhardt, M. S., and E. R. Pamuk. 2004. The importance of place of residence: Examining health in rural and nonrural areas. *American Journal of Public Health* 94(10):1682–1686.

Egerter, S., C. Barclay, R. Grossman-Kahn, and P. A. Braveman. 2011. Violence, social disadvantage and health. Princeton, NJ: Robert Wood Johnson Foundation.

Espey, D. K., M. A. Jim, N. Cobb, M. Bartholomew, T. Becker, D. Haverkamp, and M. Plescia. 2014. Leading causes of death and all-cause mortality in American Indians and Alaska Natives. *American Journal of Public Health* 104(Suppl 3):S303–S311.

Evans, B. F., E. Zimmerman, S. H. Woolf, and A. D. Haley. 2012. Social determinants of health and crime in post-Katrina Orleans Parish: Technical report. Richmond, VA: Center on Humans Needs, Virginia Commonwealth University. http://www.societyhealth.vcu.edu/media/society-health/pdf/PMReport_Orleans_Parish.pdf (accessed October 21, 2016).

Ford, C. L., T. Slavin, K. L. Hilton, and S. L. Holt. 2013. Intimate partner violence prevention services and resources in Los Angeles: Issues, needs, and challenges for assisting lesbian, gay, bisexual, and transgender clients. *Health Promotion Practice* 14(6):841–849.

Garcia, D., G. Betancourt, and L. Scaccabarrozzi. 2015. *The state of HIV/AIDS among Hispanics/Latinos in the U.S. and Puerto Rico*. New York: Latino Commission on AIDS. https://www.fpcouncil.com/sites/fpcouncil.com/files/files/HIVbrief2015_Eng.pdf (accessed October 21, 2016).

Garofalo, R., and S. Bush. 2008. Addressing LGBTQ youth in the clinical setting. In *Fenway guide to lesbian, gay, bisexual, and transgender health*, edited by H. Makadon, K. H. Mayer, J. Potter, and H. Goldhammer. Philadelphia, PA: American College of Physicians. Pp. 75–99.

Gern, J. E. 2010. The urban environment and childhood asthma study. *The Journal of Allergy and Clinical Immunology* 125(3):545–549.

GPO (Government Publishing Office). 2016a. Indian entities recognized and eligible to receive services from the United States Bureau of Indian Affairs. *Federal Register* 81(86). https://www.gpo.gov/fdsys/pkg/FR-2016-05-04/pdf/2016-10408.pdf (accessed October 21, 2016).

GPO. 2016b. Standards for maintaining, collecting, and presenting federal data on race and ethnicity. *Federal Register* 81(190):67398-67401. https://www.whitehouse.gov/sites/default/files/omb/inforeg/directive15/race-ethnicity_directive_2016FRN1.pdf (accessed October 21, 2016).

Graham, H. 2004. Social determinants and their unequal distribution: Clarifying policy understandings. *Milbank Q* 82(1):101–124.

Grant, J., L. Mottet, and J. Tanis. 2011. *National transgender discrimination survey report on health and health care*. Washington, DC: National Center for Transgender Equality and National Gay and Lesbian Task Force.

Gundersen, C. 2015. *Map the meal gap 2016: Highlights and findings for overall and child food security*. Chicago, IL: Feeding America.

Hamilton, B. E., and S. J. Ventura. 2012. Birth rates for U.S. teenagers reach historic lows for all age and ethnic groups. *NCHS data brief* 89. http://www.cdc.gov/nchs/data/databriefs/db89.pdf (accessed October 21, 2016).

Hamilton, B. E., J. A. Martin, and M. J. K. Osterman. 2016. Births: Preliminary data for 2015. *National Vital Statistics Reports* 65(3). http://www.cdc.gov/nchs/data/nvsr/nvsr65/nvsr65_03.pdf (accessed October 21, 2016).

Hansen, E., and M. Donohoe. 2003. Health issues of migrant and seasonal farmworkers. *Journal of Health Care for the Poor and Underserved* 14(2):153–164.

Healthy People 2020. 2016. *Healthypeople 2020*. https://www.healthypeople.gov (accessed October 21, 2016).

Heckler, M. M. 1985. *Report of the Secretary's Task Force on Black & Minority Health. Volume 1: Executive summary*. Washington, DC: U.S. Department of Health and Human Services.

Henning-Smith, C., G. Gonzales, and T. P. Shippee. 2015. Differences by sexual orientation in expectations about future long-term care needs among adults 40 to 65 years old. *American Journal of Public Health* 105(11):2359–2365.

Herek, G. M. 2009. Hate crimes and stigma-related experiences among sexual minority adults in the United States: Prevalence estimates from a national probability sample. *Journal of Interpersonal Violence* 24(1):54–74.

Herne, M. A., M. L. Bartholomew, and R. L. Weahkee. 2014. Suicide mortality among American Indians and Alaska Natives, 1999-2009. *American Journal of Public Health* 104(Suppl 3):S336–S342.

HHS (U.S. Department of Health and Human Services). 2011. Lesbian, gay, bisexual, and transgender health. https://www.healthypeople.gov/2020/topics-objectives/topic/lesbian-gay-bisexual-and-transgender-health?topicid=25 (accessed October 21, 2016).

HHS. 2014. Infant mortality disparities fact sheets. http://minorityhealth.hhs.gov/omh/content.aspx?ID= 6907&lvl=3&lvlID=8 (accessed October 21, 2016).

HHS. 2015. Profile: Hispanic/Latino Americans. http://minorityhealth.hhs.gov/omh/browse.aspx?lvl=3&lvlid=64 (accessed October 24, 2016).

HHS. 2016a. Disability and health. https://www.healthypeople.gov/2020/topics-objectives/topic/disability-and-health (accessed October 21, 2016).

HHS. 2016b. Heart disease and African Americans. http://minorityhealth.hhs.gov/omh/browse.aspx?lvl=4&lvlid=19 (accessed October 24, 2016).

HHS. 2016c. Profile: American Indian/Alaska Native. http://minorityhealth.hhs.gov/omh/browse.aspx?lvl=3&lvlid=62 (accessed August 25, 2016).

HHS. 2016d. Stroke and African Americans. http://minorityhealth.hhs.gov/omh/browse.aspx?lvl=4&lvlid=28 (accessed December 7, 2016).

Holland, A. T., and L. P. Palaniappan. 2012. Problems with the collection and interpretation of Asian-American health data: Omission, aggregation, and extrapolation. *Annals of Epidemiology* 22(6):397–405.

HUD (U.S. Department of Housing and Urban Development). 2016. 2016 PIT Estimate of veteran homelessness in the U.S. https://www.hudexchange.info/resource/5114/2016-pit-estimate-of-veteran-homelessness-in-the-us/ (accessed September 7, 2016).

IOM (Institute of Medicine). 2003. *Unequal treatment: Confronting racial and ethnic disparities in health care*. Washington, DC: The National Academies Press.

IOM. 2009. *Race, ethnicity, and language data: Standardization for health care quality improvement*. Washington, DC: The National Academies Press.

IOM. 2010. *Women's health research: Progress, pitfalls, and promise*. Washington, DC: The National Academies Press.

IOM. 2011. *The health of lesbian, gay, bisexual, and transgender people: Building a foundation for better understanding*. Washington, DC: The National Academies Press.

IOM. 2012. *Treatment for posttraumatic stress disorder in military and veteran populations: Initial assessment*. Washington, DC: The National Academies Press.

James, M. 2016. Race. In *The Stanford encyclopedia of philosophy*, edited by E. N. Zalta. Stanford, CA: Stanford University.

Jernigan, V. B. B., M. Peercy, D. Branam, B. Saunkeah, D. Wharton, M. Winkleby, J. Lowe, A. L. Salvatore, D. Dickerson, A. Belcourt, E. D'Amico, C. A. Patten, M. Parker, B. Duran, R. Harris, and D. Buchwald. 2015. Beyond health equity: Achieving wellness within American Indian and Alaska Native communities. *American Journal of Public Health* 105(S3):S376–S379.

Jim, M. A., E. Arias, D. S. Seneca, M. J. Hoopes, C. C. Jim, N. J. Johnson, and C. L. Wiggins. 2014. Racial misclassification of American Indians and Alaska Natives by Indian Health Service contract health service delivery area. *American Journal of Public Health* 104(Suppl 3):S295–S302.

JSRI (Jesuit Social Research Institute). 2016. Inaugural JustSouth index 2016. http://www.loyno.edu/jsri/news/inaugural-justsouth-index-2016 (accessed October 21, 2016).

Kang, H. K., T. A. Bullman, D. J. Smolenski, N. A. Skopp, G. A. Gahm, and M. A. Reger. 2015. Suicide risk among 1.3 million veterans who were on active duty during the Iraq and Afghanistan Wars. *Annals of Epidemiology* 25(2):96–100.

Kaufman, R. 2008. Introduction to transgender identity and health. In *Fenway guide to lesbian, gay, bisexual, and transgender health*, edited by H. J. Makadon, K. H. Mayer, J. Potter, and H. Goldhammer. Philadelphia, PA: American College of Physicians.

Keet, C. A., M. C. McCormack, C. E. Pollack, R. D. Peng, E. McGowan, and E. C. Matsui. 2015. Neighborhood poverty, urban residence, race/ethnicity, and asthma: Rethinking the inner-city asthma epidemic. *Journal of Allergy and Clinical Immunology* 135(3):655–662.

Kelley, A., A. Belcourt-Dittloff, C. Belcourt, and G. Belcourt. 2013. Research ethics and indigenous communities. *American Journal of Public Health* 103(12):2146–2152.

Kindig, D. A., and E. R. Cheng. 2013. Even as mortality fell in most U.S. counties, female mortality nonetheless rose in 42.8 percent of counties from 1992 to 2006. *Health Affairs* 32(3):451–458.

Klingensmith, K., J. Tsai, N. Mota, S. M. Southwick, and R. H. Pietrzak. 2014. Military sexual trauma in U.S. veterans: Results from the National Health and Resilience in Veterans Study. *Journal of Clinical Psychiatry* 75(10):e1133–e1139.

Kozyrskyj, A. L., C. A. Mustard, and A. B. Becker. 2004. Identifying children with persistent asthma from health care administrative records. *Canadian Respiratory Journal* 11(2):141–145.

Krahn, G. L., D. K. Walker, and R. Correa-De-Araujo. 2015. Persons with disabilities as an unrecognized health disparity population. *American Journal of Public Health* 105(Suppl 2):S198–S206.

Kulkarni, S. C., A. Levin-Rector, M. Ezzati, and C. J. Murray. 2011. Falling behind: Life expectancy in U.S. counties from 2000 to 2007 in an international context. *Population Health Metrics* 9(1):16.

Landen, M., J. Roeber, T. Naimi, L. Nielsen, and M. Sewell. 2014. Alcohol-attributable mortality among American Indians and Alaska Natives in the United States, 1999-2009. *American Journal of Public Health* 104(S3):S343–S349.

Lara, M., R. Health, and C. Rand. 2005. *Acculturation and Latino health in the United States: A review of the literature and its sociopolitical context*. Santa Monica, CA: RAND Corporation.

LaVeist, T., K. Pollack, R. Thorpe, Jr., R. Fesahazion, and D. Gaskin. 2011. Place, not race: Disparities dissipate in southwest Baltimore when blacks and whites live under similar conditions. *Health Affairs* 30(10):1880–1887.

Lawrence, A. A. 2007. Transgender health concerns. In *The health of sexual minorities: Public health perspectives on lesbian, gay, bisexual and transgender populations*, edited by I. H. Meyer and M. E. Northridge. New York: Springer. Pp. 355–374.

Levi, J., L. M. Segal, and A. Martin. 2015a. *The facts hurt: A state-by-state injury prevention policy report*. Washington, DC: Trust for America's Health.

Levi, J., L. M. Segal, J. Rayburn, and A. Martin. 2015b. *The state of obesity: Better policies for a healthier America 2015*. Washington, DC: Trust for America's Health and Robert Wood Johnson Foundation.

Levine, R. S., J. E. Foster, R. E. Fullilove, M. T. Fullilove, N. C. Briggs, P. C. Hull, B. A. Husaini, and C. H. Hennekens. 2001. Black-white inequalities in mortality and life expectancy, 1933-1999: Implications for Healthy People 2010. *Public Health Reports* 116:474–483.

Levine, R. S., N. C. Briggs, B. S. Kilbourne, W. D. King, Y. Fry-Johnson, P. T. Baltrus, B. A. Husaini, and G. S. Rust. 2007. Black-white mortality from HIV in the United States before and after introduction of highly active antiretroviral therapy in 1996. *American Journal of Public Health* 97(10):1884–1892.

Makadon, H. J., K. H. Mayer, J. Potter, and H. Goldhammer. 2008. *Fenway guide to lesbian, gay, bisexual, and transgender health.* Philadelphia, PA: American College of Physicians.

Mathews, T. J., M. F. MacDorman, and M. E. Thoma. 2015. Infant mortality statistics from the 2013 period linked birth/infant death data set. *National Vital Statistics Reports* 64(9). Hyattsville, MD: National Center for Health Statistics.

McGarvey, E. L., M. Leon-Verdin, L. F. Killos, T. Guterbock, and W. F. Cohn. 2011. Health disparities between Appalachian and non-Appalachian counties in Virginia USA. *Journal of Community Health* 36(3):348–356.

Mondragon, S. A., D. Wang, L. Pritchett, D. P. Graham, M. L. Plasencia, and E. J. Teng. 2015. The influence of military sexual trauma on returning OEF/OIF male veterans. *Psychological Services* 12(4):402–411.

NASEM (National Academies of Sciences, Engineering, and Medicine). 2015. *The growing gap in life expectancy by income: Implications for federal programs and policy responses.* Washington, DC: The National Academies Press.

NASEM. 2016a. *Improving the health of women in the United States: Workshop summary.* Washington, DC: The National Academies Press.

NASEM. 2016b. Workshop on the intersections among health disparities, disabilities, health equity, and health literacy. http://www.nationalacademies.org/hmd/Activities/PublicHealth/HealthLiteracy/2016-JUN-14.aspx (accessed October 21, 2016).

National Equity Atlas. 2016. National Equity Atlas. http://nationalequityatlas.org (accessed October 21, 2016).

NCFH (National Center for Farmworker Health). 2009. Migrant and seasonal farmworker demographics. http://www.unctv.org/content/sites/default/files/0000011508-fs-Migrant%20Demographics.pdf (accessed October 21, 2016).

NCHS (National Center for Health Statistics). 2016. Health, United States, 2015: With special feature on racial and ethnic health disparities. Hyattsville, MD: National Center for Health Statistics.

NIH (National Institutes of Health). 2014. Health disparities. http://www.nhlbi.nih.gov/health/educational/healthdisp (accessed November 2, 2016).

Norris, T., P. L. Vines, and E. M. Hoeffel. 2012. The American Indian and Alaska Native population: 2010 census brief. Washington, DC: U.S. Census Bureau.

NRC and IOM (National Research Council and Institute of Medicine). 2013. *U.S. health in international perspective: Shorter lives, poorer health.* Washington, DC: The National Academies Press.

O'Brien, B. S., and L. Sher. 2013. Military sexual trauma as a determinant in the development of mental and physical illness in male and female veterans. *International Journal of Adolescent Medicine and Health* 25(3):269–274.

Office for Victims of Crime. n.d. Responding to transgender victims of sexual assault. https://www.ovc.gov/pubs/forge/sexual_numbers.html (accessed December 7, 2016).

O'Hanlan, K. A., and C. M. Isler. 2007. Health care of lesbian and bisexual women. In *The health of sexual minorities: Public health perspectives on lesbian, gay, bisexual and transgender populations,* edited by I. H. Meyer and M. E. Northridge. New York: Springer. Pp. 506–522.

Opportunity Index. 2016. Opportunity Index. http://opportunityindex.org (accessed October 21, 2016).

Oreskovich, J., and H. Zimmerman. 2012. Defining disability: A comparison of disability prevalence estimates produced by BRFSS and other data sources. *Montana Fact[or]s* (1). https://dphhs.mt.gov/Portals/85/publichealth/documents/BRFSS/Factors/2012Factors1.pdf (accessed Ocrober 21, 2016).

Pinderhughes, H., R. A. Davis, and M. Williams. 2015. *Adverse community experiences and resilience: A framework for addressing and preventing community trauma.* Oakland, CA: Prevention Institute.

Pollard, K., and L. A. Jacobsen. 2016. The Appalachian region: A data overview from the 2010–2014 American Community Survey chartbook. Appalachian Regional Commission and Population Reference Bureau.

Prevention Institute. 2011. Fact sheet: Links between violence and health equity. Oakland, CA: Prevention Institute. https://www.preventioninstitute.org/sites/default/files/publications/Fact%20Sheet--Links%20Between%20Violence%20and%20Health%20Equity.pdf (accessed October 12, 2016).

Reichard, A., and H. Stolzle. 2011. Diabetes among adults with cognitive limitations compared to individuals with no cognitive disabilities. *Intellectual and Developmental Disabilities* 49(3):141–154.

Reichard, A., H. Stolzle, and M. H. Fox. 2011. Health disparities among adults with physical disabilities or cognitive limitations compared to individuals with no disabilities in the United States. *Disability and Health Journal* 4(2):59–67.

Reisner, S. L., Z. Bailey, and J. Sevelius. 2014. Racial/ethnic disparities in history of incarceration, experiences of victimization, and associated health indicators among transgender women in the U.S. *Women's Health* 54(8):750–767.

Rhoades, E. R., and D. A. Rhoades. 2014. The public health foundation of health services for American Indians and Alaska Natives. *American Journal of Public Health* 104(S3): S278–S285.

Roberts, S. J., E. M. Stuart-Shor, and R. A. Oppenheimer. 2010. Lesbians' attitudes and beliefs regarding overweight and weight reduction. *Journal of Clinical Nursing* 19(13–14): 1986–1994.

Robinson, J. P., and D. L. Espelage. 2013. Peer victimization and sexual risk differences between lesbian, gay, bisexual, transgender, or questioning and nontransgender heterosexual youths in grades 7–12. *American Journal of Public Health* 103(10):1810–1819.

Rothman, E. F., D. Exner, and A. L. Baughman. 2011. The prevalence of sexual assault against people who identify as gay, lesbian, or bisexual in the United States: A systematic review. *Trauma, Violence & Abuse* 12(2):55–66.

Ruble, M. W., and M. Forstein. 2008. Mental health: Epidemiology, assessment and treatment. In *Fenway guide to lesbian, gay, bisexual, and transgender health*, edited by H. J. Makadon, K. H. Mayer, J. Potter, and H. Goldhammer. Philadelphia, PA: American College of Physicians. Pp. 75–99.

RWJF (Robert Wood Johnson Foundation). 2013a. Metro map: Kansas City, Missouri. http://www.rwjf.org/en/library/infographics/kansas-city-map.html (accessed October 21, 2016).

RWJF. 2013b. Metro map: New Orleans, Louisiana. http://www.rwjf.org/en/library/infographics/new-orleans-map.html (accessed October 21, 2016).

RWJF. 2015. Menominee Nation, WI: 2015 culture of health prize winner. http://www.rwjf.org/en/library/articles-and-news/2015/10/coh-prize-menominee-wi.html (accessed October 21, 2016).

RWJF. 2016a. County Health Rankings & Roadmaps: Our approach. http://www.countyhealthrankings.org/our-approach (accessed October 21, 2016).

Ryan, C. L., and K. Bauman. 2016. Educational attainment in the United States: 2015. Current Population Reports. P20-578. March 2016. http://www.census.gov/content/dam/Census/library/publications/2016/demo/p20-578.pdf (accessed October 21, 2016).

Saha, S., M. Freeman, J. Toure, K. M. Tippens, and C. Weeks. 2007. VA evidence-based synthesis program reports. In *Racial and ethnic disparities in the VA healthcare system: A systematic review*. Washington, DC: U.S. Department of Veterans Affairs.

SAMHSA (Substance Abuse and Mental Health Services Administration). 2015a. 2014 National Survey on Drug Use and Health: Detailed tables: Prevalence estimates, standard errors, p values, and sample sizes. Rockville, MD: Center for Behavioral Health Statistics and Quality, Substance Abuse and Mental Health Services Administration.

SAMHSA. 2015b. Behavioral health trends in the United States: Results from the 2014 National Survey on Drug Use and Health (HHS publication no. SMA 15-4927, NSDUH series H-50). Rockville, MD: Center for Behavioral Health Statistics and Quality, Substance Abuse and Mental Health Services Administration.

Sausa, L. A., J. Keatley, and D. Operario. 2007. Perceived risks and benefits of sex work among transgender women of color in San Francisco. *Archives of Sexual Behavior* 36(6):768-777.

Schulz, L. O., P. H. Bennett, E. Ravussin, J. R. Kidd, K. K. Kidd, J. Esparza, and M. E. Valencia. 2006. Effects of traditional and western environments on prevalence of type 2 diabetes in Pima Indians in Mexico and the U.S. *Diabetes Care* 29(8):1866–1871.

Singh, G. K., and M. Siahpush. 2014. Widening rural-urban disparities in life expectancy, U.S., 1969–2009. *American Journal of Preventive Medicine* 46(2):e19–e29.

Smedley, B., M. Jeffries, L. Adelman, and J. Cheng. 2008. Race, racial inequality and health inequities: Separating myth from fact. http://www.unnaturalcauses.org/assets/uploads/file/Race_Racial_Inequality_Health.pdf (accessed October 21, 2016).

Stand for the Troops Inc. 2016. Stand for the troops: Archi's Acres—sustainable employment for veterans through sustainable agriculture. http://sftt.org/blog/ptsd/archis-acres-sustainable-employment (accessed October 21, 2016).

Tjaden, P., and N. Thoennes. 2000. Extent, nature, and consequences of intimate partner violence: Findings from the National Violence Against Women Survey. NCJ 181867. https://www.ncjrs.gov/pdffiles1/nij/181867.pdf (accessed October 21, 2016).

Tsai, J., and R. A. Rosenheck. 2015. Risk factors for homelessness among U.S. veterans. *Epidemiologic Reviews* 37:177–195.

United Health Foundation. 2016. America's health rankings: Health of those who have served report: 2016. Minneapolis, MN: United Health Foundation. http://assets.americas healthrankings.org/app/uploads/htwhs_report_r3.pdf (accessed October 21, 2016).

UWPHI (University of Wisconsin Population Health Institute). 2016. County Health Rankings & Roadmaps. http://www.countyhealthrankings.org (accessed October 21, 2016).

VA (U.S. Department of Veterans Affairs). 2016. Suicide among veterans and other Americans 2001–2014. http://www.mentalhealth.va.gov/docs/2016suicidedatareport.pdf (accessed December 20, 2016).

van den Berk-Clark, C., and J. McGuire. 2013. Elderly homeless veterans in Los Angeles: Chronicity and precipitants of homelessness. *American Journal of Preventive Medicine* 103(Suppl 2):S232–S238.

VanOrman, A., and B. Jarosz. 2016. Suicide replaces homicide as second-leading cause of death among U.S. teenagers. Washington, DC: Population Reference Bureau.

VDH (Virginia Department of Health). 2016. Virginia health opportunity index (HOI). https://www.vdh.virginia.gov/OMHHE/policyanalysis/virginiahoi.htm (accessed October 21, 2016).

Veazie, M., C. Ayala, L. J. Schieb, S. Dai, J. Henderson, and P. Cho. 2014. Trends and disparities in heart disease mortality among American Indians/Alaska Natives, 1990–2009. *American Journal of Public Health* 104(S3):S359–S367.

Wallace, S. P., S. D. Cochran, E. M. Durazo, and C. L. Ford. 2011. The health of aging lesbian, gay and bisexual adults in California. Health policy research brief. UCLA Center for Health Policy Research (March):1–8.

Walters, M. L., J. Chen, and M. J. Breiding. 2013. The National Intimate Partner and Sexual Violence Survey (NISVS): 2010 findings on victimization by sexual orientation. Atlanta, GA: National Center for Injury Prevention and Control Division of Violence Prevention, U.S. Centers for Disease Control and Prevention.

White, M. C., D. K. Espey, J. Swan, C. L. Wiggins, C. Eheman, and J. S. Kaur. 2014. Disparities in cancer mortality and incidence among American Indians and Alaska Natives in the United States. *American Journal of Public Health* 104(S3):S377–S387.

WHO (World Health Organization). 2001. International classification of functioning, disability, and health. http://www.who.int/classifications/icf/en (accessed November 2, 2016).
WHO. 2016. Disability and health. http://www.who.int/mediacentre/factsheets/fs352/en (accessed December 7, 2016).
Williams, D. R., S. A. Mohammed, J. Leavell, and C. Collins. 2010. Race, socioeconomic status, and health: Complexities, ongoing challenges, and research opportunities. *Annals of the New York Academy of Sciences* 1186:69–101.
Wong, S. T., and S. Regan. 2009. Patient perspectives on primary health care in rural communities: Effects of geography on access, continuity and efficiency. *Rural and Remote Health* 9(1):1142.
Xu, J. Q., S. L. Murphy, K. D. Kochanek, and E. Arias. 2016. *Mortality in the United States, 2015. NCHS data brief, no. 267* Hyattsville, MD: National Center for Health Statistics.
Yao, N., S. A. Matthews, and M. M. Hillemeier. 2012. White infant mortality in Appalachian states, 1976-1980 and 1996-2000: Changing patterns and persistent disparities. *Journal of Rural Health* 28(2):174–182.
Zarembo, A. 2013. Death rate unusually high for young veterans. Los Angeles Times, December 17, 2013. http://www.latimes.com/local/la-me-veteran-deaths-20131217-dto-htmlstory.html (accessed December 20, 2016).
Zimmerman, E., and S. H. Woolf. 2014. *Understanding the relationship between education and health.* National Academy of Medicine Discussion Paper. https://nam.edu/perspectives-2014-understanding-the-relationship-between-education-and-health (accessed October 21, 2016).

3

The Root Causes of Health Inequity

Health inequity, categories and examples of which were discussed in the previous chapter, arises from social, economic, environmental, and structural disparities that contribute to intergroup differences in health outcomes both within and between societies. The report identifies two main clusters of root causes of health inequity. The first is the intrapersonal, interpersonal, institutional, and systemic mechanisms that organize the distribution of power and resources differentially across lines of race, gender, class, sexual orientation, gender expression, and other dimensions of individual and group identity (see the following section on such structural inequities for examples). The second, and more fundamental root cause of health inequity, is the unequal allocation of power and resources—including goods, services, and societal attention—which manifest in unequal social, economic, and environmental conditions, also called the social determinants of health. Box 3-1 includes the definitions of structural inequities and the social determinants of health.

The factors that make up the root causes of health inequity are diverse, complex, evolving, and interdependent in nature. It is important to understand the underlying causes and conditions of health inequities to inform equally complex and effective interventions to promote health equity.

The fields of public health and population health science have accumulated a robust body of literature over the past few decades that elucidates how social, political, economic, and environmental conditions and

> **BOX 3-1**
> **Definitions**
>
> *Structural inequities* refers to the systemic disadvantage of one social group compared to other groups with whom they coexist, and the term encompasses policy, law, governance, and culture and refers to race, ethnicity, gender or gender identity, class, sexual orientation, and other domains. The *social determinants of health* are the conditions in the environments in which people live, learn, work, play, worship, and age that affect a wide range of health, functioning, and quality-of-life outcomes and risks. For the purposes of this report, the social determinants of health are: education; employment; health systems and services; housing; income and wealth; the physical environment; public safety; the social environment; and transportation.

context contribute to health inequities. Furthermore, there is mounting evidence that focusing programs, policies, and investments on addressing these conditions can improve the health of vulnerable populations and reduce health disparities (Bradley et al., 2016; Braveman and Gottlieb, 2014; Thornton et al., 2016; Williams and Mohammed, 2013). This literature is discussed below in the sections on structural inequities and the social determinants of health.

HOW STRUCTURAL INEQUITIES, SOCIAL DETERMINANTS OF HEALTH, AND HEALTH EQUITY CONNECT

Health inequities are systematic differences in the opportunities groups have to achieve optimal health, leading to unfair and avoidable differences in health outcomes (Braveman, 2006; WHO, 2011). The dimensions of social identity and location that organize or "structure" differential access to opportunities for health include race and ethnicity, gender, employment and socioeconomic status, disability and immigration status, geography, and more. *Structural inequities* are the personal, interpersonal, institutional, and systemic drivers—such as, racism, sexism, classism, able-ism, xenophobia, and homophobia—that make those identities salient to the fair distribution of health opportunities and outcomes. Policies that foster inequities at all levels (from organization to community to county, state, and nation) are critical drivers of structural inequities. The *social, environmental, economic, and cultural determinants of health* are the terrain on which structural inequities produce health inequities. These multiple determinants are the conditions in which people live, including access to good food, water, and housing; the quality of schools, workplaces, and neighborhoods; and the composition of social networks and nature of social relations.

So, for example, the effect of interpersonal, institutional, and systemic biases in policies and practices (structural inequities) is the "sorting" of people into resource-rich or resource-poor neighborhoods and K–12 schools (education itself being a key determinant of health (Woolf et al., 2007) largely on the basis of race and socioeconomic status. Because the quality of neighborhoods and schools significantly shapes the life trajectory and the health of the adults and children, race- and class-differentiated access to clean, safe, resource-rich neighborhoods and schools is an important factor in producing health inequity. Such structural inequities give rise to large and preventable differences in health metrics such as life expectancy, with research indicating that one's zip code is more important to health than one's genetic code (RWJF, 2009).

The impact of structural inequities follows individuals "from womb to tomb." For example, African American women are more likely to give birth to low-birthweight infants, and their newborns experience higher infant death rates that are not associated with any biological differences, even after accounting for socioeconomic factors (Braveman, 2008; Hamilton et al., 2016; Mathews et al., 2015). Although the science is still evolving, it is hypothesized that the chronic stress associated with being treated differently by society is responsible for these persistent differential birth outcomes (Christian, 2012; El-Sayed et al., 2015; Strutz et al., 2014; Witt et al., 2015). In elementary school there are persistent differences across racial and ethnic divisions in rates of discipline and levels of reading attainment, rates that are not associated with any differences in intelligence metrics (Howard, 2010; Losen et al., 2015; Reardon et al., 2012; Skiba et al., 2011; Smith and Harper, 2015). There also are race and class differences in adverse childhood experiences and chronic stress and trauma, which are known to affect learning ability and school performance, as well as structural inequities in environmental exposures, such as lead, which ultimately can lead to differences in intelligence quotient (IQ) (Aizer et al., 2015; Bethell et al., 2014; Jimenez et al., 2016; Levy et al., 2016). One of the strongest predictors of life expectancy is high school graduation, which varies dramatically along class and race and ethnicity divisions, as do the rates of college and vocational school participation—all of which shape employment, income, and individual and intergenerational wealth (Olshansky et al., 2012). Structural inequities affect hiring policies, with both implicit and explicit biases creating differential opportunities along racial, gender, and physical ability divisions. Lending policies continue to create differences in home ownership, small business development, and other asset development (Pager and Shepherd, 2008). Structural inequities create differences in the ability to participate and have a voice in policy and political decision making, and even to participate in the arguably most fundamental aspect of our democracy, voting (Blakely et al., 2001; Carter and Reardon, 2014). And implicit biases create differential health care service offerings and delivery and affect the effectiveness of care provided, including a lack of cultural competence (IOM and NRC, 2003; Sabin et al., 2009).

For many people, the challenges that structural inequities pose limit the scope of opportunities they have for reaching their full health potential. The health of communities is dependent on the determinants of health.

STRUCTURAL INEQUITIES

As described above, *structural inequities* refers to the systematic disadvantage of one social group compared to other groups with whom they coexist that are deeply embedded in the fabric of society. In Figure 3-1,

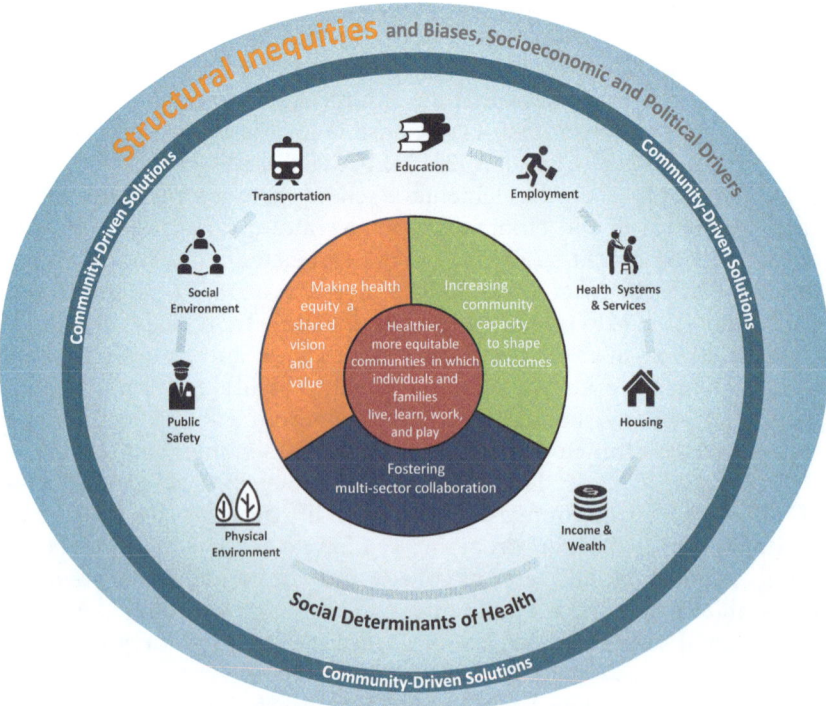

FIGURE 3-1 Report conceptual model for community solutions to promote health equity.
NOTE: Structural inequities are highlighted to convey the focus of this section.

the outermost circle and background indicate the context in which health inequities exist. Structural inequities encompass policy, law, governance, and culture and refer to race, ethnicity, gender or gender identity, class, sexual orientation, and other domains. These inequities produce systematic disadvantages, which lead to inequitable experiences of the social determinants of health (the next circle in the report model, which is discussed in detail later in this chapter) and ultimately shape health outcomes.

Historical Perspective and Contemporary Perceptions

Whether with respect to race, ethnicity, gender, class, or other markers of human difference, the prevailing American narrative often draws a sharp line between the United States' "past" and its "present," with the 1960s and 1970s marking a crucial before-and-after moment in that narrative. This narrative asserts that until the 1950s, U.S. history was shaped by the impacts of past slavery, Indian removal, lack of rights for women, Jim Crow segregation, periods of nativist restrictions on immigration and waves of mass deportation of Hispanic immigrants, eugenics, the internment of Japanese Americans, the Chinese exclusion policies, the criminalization of "homosexual acts," and more (Gee and Ford, 2011; Gee et al., 2009). White women and people of color were effectively barred from many occupations and could not vote, serve on juries, or run for office. People with disabilities suffered widespread discrimination, institutionalization, and social exclusion.

Civil rights, women's liberation, gay rights, and disability rights movements and their aftermaths may contribute to a narrative that social, political, and cultural institutions have made progress toward equity, diversity, or inclusion. Highlights of progress include the Civil Rights Act of 1964, the Voting Rights Act of 1965, the Fair Housing Act, Title IX of the Education Amendments of 1972, the Americans with Disabilities Act, the Patient Protection and Affordable Care Act, and, most recently, the Supreme Court case[1] that legalized marriage equality in the United States. With a few notable exceptions—undocumented immigrants and Muslims, for example—these advances in law and policy have been mirrored by the liberalization of attitudes toward previously marginalized identity groups.

Today, polls and surveys indicate that most Americans believe that interpersonal and societal bias on the basis of identity no longer shapes individual or group social outcomes. For example, 6 in 10 respondents to a recent national poll said they thought the country has struck a

---

[1] *Obergefell v. Hodges*, 576 U.S. (2015).

"reasonable balance" or even gone "too far" in "accepting transgender people" (Polling Report, n.d.). In 2015, 72 percent of respondents, including 81 percent of whites, said they believe that "blacks have as good a chance as white people in your community to get any kind of job for which they are qualified" (Polling Report, n.d.). In another poll, a total of 72 percent agreed that "women and men have equal trouble finding good-paying jobs" (64 percent) or that men have more trouble (8 percent) (Ms. Foundation for Women, 2015). However, when broken down by racial and ethnic categories, the polls tell a different narrative. A recent survey revealed that 70 percent of African Americans, compared with 36 percent of whites, believe that racial discrimination is a major reason that African Americans have a harder time getting ahead than whites (Pew Research Center, 2016). Furthermore, African Americans (66 percent) and Hispanics (64 percent) are more likely than whites (43 percent) to say that racism is a big problem (DiJulio et al., 2015). Here, perceptions among African Americans and whites have not changed substantially; however, Hispanics are much more likely to now say that racism is a big problem (46 percent in 1995 versus 64 percent in 2015) (DiJulio et al., 2015).

Perceptions are confirmed by the persistence of disparities along the lines of socioeconomic position, gender, race, ethnicity, immigration status, geography, and the like has been well documented. Why? For one, historical inequities continue to ramify into the present. To understand how historical patterns continue to affect life chances for certain groups, historians and economists have attempted to calculate the amount of wealth transmitted from one generation to the next (Margo, 1990). They find that the baseline inequities contribute to intergenerational transfers of disadvantage and advantage for African Americans and whites, respectively (Chetty et al., 2014; Darity et al., 2001). The inequities also reproduce the conditions in which disparities develop (Rodriguez et al., 2015).

Racism

Though inequities may occur on the basis of socioeconomic status, gender, and other factors, we illustrate these points through the lens of racism, in part because disparities based on race and ethnicity remain the most persistent and difficult to address (Williams and Mohammed, 2009). Racial factors play an important role in structuring socioeconomic disparities (Farmer and Ferraro, 2005); therefore, addressing socioeconomic factors without addressing racism is unlikely to remedy these inequities (Kaufman et al., 1997).

Racism is an umbrella concept that encompasses specific mechanisms that operate at the intrapersonal, interpersonal, institutional, and systemic levels[2] of a socioecological framework (see Figure 3-2). Because it is not possible to enumerate all of the mechanisms here, several are described below to illustrate racism mechanisms at different socioecological levels. Stereotype threat, for example, is an intrapersonal mechanism. It "refers to the risk of confirming negative stereotypes about an individual's racial, ethnic, gender, or cultural group" (Glossary of Education Reform, 2013). Stereotype threat manifests as self-doubt that can lead the individual to perform worse than she or he might otherwise be expected to—in the context of test-taking, for example. Implicit biases—unconscious cognitive biases that shape both attitudes and behaviors—operate interpersonally (discussed in further detail below) (Staats et al., 2016). Racial profiling often operates at the institutional level, as with the well-documented institutionalization of stop-and-frisk practices on Hispanic and African American individuals by the New York City Police Department (Gelman et al., 2007).

Finally, systemic mechanisms, which may operate at the community level or higher (e.g., through policy), are those whose effects are interactive, rather than singular, in nature. For example, racial segregation of neighborhoods might well be due in part to personal preferences and behavior of landlords, renters, buyers, and sellers. However, historically, segregation was created by legislation, which was reinforced by the policies and practices of economic institutions and housing agencies (e.g., discriminatory banking practices and redlining), as well as enforced by the judicial system and legitimized by churches and other cultural institutions (Charles, 2003; Gee and Ford, 2011; Williams and Collins, 2001). In other words, segregation was, and remains, an interaction and cumulative "product," one not easily located in any one actor or institution. Residential segregation remains a root cause of racial disparities in health today (Williams and Collins, 2001).

Racism is not an attribute of minority groups; rather, it is an aspect of the social context and is linked with the differential power relations among racial and ethnic groups (Guess, 2006). Consider the location of environmental hazards in or near minority communities. Placing a hazard in a minority community not only increases the risk of adverse exposures for the residents of that community, it also ensures the reduction of risk for residents of the nonminority community (Cushing et al., 2015; Taylor, 2014). Recognizing this, the two communities could work together toward an alternative that precludes having the hazard in the first place, an alternative that disadvantages neither group.

---

[2] In 2000 Dr. Camara Jones developed a theoretical framework for the multiple levels of racism and used an allegory of a garden to illustrate the mechanisms through which these levels operate (Jones, 2000).

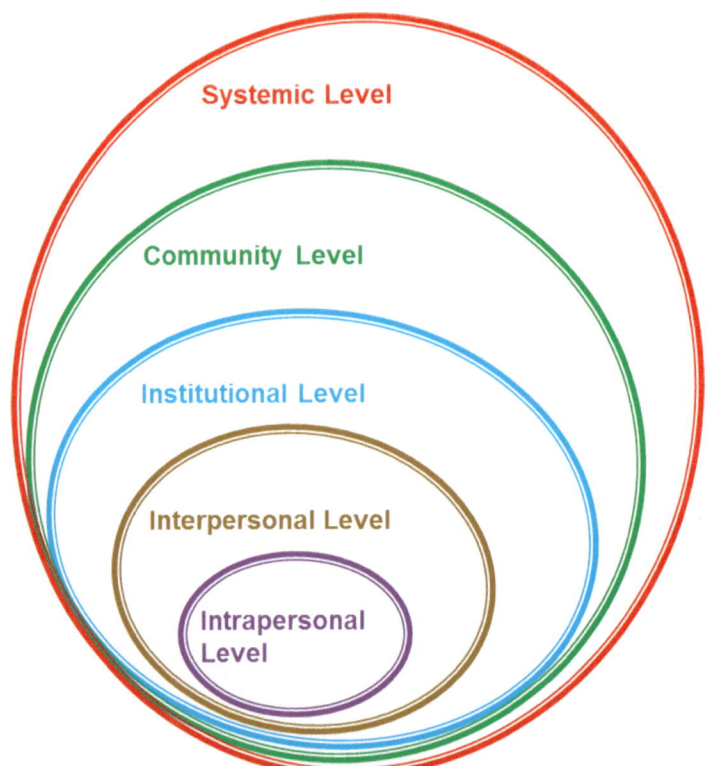

Systemic Level
- Immigration policies
- Incarceration policies
- Predatory banking

Community Level
- Differential resource allocation
- Racially or class segregated schools

Institutional Level
- Hiring and promotion practices
- Under- or over-valuation of contributions

Interpersonal Level
- Overt discrimination
- Implicit bias

Intrapersonal Level
- Internalized racism
- Stereotype threat
- Embodying inequities

FIGURE 3-2 Social ecological model with examples of racism constructs.
NOTES: The mechanisms by which the social determinants of health operate differ with respect to the level. For the intrapersonal level, these mechanisms are individual knowledge, attitudes/beliefs, and skills. At the interpersonal level, they are families, friends, and social networks. At the institutional level, they are organizations and social institutions. At the community level, they are relationships among organizations. At the systemic level, the mechanisms are national, state, and local policies, laws, and regulations.
SOURCE: Concept from McLeroy et al., 1988.

Most studies of racism are based on African American samples; however, other populations may be at risk for manifestations of racism that differ from the African American experience. Asians, Hispanics, and, more recently, Arabs and Muslims are subject to assumptions that they are not U.S. citizens and, therefore, lack the rights and social entitlements that other U.S. residents claim (Chou and Feagin, 2015; Cobas et al., 2009; Feldman, 2015; Gee et al., 2009; Johnson, 2002; Khan and Ecklund, 2013). The implications of this include threats or actual physical violence against members of these groups. For instance, researchers have found that in the months immediately following September 11, 2001, U.S. women with Arabic surnames who were residing in California experienced increases in both racial microaggressions (i.e., seemingly minor forms of "everyday racism") and in poor birth outcomes compared to the 6 months preceding 9/11, while women of other U.S. ethnic groups did not (Kulwicki et al., 2008; Lauderdale, 2006). For Native Americans, because tribes are independent nations, the issues of racism need to be considered to intersect with those of sovereignty (Berger, 2009; Massie, 2016; Sundeen, 2016).

The evidence linking racism to health disparities is expanding rapidly. A variety of both general and disease-specific mechanisms have been identified; they link racism to outcomes in mental health, cardiovascular disease, birth defects, and other outcomes (Paradies, 2006a; Pascoe and Smart Richman, 2009; Shavers et al., 2012; Williams and Mohammed, 2009). Which racism mechanisms matter most depends in part on the disease and, to a lesser degree, the population. The vast majority of studies focus on the role of discrimination; that is racially disparate treatment from another individual or, in some cases, from an institution. Among the studies not focused on discrimination, the majority examine segregation. Generally, findings show that members of all groups, including whites, report experiencing racial discrimination, with levels typically, though not always, higher among African Americans and, to a lesser degree, Hispanics than among whites. Gender differences in some perceptions about and responses to racism have also been observed (Otiniano Verissimo et al., 2014). Three major mechanisms by which systemic racism influences health equity—discrimination (including implicit bias), segregation, and historical trauma—are discussed in more detail in the following paragraphs.

Discrimination

The mechanisms by which discrimination operates include overt, intentional treatment as well as inadvertent, subconscious treatment of individuals in ways that systematically differ so that minorities are treated worse than nonminorities. Recent meta-analyses suggest that racial discrimination has deleterious effects on the physical and mental health of individuals (Gee et al., 2009; Paradies, 2006a; Pascoe and Smart Richman, 2009; Priest et al., 2013; Williams and Mohammed, 2009). Significant percentages of members of racial and ethnic minority populations report experiencing discrimination in health care and non-health care settings (Mays et al., 2007). Greater proportions of African Americans than members of other groups report either experiencing discrimination personally or perceiving it as affecting African Americans in general, even if they have not experienced it personally. Hate crimes motivated by race or ethnicity bias disproportionately affect Hispanics and African Americans (UCR, 2015) (see the public safety section in this chapter for more on hate crimes).

Discrimination is generally associated with worse mental health (Berger and Sarnyai, 2015; Gee et al., 2009; Paradies, 2006b; Williams and Mohammed, 2009); greater engagement in risky behaviors (Gee et al., 2009; Paradies, 2006b; Williams and Mohammed, 2009); decreased neurological responses (Harrell et al., 2003; Mays et al., 2007) and other biomarkers signaling the dysregulation of allostatic load; hypertension-related outcomes (Sims et al., 2012), though some evidence suggests racism does not drive these outcomes (Roberts et al., 2008); reduced likelihood of some health protecting behaviors (Pascoe and Smart Richman, 2009); and poorer birth-related outcomes such as preterm delivery (Alhusen et al., 2016). Paradoxically, despite higher levels of exposure to discrimination, the mental health consequences may be less severe among African Americans than they are among members of other groups, especially Asian populations (Gee et al., 2009; Williams and Mohammed, 2009). Researchers have suggested that African Americans draw on reserves of resilience in ways that temper the effects of discrimination on mental health (Brown and Tylka, 2011).

Though people may experience overt forms of racism (e.g., being unfairly fired on the basis of race), the adverse health effects of racism appear to stem primarily from the stress of chronic exposure to seemingly minor forms of "everyday racism" (i.e., racial microaggressions), such as being treated with less respect by others, being stopped by police for no apparent reason, or being monitored by salespeople while shopping (APA, 2016; Sue et al., 2007; Williams et al., 2003). The chronic exposure contributes to stress-related physiological effects. Thus, discrimination appears to exert its greatest effects not because of exposure to a single life traumatic incident but because people must mentally and physically contend with or be prepared to contend with seemingly minor insults and assaults on a near continual basis (APA, 2016). The implications appear to be greatest for stress-related conditions such as those tied to hypertension, mental health outcomes, substance abuse behaviors, and birth-related outcomes (e.g., low birth weight and premature birth) than for other outcomes (Williams and Mohammed, 2009).

Higher socioeconomic status (SES) does not protect racial and ethnic minorities from discriminatory exposures. In fact, it may increase opportunities for exposure to discrimination. The concept of "John Henryism" is used to describe an intensely active way of tackling racial and other life challenges (James, 1994). Though the evidence is mixed, John Henryism may contribute to worse cardiovascular outcomes among African American males who respond to racism by working even harder to disprove racial stereotypes (Flaskerud, 2012; Subramanyam et al., 2013).

Implicit bias John Dovidio defines implicit bias—a mechanism of unconscious discrimination—as a form of racial or other bias that operates beneath the level of consciousness (Dovidio et al., 2002). Research conducted over more than four decades finds that individuals hold racial biases of which they are not aware and, importantly, that discriminatory behaviors can be predicted based on this construct (Staats et al., 2016). The effects are greatest in situations marked by ambiguity, stress, and time constraints (Bertrand et al., 2005; Dovidio and Gaertner, 2000). Implicit bias is not an arbitrary personal preference that individuals hold; for example, "I just happen to prefer pears over apples." Rather, the nature and direction of individuals' biases are structured by the racial stratification and norms of society. As a result, they are predictable.

Much of the public health literature has focused on the implicit biases of health care providers, who with little time to devote to each patient can provide care that is systematically worse for African American patients than for white patients even though the health care provider never intended to do so (IOM and NRC, 2003; van Ryn and Burke, 2000). The evidence is clear that unconscious racialized perceptions contribute to differences in how various individual actors, including health care providers, perceive others and treat them. Based on psychology lab experiments, functional magnetic resonance imaging (fMRI) pictures of the brain, and other tools, researchers find that white providers hold implicit biases against African Americans and that, to a lesser degree, some minority providers may also hold these biases (Hall et al., 2015). Although not limited to health care professionals, the biases lead providers to link negative characteristics (e.g., bad) and emotions (e.g., fear) with people or images they perceive as being African American (Zestcott et al., 2016). As a result of such implicit biases, physicians treat patients differently depending on the patient's race, ethnicity, gender, or other assumed or actual characteristics (IOM and NRC, 2003; Zestcott et al., 2016).

Given the importance of implicit bias, researchers have considered the role of health care provider–patient racial and ethnic concordance. Even if patients have similar clinical profiles, their care may differ systematically based on their race or ethnicity and that of their health care provider (Betancourt et al., 2014; van Ryn and Fu, 2003; Zestcott et al., 2016). The evidence on whether and how patient–provider concordance contributes to health disparities is mixed (van Ryn and Fu, 2003). Qualitative and quantitative findings suggest that patients do not necessarily prefer providers of the same race or ethnicity; they prefer a provider who treats them with respect (Dale et al., 2010; Ibrahim et al., 2004; Schnittker and Liang, 2006; Volandes et al., 2008). Providers appear to evaluate African American patients more negatively than they do similar white patients; seem to perceive them as more likely to participate in risky health behaviors; and may be less willing to prescribe them pain medications and narcotics medications (van Ryn and Fu, 2003). In a video-based study conducted among primary care providers, the odds ratio of providers referring simulated African American patients to otherwise identical white patients for cardiac catheterization was 0.6 (Schulman et al., 1999). Some evidence suggests minority providers deliver more equitable care to their diverse patients than white providers. For instance, a longitudinal study among African American and white HIV-positive patients enrolled in HIV care found that white doctors took longer to prescribe protease inhibitors (an effective HIV medication) for their African American patients than for their clinically similar white patients. Providers prescribed them on average 162 days earlier for white patients than for comparable African American patients (King et al., 2004). Among African American providers, there was no difference between African American and white patients in how long before providers prescribed the medications.

Racial and ethnic minority providers play an important role in addressing disparities because they help bridge cultural gulfs (Butler et al., 2014; Cooper et al., 2003; Lehman et al., 2012), and greater proportions of them serve minority and socially disadvantaged communities (Cooper and Powe, 2004); however, these providers are underrepresented in the health professions, and they face challenges that may constrain their professional development and the quality of care they are able to provide (Landrine and Corral, 2009). Specifically, they are more likely to serve patients in resource-poorer areas and lack professional privileges associated with academic and other resource-rich institutions. The structural inequities have implications not only for individual clinicians but also for the patients and communities they serve. Pipeline programs that grow the numbers of minority providers may help to address underrepresentation in the health professions. The available data suggest that pipeline participants are more likely to care for poor or underserved patients when they join the workforce (McDougle et al., 2015). Supporting the professional development of and expanding the resources and tools available to providers working in resource-poor communities seems to be one option for improving access to and quality of care; however, the literature does not clearly elucidate the relationship between health care workforce pipeline programs (e.g., to grow the numbers of minority providers) and their impact on the social determinants of health for poor and underserved communities (Brown et al., 2005; Smith et al., 2009). A commitment to equity is not enough to remedy the discriminatory treatment that results from implicit biases because the inadvertent discriminatory behavior co-occurs alongside deeply held personal commitments to equity. Identifying implicit biases and acknowledging them is one of the most effective steps that can be taken to address their effects (Zestcott et al., 2016). Trainings can help health care providers identify their implicit biases. Well-planned allocations of resources, including time, may afford them sufficient opportunity to account for it while serving diverse persons/patients.

Segregation

Residential segregation—that is, the degree to which groups live separately from one another (Massey and Denton, 1988)—can exacerbate the rates of disease among minorities, and social isolation can reduce the public's sense of urgency about the need to intervene (Acevedo-Garcia, 2000; Wallace and Wallace, 1997). The effects of racial segregation differ from those of socioeconomic segregation. Lower SES whites are more likely to live in areas with a range of SES levels, which affords even the poorest residents of these communities access to shared resources (e.g., parks, schools) that buffer against the effects of poverty (APA Task Force on Socioeconomic Status, 2007; North Carolina Institute of Medicine Task Force on Prevention, 2009). By contrast, racial and ethnic minorities are more likely to live in areas of concentrated poverty (Bishaw, 2011). Indeed, if shared resources are of poor quality, they may compound the low SES challenges an individual faces. Racial segregation contributes to disparities in a variety of ways. It limits the socioeconomic resources available to residents of minority neighborhoods as employers and higher SES individuals leave the neighborhoods; it reduces health care provider density in predominately African American communities, which affects access to health care (Gaskin et al., 2012); it constrains opportunities to engage in recommended health behaviors such as walking; it may be associated with greater density of alcohol outlets, tobacco advertisements, and fast food outlets in African American and other minority neighborhoods (Berke et al., 2010; Hackbarth et al., 1995; Kwate, 2008; LaVeist and Wallace, 2000); it increases the risk for exposure to environmental hazards (Brulle and Pellow, 2006); and it contributes to the mental and physical consequences of prevalent violence, including gun violence and aggressive policing (Landrine and Corral, 2009; Massey and Denton, 1989; Polednak, 1996).

Historical Trauma

Historical trauma, "a collective complex trauma inflicted on a group of people who share a specific group identity or affiliation" (Evans-Campbell, 2008, p. 320), manifests from the past treatment of certain racial and ethnic groups, especially Native Americans. This is another form of structural (i.e., systemic) racism that continues to shape the opportunities, risks, and health outcomes of these populations today (Gee and Ford, 2011; Gee and Payne-Sturges, 2004; Heart et al., 2011). The past consignment of Native Americans to reservations with limited resources continues to constrain physical and mental health in these communities; however, the methods to support research on this topic have not yet been fully developed (Heart et al., 2011). Additional details on the health of Native Americans are presented in Chapter 2 and Appendix A.

Interventions

The literature includes a small number of tested interventions. Interventions to address the health consequences of racism need not target racism in order to address the disparities it helps to produce. Furthermore, despite the deeply rooted nature of racism, communities are taking action to address the issue. (See Box 3-2 for a brief example of a community targeting structural racism and Box 3-3 for guidance on how to start a conversation about race.) Policy interventions and multi-sectoral efforts may be necessary to address structural factors such as segregation.

Examples of interventions that target racism include the following:

- Dismantling racism by addressing factors in organizational settings and environments that "directly and indirectly contribute to racial health care disparities" (Griffith et al., 2010, p. 370); see work by Derek Griffith (Griffith et al., 2007, 2010).
- The Undoing Racism project (Yonas et al., 2006), which integrates community-based participatory research with the "undoing racism" process, which is built around community organizing.
- The Praxis Project,[3] a national organization whose mission is to build healthy communities by transforming the power relationships and structures that affect lives. The organization's comprehensive strategy for change includes policy advocacy, local organizing, strategic communications, and community research.

---

[3] For more information, see http://www.thepraxisproject.org (accessed October 20, 2016).

BOX 3-2
Addressing Structural Racism in Everett, Massachusetts, Through Improving Community–Police Interactions

Everett is a small city of 42,000 near Boston which has experienced a dramatic demographic change in the past 25 years. In 1990 foreign-born residents accounted for 11 percent of the population; by 2013 they made up 41 percent. Motivated by tragedy—a 12-year-old Spanish-speaking girl drowned in 2004 in the Mystic River because she was unable to read the swimming safety signs—Everett has taken on the difficult issues related to structural racism for over a decade. The mayor's office established a multi-sector multicultural alliance to begin hashing out issues. At the top of the list for immigrants were police interactions. Through the years, multiple strategies have been taken to mitigate structural racism and enhance the relationship between the community and police; all are based on creating a safe place for dialogue and for trust to grow.

Racial Profiling by Police Force. As a result of multiple meetings between the police chief and the community, the department put down in writing—in Spanish, Portuguese, Arabic, and Haitian Creole—what people should expect when stopped by police. The police chief also dispatched officers for crash courses in Spanish and Portuguese.

Police Department Hiring Practices. The police department and Zion Church Ministries convened a forum to address police relations. In response to the community's concerns regarding department hiring practices and lack of diversity in the police force, the Police Chief explained how officers were selected and pledged to increase the diversity of the police force.

Youth Perceptions About Police. Facilitated by the coordinator of the Everett Community Health Partnership's Substance Abuse Coalition, about 50 teens from the Everett Teen Center and Teens in Everett Against Substance Abuse interacted with 7 police officers including the police chief. The conversations started with focusing on commonalities as members of the Everett community through an initial warm-up session, followed by small self-organized "affinity" groups in which each officer interacted with each group of teens. With this grounding, a baseline of trust was established, and further dialogue revealed misperceptions that can serve as the foundation for solutions. Additional meetings followed. The facilitator summarized the process as follows: "We've started a conversation where particularly for youth, they feel they can talk about race and the concerns they have and interact with adults in a different way."

SOURCE: RWJF, 2015a.

> **BOX 3-3**
> **How to Start a Conversation on Race and Health**
> **(Excerpted from Culture of Health Prize**
> **Winner, Everett, Massachusetts)**
>
> 1. Recognize the connections among race, police practices, and health.
> 2. Create a safe place for the conversation and for trust to grow.
> 3. Ask and answer the tough questions.
> 4. Wrap it in a larger effort to confront and change health inequities.
>
> SOURCE: RWJF, 2015a.

Although there is not a robust evidence base from which to draw solutions for implicit bias and its effects, there are promising strategies. For example, there is emerging evidence that mindfulness-based interventions have the potential to reduce implicit bias (Kang et al., 2014; Levesque and Brown, 2007; Lueke and Gibson, 2014). One promising avenue of research involves models of self-regulation and executive control on interracial interaction (Richeson and Shelton, 2003). Mindfulness has been shown to work on the cognitive brain function attentional processes involved in executive function, which is involved in decision making (Lueke and Gibson, 2014; Malinowski, 2013). A key component of mindfulness is paying attention with intention and without judgment.

There is also existing literature that points to the need for community-based interventions to mitigate implicit bias within the context of criminal justice and community safety (Correll et al., 2002, 2007; La Vigne et al., 2014; Richardson and Goff, 2013). According to the National Initiative for Building Community Trust and Justice, implicit bias can shape the outcomes of interactions between police and residents, which in turn result in pervasive practices that focus suspicion on specific populations (National Initiative for Building Community Trust and Justice, 2015). As discussed later in this chapter, the criminal justice system is a key actor and setting in shaping health inequity (see also Chapters 6 and 7 for more on criminal justice system as policy context and as a partner, respectively). Law enforcement agencies in communities around the country have employed strategies such as "principled policing" and policy changes and trainings to strengthen police–community relations (Gilbert et al., 2016; Jones, 2016).

The Perception Institute,[4] an organization committed to generating evidence-based solutions for bias in education, health care, media, workplace, law enforcement, and civil justice, published a report authored by Godsil et al. (2014) in which promising interventions for implicit bias are highlighted (Godsil et al., 2014). Among these interventions was a multi-pronged approach to reducing implicit bias that Devine and colleagues (2012) found to be successful and the "first evidence that a controlled, randomized intervention can produce enduring reductions in implicit bias" (Devine et al., 2012, p. 1271). The multiple strategies of the intervention tested included stereotype replacement, counter-stereotype imaging, individuation, perspective taking, and increasing opportunities for contact. As discussed above, there is an emerging body of literature that is beginning to highlight promising solutions for implicit bias; however, that research base needs to be expanded further.

Recommendation 3-1: The committee recommends that research funders[5] support research on (a) health disparities that examines the multiple effects of structural racism (e.g., segregation) and implicit and explicit bias across different categories of marginalized status on health and health care delivery; and (b) effective strategies to reduce and mitigate the effects of explicit and implicit bias.

This could include implicit and explicit bias across race, ethnicity, gender identity, disability status, age, sexual orientation, and other marginalized groups.

There have been promising developments in the search for interventions to address implicit bias, but more research is needed, and engaging community members in this and other aspects of research on health disparities is important for ethical and practical reasons (Minkler et al., 2010; Mosavel et al., 2011; Salway et al., 2015). In the context of implicit bias in workplaces and business settings, including individuals with relevant expertise in informing and conducting the research could also be helpful. Therefore, teams could be composed of such nontraditional participants as community members and local business leaders, in addition to academic researchers.

Conclusion 3-1: To reduce the adverse effects and the level of implicit bias among stakeholders in the community (such as health care workers,

---

[4] For more information, see https://perception.org (accessed October 18, 2016).
[5] Funders include government agencies, private foundations, and other sources such as academic centers of higher education.

social service workers, employers, police officers, and educators), the committee concludes, based on its judgment, that community-based programs are best suited to mitigate the adverse effects of implicit bias. Successful community programs would be tailored to the needs of the community. However, proven strategies and efficacious interventions to reduce the effects of or mitigate effects of implicit bias are lacking. Therefore:

Recommendation 3-2: The committee recommends that research funders support and academic institutions convene multidisciplinary research teams that include nonacademics to (a) understand the cognitive and affective processes of implicit bias and (b) test interventions that disrupt and change these processes toward sustainable solutions.

SOCIAL DETERMINANTS OF HEALTH

As described earlier, structural inequities are produced on the basis of social identity (e.g., race, gender, and sexual orientation), and the social determinants of health are the "terrain" on which the effects play out. Traditionally, the most well-known and cited of the factors that shape health outcomes are the individual-level behavioral factors (e.g., smoking, physical activity, nutrition habits, and alcohol and drug use) that the evidence shows are proximally associated with individual health status and outcomes. As stated in Chapter 1, understanding the social determinants of health requires a shift toward a more upstream perspective (i.e., the conditions that provide the context within which an individual's behaviors are shaped). Again, consider the metaphor of a fish, and the role of the conditions of the fishbowl in influencing the fish's well-being, and the analogy to human beings and conditions in which people live, learn, work, play, worship, and age that affect a wide range of health, functioning, and quality-of-life outcomes and risks. These environments and settings (e.g., school, workplace, neighborhood, and church) have been referred to as "place." In addition to the more material attributes of "place," the patterns of social engagement, social capital, social cohesion, and sense of security and well-being are also affected by where people live (Braveman and Gottlieb, 2014; Healthy People 2020, 2016). Although the term "social determinants of health" is widely used in the literature, the term may incorrectly suggest that such factors are immutable. It is important to note that the factors included among the social determinants of health are indeed modifiable and that they can be influenced by social, economic, and political processes and policies. In fact, there are communities throughout the United States that have prioritized

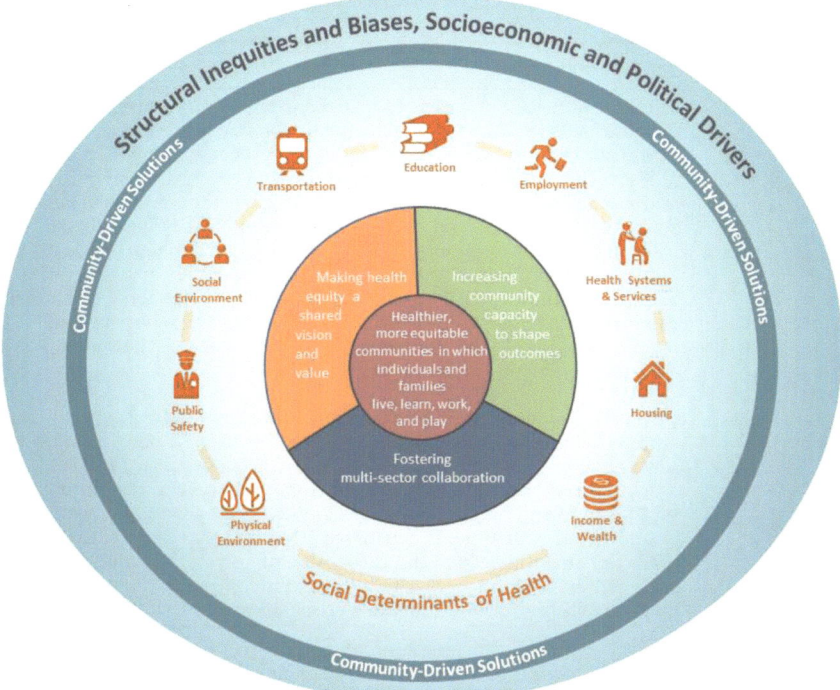

FIGURE 3-3 Report framework for community solutions to promote health equity.
NOTE: The social (and other) determinants of health are highlighted to convey the focus of this section.

addressing the social determinants of health and are demonstrating how specific upstream strategies lead to improved community conditions and health-related outcomes. (See Chapter 5 for an in depth examination of nine community examples.) Although it might be more accurate to refer to social "contributing factors" for health, the committee continues to use the widely accepted word "determinants" in this report.

For the purposes of this report, the committee has identified nine social determinants of health (see report conceptual model, Figure 3-3) that the literature shows fundamentally influence health outcomes at the community level. These determinants are education, income and wealth, employment, health systems and services, housing, the physical environment, transporation, the social environment, and public safety (Table 3-1 provides a brief definition of each).

There is a vast and growing body of literature on the social, economic, and environmental determinants of health and their impacts on health

TABLE 3-1 The Social (and Other) Determinants of Health[a]

Determinant of Health	Explanation
Education	The access or lack of access to learning opportunities and literacy development for all ages which effectively serves all learners. Education is a process and a product: as a process, education occurs at home, in school, and in the community. As a product, an education is the sum of knowledge, skills, and capacities (i.e., intellectual, socio-emotional, physical, productive, and interactive) acquired through formal and experiential learning. Educational attainment is a dynamic, ever-evolving array of knowledge, skills, and capacities. Education can influence health in many ways. Educational attainment can influence health knowledge and behaviors, employment and income, and social and psychological factors, such as the sense of control, social standing, and social networks.
Income and Wealth	Income is the amount of money earned in a single year from employment, government assistance, retirement and pension payments, and interest or dividends from investments or other assets. Income can fluctuate greatly from year to year, depending on life stage and employment status. Wealth, or economic assets accumulated over time, is calculated by subtracting outstanding debts and liabilities from the cash value of currently owned assets—such as houses, land, cars, savings accounts, pension plans, stocks and other financial investments, and businesses. Wealth measured at a single point in time may provide a more complete picture of a person's economic resources. Access to financial resources, be it income or wealth, affects health by safeguarding individuals against large medical bills while also making available more preventive health measures such as access to healthy neighborhoods, homes, land uses, and parks.
Employment	The level or absence of adequate participation in a job or the workforce, including occupation, unemployment, and underemployment. Work influences health not only by exposing employees to physical environments, but also by providing a setting where healthy activities and behaviors can be promoted (An et al., 2011). The features of a worksite, the nature of the work, and how the work is organized can affect worker mental and physical health (Clougherty et al., 2010). Many Americans also obtain health insurance through their workplace, another potential impact on health and well-being. Health also affects one's ability to maintain stable employment (Davis et al., 2016; Goodman, 2015). For most working adults, employment is the main source of income, providing access to homes, neighborhoods, and other goods and services that promote health.
Health Systems and Services	The access or lack of access to effective, affordable, culturally and linguistically appropriate, and respectful preventative care, chronic disease management, emergency services, mental health services, and dental care and the promotion of better community services and community conditions that promote health over the lifespan, including population health outcomes. It also refers to a paradigm shift that reflects *health* care over *sick* care and that promotes prevention.

TABLE 3-1 Continued

Determinant of Health	Explanation
Housing	The availability or lack of availability of high-quality, safe, and affordable housing that is accessible for residents with mixed income levels. Housing also refers to the density within a housing unit and within a geographic area, as well as the overall level of segregation/diversity in an area based on racial and ethnic and/or socioeconomic status. Housing affects health because of the physical conditions within homes, the conditions in the neighborhoods surrounding homes, and housing affordability, which affects the overall ability of families to make healthy choices.
Physical Environment	The physical environment reflects the place, including the human-made physical components, design, permitted use of space, and the natural environment. It includes, for example, transportation/getting around, what's sold and how it's promoted, parks and open space, look and feel, air/water/soil, and arts and cultural expression.
Transportation	Transportation consists of the network, services, and infrastructure necessary for residents to get from one place to another. If designed and maintained properly, transportation promotes safe mobility and is accessible to all residents, regardless of geographic location, age or disability status. Unsafe transportation can result in unintentional injuries or death. Access or lack of access to quality transportation at the community level affects opportunity for employment and vital services such as health care, education, and social services. Active transportation—the promotion of walking and cycling for transportation, complemented by public transportation or any other active mode—is a form of transportation that reduces environmental barriers to physical activity and promotes positive health outcomes. Transportation can also have negative environmental impacts, such as air pollution, which can affect health.
Social Environment	The social environment, sometimes referred to as social capital, reflects the individuals, families, and businesses within a community, the interactions and kinship ties between them, and norms and culture. It also includes social networks and trust as well as civic participation and willingness to act for the common good.
Public Safety	Public safety refers to the safety and protection of the general public. Here it is characterized by the absence of violence in public settings and the role of the justice system. Violence is the intentional use of physical force or power, threatened or actual, against oneself, another person, or against a group or community that either results in or has a high likelihood of resulting in injury, death, psychological or emotional harm, maldevelopment or deprivation, and trauma from actual and/or threatened, witnessed and/or experienced violence.

[a] Determinants are listed in the order in which they are discussed in this section.
SOURCES: Davis et al., 2016; Mueller et al., 2015.

outcomes (Braveman and Gottlieb, 2014; Braveman et al., 2011; CSDH, 2008; Marmot et al., 2010). Often, the evidence is in the form of cross-sectional analyses, and the pathways to health outcomes are not always clearly delineated, in part due to the complexity of the mechanisms and the long time periods it takes to observe outcomes (Braveman and Gottlieb, 2014). Therefore, the literature is not sufficient to establish a causal relationship between each of these determinants and health, but the determinants certainly are correlated with and contribute to health outcomes. While this report focuses on the community level, it should be made clear that the social determinants of health operate at multiple levels throughout the life course (IOM, 2006). This includes the individual level (knowledge, attitudes/beliefs, skills), family and community level (friends and social networks), institutional level (relationships among organizations), and systemic level (national, state, and local policies, laws, and regulations) (see Figure 3-2, the social ecological model adapted from McLeroy et al. [1988]). Furthermore, the various levels of influence that the social determinants of health have can occur simultaneously and interact with one another (IOM, 2006). In addition to the multiple levels of influence, there is a diversity of actors, sectors, settings, and stakeholders that interact with and shape the social determinants of health. This adds an additional layer of complexity to the factors that shape health disparities.

The following sections describe each of these nine determinants and how they shape health outcomes, as well as the disparities within these social determinants of health that contribute to health inequity. To highlight the ongoing work of communities that seek to address the conditions in which members live, learn, work, and play, this section will feature brief examples of communities for each determinant of health.

Education

Education, as it pertains to health, can be conceptualized as a process and as an outcome. The process of educational attainment takes place in many settings and levels (e.g., the home/family, school, and community), while the outcome can be described as a sum of knowledge, skills, and capacities that can influence the other social determinants of health, or health, more directly (Davis et al., 2016). Within the current social determinants of health literature, the primary focus on education is on educational attainment as an outcome (i.e., years of schooling, high school completion, and number of degrees obtained) and how it relates to health outcomes.

There is an extensive body of research that consistently demonstrates a positive correlation between educational attainment and health status indicators, such as life expectancy, obesity, morbidity from acute and chronic diseases, health behaviors (e.g., smoking status, heavy drinking physical activity, preventive services or screening behavior, automobile and home safety) and more (Baum et al., 2013; Cutler and Lleras-Muney, 2006, 2010; Feinstein et al., 2006; Krueger et al., 2015; Rostron et al., 2010). Educational attainment also has an intergenerational effect, in which the education of the parents, particularly maternal education, is linked to their children's health and well-being (Cutler and Lleras-Muney, 2006). For example, research suggests that babies born to mothers who have not completed high school are twice as likely to die before their first birthday as babies who are born to college graduates (Egerter et al., 2011b; Mathews and MacDorman, 2007). Death rates are declining among the most-educated Americans, accompanied by steady or increasing death rates among the least educated (Jemal et al., 2008). The findings on the association between education and health are consistent with population health literature within the international context as well (Baker et al., 2011; Furnee et al., 2008; Marmot et al., 2010).

Even more noteworthy about the education and health relationship is the graded association that is observed across populations with varying education levels, commonly referred to as the "education gradient." In the United States the gradient in health outcomes by educational attainment has steepened over the last four decades in all regions of the United States (Goldman and Smith, 2011; Montez and Berkman, 2014; Olshansky et al., 2012), producing a larger gap in health status between Americans with high and low education. Specifically, trends in data suggest that, over time, the disparities in mortality and life expectancy by education level have been increasing (Meara et al., 2008; Olshansky et al., 2012). Meara et al. found that approximately 20 percent of this trend was attributable to differential trends in smoking-related diseases in the 1980s and 1990s, despite the overall population increases in life expectancy during these two decades (Meara et al., 2008). Economic trends and shifting patterns of employment, in which skilled jobs linked to educational attainment are associated with increased income, also have implications for health (NRC, 2012). This makes the connection between education and health, mediated by employment opportunities, even more important and worth exploring.

Data from the Behavioral Risk Factor Surveillance System reveal that across all racial groups, adults with higher levels of educational attainment are less likely to rate their own health as less than very good (Egerter et al., 2011b). While the education gradient is present across racial and ethnic groups, it is important to keep in mind that the rates of educational attainment vary across different racial and ethnic groups. For the 2013–2014 academic year, the high school graduation rate for white students was 87.2 percent as compared with 76.3 percent among Hispanics, 72.5 percent among African Americans, and 70 percent among Native

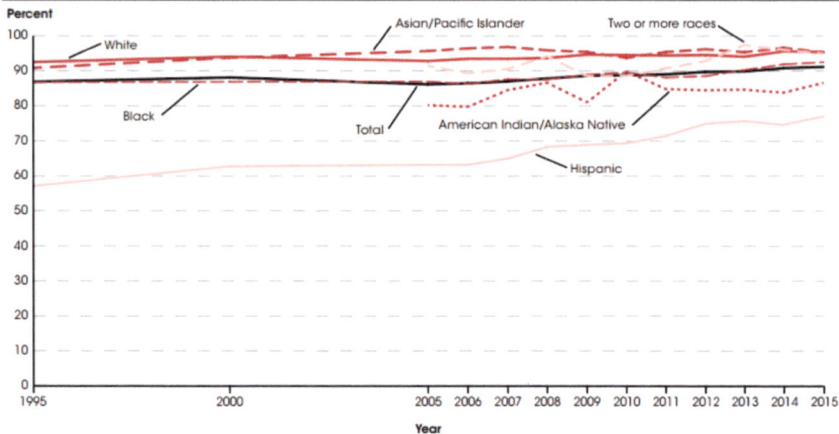

FIGURE 3-4 Percentage of 25- to 29-year-olds who completed at least a high school diploma or its equivalent, by race and ethnicity: Selected years, 1995–2015. NOTE: Race categories exclude persons of Hispanic ethnicity. Prior to 2005, separate data on persons of two or more races were not available; data for American Indians/Alaska natives are not shown prior to 2005.
SOURCE: Kena et al., 2016.

Americans (Kena et al., 2016). These rates are consistent with high school diploma and bachelor degree achievement gaps that have persisted since the late 1990s (see Figures 3-4 and 3-5).

Although the literature linking education and health is robust, there is still some debate as to whether or not this relationship is a causal one (Baker et al., 2011; Fujiwara and Kawachi, 2009; Grossman, 2015). Issues that have been raised in the course of this debate include the role of reverse causation and the potential influence of any unobserved third variables (Grossman, 2015). The association between education and health is clearly bidirectional. Education outcomes are substantially affected by health (Cutler and Lleras-Muney, 2006). Students living in community conditions that contribute to hunger, chronic stress, or lack of attention to visual or hearing needs are likely to have problems concentrating in class (Evans and Schamberg, 2009). Unmanaged health conditions (e.g., asthma, dental pain, acute illnesses, mental health issues, etc.) give rise to chronic absenteeism, which in turn is highly correlated with underachievement (Ginsburg et al., 2014). In short, health issues are much more than minor distractions in the lives of students, especially students living in low-income communities.

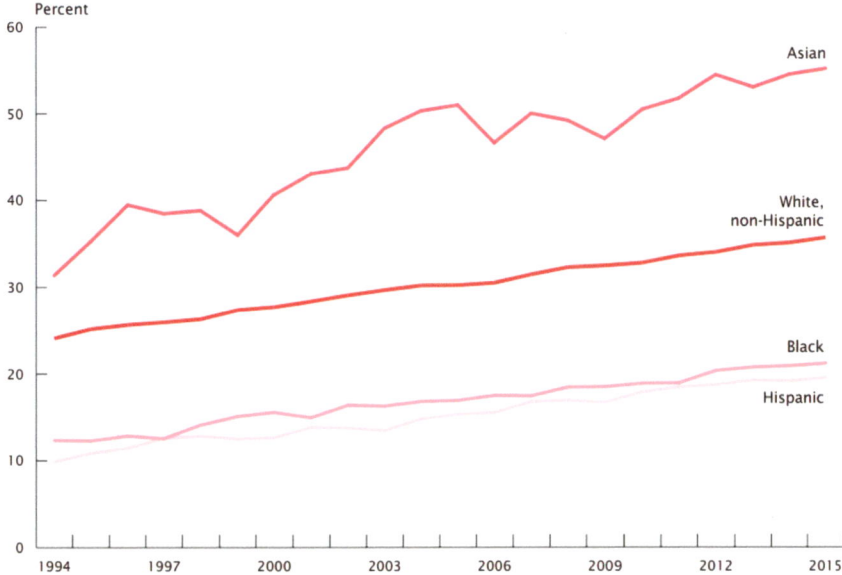

FIGURE 3-5 Percentage of U.S.-born population ages 25 years and older with a bachelor's degree or higher by race and Hispanic origin, 1988–2015.
SOURCE: Ryan and Bauman, 2016.

Disparities in Education

Educational attainment, common measures of which include high school diploma or bachelor's degree, has increased for all race groups and Hispanics since 1988, according to U.S. Census estimates (Ryan and Bauman, 2016). Despite this overall progress, the gaps between these groups have remained the same for some and increased for others. For example, in 1988 African Americans and Hispanics attained bachelor's degrees at very similar rates; however, by 2015 the percentage gap between African Americans and Hispanics had reached 7 percent, with rates of completion at 22 percent and 15 percent, respectively (Ryan and Bauman, 2016). Furthermore, there has been little to no progress in closing the gap of achievement between whites and African Americans (Ryan and Bauman, 2016).

A recent study of school trends conducted by the U.S. Government Accountability Office (GAO) found that there has been a large increase in schools that are distinguished by the poverty and race of their student bodies (GAO, 2016). The percent of K–12 schools with students who are poor and are mostly African American or Hispanic grew from 9 percent to 16 percent from 2000 to 2013. These schools were the most racially and economically concentrated among all schools, with 75 to 100 percent of the students African American or Hispanic and eligible for free or reduced-price lunch—a commonly used indicator of poverty. Moreover, compared with other schools, these schools offered disproportionately fewer math, science, and college preparatory courses and had disproportionately higher rates of students who were held back in 9th grade, suspended, or expelled (GAO, 2016).

One gap in educational achievement that has successfully been narrowed over the past five decades is the gender disparity in bachelor's degree attainment, in which men historically had higher achievement rates (Crissey et al., 2007). In 2015 the percentage of men ages 25 or older with a bachelor's degree or higher was not statistically different from that of women, with women leading by one percentage point (Ryan and Bauman, 2016).

The evidence suggests that disparities in education are apparent early in the life course, which reflects broader societal inequities (Garcia, 2015). In education, these early disparities are evidenced by wide gaps in vocabulary between children from low-income and those from middle- or upper-income families. Children from low-income families may have 600 fewer words in their vocabulary by age 3, a gap that grows to as many as 4,000 words by age 7 (Christ and Wang, 2010). These word gaps directly affect literacy levels and reading achievement (Marulis and Neuman, 2010). There is substantial evidence that children who do not read at grade level by 7 or 8 years of age are much more likely to struggle academically (Chall et al., 1990). Both high school graduation rates and participation in postsecondary education opportunities are correlated with early literacy levels. Hence, attention to and investments in early childhood education are generally viewed as an important way to reduce disparities in education (Barnett, 2013).

Mechanisms

Although the association between education and health is clear, the mechanisms by which educational attainment might improve health are not so clearly understood. A keen understanding of the mechanisms could help to inform the most cost-effective and targeted policies or solutions that seek to improve health and, ultimately, promote health equity (Picker, 2007). Egerter et al. (2011b) identified multiple interrelated pathways through which education can affect health, based on the literature (see Figure 3-6). The three major pathways are the following:

- Education increases health knowledge, literacy, coping, and problem solving, thereby influencing health behaviors;

THE ROOT CAUSES OF HEALTH INEQUITY 125

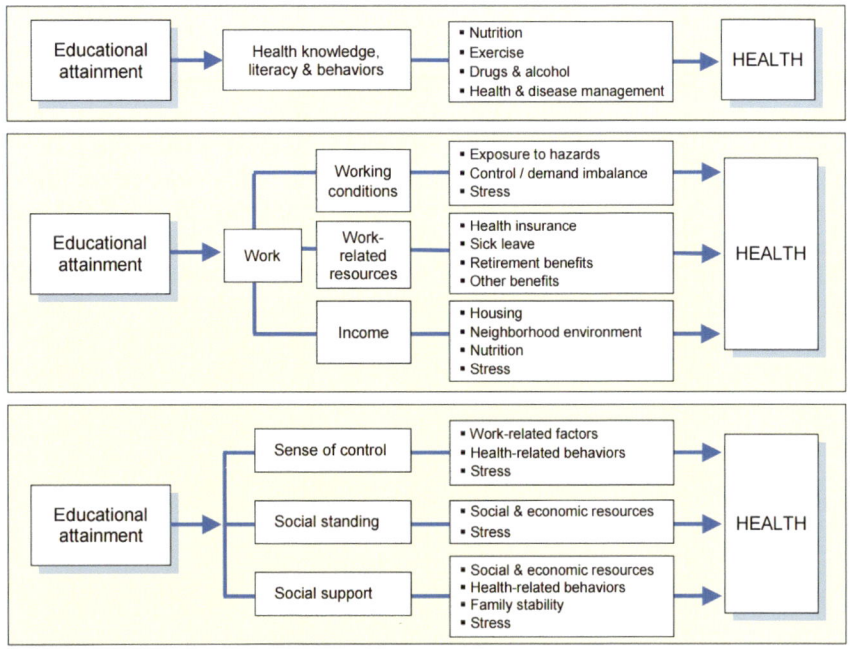

FIGURE 3-6 Pathways through which education can affect health.
SOURCE: Egerter et al., 2011b. Used with permission from the Robert Wood Johnson Foundation.

- Educational attainment shapes employment opportunities and related benefits, such as income, working conditions, and other resources; and
  - Research indicates that each additional year of education leads to almost 11 percent more income annually (Rouse and Barrow, 2006), which can secure safer working environments and benefits such as health insurance and sick leave.
- Education affects social and psychological factors that influence health (e.g., self-efficacy, social status, and social networks) (Egerter et al., 2011b).
  - Education has also been linked to human capital, a systematic way of thinking that benefits every decision, which could positively affect health decisions (Cutler and Lleras-Muney, 2006; Lundborg et al., 2012, 2016).

In this framework, note that educational attainment is a predictor of health and can either improve or hinder health outcomes depending on educational attainment. This suggests that policies and practices proven to increase academic performance and reduce education disparities are important to reducing health disparities. (See Box 3-4 for an example of a community school working to improve educational outcomes.) Intervening early is generally considered a high-impact strategy (Barnett, 2013). However, interventions that support academic achievement in high schools and in postsecondary settings are also important to increasing educational attainment (Balfanz et al., 2007; Carnahan, 1994; Kirst and Venezia, 2004; Louie, 2007). One of the key factors in both high school and college completion rates has to do with how well students transition from one level of the education system to another (Rosenbaum and Person, 2003).

BOX 3-4
Reagan High School: A Community School

A community school is both a place and a set of partnerships between the school and other community resources. Partners work together to achieve a set of results: (1) children are ready to enter school; (2) students attend school consistently; (3) students are actively involved in their learning and in their community; (4) families are increasingly involved with their children's education; (5) schools are engaged with families and communities; (6) students succeed academically; (7) students are healthy—physically, socially, and emotionally; (8) students live and learn in a safe, supportive, and stable environment; and (9) communities are desirable places to live (IEL, n.d.).

Reagan High School, now known as John H. Reagan Early College High School, is a community school in northeast Austin that was "saved" through community-driven processes. In the late 1990s and early 2000s, Reagan's student body became increasingly poor as middle-class families left the area. In 2003, a student was stabbed to death by her former boyfriend in a hallway of the school. The incident made headlines and students left Reagan in droves. Enrollment at Reagan dropped from more than 2,000 students to a new low of 600 students, and the graduation rate hovered just below 50 percent. In 2008 the district threatened to close Reagan. In reaction, a committee of parents, teachers, and students brought together by Austin Voices for Education and Youth formulated a plan to turn Reagan into a community school. The district accepted their plan.

Reagan's student population is close to 80 percent Latino and about 18 percent African American. Eighty percent are identified by the state's indicator of poverty, and 30 percent are English language learners. In 2010, before becoming a com-

Income and Wealth

Income can be defined broadly as the amount of money earned in a single year from employment, government assistance, retirement and pension payments, and interest or dividends from investments or other assets (Davis et al., 2016). Income can fluctuate greatly from year to year depending on life stage and employment status. Wealth, or economic assets accumulated over time, is calculated by subtracting outstanding debts and liabilities from the cash value of currently owned assets—such as houses, land, cars, savings accounts, pension plans, stocks and other financial investments, and businesses. Wealth measured at a single time period may provide a more complete picture than income of a person's economic resources. Moreover, wealth has an intergenerational component, which can have implications for who has access to wealth and who does not (De Nardi, 2002).

---

munity school, 25 percent of female students were pregnant or parenting, among whom barely any graduated.

Noteworthy aspects of Reagan's approach include

- The community school coordinator works with both academic and non-academic leadership teams to ensure alignment between students' needs and the services and programs provided
- The school engages with the legal system (local civil courts) to better address student discipline, and a student-led youth court was established in partnership with The University of Texas at Austin Law School
- On-site daycare and clinic services are offered for student mothers and their babies
- The school has partnered with the local community college to provide cost-free higher education

Based on 2013–2014 data, Reagan is graduating 87 percent of its students, enrollment has more than doubled, and a new Early College High School program has allowed many of Reagan's students to earn their associate's degree from a nearby community college during their time as Reagan students. In 2014, 61 percent of students took advanced placement tests and 18 percent passed (*U.S. News & World Report*, n.d.), a dozen students received associate degrees, and another 150 took college classes. Additionally, Reagan now has a 100 percent graduation rate among pregnant and parenting teens.

SOURCES: IEL, n.d.; *U.S. News & World Report*, n.d.

Access to financial resources, be it income or wealth, affects health by buffering individuals against the financial threat of large medical bills while also facilitating access to health-promoting resources such as access to healthy neighborhoods, homes, land uses, and parks (Davis et al., 2016). Income can predict a number of health outcomes and indicators, such as life expectancy, infant mortality, asthma, heart conditions, obesity, and many others (Woolf et al., 2015).

Income Inequality and Concentration of Poverty

Income inequality is rising in the United States at a rate that is among the highest in the economically developed countries in the north (OECD, 2015). The past few decades have seen dramatic rises in income inequality. In 1970, 17 percent of families lived in upper-income areas, 65 percent in middle-income areas, and 19 percent in lowest-income areas; in 2012, 30 percent of families lived in upper-income areas, 41 percent in middle-income areas, and 30 percent in lowest-income areas (Reardon and Bischoff, 2016). In 2013, the top 10 percent of workers earned an average income 19 times that of the average income earned by the bottom 10 percent of workers; in the 1990s and 1980s, this ratio was 12.5 to 1 and 11 to 1, respectively (OECD, 2015). Furthermore, households earning in the bottom 10 percent have not benefited from overall increases in household income over the past few decades; the average inflation-adjusted income for this population was 3.3 percent lower in 2012 than in 1985 (OECD, 2015). Disparities in life expectancy gains have also increased alongside the rise in income inequality. From 2001 to 2014, life expectancy for the top 5 percent of income earners rose by about 3 years while life expectancy for the bottom 5 percent of income earners saw no increase (Chetty et al., 2016).

Not only are income and wealth determinants of health, but the concentration of poverty in certain neighborhoods is important to recognize as a factor that shapes the conditions in which people live. *Concentrated poverty*, measured by the proportion of people in a given geographic area living in poverty, can be used to describe areas (e.g., census tracts) where a high proportion of residents are poor (Shapiro et al., 2015). Concentrated poverty disproportionately affects racial and ethnic minorities across all of the social determinants of health. For example, National Equity Atlas data reveal that in about half of the largest 100 cities in the United States, most African American and Hispanic students attend schools where at least 75 percent of all students qualify as poor or low-income under federal guidelines (Boschma, 2016). Given that concentrated poverty is tightly correlated with gaps in educational achievement, this has implications for educational outcomes and health (Boschma and Brownstein, 2016).

Disparities Related to Income Inequality

In 2012, of the 12 million full-time low-income workers between the ages of 25 and 64, 56 percent were racial and ethnic minorities (Ross, 2016b). Regional percentages varied from 23 percent in Honolulu, Hawaii, to 65 percent in Brownsville, Texas (Ross, 2016a). Figure 3-7 shows the proportion of low-income workers of racial and ethnic minority groups across different regions of the United States. The burden faced by low-income people suggests that efforts to advance health equity through income and wealth will need to take into consideration rising income inequality as well as significant geographic variation.

Chetty and colleagues published the largest study of its kind, using 1.4 billion income tax and Social Security records to report the association between income level and life expectancy from 1999 through 2014 (Chetty et al., 2016). Consistent with previous findings (NASEM, 2015; Waldron, 2007; Woolf et al., 2015), they found that higher income is related to higher life expectancy and that lower income is related to lower life expectancy. The gap in life expectancy for the richest and poorest 1 percent of individuals was 14.6 years for men and 10.1 years for women. A novel contribution of the study is its examination of the income–longevity relationship

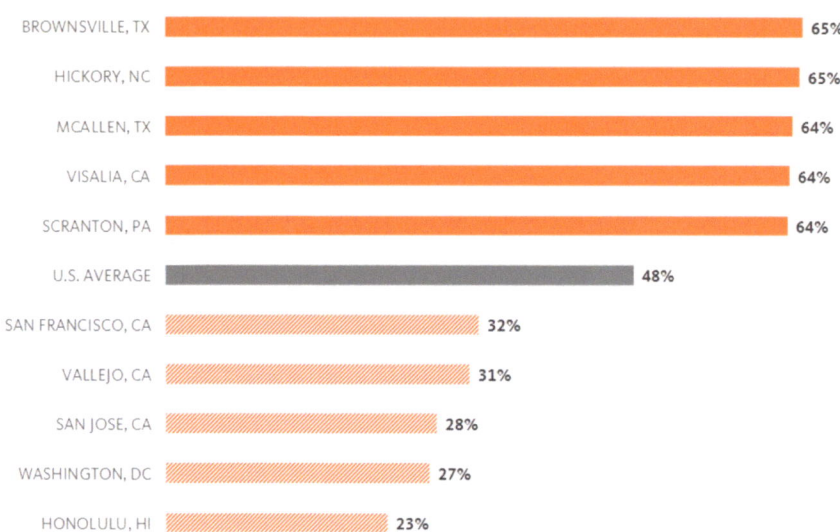

FIGURE 3-7 The share of people of color below 200 percent of poverty ranges. SOURCE: Woolf et al., 2015. Used with permission from PolicyLink, figure from article by Angel Ross, *New Data Highlights Vast and Persistent Racial Inequities in Who Experiences Poverty in America*, http://nationalequityatlas.org/data-in-action/racial-inequitiespoverty-in-america (accessed December 27, 2016).

across time and local areas. In certain local areas, the effect of being at the bottom of the income gradient is more pronounced than in others, with four- to five-fold differences. This strong local component reinforces the notion suggested by the literature that place matters. Trends in life expectancy also varied geographically, with some areas experiencing improvements and others declines. Others have commented on the limitations of the study (Deaton, 2016; McGinnis, 2016; Woolf and Purnell, 2016).

Zonderman et al. take the findings of this study a step further by considering the role of race and gender differences in the relationship between poverty and mortality. They found that while African American men below poverty status had 2.66 times higher risk of mortality than African American men living above poverty status, white men below poverty status had approximately the same risk as white men living above poverty status (Zonderman et al., 2016). Both African American women and white women living below poverty status were at an increased mortality risk relative to those living above poverty status (Zonderman et al., 2016).

Infant mortality rates in the United States rank among the highest for developed nations (NRC and IOM, 2013), and mortality rates for infants born to low-income mothers are even higher. Studies have shown an inverse correlation between family income and infant mortality (Singh and Yu, 1995) as well as a positive correlation between income inequality (measured with the Gini coefficient) and infant mortality (Olson et al., 2010). Infants born to low-income mothers have the highest rates of low birth weight (Blumenshine et al., 2010; Dubay et al., 2001).

Chronic diseases are more prevalent among low-income people than among the overall U.S. population. Low-income adults have higher rates of heart disease, diabetes, stroke, and other diseases and conditions relative to adults earning higher levels of income (Woolf et al., 2015).

Mechanisms

Researchers have offered various hypotheses about the multiple mechanisms by which income can affect health. Woolf et al. suggest that among others, these mechanisms include more income providing the opportunity to afford health care services and health insurance; greater resources affording a healthy lifestyle and access to place-based benefits known as the social determinants of health; and economic disadvantage and hardship leading to stress and harmful physiological effects on the body (Woolf et al., 2015). Evans and Kim identify "multiple risk exposure" as a potential mechanism for the socioeconomic status and health gradient. This is the convergence among populations with low socioeconomic status of multiple physical and psychosocial risk factors such as poor housing and neighborhood quality, pollutants and toxins, crowding and congestion, noise exposure, and adverse interpersonal relationships (Evans and Kim, 2010).

Wealth affects health through mechanisms that are not necessarily monetary, such as power and prestige, attitudes and behavior, and social capital (Pollack et al., 2013). Even in the absence of income, wealth can provide resources and a safety net that is not available to those without it. (See Box 3-5 for an example of an initiative seeking to build income and wealth in communities around the country.)

Employment

Employment is the level or absence of adequate participation in a job or workforce, including the range of occupation, unemployment, and underemployment. Work influences health not only by exposing employees to certain physical environments but also by providing a setting where healthy activities and behaviors can be promoted (An et al., 2011). For most adults, employment is the main source of income, thus providing access to homes, neighborhoods, and other conditions or services that promote health. The features of a worksite, the nature of the work, the amount of earnings or income, and how the work is organized can affect worker mental and physical health (An et al., 2011; Clougherty et al., 2010). Many Americans also obtain health insurance through their workplace, accounting for another potential impact on health and well-being. While the correlation between employment and health has been well established, there appears to be a bidirectional relationship between employment and health, as health also affects one's ability to participate in and maintain stable employment (Davis et al., 2016; Goodman, 2015). Not only that, but a healthy workforce is a prerequisite for economic success in any industry (Doyle et al., 2005).

The existing literature on the social determinants of health makes it clear that there is a positive correlation between SES and health (Adler and Stewart, 2010a; Braveman et al., 2005; Conti et al., 2010; Dow and Rehkopf, 2010; Pampel et al., 2010; Williams et al., 2010). Occupational status, a composite of the power, income, and educational requirements associated with various positions in the occupational structure, is a core component of a person's SES (Burgard and Stewart, 2003; Clougherty et al., 2010). Occupational status can be indicative of the types of tangible benefits, hazards, income, fringe benefits, degree of control over work, and level of exposure to harmful physical environments associated with a job (Clougherty et al., 2010). While the mechanisms by which occupational status influences health have not clearly been delineated, there is evidence that the type of job does affect such health outcomes as hypertension risk and obesity (An et al., 2011; Clougherty et al., 2010).

BOX 3-5
Family Independence Initiative: The Power of Information and Investment in Families Who Take Initiative

The Family Independence Initiative (FII) envisions a future in which each person and family recognizes their self-determination and has access to the resources and community that they need to thrive. An alternative to the traditional American social service model, FII is a national nonprofit which leverages the power of information to illuminate and accelerate the initiative low-income families take to improve their lives. FII approaches address two major challenges to upward mobility: (1) lack of information, and therefore lack of investment, in the initiatives low-income families take on their own or collectively; and (2) negative stereotypes and the focus on individualism that have led to government and charitable practices that discourage families from turning to one another (FII, n.d.-a,b).

FII has launched demonstration projects in six cities across the United States: Boston, Detroit, Fresno, New Orleans, Oakland, and San Francisco. Approaches take advantage of connections, choice, and capital through four major components:

- **Strengthening Connections:** Demonstration projects are built to strengthen the relationships people have with their friends and families. They use their time together as an opportunity to support each other, hold each other accountable, and share resources, ideas, and advice.
- **Stepping Back So Families Step Forward:** Based on the belief that families have the knowledge, initiative, and the capacity to lead themselves, families set their own direction and actions. Rather than providing directions or advice, liaisons listen and sometimes ask questions.
- **Data Tracking Through an Online Journal:** Each family has access to FII's online data system which serves the dual purposes of collecting a rich body of data on the initiative of each household (e.g., income and savings, health, education and skills, housing, leadership, and connections) and providing each family a tool for self-reflection. Families are paid for sharing their data with FII.
- **Resources That Leverage Family Initiative:** FII analyzes the data from the online data system to gain insights about family needs and match them to resources that can be leveraged (FII, n.d.-c). This has led to innovations such as character-based underwriting criteria, credit-building lending circles, and "UpTogether," a community-building website using social networking technology through which families can identify and track progress against their priorities as well as form groups around common interests to share information, get support, and hold each other accountable (FII, n.d.-d).

On the other end of the spectrum, unemployment is associated with poor psychological well-being (McKee-Ryan et al., 2005; Paul and Moser, 2009). Zhang and Bhavsar (2013) examined the literature to illuminate the causality, effect size, and moderating factors of the relationship between unemployment as a risk factor and mental illness as an outcome. The authors reported that unemployment does precede mental illness, but more research is required to determine the effect size (Zhang and Bhavsar, 2013). There is also evidence to suggest that emerging adults who are unemployed are three times as likely to suffer from depression as their employed counterparts (McGee and Thompson, 2015). Burgard and colleagues found that even after controlling for significant social background factors (e.g., gender, race, education, maternal education, income, and more), involuntary job loss was associated with poorer overall self-rated health and more depressive symptoms (Burgard et al., 2007).

Disparities in Employment

Employment data show disparities in unemployment rates across various racial and ethnic groups and geographic regions, despite the overall progress that has been made in reducing unemployment nationally (Wilson, 2016). During the fourth quarter of 2015, the highest state-level unemployment rate was 13.1 percent for African Americans (Illinois), 11.9 percent for Hispanics (Massachusetts), 6.7 percent for whites (West Virginia), and 4.3 percent for Asians (New York) (Wilson, 2016). Figure 3-8 shows how disparities in unemployment by race and ethnicity have persisted for more than 40 years, with the exception of whites and Asians. Disparities in employment between African Americans and whites persist even when level of education, a major predictor of employment, is held equal between the two groups (Buffie, 2015).

Among the employed, there are systematic differences in wages and earnings by race, ethnicity, and gender. According to the U.S. Bureau of Labor Statistics, in 2013 the median usual weekly earnings[6] were $578 for Hispanics, $629 for African Americans, $802 for whites, and $942 for Asians (BLS, 2014). These disparities are consistent across almost all occupational groups. The widest gap in median usual weekly earnings was found between Hispanic women and Asian men, who made $541 and $1,059, respectively (BLS, 2014).

As with income, the distribution of occupations tends to differ across racial and ethnic groups (see Figure 3-9). Whereas half of Asians worked in management, professional, and related occupations in 2013, only 29

---

[6] These represent earnings for full-time wage and salary workers only.

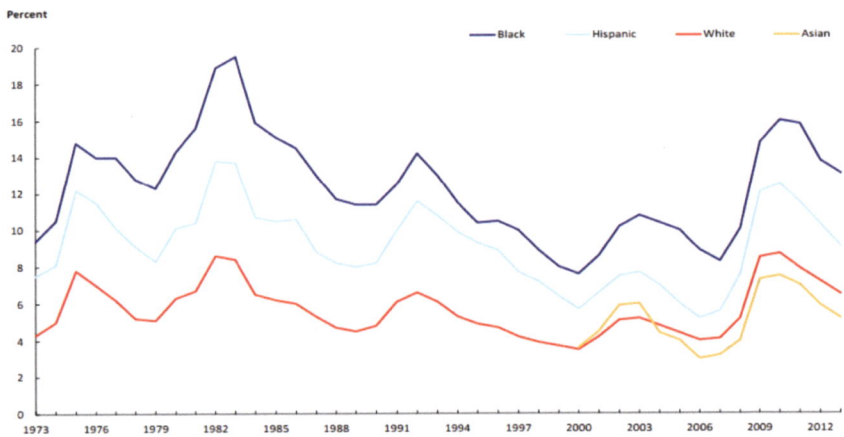

FIGURE 3-8 Unemployment rates by race and Hispanic or Latino ethnicity, 1973–2013 annual averages.
NOTE: People whose ethnicity is identified as Hispanic or Latino may be of any race. Data for Asians are only available since 2000.
SOURCE: BLS, 2014.

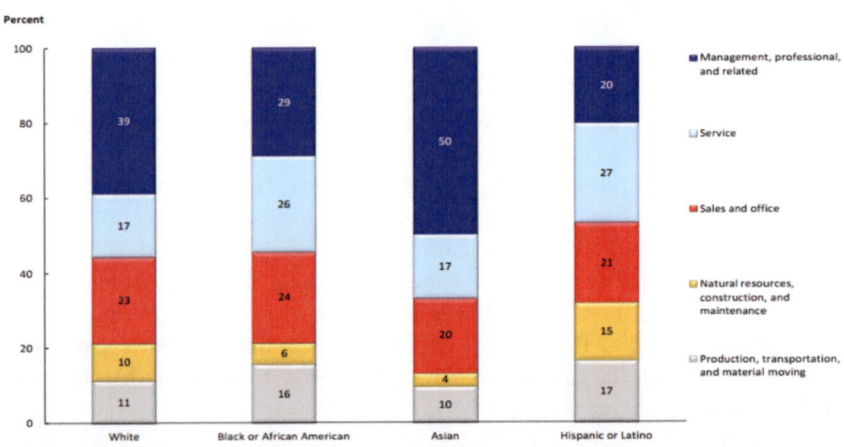

FIGURE 3-9 Employed people by occupation, race, and Hispanic or Latino ethnicity, 2013 annual averages.
NOTE: People whose ethnicity is identified as Hispanic or Latino may be of any race. Data may not sum to 100 percent due to rounding.
SOURCE: BLS, 2014.

and 20 percent of African Americans and Hispanics, respectively, worked in those professions (BLS, 2014).

Mechanisms

The literature suggests that there are three potential mechanisms through which employment affects health:

1. Physical aspects of work and the workplace
2. Psychosocial aspects of work and how work is organized
3. Work-related resources and opportunities (An et al., 2011; Clougherty et al., 2010)

The nature of work and the conditions of a workplace can increase the risk of injury or illness depending on the type of job. For employees in specific sectors (e.g., air transportation, nursing facilities, using motorized vehicles and equipment, trucking services, hospitals, grocery stores, department stores, food services), the risk of occupational injury is higher (An et al., 2011). This is especially true for operators, laborers, fabricators, and laborers (An et al., 2011). Occupational health can also be shaped by the physical nature of the tasks involved in a given work setting. For example, the health impact of a job that requires intense, laborious physical activity will be different than of a job in which the tasks are primarily sedentary. There is also emerging evidence suggesting that women working hourly jobs bear a larger burden due to hazardous conditions in the workplace than their male counterparts on outcomes such as hypertension, the risk of injury, injury severity, rates of absenteeism, and the time to return to work after illness (Clougherty et al., 2010; Hill et al., 2008).

The psychosocial aspects and organization of one's job can influence both mental and physical health. The factors that make up this pathway can include work schedules, commute to work, degree of control in work, the balance between effort and rewards, organizational justice, social support at work, and gender and racial discrimination (An et al., 2011). Longer commute times specifically affect low-income populations, as the cost burden of commuting for the working poor is much higher than for other workers and makes up a larger portion of their household budgets (Roberto, 2008).

The resources and opportunities associated with work can have lasting implications for health. Higher-paying jobs are more likely than lower-paying jobs to provide workers with safe work environments and offer benefits such as health insurance, workplace health promotion programs, and sick leave (An et al., 2011). Box 3-6 briefly describes a program

BOX 3-6
Green Jobs Central Oklahoma

Green Jobs Central Oklahoma (GJCO) is a U.S. Department of Labor–funded, comprehensive evidence-based program aimed at moving low-income individuals, including veterans and those with a criminal record, toward greater economic stability and security.[a] The program's activities leverage relationships with employer partners to ensure that trainings meet industry standards and company needs as well as to provide GJCO participants with access to jobs. Training is complemented by a range of supportive services (e.g., case management, career coaching and development) to help participants remove barriers to training completion and success. Training combines general skills that affect job success and participation in one of three "green" areas: recycling, wind energy, or green transportation. The former, Training Opportunity Preparation Services sessions, focus on communication and relationship skill-building in the workplace, understanding work cultures, leadership and success strategies, and financial literacy/competency. Trainees also complete a personality inventory, create a resume, and prepare for a job interview.

The length of specialty training varies by content area, and the training results in industry and nationally recognized certificates that enhance employment opportunities.

- **Recycle Training:** Up to 160 hours of classroom instruction based on the nationally renowned Roots of Success curriculum, a comprehensive environmental literacy and job readiness curriculum designed to prepare participants for work in the green industry. Modules include Fundamentals of Environmental Literacy, Water, Waste, Transportation, Energy, and Building. The didactic training is complemented by hands-on instruction provided by Goodwill Industries. Participants who complete training are awarded four industry or nationally recognized certificates.
- **Wind Industry Training:** A 100-hour course provided by Oklahoma City Community College. The program consists of the following trainings: Enhanced Occupational Safety Health Administration 10 Hour/First Aid-cardiopulmonary resuscitation (CPR), Intro to Wind Industry, Intro to AC/DC Fundamentals, Crane and Rigging, Confined Space, Torque Tool Safety, and Tower Safety.
- **Green Transportation Training:** A 160-hour training provided by the Center for Transportation Safety. This includes 40 hours learning the U.S. Department of Transportation rules and regulations, 40 hours learning driving fundamentals, and 80 hours of on-the-road driving time to practice the skills they learned.

Program outcomes have been positive with 190 of 250 participants placed in unsubsidized employment.

---

[a] For more information, see http://www.itsmycommunity.org/green-jobs.php (accessed December 5, 2016).

that aims to increase "green" employment opportunities for underserved individuals in a community.

Health Systems and Services

Health care is arguably the most well-known determinant of health, and it is traditionally the area where efforts to improve health have been focused (Heiman and Artiga, 2015). Over the past few decades there has been a paradigm shift that reflects "health" care over "sick" care. The idea is to promote access to effective and affordable care that is also culturally and linguistically appropriate. Health care spans a wide range of services, including preventative care, chronic disease management, emergency services, mental health services, dental care, and, more recently, the promotion of community services and conditions that promote health over the lifespan.

Although screening, disease management, and clinical care play an integral role in health outcomes, social and economic factors contribute to health outcomes almost twice as much as clinical care does (Heiman and Artiga, 2015; Hood et al., 2016; McGinnis et al., 2002; Schroeder, 2007). For example, by some estimates, social and environmental factors proportionally contribute to the risk of premature death twice as much as health care does (Heiman and Artiga, 2015; McGinnis et al., 2002; Schroeder, 2007). That being said, in March 2002, the Institute of Medicine released a report that demonstrated that even in the face of equal access to health care, minority groups suffer differences in quality of health. The noted differences were lumped into the categories of patient preferences and clinical appropriateness, the ecology of health systems and discrimination, bias, and stereotyping (IOM and NRC, 2003). Our health systems are working to better understand and address these differences and appreciate the importance of moving beyond individualized care to care that affects families, communities, and populations (Derose et al., 2011). This new focus on improving the health of populations has been accompanied by a welcome shift from siloed care to a health care structure that is interprofessional, multisectoral and considers social, economic, structural and other barriers to health (NASEM, 2016).

Arriving at the place of shared understanding concerning the health care needs of individuals, families, and communities has required taking a broader look at health. The triple aim, a framework that aims to optimize health system performance, has helped conceptualize this look, bringing to the forefront the elements that matter most, considering per capita cost, improving the health care experience for patients, and focusing on population health (Stiefel and Nolan, 2012). In addition to helping create new health care opportunities, the Patient Protection and Affordable Care Act

(ACA) has helped mitigate the challenge of access to care. According to the U.S. Centers for Disease Control and Prevention (CDC), the proportion of people in 2015 without health insurance had dropped below 10 percent (Cohen et al., 2016c).

Continuing the momentum of improving access to culturally competent and linguistically appropriate care will be a crucial step to improving the health of populations. Culturally and linguistically appropriate care includes high-quality care and clear communication regardless of socioeconomic or cultural background (Betancourt and Green, 2010). There is limited research studying whether there is a link between culturally appropriate care and health outcomes, but data do exist that indicate that behavioral and attitudinal elements of cultural competence facilitate higher-quality relationships between physicians and patients (Paez et al., 2009). Making cultural competency training a part of the all types of providers' (e.g., physicians, nurses, medical assistants, dentists, pharmacists, social workers, psychologists) education experience, as well as making it a requirement for licensure for providers (Like, 2011), may have the potential to link quality and safety. Continued work is needed to figure out how to translate increased access to care into improved health outcomes and increased health equity.

In light of the ACA's emphasis on access to improving quality, health outcomes, and population health, it makes sense to look at the environments in which patients live.[7] If the social determinants of health are not addressed in a multi-sectoral approach by educational systems, health systems, communities and others, the country will fall short of the triple aim. The Robert Wood Johnson Foundation's Culture of Health Action Framework has identified action areas meant to work together to address issues of equity, well-being, and improved population health (RWJF, 2015b). Social determinants of health are woven through these action areas. In fact, research shows that social determinants of health play a larger role in health outcomes than do medical advances (Hood et al., 2016; Woolf et al., 2007).

Disparities

While some disparities in access to care have been narrowing, gaps persist among certain groups of the population. For example, the gaps in insurance that existed between poor and nonpoor households and between African Americans and whites or Hispanics and whites decreased

---

[7] As access to care improves, it will be increasingly important to monitor potential disparities with respect to the nature of care that people receive. This is especially true for chronic conditions that require long-term engagement with the health care system.

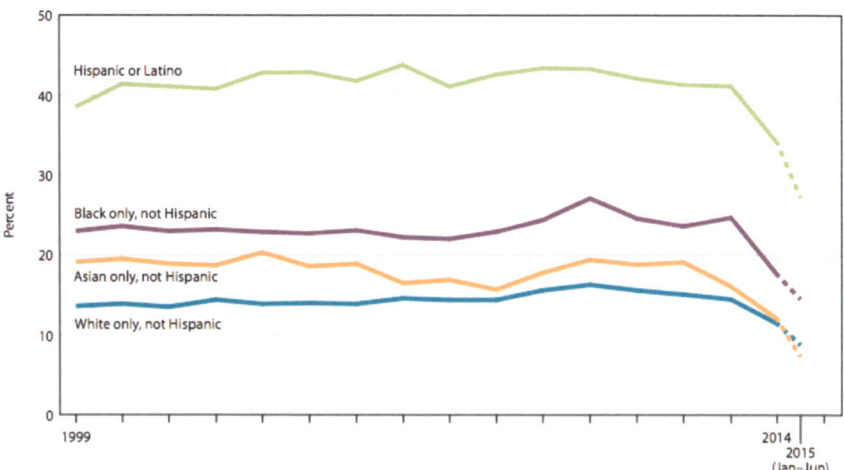

FIGURE 3-10 Percent of adults ages 18–64 with no health insurance coverage by race and Hispanic origin: United States, 1999–June 2015.
SOURCE: NCHS, 2016.

between 2010 and 2015 (AHRQ, 2016). However, systematic differences in access to care still exist and negatively affect poor households and racial and ethnic minority groups, including Hispanics and African Americans (NCHS, 2016) (see Figure 3-10). In fact, in 2013 people living below the federal poverty level had worse access to care than people in high-income households across all access measures[8] (NCHS, 2016). People living in low-income households are at an elevated risk of poor health, and access to care is vital for this vulnerable population. The ACA authorized states to expand Medicaid coverage to adults with low incomes up to 138 percent of the poverty level. From 2013 to 2014, the percent of adults who were uninsured declined in all states, with the decline in the number of uninsured being greater in the states that opted to expand their Medicaid programs (NCHS, 2016).

Racial and ethnic disparities in mental health services exist as well. Members of racial and ethnic minority groups are less likely than whites to receive necessary mental health care and more likely to receive poor-quality care when treated. Specifically, minority patients are less likely than whites to receive the best available treatments for depression and anxiety (McGuire and Miranda, 2008). Among the barriers to access to care, the

---

[8] Measures of access to care tracked in the 2015 National Healthcare Quality and Disparities Report include having health insurance, having a usual source of care, encountering difficulties when seeking care, and receiving care as soon as wanted.

lack of culturally competent care can be a barrier for specific racial and ethnic groups who face stigma due to cultural norms (Wahowiak, 2015).

The health care system has an important role to play in addressing the social determinants of health. At the community level, it can partner with community-based organizations and explore locally based interventions (Heiman and Artiga, 2015), creating payment models that take into account social determinants and implementing service delivery models that lend themselves to more community engagement and intervention. Health care systems can center equity by involving the community in decision making, allocating resources to act on the determinants of health in mind, and increasing community-based spending (Baum et al., 2009). Communities can be viewed as places of change for health systems, allowing for work both at micro and macro levels. (See Box 3-7 for an example of a community-based health system.) Cost-effective interventions to reduce health disparities and promote health equity should be recognized and explored, including attention to the structural barriers that affect access to health services.

Housing

Housing, as a social determinant of health, refers to the availability or lack of availability of high-quality, safe, and affordable housing for residents at varying income levels. Housing also encompasses the density within a housing unit and within a geographic area, as well as the overall level of segregation and diversity in an area based on racial and ethnic classifications or SES. Housing affects health because of the physical conditions within homes (e.g., lead, particulates, allergens), the conditions in a multi-residence structure (an apartment building or town home), the neighborhoods surrounding homes, and housing affordability, which affects financial stability and the overall ability of families to make healthy choices (Krieger and Higgins, 2002). The Center for Housing Policy has outlined 10 hypotheses on how affordable housing can support health improvement (Maqbool et al., 2015). These range from affordable housing freeing up resources for better nutrition and health care spending to stable housing reducing stress and the likelihood of poor health outcomes (e.g., for mental health or the management of chronic disease).

There is substantive evidence that the physical conditions in homes are important contributors to health outcomes (Cox et al., 2011; WHO, 2006). The World Health Organization (WHO) assessed the evidence in 2005 and found that sufficient evidence was available to estimate the burden of disease for physical factors, such as temperature extremes; chemical factors, such as environmental tobacco smoke and lead; biological factors, such as mold and dust mites; and building factors associated

> **BOX 3-7**
> **Kokua Kalihi Valley Comprehensive Family Services**
>
> Founded in 1972, Kohua Kahlihi Valley (KKV) Comprehensive Family Services is a nonprofit organization that is guided by a strong set of beliefs and culture and located in Honolulu, Hawaii. The guiding principles of KKV are:
>
> - Relationships are fundamental to us
> - We have a genuine commitment to our community and its diversity
> - We strive for programs and services that are extraordinary
> - We work collaboratively
> - We honor our heritage and traditions
>
> The services provided include
>
> - Primary medical care
> - Dental services
> - Behavioral health and quit tobacco services
> - Maternal and child health
> - Elder care
> - Public housing and enabling services
> - Medical–Legal Partnership for Children, Youth & Family
> - Returning to Our Roots, Ho`oulu `Āina
>
> Services are also provided on site at five local elementary and secondary schools. At Ho`oulu `Āina (the Kalihi Valley Nature Preserve), the KKV offers opportunities for community gardening, reforestation, environmental education, and the preservation of land-based cultural knowledge. This supports the reciprocal relationship between healing the land and fostering a healthy, resilient Kalihi Valley Community.
>
> SOURCE: Kokua Kalihi Valley, n.d.

with injuries and accidents. Since 2005 research has added to the areas where the WHO found some, but not sufficient, evidence to estimate the burden of disease, including more clarity on the relationship between rodent allergens and asthma (Ahluwalia et al., 2013; American College of Allergy Asthma and Immunology, 2014; Sedaghat et al., 2016). Data from the National Health and Nutrition Examination Survey show a decrease in blood lead levels between 1976 and 2002, with a steep drop between 1978 and 1988, probably due to lead being phased out of gasoline, and later a more gradual decrease, perhaps due to a reduction in the use of lead-based paint in housing (Jacobs et al., 2009). Conditions in multiunit residential buildings, including whether indoor smoking is permitted, are another dimension of housing that can affect health outcomes. Box 3-8

> **BOX 3-8**
> **Renovating the Rolling Hills Apartment Complex,
> St. Paul, Minnesota**
>
> St. Paul's East Side is home to a broad mix of immigrants, including Hmong, Somali, Karin, Bhutanese, Sudanese, Latinos, and African Americans and Native Americans. In 2012 Lutheran Social Services (LSS) and for-profit developers partnered to renovate the Rolling Hills Apartment Complex and convert it into official affordable housing. In doing so, the project addressed multiple social determinants of health, including education, health and health services, housing, income and wealth, the physical environment, and the social environment, resulting in the following enhancements to the Rolling Hills Apartment Complex:
>
> - Renovated apartments designed to serve families.
> - An LSS refugee and immigrant services office.
> - Emergency housing for arriving refugee families.
> - A clinic exam room operated by West Side Community Health Services, a federally qualified health center, and open to residents of both Rolling Hills Apartments and the surrounding community.
> - A community multipurpose room for community activities including community meetings, ESL classes, and support groups.
> - A community garden expansion.
> - Support for resident leadership of activities.
>
> Key factors to success were incentivizing funding, the involvement of partners willing to stretch from where they had gone before, and Twin Cities Local Initiatives Support Corporation's coordination and technical assistance in bringing all the pieces together. The last, a community health advocate model, is often difficult to fund, but was done so through a grant from the corporation's Healthy Futures Fund. Total project costs for the Rolling Hills Apartment Complex renovations were $14.8 million, including $9.5 million in [Low-Income Housing Tax Credit] equity and $4.8 million in bank and other loans, as well as city and state funding.
>
> SOURCE: Miller, 2015.

introduces the revitalization efforts of one multiunit apartment complex in a community in Minnesota.

Neighborhoods matter for a number of reasons, including their influence on physical safety and access to opportunity. The U.S. Department of Housing and Urban Development's (HUD's) Moving to Opportunity program was a 10-year demonstration program, which provided grants to public housing authorities in Baltimore, Boston, Chicago, Los Angeles, and New York City to implement an experimental study—a randomized controlled trial of a housing intervention. Housing authorities randomly selected experimental groups of households with children [to] receive housing counseling and vouchers that must be used in areas with less than 10 percent poverty. Families chosen for the experimental group receive tenant-based Section 8 rental assistance that helps pay their rent, as well as housing counseling to help them find and successfully use housing in low-poverty areas. Two control groups are included to test the effects of the program: one group already receiving Section 8 assistance and another just coming into the Section 8 program. (HUD, n.d.)

Homeless Populations

For homeless people, a lack of stable housing contributes to disparities in the social determinants. In addition to having direct ties with lack of employment and income, a lack of housing is also associated with greater barriers to education, lower levels of food security, and reduced public safety. Compared to the overall population, homeless people have shorter life expectancies, which are attributable to higher rates of substance abuse, infectious disease, and violence (Baggett et al., 2013). Infectious diseases—including HIV, tuberculosis, and heart disease—have all been linked to shorter life expectancies among homeless people (Fazel et al., 2014). Other studies have found drug overdose, cancer, and heart disease to be the greatest causes of death among the homeless, with greater barriers to and lower rates of screening, diagnosis, and treatment as contributing factors (Baggett et al., 2013).

The Changing American City

Neighborhoods generally change slowly, but urban neighborhoods are seeing dramatic shifts in demographics and property value and over time are becoming more segregated by income (Zuk et al., 2015). Gentrification—the process of renewal and rebuilding, which precedes the influx of new, more affluent residents—is a trend that is being observed in urban centers around the country (McKinnish et al., 2010; Phillips et al., 2014; Sturtevant, 2014). While the literature linking the process of gentrification to health outcomes is not definitive, there is substantial evidence that connects displacement and health outcomes (Zuk et al., 2015). Displacement can occur as a direct result of a policy or program (Freeman and Braconi, 2002), because of recent development and property value increases in an area, or as a result of exclusion from a property for various reasons (Levy et al., 2006).

Displacement has major implications for housing, other social determinants, and the health of communities. According to the CDC, displacement exacerbates health disparities by limiting access to healthy housing, healthy food options, transportation, quality schools, bicycle and walk paths, exercise facilities, and social networks (CDC, 2013). Displacement leads to poor housing conditions, including overcrowding and exposure to substandard housing with hazardous conditions (e.g., lead, mold, pests) (Phillips et al., 2014). Displacement can result in financial hardship, reducing disposable income for essential goods and services. This can have a negative impact on the health of the displaced population, with income being a significant determinant of health (CDC, 2013).

Physical Environment

The physical environment reflects the place, including the human-made physical components, design, permitted use of space, and the natural environment. Specific features of the physical or built environment include, but are not limited to, parks and open space, what is sold and how it is promoted, how a place looks and feels, air, water, soil, and arts and cultural expression (Davis et al., 2016). All of these physical factors shape the safety, accessibility, and livability of any locale, thus providing the context in which people live, learn, work, and play. This has direct implications for health. The physical environment contributes to 10 percent of health outcomes (Remington et al., 2015). Additionally, 40 percent of health outcomes depend on social and economic factors, which are intricately tied to the features of the physical environment (Remington et al., 2015). Inequities observed between the different physical environments of states, towns, and neighborhoods contribute to disparate health outcomes among their populations.

Exposure to a harmful physical environment is a well-documented threat to community health. Such threats include environmental exposures such as lead, particulate matter, proximity to toxic sites, water contamination, air pollution, and more—all of which are known to increase the incidence of respiratory diseases, various types of cancer, and negative birth outcomes and to decrease life expectancy (Wigle et al., 2007). Low-income communities and communities of color have an elevated risk of exposure to environmental hazards (Evans and Kantrowitz, 2002). In response to these inequities, the field of environmental justice seeks to achieve the "fair treatment and meaningful involvement of all people regardless of race, color, national origin, or income, with respect to the development, implementation, and enforcement of environmental laws, regulations, and policies" (EPA, 2016). Emerging considerations for low-income communities include the resulting gentrification and potential displacement of families when neighborhoods undergo revitalization that is driven by environmental clean-up efforts (Anguelovski, 2016).

Built Environment: Parks and Green Space

Access to green space has been demonstrated to positively affect health in many contexts. Such green space includes both parks and observable greenery. Living in the presence of more green space is associated with a reduced risk of mortality (Villeneuve et al., 2012). Nature has been shown to relieve stress and refocus the mind. Spending time in parks has been shown to improve mental health (Cohen et al., 2016a; Sturm and Cohen, 2014).

Beyond their benefits to mental health and reductions in stress, parks provide opportunities for increased physical activity. Local parks departments manage more than 108,000 outdoor public park facilities across the nation, many of them containing open space, jogging paths, and exercise equipment (Cohen et al., 2016b). According to Cohen et al., the average neighborhood park of 8.8 acres averaged 1,533 hours of active use per week (Cohen et al., 2016b). Individuals who are not as physically active face a greater risk of heart disease, diabetes, and cancer (James et al., 2016). In fact, about 9 percent of premature deaths in the United States are attributable to inactivity (Lee et al., 2012).

The usage of neighborhood parks and the associated health benefits are not equally distributed across communities. Research shows that recreational facilities are much less common in low-income and minority communities, though parks are more evenly distributed (Diez Roux et al., 2007). Moreover, the size and quality of park facilities vary based on race and income (Abercrombie et al., 2008). Accordingly, in low-income communities, residents are less likely to use parks (Cohen et al., 2016a). Beyond race and income, other disparities exist in park use. While seniors represent 20 percent of the population, they account for only 4 percent of park users (Cohen et al., 2016a). Proximity to park facilities also matters, as evidenced by a decrease in physical activity by more than half when distance between one's home and the park doubles (Giles-Corti and Donovan, 2002).

Food Environment

The food environment refers to the availability of food venues such as supermarkets, grocery stores, corner stores, and farmer's markets, including food quality and affordability. In communities described as food deserts, there is limited access to affordable and quality food. When there are fewer supermarkets, fruit and vegetable intake is lower, and prices are higher (Powell et al., 2007). This makes achieving a healthy diet difficult for local residents. Research indicates that a poor diet is associated with the development of cancer, diabetes, hypertension, birth defects, and heart disease (Willett et al., 2006).

The distribution of supermarkets is not equitable in the United States. Neighborhoods housing residents of lower socioeconomic status often have fewer supermarkets. Discrepancies also exist between racial and ethnic groups (Powell et al., 2007). Underserved communities turn to small grocery or corner stores to serve their food needs, but these businesses rarely provide the healthy selection offered by larger supermarkets. Moreover, food is most often higher priced in such stores.

Access to and the density of alcohol outlets are also associated with health outcomes in communities. In local areas where liquor store density is higher, alcohol consumption rates in the community are also higher (Pereiram et al., 2013). Alcoholism has been linked to diseases such as cancer, anemia, and mental illnesses. Moreover, alcohol outlets can serve as nuisance businesses, with their clientele bothering others in the neighborhood, decreasing the sense of security, and detracting from social cohesion. There is also evidence that links high-density alcohol outlet areas with higher rates of crime and substance use. In urban environments, a higher concentration of liquor stores is found in low-income, African American, and Hispanic communities, contributing to an elevated risk of alcohol-associated disorders in these neighborhoods (Berke et al., 2010).

A Changing Climate

Climate change has become a public health concern (Wang and Horton, 2015). There is a growing recognition that the physical environment is undergoing changes caused by human activity, such as through the production of greenhouse gases (IPCC, 2014). Human health is intricately linked to the places where we live, learn, work, and play. The air we breathe, the surrounding temperature, the availability of food, and whether there is access to clean water are all important ingredients to a healthy life, and the changing climate will affect all of these areas (Luber et al., 2014).

Not only do polluting emissions make air quality worse in the short term, but climate change itself will worsen air quality. Poor air quality exacerbates previous health conditions such as asthma and chronic obstructive pulmonary disease, and air pollution is associated with cardiovascular disease and many other illnesses. The changing climate is also causing a shift in seasons, which can affect pollen production and therefore seasonal allergies. Overall, with the changing climate there will be more extreme weather events such as increasing drought, vulnerability to wildfires, floods, hurricanes, and winter storms—all with subsequent health impacts from displacement, stress, or primary physical harm. The changing temperature is even having an impact on infectious diseases. New infectious diseases that spread via a vector, such as a tick or mosquito, have the potential to emerge in previously non-affected areas. There is also a risk for an increase in food-related and waterborne illness caused by the changing temperatures and the survival of various infectious agents. Food insecurity, which is already a challenge in many locations, is at risk of worsening due to higher food prices, poorer nutritional content, and new challenges with distribution.

Although climate change will affect everyone, certain communities and groups will be more vulnerable to these effects. People with preexisting medical conditions, children, elderly populations, and low-income groups are at increased risk for poor outcomes. Existing health disparities that are due to social, economic, and environmental factors have the potential to be even more affected by climate change.

However, climate change also presents a significant opportunity. Given the existential threat to humanity, there is now a great deal of momentum to mitigate and adapt to climate change. Companies are pursuing new business opportunities, governments are forming international agreements, and policies are being implemented at the national, subnational, state, regional, and local levels to affect change. Many of these policies to adapt to and mitigate climate change are also the key components in creating healthier, more equitable, and resilient communities. There are many co-benefits, and the policies, if implemented correctly, have the potential to significantly improve health outcomes and reduce health disparities (Rudolph et al., 2015). Examples of climate change mitigation and adaptation policies with co-benefits to build healthier, more equitable places include

- Improving access to public transit;
- Promoting flexible workplace transit;
- Creating more complete streets for better pedestrian and bicycle use;
- Implementing urban greening programs;
- Reducing urban heat islands through green space, cool roofs, and cool pavements;
- Promoting sustainable food systems and improved access;
- Building more walkable, dense, affordable housing and amenities;
- Reducing greenhouse gases;
- Promoting weatherizing homes, energy efficiency, and green buildings; and
- Greening fleets and reducing emissions.

Climate change will affect the physical environment in unprecedented ways. To mitigate and adapt to climate change will require multi-sector collaboration and approaches to effect systems change. Many of the same

> **BOX 3-9**
> **A Community Addressing Climate Change, Food Insecurity, and Improving Health Equity—Achieving Co-Benefits**
>
> **The Context**
>
> The City of Fresno is located in the heart of the Central Valley in California. It is a community with great diversity and is home to significant Hispanic/Latino (46.9 percent), Asian American (12.6 percent), and African American (8.3 percent) populations. In Fresno County alone there are more than 26,000 farmworkers, the majority being Hispanic/Latino and foreign born.
>
> **The Challenge and Opportunity**
>
> Fresno is the second most food insecure city in the United States, according to the 2014 Food Research and Action Center. At a county level, the statistics were just as concerning. As measured by the U.S. Department of Agriculture in 2011, 12 areas in Fresno County are classified as a food desert.
>
> - In 2014, 16 percent of Fresno County residents faced food insecurity, totaling more than 155,000 people (Feeding America, 2014b; U.S. Census Bureau, 2015).
> - In the cities of Fresno and Clovis alone, more than 64,000 people are food insecure; 80 percent do not have enough meat, bread, fruits and vegetables, and 71 percent of them have small children and do not have enough milk (Erro, n.d.).
> - One in three children in Fresno County struggles with hunger on a regular basis (Feeding America, 2014a).
> - In 2014, there were 81,200 food-insecure children in Fresno County (Feeding America, 2014b).
>
> At the same time, more globally, approximately 40 percent of food that is grown, processed, and transported in the United States is wasted. Food waste that goes

multi-sector partners required to address the social determinants of health also are already partnering on related climate change work in their communities, creating a substantial opportunity for change (see Box 3-9 for an example of a community engaged in climate change–related work).

Transportation

In the social determinants of health literature, transportation is typically discussed as a feature of the physical (or built) environment (TRB and IOM, 2005). This report highlights transportation as a separate determinant of health because of its multifaceted nature: pollution and to landfills emits gas that is bad for air quality and contributes to climate change. Working through multiple sectors with diverse partners, there is an unmet need and unique opportunity to tackle climate change and health equity by addressing both issues at the same time.

The Community-Driven Solution

Founded in 1970, Fresno Metro Ministry is a 501(c)(3) community-benefit organization started by churches to address the social, economic, health, and safety issues experienced by children and families that remained in neglected and disinvested neighborhoods. Metro evolved to become a multi-faith and multi-cultural organization dedicated to improving the health, environmental quality, economic development, and overall resiliency of the San Joaquin Valley.

In collaboration with many partners and driven by community priorities, Metro created the Food to Share program in 2015. Food to Share is a community food system partnership that works to fight against food insecurity and environmental issues. Food to Share has three main goals: to address hunger, reduce waste, and generate energy. They start by collecting excess food from schools, farmer's markets, food service facilities, restaurants, supermarkets, food distributors, hospitals, institutional cafeterias, growers and packers, gleanings, and food institutions. Once they have collected the food, they share it with churches, food kitchens, pantries, and distribution centers. These organizations then get the food out to the community in need. In the near future, the food that is unable to be used for healthy consumption will go to an anaerobic digester which is better for the environment and air quality and creates a low-carbon renewable source of energy. Over a period of 4 months, Food to Share has distributed nearly 180,000 pounds of donated and recovered food to neighborhoods in need, reducing greenhouse gas emissions by 396,000 pounds. This food reaches disadvantaged communities through Food to Share's food distribution events in six food desert neighborhoods in Fresno, in collaboration with the Fresno Public Health Department's Partnerships to Improve Community Health Farm-to-Table initiative.

---

greenhouse gas production; motor vehicle–related deaths and injuries; mobility and access to employment and vital goods and services; and active transportation. Transportation consists of the network, services, and infrastructure necessary to provide residents with the means to get from one place to another (Davis et al., 2016), and it is also vital to accessing goods, services (including health and social services), social networks, and employment. If designed and maintained properly, transportation facilitates safe mobility and is accessible to all residents, regardless of geographic location, age, or disability status. However, current research suggests that transportation costs are a barrier to mobility for households in poverty, which are disproportionately represented by African

Americans and Hispanics (FHWA, 2014). Long commute times and high transportation costs are significant barriers to employment and financial stability (Roberto, 2008). Brookings researchers have concluded, based on analyses of census data, that the suburbanization of poverty is disproportionately affecting proximity to jobs for poor and minority populations as compared with their nonpoor and white peers (Kneebone and Holmes, 2015; Zimmerman et al., 2015).

Transportation presents unevenly distributed negative externalities, including air pollution, noise, and motor vehicle–related injuries and deaths that are more prevalent in low-income and minority communities with poor infrastructure (Bell and Cohen, 2014; US DOT, 2015). Low-income and minority populations are more likely to live near environmental hazards, including transportation-related sources of pollution and toxic emissions such as roadways, bus depots, and ports (McConville, 2013; NEJAC, 2009; Perez et al., 2012). See, for example, Shepard (2005/2006) on the high concentration of bus depots in West Harlem, which also has one of the highest rates of asthma in the nation. The Regional Asthma Management and Prevention collaborative, in Oakland, California, and the California Environmental Protection Agency's Air Resources Board, among others, have described the evidence on the relationship between asthma and exposures to diesel and other air pollution (California EPA, 2016; RAMP, 2009).

Active transportation—the promotion of walking and cycling for transportation complemented by public transportation or any other active mode—is a form of transportation that reduces environmental barriers to physical activity and can improve health outcomes (Besser and Dannenberg, 2005; Dannenberg et al., 2011). Since the mid-20th century, road design and transportation planning have centered on the automobile, with multiple and interconnected consequences for health and equity (IOM, 2014).

The relationship between physical activity and health is well established and was summarized by the U.S. Surgeon General's 1996 report *Physical Activity and Health* (HHS, 1996) and the U.S. Task Force on Community Preventive Services (U.S. Task Force on Community Preventive Services, 2001). The evidence on the relationship among active transportation, physical activity, and health has been accumulating more recently. In a 2005 report from the Transportation Research Board and the Institute of Medicine, the authoring committee stated that "[r]esearch has not yet identified causal relationships to a point that would enable the committee to provide guidance about cost beneficial investments or state unequivocally that certain changes to the built environment would lead to more physical activity or be the most efficient ways of increasing such activity" (TRB and IOM, 2005, p. 10). Since then, Pucher et al. (2010) found "statistically significant negative relationships" between active travel (walking and cycling) and self-reported obesity as well as between active travel and diabetes (Pucher et al., 2010).

McCormack and Shiell conducted a systematic review of 20 cross-sectional studies and 13 quasi-experimental studies and concluded that most associations "between the built environment and physical activity were in the expected direction or null" (McCormack and Shiell, 2011). They also found that physical activity was considerably influenced by "land use mix, connectivity and population density and overall neighborhood design" and that "the built environment was more likely to be associated with transportation walking compared with other types of physical activity including recreational walking" (McCormack and Shiell, 2011).

CDC has developed a set of transportation recommendations that address all of the facets described above and has also developed a Transportation Health Impact Assessment Toolkit.[9] The CDC and the U.S. Department of Transportation (DOT) have also developed a Transportation and Health Tool to share indicator data on transportation and health.[10]

There have been multiple national initiatives in the past two to three decades aiming to improve livability and sustainability in places across the United States, and transportation equity is a mainstay of much of this work. (See Box 3-10 for an example of a regional transportation planning agency that seeks to improve access to transportation.) Initiatives have ranged from the federal Sustainable Communities Partnership,[11] launched by the DOT, HUD, and the U.S. Environmental Protection Agency in 2009 to help U.S. communities "improve access to affordable housing, increase transportation options, and lower transportation costs while protecting the environment," to Safe Routes to School, which aims to improve children's safety while walking and riding bicycles.[12]

Social Environment

How the social environment is conceptualized varies depending on the source (Barnett and Casper, 2001; HealthyPeople 2020, 2016). However, there are common elements identified by the literature that collectively shape a community's social environment as a determinant of health.

---

[9] For more information, see https://www.cdc.gov/healthyplaces/transportation/hia_toolkit.htm (accessed September 21, 2016).

[10] For more information, see https://www.transportation.gov/transportation-health-tool (accessed September 21, 2016).

[11] For more information, see https://www.sustainablecommunities.gov/mission/about-us (accessed September 21, 2016).

[12] For more information, see http://www.saferoutesinfo.org (accessed September 21, 2016).

> **BOX 3-10**
> **The Nashville Metropolitan Planning Organization**
>
> The Nashville Metropolitan Planning Organization (MPO) is a local planning agency for seven counties in Tennessee. The MPO also functions as a convener for local communities and state leaders to collaborate on strategic planning for the region's multi-modal transportation system. The mission of the organization is to "develop policies and programs that direct public funds to transportation projects that increase access to opportunity and prosperity, while promoting the health and wellness of Middle Tennesseans and the environment."
>
> The Nashville MPO developed a regional transportation plan in 2015 and outlined the following objectives to help communities grow in a healthy and sustainable way by:
>
> - Aligning transportation decisions with economic development initiatives, land use planning, and open-space conservation efforts;
> - Integrating healthy community design strategies and promoting active transportation to improve the public health outcomes of the built environment;
> - Encouraging the deployment of context-sensitive solutions to ensure that community values are not sacrificed for mobility improvement;
> - Incorporating the arts and creative place-making into planning and public works projects to foster innovative solutions and to enhance the sense of place and belonging;
> - Pursuing solutions that promote social equity and contain costs for transportation and housing; and
> - Minimizing the vulnerability of transportation assets to extreme weather events.
>
> The criteria by which the MPO plans to evaluate its projects include indicators related to health, such as physical activity, air quality, and traffic collisions.
>
> SOURCE: Nashville Area Metropolitan Planning Organization, n.d.

For the purposes of this report, the social environment can be thought of as reflecting the individuals, families, businesses, and organizations within a community; the interactions among them; and norms and culture. It can include social networks, capital, cohesion, trust, participation, and willingness to act for the common good in relation to health. *Social cohesion* refers to the extent of connectedness and solidarity among groups in a community, while *social capital* is defined as the features of social structures (e.g., interpersonal trust, norms of reciprocity, and mutual aid) that serve as resources for individuals and facilitate collective action (Kawachi and Berkman, 2000).

A 2008 systematic review found associations between trust as an indicator of social cohesion and better physical health, especially with respect to self-rated health. Furthermore, it revealed a pattern in which the association between social capital and better health outcomes was especially salient in inegalitarian countries (i.e., countries with a high degree of economic inequity), such as the United States, as opposed to more egalitarian societies (Kim et al., 2008).

The social environment in a community is often measured as it relates to mental health outcomes. For example, social connections between neighbors (i.e., greater social cohesion, social capital, and reciprocal exchanges between neighbors) are protective against depression (Diez Roux and Mair, 2010). Factors such as exposure to violence, hazardous conditions, and residential instability are all associated with depression and depressive symptoms (Diez Roux and Mair, 2010).

It is important to note that high levels of social capital and a strong presence of social networks are not necessarily guarantors of a healthy community. In fact, they can be sources of strain as well as support (Pearce and Smith, 2003). Some studies explore the potential drawbacks of social capital, such as the contagion of high-risk behaviors (e.g., suicidal ideation, injection drug use, alcohol and drug use among adolescents, smoking, and obesity) (Bearman and Moody, 2004; Christakis and Fowler, 2007; Friedman and Aral, 2001; Valente et al., 2004).

Mechanisms

McNeill et al. (2006) postulate that the following are mechanisms by which features of the social environment influence health behaviors:

- Social support and social networks enable or constrain the adoption of health-promoting behaviors; provide access to resources and material goods; provide individual and coping responses; buffer negative health outcomes; and restrict contact to infectious diseases.
- Social cohesion and social capital shape the ability to enforce and reinforce group or social norms for positive health behaviors and the provision of tangible support (e.g., transportation).

The social environment interacts with features of the physical environment at the neighborhood level to shape health behaviors, stress, and, ultimately, health outcomes (Diez Roux and Mair, 2010). For example, a built environment that is poor in quality (i.e., low walkability, fewer parks or open space, unsafe transportation) can contribute to a lack of structural opportunities for social interactions, resulting in limited social networks in a community (Suglia et al., 2016). Other research points to the role of physical activity as a potential pathway by which the social environment affects health outcomes such as obesity (Suglia et al., 2016).

At the community level, an important element of the social environment that can mediate health outcomes is the presence of neighborhood stressors. While the occurrence of stress is a daily facet of life that all people experience, chronic or toxic stress, in which the burden of stress accumulates, is a factor in the expression of disease (McEwen, 2012). Stressful experiences are particularly critical during early stages of life, as evidenced by the adverse childhood experiences study (Felitti et al., 1998), and are associated with abnormal brain development (IOM, 2000; Shonkoff and Garner, 2012). For low-income communities, stressors are salient because of the lack of resources, the presence of environmental hazards, unemployment, and exposure to violence, among other factors (McEwen, 2012; Steptoe and Feldman, 2001). (See Box 3-11 for an example of a community working to combat these stressors.) This applies as well to children in low-income households, who are more likely to experience multiple stressors that can harm health and development (Evans and Kim, 2010), mediated by chronic stress (Evans et al., 2011).

Chronic stress due to adverse neighborhood and family conditions has been linked to the academic achievement gap, in which children living in poverty fall behind those in better-resourced neighborhoods (Evans et al., 2011; Zimmerman and Woolf, 2014). Furthermore, stress and poor health in childhood are associated with decreased cognitive development, increased tobacco and drug use, and a higher risk of cardiovascular disease, diabetes, depression, and other conditions (County Health Rankings, 2016).

Public Safety

Public safety and violence are significant, intertwined social determinants of health, but they are also each significant indicators of health and community well-being in their own right. Public safety refers to the safety and protection of the public, and it is often characterized as the absence of violence in public settings (Davis et al., 2016). Since the late 1960s, homicide and suicide (another form of violence) have consistently ranked among the top leading causes of death in the United States (Dahlberg and Mercy, 2009).

Violent victimization affects health by causing psychological and physical injury, which can lead to disability and, in some cases, premature death. Beyond the risk of injury and death, violent victimization also has far-reaching health consequences for individuals, families, and neighborhoods. Furthermore, research shows that simply being exposed

> **BOX 3-11**
> **Cowlitz Community Network**
>
> From 1994 to 2012, 53 communities across Washington State set up networks to address youth violence. The Family Policy Council helped these groups establish processes to cultivate leadership and broad partnerships, work with local citizens to set priorities and goals, use evidence to make decisions, and continue educating themselves. Over the years, the Family Policy Council also disseminated research about the connections between adverse childhood experiences and associate risks for social and health problems such as academic failure, mental and physical illness, substance abuse, and violence.[a]
>
> One such network is the Cowlizt Community Network, which was formed in 1995 and whose mission is to bring the community together and create opportunities to help at-risk youth and families succeed. Its initiatives focus on improving the child maternal health system in Cowlitz County and connecting young, at-risk mothers to the resources they need to help them and their children. In addition, through collaboration with Longview Anti-Drug Coalition, it is expanding the Community Resource Directory to include comprehensive information about services offered in Cowlitz and surrounding counties to help individuals and families in need. Another aspect of its work is hosting conversations on neuroscience, epigenetics, adverse childhood experiences, and resiliency—a holistic perspective of a person's experiences over a lifetime.
>
> An evaluation of the Washington State networks found that the work of funded community networks had a positive effect in reducing county level health and safety problems and that community capacity development processes led by funded community networks were a key to success.
>
> ---
> [a] For more information, see http://www.cowlitzcommunitynetwork.com (accessed October 20, 2016).
> SOURCE: Hall et al., 2012.

to violence can have detrimental effects on physical and psychological well-being (Felitti et al., 1998; Pinderhughes et al., 2015). Violent victimization and exposure to violence have been linked to poor health outcomes, including chronic diseases (e.g., ischemic heart disease, cancer, stroke, chronic obstructive lung disease, diabetes, and hepatitis), asthma-related symptoms, obesity, posttraumatic stress disorder, depression, and substance abuse (Prevention Institute, 2011). For youth in schools, the data suggest that there is a cumulative effect of exposure to violence, with multiple exposures to violence being associated with higher rates of youth reporting their health as "fair" or "poor" (Egerter et al., 2011a). There is also research that indicates a link between neighborhood crime rates and adverse birth outcomes such as preterm birth and low birth weight (Egerter et al., 2011a).

Violence and the fear of violence can negatively affect other social determinants that further undermine community health. Violence rates can lead to population loss, decreased property values and investments in the built environment, increased health care costs, and the disruption of the provision of social services (Massetti and Vivolo, 2010; Velez et al., 2012). In addition, violence in communities is associated with reduced engagement in behaviors that are known to promote health, such as physical activity and park use (Cohen et al., 2010).

The perception of safety is a key indicator of violence in a community that is associated with health. For example, people who describe their neighborhoods as not safe are almost three times more likely to be physically inactive than those who describe their neighborhood as extremely safe (Prevention Institute, 2011). The perception of safety is also important for mental health. There is research that suggests that perceived danger and the fear of violence can influence stress, substance use, anger, anxiety, and feelings of insecurity—all of which compromise the psychological well-being of a community (Moiduddin and Massey, 2008; Perkins and Taylor, 1996). At the community level, fear of crime and violence can undermine social organization, social cohesion, and civic participation—all key elements in a social environment that is conducive to optimal health (Perkins and Taylor, 1996). Low perception of safety can also undermine the efforts of a community to improve the built environment through the availability of parks and open space to promote physical activity (Cohen et al., 2016a; Weiss et al., 2011).

Violence is not a phenomenon that affects all communities equally, nor is it distributed randomly. The widespread disparity in the occurrence of violence is a major facet of health inequity in the United States. Low-income communities are disproportionately affected by violence and by the many effects that it can have on physical and mental well-being. The conditions of low-income communities (concentrated poverty, low housing values, and high schools with low graduation rates among others), foster violence and put residents at an increased risk of death from homicide (Prevention Institute, 2011). This holds true for other types of violence as well. Living in poor U.S. neighborhoods puts African American and white women at an increased risk for intimate partner violence compared with women who reside in areas that are not impoverished (Prevention Institute, 2011).

Criminologists attribute the disparities in neighborhood violence not to the kinds of people living in certain neighborhoods but to the vast differences in social and economic conditions that characterize communities in the United States. Some refer to these differences as "divergent social worlds" and the "racial–spatial divide" (Peterson and Krivo, 2010). This is because there are specific racial and ethnic groups, such as African Americans, Hispanics, and Native Americans, who are vastly overrepresented in communities that are at risk for violence because of the social and economic conditions. Residential segregation, which has been perpetuated by discriminatory housing and mortgage market practices, affects the quality of neighborhoods by increasing poverty, poor housing conditions, and social disorder and by limiting economic opportunity for residents (Prevention Institute, 2011).

As a result of the racial–spatial divide in community conditions, the violent crime rate in majority nonwhite neighborhoods is two to five times higher than in majority white neighborhoods. This is especially true for youth of color, particularly males. Overall homicide rates among 10- to 24-year-old African American males (60.7 per 100,000) and Hispanic males (20.6 per 100,000) exceed that of white males in the same age group (3.5 per 100,000) (Prevention Institute, 2011). African American males 15 to 19 years old are six times as likely to be homicide victims as their white peers (Prevention Institute, 2011). More specifically, African American males ages 15 to 19 are almost four times as likely to be victims of firearm-related homicides as white males (Prevention Institute, 2011). In terms of exposure to violence, African American and Hispanic youth are more likely to be exposed to shootings, riots, domestic violence, and murder than their white counterparts (Prevention Institute, 2011). This has major implications for trauma in communities that are predominantly African American or Hispanic. Native American communities also suffer from a disproportionately high violent crime rate that is two to three times higher than the national average (Prevention Institute, 2011). Box 3-12 briefly describes a public health–oriented model to address violence in communities.

BOX 3-12
The Cure Violence Health Model

The Cure Violence Health model applies principles drawn from epidemic disease outbreak control. The model uses three components: (a) identifying and preventing transmission, (b) reducing the risk of the highest risk, and (c) changing community norms (Cure Violence, n.d.-a). The model has been implemented in several U.S. cities including Baltimore, Chicago, Kansas City, New Orleans, New York, and Philadelphia as well as internationally. The model is characterized by the use of trained violence interrupters and culturally appropriate outreach workers to implement the model, partnerships with local hospitals, and continual data collection and monitoring.

continued

BOX 3-12 Continued

Identifying and Preventing Transmission

- Prevent retaliations: At the time of a shooting, workers immediately work in the community and at the hospital with victims and others related to the event to cool down emotions and prevent retaliations.
- Mediate ongoing conflicts: Through talking to key people in the community about situations (e.g., ongoing disputes, recent arrests, recent prison releases), workers identify ongoing conflicts and use mediation techniques to resolve them without violence.
- Keep conflicts "cool": Workers follow up with conflicts for as long as needed to ensure that the conflict does not become violent.

Reducing Risk of the Highest Risk

- Access highest risk: Building upon their trust with high-risk individuals, workers establish contact, develop relationships, and begin to work with the people most likely to be involved in violence.
- Change behaviors: Workers engage with high-risk individuals to convince them to reject the use of violence by discussing the cost and consequences of violence and teaching alternative responses to potentially violent situations.
- Provide treatment: Workers engage intensively with a caseload of clients and assist them with their needs such as drug treatment, employment, leaving gangs.

Changing Community Norms

- Respond to every shooting: Whenever a shooting occurs, workers organize a response where dozens of community members (e.g., local business owners, faith leaders, service providers) voice their objection to the shooting.
- Organize community: Workers coordinate with existing and establish new block clubs, tenant councils, and neighborhood associations to assist with changing community norms.
- Spread positive norms: To convey the message that violence is not acceptable, the program distributes materials and hosts events.

The model's apparent effectiveness has been documented in multiple communities (Blount-Hill and Butts, 2015; Butts et al., 2015; Cure Violence, n.d.-b; Picard-Fritsche and Cerniglia, 2013). Changes include decreased shootings, decreased killings, reduction in retaliations, improved attitudes toward violence, and evidence of norm change that violence is not acceptable.

SOURCES: Cure Violence, n.d.-a,b.

Child Abuse and Neglect

Child abuse and neglect are two important measures of community violence that can affect physical and mental health. The Institute of Medicine and the National Research Council published a report (2014) that cited abuse and neglect during childhood as a contributor to the following health-related outcomes: problems with growth and motor development, lower self-reported health, gastrointestinal symptoms, obesity, delinquency and violence, and alcohol abuse (IOM and NRC, 2014).

In 1998, Felitti and colleagues published a pivotal study which demonstrated a link between adverse childhood experiences and the leading causes of death in adults at the time. The authors found a strong, graded association between the amount of exposure to abuse or household dysfunction and multiple risk factors (e.g., smoking, severe obesity, physical inactivity, depressed mood, and suicide attempts) for several leading causes of death (Felitti et al., 1998). Child abuse and neglect not only affect health directly, they also affect outcomes within the other social determinants of health, such as education, work, and social relationships (IOM and NRC, 2014). While the overall rates of child maltreatment have been declining since 2002, rates are still much higher for African American (14.3 per 1,000), Native American (11.4 per 1,000), multiracial (10.1 per 1,000), and Hispanic (8.6 per 1,000) children than for white children (7.9 per 1,000) (IOM and NRC, 2014; Prevention Institute, 2011). Child abuse and neglect are often accompanied by family stressors and other forms of family violence (IOM and NRC, 2014). As discussed above, the conditions of concentrated poverty in a neighborhood are associated with violence incidence. According to the Prevention Institute, the higher the percentage of families living below the federal poverty level in a neighborhood, the higher the rate of child maltreatment (Prevention Institute, 2011).

Hate Crimes

Hate crimes, which may or may not involve physical violence, are often motivated by some bias against a perceived characteristic.[13] An FBI analysis of single-bias hate crime incidents revealed that in 2014, 48.3 percent of victims were targeted because of the offender's bias against race, and 62.7 percent of those victims were targeted because of anti-African American bias (UCR, 2015). Among hate crimes motivated by bias toward a particular ethnicity in 2014, almost 48 percent of the victims were targeted because of anti-Hispanic bias (UCR, 2015).

---

[13] The Hate Crimes Statistics Act (28 U.S.C. § 534) defines hate crimes as "crimes that manifest evidence of prejudice based on race, gender or gender identity, religion, disability, sexual orientation, or ethnicity."

As is the case with other types of violence, exposure to hate crime violence can have pernicious effects on health. For lesbian, gay, bisexual, and transgender (LGBT) persons specifically, exposure to hate crimes at the community level has been linked to increased rates of suicide among youth, marijuana use, and all-cause mortality (Duncan and Hatzenbuehler, 2014; Duncan et al., 2014; Hatzenbuehler et al., 2014). Discrimination in general, which by definition is the driving factor behind the perpetration of hate crimes, has been shown to affect the health of individuals and communities. Whether it be perceived discrimination in everyday encounters or systemic discrimination in housing policies, this type of unequal treatment has been associated with major depression, psychological distress, stress, increased pregnancy risk, mortality, hypertension, and more health-related outcomes (Dolezsar et al., 2014; Galea et al., 2011; Kessler et al., 1999; Padela and Heisler, 2010; Sims et al., 2012).

Criminal Justice System

The criminal justice system is a key actor, setting, and driver of public safety as it relates to health equity. Specifically, the criminal justice system's role in the mass incarceration of racial and ethnic minorities is an important factor when examining the social determinants of health (NRC, 2014). The past 40–50 years have seen a large-scale expansion of incarceration, which has had lasting effects on families and communities (Cloud, 2014; Drake, 2013). This expansion has affected racial and ethnic minority groups, and particularly men (Drake, 2013). Research suggests that disproportionately more Hispanics and African Americans are confined in jails and prisons than would be predicted by their arrest rates and that Hispanic and African American juveniles are more likely than white juveniles to be referred to adult court rather than juvenile court (Harris, 2009).

When those who were formerly incarcerated are released back into their communities, successful reentry is hindered by a number of obstacles, such as stigma, limited employment and housing opportunities, and the lack of a cohesive social network (Lyons and Pettit, 2011). All of these factors are vital to achieving optimal health, and for communities with high rates of incarceration, the absence of these opportunities can lead to a diminished capacity to combat crime and mobilize for resources (Clear, 2008). It is important to examine the patterns and effects of mass incarceration because it not only affects the health of incarcerated populations but also has a detrimental effect on multiple determinants of health in communities. Mass incarceration has contributed to the breakdown of educational opportunities, family structures, economic mobility, housing options, and neighborhood cohesion, especially in low-income communities of color (Cloud, 2014). Neal and Rick examined U.S. Census data from

1960 to 2010 and found that although great progress was made in closing the black–white education and employment gap up until the 1980s, that progress then came to a halt in large part due to rising incarceration rates (Neal and Rick, 2014). In addition, communities with high levels of incarceration have higher rates of lifetime major depressive disorder and generalized anxiety disorder (Hatzenbuehler et al., 2015).

Wildeman estimated the effects of incarceration on population-level infant mortality rates, and his findings suggest that if incarceration rates remained the same as they were in 1973, the infant mortality rate in 2003 would have been 7.8 percent lower and the absolute African American–white disparity in infant mortality would have been 14.8 percent lower (Wildeman, 2012). A keen understanding of the precise mechanisms by which incarceration affects the health of specific populations and contributes to health inequity is needed to reduce disparities in key health outcomes such as infant mortality.

CONCLUDING OBSERVATIONS

The root causes of health inequity begin with historical and contemporary inequities that have been shaped by institutional and societal structures, policies, and norms in the United States. As discussed in this chapter, these deeply rooted inequities have shaped inequitable experiences of the social and other determinants of health: education, income and wealth, employment, health systems and services, housing, the physical environment, transportation, the social environment, and public safety.

Conclusion 3-2: Based on its review of the evidence, the committee concludes that health inequities are the result of more than individual choice or random occurrence. They are the result of the historic and ongoing interplay of inequitable structures, policies, and norms that shape lives.

These structures, policies, and norms—such as segregation, redlining and foreclosure, and implicit bias—play out on the terrain of the social, economic, environmental, and cultural determinants of health.

What Can Academic Research Do?

The current public health interest in the role of place, including communities, stems from significant empirical epidemiological evidence. As discussed in this chapter, there are a range of factors that contribute to health and that need to be more extensively studied. These include factors beyond the individual domain, such as living and working conditions and economic policies at the local, state, and national levels that are intimately connected to health and well-being. Likewise, the American Public Health Association's (APHA's) 2014 and 2015 conference themes on the geography of health and health in all policies, respectively, reflect a growing recognition of the need for action on social and environmental factors in order to achieve the goal of becoming the healthiest nation in one generation (APHA, 2016).

At a meeting of the National Academies of Sciences, Engineering, and Medicine's Roundtable on Population Health Improvement in 2013, David Williams asked, "How could we expect that the lives and health of our patients would improve if they continued to live in the same conditions that contributed to their illness?" (IOM, 2013). His question points to a fundamental challenge to improving the public's health and promoting health equity. This recognition that inequities in social arrangements and community factors shape life opportunities is not new; it was asserted as early as 1906 by W. E. B. Du Bois in his address regarding the role of social status and life conditions in shaping health and inequities. Du Bois reported findings from the 11th Atlanta Conference on the Study of the Negro Problem held at Atlanta University, which in part concluded that "the present difference in mortality seems to be sufficiently explained by conditions of life" (DuBois, 1906).

Despite the increasingly widespread recognition in the field, many public health efforts continue to target individuals and are most often disease specific. The existing approaches to prevention and health promotion are still "catching up" with what is known about the social determinants of health and population health. Kindig and Stoddart pointed out that "much of public health activity, in the United States at least, does not have such a broad mandate" (Kindig and Stoddart, 2003, p. 382). Building the science base for how to move upstream to improve population health has begun. While our understanding of the role of the social determinants of health, including features of the physical and social environments, has greatly improved over the last several decades, the scientific progress has not been so great on how, when, and where to intervene. Progress on how to move upstream in taking action has developed much more slowly than progress in the ability to describe the role of context and community-level factors that shape the major causes of morbidity, mortality, and well-being (Amaro, 2014).

Improving the science of population health interventions, place-based approaches, and strategies to improve health equity will require a workforce of scientists and practitioners equipped to develop the requisite knowledge base and practice tools. As Kindig and Stoddart noted, social epidemiology has made highly important contributions to our understanding of the social determinants of health and population health but "does not have the breadth, or imply all of the multiple interactions and pathways" involved in population health (Kindig and Stoddart, 2003, p. 382). Diez Roux and Mair describe social epidemiology's most critical conceptual and methodological challenges as well as promising directions in studying neighborhood health effects (Diez Roux and Mair, 2010). Specifically, models for the training of population and place-based scientists and practitioners are needed to develop the research required to guide upstream approaches—including place-based interventions—that will address the contextual factors that shape major public health problems such as obesity, interpersonal violence, infant and maternal health, cardiovascular diseases, infectious diseases, substance abuse, and mental health disorders. For example, training models such as the interdisciplinary team science McArthur Model described by Adler and Stewart could be expanded to integrate public health practitioners and community leaders alongside research leaders (Adler and Stewart, 2010b).

Translating knowledge on the social determinants of health into practice requires at least four essential areas of expertise:

1. An understanding of theories that articulate the complex mechanisms of action in the social determinants of health and how place influences health.
2. Expertise in the design of community-level interventions and in models of community–academic partnerships.
3. Expertise in the complex issues of study design, measurement, and analytic methods in assessing changes resulting from interventions focused on population-level impacts and community-level health improvement.
4. Expertise and understanding of various socio-demographic groups, cultures, and varied sector stakeholders and drivers that shape sustained stakeholder engagement in improving population health and community conditions.

Considering the distinct fields of expertise required for these components and theory, the approaches to intervention and measurement stem from different disciplines and have often been developed without significant interchange. Researchers face significant challenges. Thus, academic institutions involved in the training of population and place-based scientists need to integrate these diverse bodies of knowledge—including theory, methods, and tools from diverse disciplines. Models for the transdisciplinary training of researchers, practitioners, and community partners are needed. Academic institutions need to develop models for intra-professional workforce training on place-based and community-level implementation science and evaluation that target improving population health and addressing health inequities. See Chapter 7 for more on the role of academic research in community solutions to promote health equity.

The social determinants of health, while interdependent and complex, are made up of mutable factors that shape the conditions in which one lives, learns, works, plays, worships, and ages. As highlighted in the boxes throughout this chapter, communities around the country are taking it upon themselves to address these conditions. Chapter 4 will discuss why communities are powerful agents of change, along with discussing the conditions necessary for successful and sustainable outcomes. Chapter 5 will provide an in-depth overview of nine communities that are addressing the root causes of health inequities.

REFERENCES

Abercrombie, L. C., J. F. Sallis, T. L. Conway, L. D. Frank, B. E. Saelens, and J. E. Chapman. 2008. Income and racial disparities in access to public parks and private recreation facilities. *American Journal of Preventive Medicine* 34(1):9–15.

Acevedo-Garcia, D. 2000. Residential segregation and the epidemiology of infectious diseases. *Social Science & Medicine* 51(8):1143–1161.

Adler, N. E., and J. Stewart. 2010a. Preface to the biology of disadvantage: Socioeconomic status and health. *Annals of the New York Academy of Sciences* 1186(1):1–4.

Adler, N. E., and J. Stewart. 2010b. Using team science to address health disparities: MacArthur network as case example. *Annals of the New York Academy of Sciences* 1186: 252–260.

Ahluwalia, S. K., R. D. Peng, P. N. Breysse, G. B. Diette, J. Curtin-Brosnan, C. Aloe, and E. C. Matsui. 2013. Mouse allergen is the major allergen of public health relevance in Baltimore City. *Journal of Allergy and Clinical Immunology* 132(4):830–835, e831–e832.

AHRQ (Agency for Healthcare Research and Quality). 2016. 2015 National Healthcare Quality and Disparities Report and 5th anniversary update on the National Quality Strategy. AHRQ Pub., No. 16-0015. Rockville, MD: U.S. Department of Health and Human Services.

Aizer, A., J. Currie, P. Simon, and P. Vivier. 2015. Inequality in lead exposure and the blackwhite test score gap. Institute for Public Policy and Social Research. https://www.ippsr.msu.edu/research/inequality-lead-exposure-and-black-white-test-score-gap (accessed December 9, 2016).

Alhusen, J. L., K. M. Bower, E. Epstein, and P. Sharps. 2016. Racial discrimination and adverse birth outcomes: An integrative review. *Journal of Midwifery and Women's Health* October:1–14.

Amaro, H. 2014. The action is upstream: Place-based approaches for achieving population health and health equity. *American Journal of Public Health* 104(6):964.

American College of Allergy Asthma and Immunology. 2014. Mouse infestations cause more asthma symptoms than cockroach exposure. https://www.sciencedaily.com/releases/2014/11/141107091226.htm (accessed September 21, 2016).

An, J., P. Braveman, M. Dekker, S. Egerter, and R. Grossman-Kahn. 2011. Work, workplaces, and health. Princeton, NJ: Robert Wood Johnson Foundation.

Anguelovski, I. 2016. From toxic sites to parks as (green) LULUs? New challenges of inequity, privilege, gentrification, and exclusion for urban environmental justice. *Journal of Planning Literature* 31(1):23–36.

APA (American Psychological Association). 2016. Stress in America: The impact of discrimination. Stress in America™ Survey. Washington, DC: American Psychological Association.
APA Task Force on Socioeconomic Status. 2007. Report of the APA Task Force on Socioeconomic Status. Washington, DC: American Psychological Association.
APHA (American Public Health Association). 2016. Past and future annual meetings. American Public Health Association. https://www.apha.org/events-and-meetings/annual/past-and-future-annual-meetings (accessed December 12, 2016).
Baggett, T. P., S. W. Hwang, J. J. O'Connell, B. C. Porneala, E. J. Stringfellow, E. J. Orav, D. E. Singer, and N. A. Rigotti. 2013. Mortality among homeless adults in Boston: Shifts in causes of death over a 15-year period. *JAMA Internal Medicine* 173(3):189–195.
Baker, D. P., J. Leon, E. G. Smith Greenaway, J. Collins, and M. Movit. 2011. The education effect on population health: A reassessment. *Population and Development Review* 37(2):307–332.
Balfanz, R., L. Herzog, and D. J. Mac Iver. 2007. Preventing student disengagement and keeping students on the graduation path in urban middle-grades schools: Early identification and effective interventions. *Educational Psychologist* 42(4):223–235.
Barnett, E., and M. Casper. 2001. A definition of "social environment." *American Journal of Public Health* 91(3):465.
Barnett, W. S. 2013. Getting the facts right on pre-K and the President's pre-K proposal. New Brunswick, NJ: National Institute for Early Education Research.
Baum, F. E., M. Begin, T. A. J. Houweling, and S. Taylor. 2009. Changes not for the fainthearted: Reorienting health care systems toward health equity through action on the social. *American Journal of Public Health* 99(11):1967–1974.
Baum, S., J. Ma, and K. Payea. 2013. Education pays: The benefits of higher education for individuals and society. Trends in Higher Education. The College Board. http://trends.collegeboard.org/sites/default/files/education-pays-2013-full-report.pdf (accessed October 31, 2016).
Bearman, P. S., and J. Moody. 2004. Suicide and friendships among American adolescents. *American Journal of Public Health* 94(1):89–95.
Bell, J., and L. Cohen. 2014. The transportation prescription: Bold new ideas for healthy, equitable transportation reform in America. Oakland, CA: PolicyLink and Prevention Institute.
Berger, B. R. 2009. Red: Racism and the American Indian. *UCLA Law Review* 56(3):591–656.
Berger, M., and Z. Sarnyai. 2015. "More than skin deep": Stress neurobiology and mental health consequences of racial discrimination. *Stress* 18(1):1–10.
Berke, E. M., S. E. Tanski, E. Demidenko, J. Alford-Teaster, X. Shi, and J. D. Sargent. 2010. Alcohol retail density and demographic predictors of health disparities: A geographic analysis. *American Journal of Public Health* 100(10):1967–1971.
Bertrand, M., D. Chugh, and S. Mullainathan. 2005. Implicit discrimination. *American Economic Review* 95(2):94–98.
Besser, L. M., and A. L. Dannenberg. 2005. Walking to public transit: Steps to help meet physical activity recommendations. *American Journal of Preventive Medicine* 29(4):273–280.
Betancourt, J. R., and A. R. Green. 2010. Linking cultural competence training to improved health outcomes: Perspectives from the field. *Academic Medicine* 85(4):583–585.
Betancourt, J. R., J. Corbett, and M. R. Bondaryk. 2014. Addressing disparities and achieving equity: Cultural competence, ethics, and health-care transformation. *Chest* 145(1):143–148.
Bethell, C. D., P. Newacheck, E. Hawes, and N. Halfon. 2014. Adverse childhood experiences: Assessing the impact on health and school engagement and the mitigating role of resilience. *Health Affairs* 33(12):2106–2115.

Bishaw, A. 2011. Areas with concentrated poverty: 2006–2010. U.S. Cenus Bureau. http://www.census.gov/prod/2011pubs/acsbr10-17.pdf (accessed November 21, 2016).

Blakely, T. A., B. P. Kennedy, and I. Kawachi. 2001. Socioeconomic inequality in voting participation and self-rated health. *American Journal of Public Health* 91(1):99–104.

Blount-Hill, K.-L., and J. A. Butts. 2015. Respondent-driven sampling: Evaluating the effects of the Cure Violence model with neighborhood surveys. New York: John Jay College of Crimincal Justice, City University of New York.

BLS (U.S. Bureau of Labor Statistics). 2014. Labor force characteristics by race and ethnicity, 2013. Report 1050. U.S. Bureau of Labor Statistics.

Blumenshine, P., S. Egerter, C. J. Barclay, C. Cubbin, and P. A. Braveman. 2010. Socioeconomic disparities in adverse birth outcomes: A systematic review. *American Journal of Preventive Medicine* 39(3):263–272.

Boschma, J. 2016. Separate and still unequal. *The Atlantic*, March 1. http://www.theatlantic.com/education/archive/2016/03/separate-still-unequal/471720 (accessed December 12, 2016).

Boschma, J., and R. Brownstein. 2016. The concentration of poverty in American schools. *The Atlantic*. February 29. http://www.theatlantic.com/education/archive/2016/02/concentration-poverty-american-schools/471414 (accessed December 2, 2016).

Bradley, E. H., M. Canavan, E. Rogan, K. Talbert-Slagle, C. Ndumele, L. Taylor, and L. A. Curry. 2016. Variation in health outcomes: The role of spending on social services, public health, and health care, 2000–09. *Health Affairs* 35(5):760–768.

Braveman, P. 2006. Health disparities and health equity: Concepts and measurement. *Annual Review of Public Health* 27:167–194.

Braveman, P. 2008. Racial disparities at birth: The puzzle persists. *Issues in Science and Technology* 24(2):23–30.

Braveman, P., and L. Gottlieb. 2014. The social determinants of health: It's time to consider the causes of the causes. *Public Health Reports* 129(Suppl 2):19–31.

Braveman, P. A., C. Cubbin, S. Egerter, S. Chideya, K. S. Marchi, M. Metzler, and S. Posner. 2005. Socioeconomic status in health research: One size does not fit all. *JAMA* 294(22):2879–2888.

Braveman, P., S. Egerter, and D. R. Williams. 2011. The social determinants of health: Coming of age. *Annual Review of Public Health* 32:381–398.

Brown, D., and T. Tylka. 2011. Racial discrimination and resilience in African American young adults: Examining racial socialization as a moderator. *Journal of Black Psychology* 37(3):259–285.

Brown, D. J., A. L. DeCorse-Johnson, M. Irving-Ray, and W. W. Wu. 2005. Performance evaluation for diversity programs. *Policy, Politics & Nursing Practice* 6(4):331–344.

Brulle, R. J., and D. N. Pellow. 2006. Environmental justice: human health and environmental inequalities. *Annual Review Public Health* 27:103–124.

Buffie, N. 2015. The problem of black unemployment: Racial inequalities persist even amongst the unemployed. CEPR Blog, November 4. Washington, DC: Center for Economic and Policy Research. http://cepr.net/blogs/cepr-blog/the-problem-of-black-unemployment-racial-inequalities-persist-even-amongst-the-unemployed (accessed October 31, 2016).

Burgard, S., and J. Stewart. 2003. Occupational status. MacArthur Research Network on SES & Health. http://www.macses.ucsf.edu/research/socialenviron/occupation.php (accessed December 2, 2016).

Burgard, S., J. E. Brand, and J. S. House. 2007. Toward a better estimation of the effect of job loss on health. *Journal of Health and Social Behavior* 48(December):369–384.

Butler, M., E. McCreedy, N. Schwer, D. Burgess, K. Call, J. Przedworski, S. Rosser, S. Larson, M. Allen, S. Fu, and R. L. Kane. 2014. Improving cultural competence to reduce health disparities. AHRQ Publication No. 16-EHC006-EF. Prepared by Minnesota Evidence-based Practice Center for Agency for Healthcare Research and Quality. https://effectivehealthcare.ahrq.gov/ehc/products/573/2206/cultural-competence-report-160327.pdf (accessed December 2, 2016).

Butts, J. A., C. G. Roman, L. Bostwick, and J. R. Porter. 2015. Cure Violence: A public health model to reduce gun violence. *Annual Review of Health* 36:39–53.

California EPA (Environmental Protection Agency). 2016. Asthma and air pollution. https://www.arb.ca.gov/research/asthma/asthma.htm (accessed September 21, 2016).

Carnahan, S. 1994. Preventing school failure and dropout. In *Risk, resilience, and prevention: Promoting the well-being of all children*, edited by R. Simeonsson. Baltimore, MD: Brookes. Pp. 103–123.

Carter, P. L., and S. F. Reardon. 2014. Inequality matters. William T. Grant Foundation.

CDC (U.S. Centers for Disease Control and Prevention). 2013. Health effects of gentrification. http://www.cdc.gov/healthyplaces/healthtopics/gentrification.htm (accessed October 31, 2016).

Chall, J. S., V. A. Jacobs, and L. E. Baldwin. 1990. The reading crisis: Why poor children fall behind. Cambridge, MA: Harvard University Press.

Charles, C. Z. 2003. The dynamics of racial residential segregation. *Annual Review of Sociology* 29(1):167–207.

Chetty, R., N. Hendren, R. Chetty, N. Hendren, P. Kline, E. Saez, P. Kline, and E. Saez. 2014. Where is the land of opportunity? The geography of intergenerational mobility in the United States. *Quarterly Journal of Economics* 129(4):1553–1623.

Chetty, R., M. Stepner, S. Abraham, S. Lin, B. Scuderi, N. Turner, A. Bergeron, and D. Cutler. 2016. The association between income and life expectancy in the United States, 2001–2014. *JAMA* 315(16):1750–1766.

Chou, R. S., and J. R. Feagin. 2015. Myth of the model minority: Asian Americans facing racism, second edition. Boulder, CO: Paradigm Publishers..

Christ, T., and X. C. Wang. 2010. Bridging the vocabulary gap: What the research tells us about vocabulary instruction in early childhood. *Young Children*, 84–91.

Christakis, N. A., and J. H. Fowler. 2007. The spread of obesity in a large social network over 32 years. *The New England Journal of Medicine* 357(4):370–379.

Christian, L. M. 2012. Psychoneuroimmunology in pregnancy: Immune pathways linking stress with maternal health, adverse birth outcomes, and fetal development. *Neuroscience & Biobehavioral Reviews* 36(1):350–361.

Clear, T. R. 2008. The effects of high imprisonment rates on communities. *Crime and Justice* 37(1):97–132.

Cloud, D. 2014. On life support: Public health in the age of mass incarceration. New York: Vera Institute of Justice.

Clougherty, J. E., K. Souza, and M. R. Cullen. 2010. Work and its role in shaping the social gradient in health. *Annals of the New York Academy of Sciences* 1186:102–124.

Cobas, J. A., J. Duany, and J. R. Feagin. 2009. How the United States racializes Latinos: White hegemony and its consequences. Boulder, CO: Paradigm.

Cohen, D. A., B. Han, K. P. Derose, S. Williamson, T. Marsh, L. Raaen, and T. L. McKenzie. 2016a. The paradox of parks in low-income areas: Park use and perceived threats. *Environment and Behavior* 48(1):230–245.

Cohen, D. A., B. Han, C. J. Nagel, P. Harnik, T. L. McKenzie, K. R. Evenson, T. Marsh, S. Williamson, C. Vaughan, and S. Katta. 2016b. The first national study of neighborhood parks. *American Journal of Preventive Medicine* 51(4):419–426.

Cohen, L., R. Davis, V. Lee, and E. Valdovinos. 2010. Addressing the intersection: Preventing violence and promoting healthy eating and active living. Oakland, CA: Prevention Institute.

Cohen, R. A., M. E. Martinez, and E. P. Zammitti. 2016c. Health insurance coverage: Early release of estimates from the National Health Interview Survey, 2015. Hyattsville, MD: National Center for Health Statistics.

Conti, G., J. Heckman, and S. Urzua. 2010. The education-health gradient. *American Journal of Economic Review* 100(2):234–238.

Cooper, L. A., and N. R. Powe. 2004. Disparities in patient experiences, health care processes, and outcomes: The role of patient-provider racial, ethnic, and language concordance. New York: The Commonwealth Fund.

Cooper, L. A., D. L. Roter, R. L. Johnson, D. E. Ford, D. M. Steinwachs, and N. R. Powe. 2003. Patient-centered communication, ratings of care, and concordance of patient and physician race. *Annals of Internal Medicine* 139(11):907–915.

Correll, J., B. Park, C. M. Judd, and B. Wittenbrink. 2002. The police officer's dilemma: Using ethnicity to disambiguate potentially threatening individuals. *Journal of Personality and Social Psychology* 83(6):1314–1329.

Correll, J., B. Park, C. M. Judd, and B. Wittenbrink. 2007. The influence of stereotypes on decisions to shoot. *European Journal of Social Psychology* 37:1102–1117.

County Health Rankings. 2016. Health factors. http://www.countyhealthrankings.org/our-approach/health-factors (accessed October 11, 2016).

Cox, D. C., G. Dewalt, G. O'Haver, and B. Salatino. 2011. American healthy homes survey: Lead and arsenic findings. U.S. Department of Housing and Urban Development. http://portal.hud.gov/hudportal/documents/huddoc?id=AHHS_Report.pdf (accessed October 31, 2016).

Crissey, S., N. Scanniello, and H. B. Shin. 2007. The gender gap in educational attainment: Variation by age, race, ethnicity, and nativity in the United States. Housing and Household Economic Statistics Division, U.S. Census Bureau. Presented at the Annual Meeting of the Population Association of America, New York, NY, March 29–31, 2007. https://www.census.gov/hhes/socdemo/education/data/acs/CrisseyScannielloShin_poster.pdf (accessed December 12, 2016).

CSDH (Commission on Social Determinants of Health). 2008. Closing the gap in a generation: Health equity through action on the social determinants of health. Final report of the Commission on Social Determinants of Health. Geneva, Switzerland: World Health Organization.

Cure Violence. n.d.-a. The Cure Violence health model. http://cureviolence.org/the-model/essential-elements (accessed December 2, 2016).

Cure Violence. n.d.-b. Summary of findings on Cure Violence. http://cureviolence.org/results/summary-of-findings (accessed December 2, 2016).

Cushing, L., R. Morello-Frosch, M. Wander, and M. Pastor. 2015. The haves, the have-nots, and the health of everyone: The relationship between social inequality and environmental quality. *Annual Review of Public Health* 36:193–209.

Cutler, D. M., and A. Lleras-Muney. 2006. Education and health: Evaluating theories and evidence. National Bureau of Economic Research working paper no. 12352. http://www.nber.org/papers/w12352 (accessed October 31, 2016).

Cutler, D. M., and A. Lleras-Muney. 2010. Understanding differences in health behaviors by education. *Journal of Health Economics* 29(1):1–28.

Dahlberg, L. L., and J. A. Mercy. 2009. History of violence as a public health problem. *American Medical Association Journal of Ethics* 11(2):167–172.

Dale, H. E., B. J. Polivka, R. V. Chaudry, and G. C. Simmonds. 2010. What young African American women want in a health care provider. *Qualitative Health Research* 20(11):1484–1490.

Dannenberg, A. L., H. Frumkin, and R. J. Jackson. 2011. Making healthy places: Designing and building for health, well-being, and sustainability. Washington, DC: Island Press.

Darity, W. A., J. Dietrich, and D. Guilkey. 2001. Persistent advantage or disadvantage?: Evidence in support of the intergenerational drag hypothesis. *American Journal of Economics and Sociology* 60(2):435–470.

Davis, R., S. Savannah, M. Harding, A. Macaysa, and L. F. Parks. 2016. Countering the production of inequities: An emerging systems framework to achieve an equitable culture of health. Oakland, CA: Prevention Institute.

De Nardi, M. 2002. Wealth inequality and intergenerational links. Minneapolis: Federal Reserve Bank of Minneapolis.

Deaton, A. 2016. On death and money: History, facts, and explanations. *JAMA* 315(16):1703–1705.

Derose, K. P., C. R. Gresenz, and J. S. Ringel. 2011. Understanding disparities in health care access—and reducing them—through a focus on public health. *Health Affairs* 30(10):1844–1851.

Devine, P. G., P. S. Forscher, A. J. Austin, and W. T. Cox. 2012. Long-term reduction in implicit race bias: A prejudice habit-breaking intervention. *Journal of Experimental Social Psychology* 48(6):1267–1278.

Diez Roux, A. V., and C. Mair. 2010. Neighborhoods and health. *Annals of the New York Academy of Sciences* 1186(1):125–145.

Diez Roux, A. V., K. R. Evenson, A. P. McGinn, D. G. Brown, L. Moore, S. Brines, and D. R. Jacobs. 2007. Availability of recreational resources and physical activity in adults. *American Journal of Public Health* 97(3):493–499.

DiJulio, B., M. Norton, S. Jackson, and M. Brodie. 2015. Kaiser Family Foundation/CNN survey of Americans on race. Washington, DC: The Henry J. Kaiser Family Foundation.

Dolezsar, C. M., J. J. McGrath, A. J. Herzig, and S. B. Miller. 2014. Perceived racial discrimination and hypertension: A comprehensive systematic review. *Health Psychology* 33(1):20–34.

Dovidio, J., and S. L. Gaertner. 2000. Aversive racism and selection decisions: 1989 and 1999. *Psychological Science* 11(4):315–319.

Dovidio, J., S. L. Gaertner, K. Kawakami, and G. Hodson. 2002. Why can't we just get along? Interpersonal biases and interracial distrust. *Cultural Diversity and Ethnic Minority Psychology* 8(2):88–102.

Dow, W. H., and D. H. Rehkopf. 2010. Socioeconomic gradients in health in international and historical context. *Annals of the New York Academy of Sciences* 1186:24–36.

Doyle, C., P. Kavanagh, O. Metcalfe, and T. Lavin. 2005. Health impacts of employment: A review. Dublin, IE: The Institute of Public Health in Ireland.

Drake, B. 2013. Incarceration gap widens between whites and blacks. Pew Research Center, September 6. http://www.pewresearch.org/fact-tank/2013/09/06/incarceration-gap-between-whites-and-blacks-widens (accessed September 6, 2016).

Dubay, L., T. Joyce, R. Kaestner, and G. M. Kenney. 2001. Changes in prenatal care timing and low birth weight by race and socioeconomic status: Implications for the Medicaid expansions for pregnant women. *Health Services Research* 36(2):373–398.

DuBois, W. E. B. 1906. Report of a social study made under the direction of Atlanta University. Paper read at The Eleventh Conference for the Study of the Negro Problems, Atlanta, GA.

Duncan, D. T., and M. L. Hatzenbuehler. 2014. Lesbian, gay, bisexual, and transgender hate crimes and suicidality among a population-based sample of sexual-minority adolescents in Boston. *American Journal of Public Health* 104(2):272–278.

Duncan, D. T., M. L. Hatzenbuehler, and R. M. Johnson. 2014. Neighborhood-level LGBT hate crimes and current illicit drug use among sexual minority youth. *Drug and Alcohol Dependence* 135:65–70.

Egerter, S., C. Barclay, R. Grossman-Kahn, and P. A. Braveman. 2011a. Violence, social disadvantage and health. Princeton, NJ: Robert Wood Johnson Foundation.

Egerter, S., P. Braveman, T. Sadegh-Nobari, R. Grossman-Kahn, and M. Dekker. 2011b. Education and health. Princeton, NJ: Robert Wood Johnson Foundation.

El-Sayed, A. M., D. W. Finkton, M. Paczkowski, K. M. Keyes, and S. Galea. 2015. Socioeconomic position, health behaviors, and racial disparities in cause-specific infant mortality in Michigan, USA. *Preventive Medicine* 76:8–13.

EPA (U.S. Environmental Protection Agency). 2016. Environmental justice. https://www.epa.gov/environmentaljustice (accessed October 11, 2016).

Erro, P. n.d. Fresno Hunger Count: Survey methodology. Fresno Hunger Count. http://www.hunger-count.org/uploads/1/3/5/7/13572364/fhc_survey_methodology.pdf (accessed December 12, 2016).

Evans, G. W., and E. Kantrowitz. 2002. Socioeconomic status and health: The potential role of environmental risk exposure. *Annual Review of Public Health* 23:303–331.

Evans, G. W., and P. Kim. 2010. Multiple risk exposure as a potential explanatory mechanism for the socioeconomic status-health gradient. *Annals of the New York Academy of Sciences* 1186:174–189.

Evans, G. W., and M. A. Schamberg. 2009. Childhood poverty, chronic stress, and adult working memory. *Proceedings of the National Academy of Sciences* 106(16):6545–6549.

Evans, G. W., J. Brooks-Gunn, and P. K. Klebanov. 2011. Stressing out the poor: Chronic physiological stress and the income-achievement gap. Pathways. Stanford, CA: Stanford Center on Poverty and Inequality Winter. Pp. 17–21.

Evans-Campbell, T. 2008. Historical trauma in American Indian/Native Alaska communities: A multilevel framework for exploring impacts on individuals, families, and communities. *Journal of Interpersonal Violence* 23(3):316–338.

Farmer, M. M., and K. F. Ferraro. 2005. Are racial disparities in health conditional on socioeconomic status? *Social Science & Medicine* 60(1):191–204.

Fazel, S., J. R. Geddes, and M. Kushel. 2014. The health of homeless people in high-income countries: Descriptive epidemiology, health consequences, and clinical and policy recommendations. *The Lancet* 384(9953):1529–1540.

Feeding America. 2014a. Hunger in America 2015: Executive summary. Feeding America. http://www.feedingamerica.org/hunger-in-america/our-research/hunger-in-america/hia-2014-executive-summary.pdf (accessed December 12, 2016).

Feeding America. 2014b. Map the meal gap 2016: Child food insecurity in California by county in 2014. http://www.feedingamerica.org/hunger-in-america/our-research/map-the-meal-gap/2014/CA_AllCounties_CDs_CFI_2014.pdf (accessed December 12, 2016).

Feinstein, L., R. Sabates, T. M. Anderson, A. Sorhaindo, and C. Hammond. 2006. What are the effects of education on health? Paper presented at Social Outcome of Learning Project Symposium, Copenhagen, Denmark.

Feldman, K. P. 2015. A shadow over Palestine: The imperial life of race in America. Minneapolis: University of Minnesota Press.

Felitti, V. J., R. F. Anda, D. Nordenberg, D. F. Williamson, A. M. Spitz, V. Edwards, M. P. Koss, and J. S. Marks. 1998. Relationship of childhood abuse and household dysfunction to many of the leading causes of death in adults: The Adverse Childhood Experiences (ACE) Study. *American Journal of Preventive Medicine* 14(4):245–258.

FHWA (Federal Highway Administration). 2014. Mobility challenges for households in poverty: 2009 National household travel survey. U.S. Department of Transportation, Federal Highway Administration.

FII (Family Independence Initiative). n.d.-a. About. http://www.fii.org/about (accessed December 2, 2016).

FII. n.d.-b. Mission and vision. http://www.fii.org/mission-and-vision (accessed December 2, 2016).
FII. n.d.-c. Our approach in action. http://www.fii.org/our-approach-in-action (accessed December 2, 2016).
FII. n.d.-d. Resource bank. http://www.fii.org/resource-bank (accessed December 2, 2016).
Flaskerud, J. H. 2012. Coping and health status: John Henryism. *Issues in Mental Health Nursing* 33(10):712–715.
Freeman, L., and F. Braconi. 2002. Gentrification and displacement. *The Urban Prospect* 8(1):1–4.
Friedman, S. R., and S. Aral. 2001. Social networks, risk-potential networks, health, and disease. *Journal of Urban Health* 78(3):411–418.
Fujiwara, T., and I. Kawachi. 2009. Is education causally related to better health? A twin fixed-effect study in the USA. *International Journal of Epidemiology* 38(5):1310–1322.
Furnee, C. A., W. Groot, and H. M. van den Brink. 2008. The health effects of education: A meta-analysis. *European Journal of Public Health* 18(4):417–421.
Galea, S., M. Tracy, K. J. Hoggat, C. DiMaggio, and A. Karpati. 2011. Estimated deaths attributable to social factors in the United States. *American Journal of Public Health* 101(8):1456–1465.
GAO (U.S. Government Accountability Office). 2016. K-12 education: Better use of information could help agencies identify disparities and address racial discrimination. GAO-16-345. U.S. Government Accountability Office. http://www.gao.gov/products/GAO-16-345 (accessed October 31, 2016).
Garcia, E. 2015. Inequalities at the starting gate: Cognitive and noncognitive skills gaps between 2010-2011 kindergarten classmates. Washington, DC: Economic Policy Institute.
Gaskin, D. J., G. Y. Dinwiddie, K. S. Chan, and R. R. McCleary. 2012. Residential segregation and the availability of primary care physicians. *Health Services Research* 47(6):2353–2376.
Gee, G. C., and C. L. Ford. 2011. Structural racism and health inequities: Old issues, new directions. *Du Bois Review: Social Science Research on Race* 8(1):115–132.
Gee, G. C., and D. C. Payne-Sturges. 2004. Environmental health disparities: A framework integrating psychosocial and environmental concepts. *Environmental Health Perspectives* 112(17):1645–1653.
Gee, G. C., A. Ro, S. Shariff-Marco, and D. Chae. 2009. Racial discrimination and health among Asian Americans: Evidence, assessment, and directions for future research. *Epidemiology* 31:130–151.
Gelman, A., J. Fagan, and A. Kiss. 2007. An analysis of the New York City police department's "stop-and-frisk" policy in the context of claims of racial bias. *Journal of the American Statistical Association* 102(479):813–823.
Gilbert, D., S. Wakeling, and V. Crandall. 2016. Strengthening community-police relationships: Training as a tool for change. Oakland: California Partnership for Safe Communities.
Giles-Corti, B., and R. J. Donovan. 2002. The relative influence of individual, social and physical environment determinants of physical activity. *Social Science & Medicine* 54(12):1793–1812.
Ginsburg, A., P. Jordan, and H. Chang. 2014. Absences add up: How school attendance influences student success. Attendance Works. http://www.attendanceworks.org/research/absences-add (accessed October 19, 2016).
Glossary of Education Reform. 2013. Stereotype threat. http://edglossary.org/stereotype-threat (accessed December 2, 2016).
Godsil, R. D., L. R. Tropp, P. A. Goff, and j. a. powell. 2014. Addressing implicit bias, racial anxiety, and stereotype threat in education and health care. The Perception Institute. http://perception.org/wp-content/uploads/2014/11/Science-of-Equality.pdf (accessed October 31, 2016).

Goldman, D., and J. P. Smith. 2011. The increasing value of education to health. *Social Science & Medicine* 72(10):1728–1737.

Goodman, N. 2015. The impact of employment on the health status and health care costs of working-age people with disabilities. The National Center on Leadership for the Employment and Economic Advancement of People with Disabilities. http://www.leadcenter.org/system/files/resource/downloadable_version/impact_of_employment_health_status_health_care_costs_0.pdf (accessed October 31, 2016).

Griffith, D. M., M. Mason, M. Yonas, E. Eng, V. Jeffries, S. Plihcik, and B. Parks. 2007. Dismantling institutional racism: Theory and action. *American Journal of Community Psychology* 39(3–4):381–392.

Griffith, D. M., M. Yonas, M. Mason, and B. E. Havens. 2010. Considering organizational factors in addressing health care disparities: Two case examples. *Health Promotion Practice* 11(3):367–376.

Grossman, M. 2015. The relationship between health and schooling: What's new? Cambridge, MA: National Bureau of Economic Research.

Guess, T. J. 2006. The social construction of whiteness: Racism by intent, racism by consequence. *Critical Sociology* 32(4):649–673.

Hackbarth, D. P., B. Silvestri, and W. Cosper. 1995. Tobacco and alcohol billboards in 50 Chicago neighborhoods: Market segmentation to sell dangerous products to the poor. *Journal of Public Health Policy* 16(2):213–230.

Hall, J., L. Porter, D. Longhi, J. Becker-Green, and S. Dreyfus. 2012. Reducing adverse childhood experiences (ACE) by building community capacity: A summary of Washington Family Policy Council research findings. *Journal of Prevention & Intervention in the Community* 40(4):325–334.

Hall, W. J., M. V. Chapman, K. M. Lee, Y. M. Merino, T. W. Thomas, B. K. Payne, E. Eng, S. H. Day, and T. Coyne-Beasley. 2015. Implicit racial/ethnic bias among health care professionals and its influence on health care outcomes: A systematic review. *American Journal of Public Health* 105(12):e60–e76.

Hamilton, B. W., J. A. Martin, and M. J. K. Osterman. 2016. National vital statistics reports. Hyattsville, MD: National Center for Health Statistics 65(3).

Harrell, J. P., S. Hall, and J. Taliaferro. 2003. Physiological responses to racism and discrimination: An assessment of the evidence. *American Journal of Public Health* 93(2):243–248.

Harris, A. 2009. Attributions and institutional processing: How focal concerns guide decision-making in the juvenile court. *Race and Social Problems* 1(4):243–256.

Hatzenbuehler, M. L., A. Bellatorre, Y. Lee, B. K. Finch, P. Muennig, and K. Fiscella. 2014. Structural stigma and all-cause mortality in sexual minority populations. *Social Science & Medicine* 103:33–41.

Hatzenbuehler, M. L., K. Keyes, A. Hamilton, M. Uddin, and S. Galea. 2015. The collateral damage of mass incarceration: Risk of psychiatric morbidity among nonincarcerated residents of high-incarceration neighborhoods. *American Journal of Public Health* 105(1):138–143.

Healthy People 2020. 2016. Social determinants of health. https://www.healthypeople.gov/2020/topics-objectives/topic/social-determinants-of-health (accessed October 24, 2016).

Heart, M. Y., J. Chase, J. Elkins, and D. B. Altshul. 2011. Historical trauma among Indigenous Peoples of the Americas: Concepts, research, and clinical considerations. *Journal of Pyschoactive Drugs* 43(4):282–290.

Heiman, H. J., and S. Artiga. 2015. Beyond health care: The role of social determinants in promoting health and health equity. Menlo Park, CA: The Henry J. Kaiser Family Foundation.

HHS (U.S. Department of Health and Human Services). 1996. Physical activity and health: A report of the Surgeon General. Atlanta, GA: U.S. Department of Health and Human Services, U.S. Centers for Disease Control and Prevention, National Center for Chronic Disease Prevention and Health Promotion.

Hill, J. J., 3rd, M. D. Slade, L. Cantley, S. Vegso, M. Fiellin, and M. R. Cullen. 2008. The relationships between lost work time and duration of absence spells: Proposal for a payroll driven measure of absenteeism. *Journal of Occupational and Environmental Medicine* 50(7):840–851.

Hood, C. M., K. P. Gennuso, G. R. Swain, and B. B. Catlin. 2016. County Health Rankings: Relationships between determinant factors and health outcomes. *American Journal of Preventive Medicine* 50(2):129–135.

Howard, T. C. 2010. Why race and culture matter in schools: Closing the achievement gap in America's classrooms. New York: Teachers College Press.

HUD (U.S. Department of Housing and Urban Development). n.d. Moving to opportunity for fair housing. http://portal.hud.gov/hudportal/HUD?src=/programdescription/mto (accessed September 21, 2016).

Ibrahim, S. A., A. Zhang, M. B. Mercer, M. Baughman, and C. K. Kwoh. 2004. Inner city African-American elderly patients' perceptions and preferences for the care of chronic knee and hip pain: Findings from focus groups. *Journals of Gerontology* 59(12):1318–1322.

IEL (Institute for Educational Leadership). n.d. What is a community school? Coalition for Community Schools, Institute for Educational Leadership. http://www.communityschools.org/aboutschools/what_is_a_community_school.aspx (accessed December 12, 2016).

IOM (Institute of Medicine). 2003. *Unequal treatment: Confronting racial and ethnic disparities in health care*. Washington, DC: The National Academies Press.

IOM. 2006. *Genes, behavior, and the environment: Moving beyond the nature/nurture debate*. Washington, DC: The National Academies Press.

IOM. 2013. Roundtable on Population Health Improvement: April 2013. http://nationalacademies.org/hmd/Activities/PublicHealth/PopulationHealthImprovementRT/2013-APR-09/Videos/Panel%20Presentations%20and%20Discussion/8-Williams-Video.aspx (accessed December 14, 2016).

IOM. 2014. *Applying a health lens to decision making in non-health sectors: Workshop summary*. Washington, DC: The National Academies Press.

IOM and NRC (Institute of Medicine and National Research Council). 2000. *From neurons to neighborhoods: The science of early childhood development*. Washington, DC: National Academy Press.

IOM and NRC. 2014. *New directions in child abuse and neglect research*. Washington, DC: The National Academies Press.

IPCC (Intergovernmental Panel on Climate Change). 2014. Climate change 2014 synthesis report: Summary for policy. Geneva, Switzerland: Intergovernmental Panel on Climate Change.

Jacobs, D. E., J. Wilson, S. L. Dixon, J. Smith, and A. Evens. 2009. The relationship of housing and population health: A 30-year retrospective analysis. *Environmental Health Perspectives* 117(4):597–604.

James, P., J. E. Hart, R. F. Banay, and F. Laden. 2016. Exposure to greenness and mortality in a nationwide prospective cohort study of women. *Environmental Health Perspectives* 124(9):1344–1352.

James, S. A. 1994. John Henryism and the health of African-Americans. *Culture, Medicine & Psychiatry* 18(2):163–182.

Jemal, A., E. Ward, R. N. Anderson, T. Murray, and M. J. Thun. 2008. Widening of socioeconomic inequalities in U.S. death rates, 1993-2001. *PLOS One* 3(5):e2181.

Jimenez, M. E., N. E. Reichman, R. Wade, Y. Lin, and L. M. Morrow. 2016. Adverse experiences in early childhood and kindergarten outcomes. *Pediatrics* 137(2).

Johnson, K. R. 2002. Race and the immigration laws: The need for critical inquiry. In *Crossroads, directions and a new critical race theory*, edited by F. Valdes, J. M. Culp, and A. P. Harris. Philadelphia, PA: Temple University Press. Pp. 187–198.

Jones, C. P. 2000. Levels of racism: A theoretic framework and a gardener's tale. *American Journal of Public Health* 90(8):1212–1215.

Jones, E. 2016. Principled policing. *California Police Chief* Spring:40–41.

Kang, Y., J. R. Gray, and J. F. Dovidio. 2014. The nondiscriminating heart: Lovingkindness meditation training decreases implicit intergroup bias. *Journal of Experimental Psychology* 143(3):1306–1313.

Kaufman, J. S., R. S. Cooper, and D. L. Mcgee. 1997. Socioeconomic status and health in blacks and whites: The problem of residual confounding and the resiliency of race. *Epidemiology* 8:621–628.

Kawachi, I., and L. Berkman. 2000. Social cohesion, social capital, and health. In *Social epidemiology*, edited by I. Kawachi and L. Berkman. New York: Oxford University Press. Pp. 174–190.

Kena, G., W. Hussar, M. J., C. de Brey, L. Musu-Gillette, X. Wang, J. Zhang, A. Rathbun, S. Wilkinson-Flicker, M. Diliberti, A. Barmer, F. Bullock Mann, and E. Dunlop Velez. 2016. The condition of education 2016 (NCES 2016-144). Washington, DC: U.S. Department of Education, National Center for Education Statistics.

Kessler, R. C., K. D. Mickelson, and D. R. Williams. 1999. The prevalence, distribution, and mental health correlates of perceived discrimination in the United States. *Journal of Health and Social Behavior* 40:208–230.

Khan, M., and K. Ecklund. 2013. Attitudes toward Muslim Americans post-9/11. *Journal of Muslim Mental Health* 7(1).

Kim, D., S. Subramanian, and I. Kawachi. 2008. Social capital and physical health: A systematic review of the literature. In *Social capital and health*, edited by I. Kawachi, S. Subramanian, and D. Kim. New York: Springer Science + Business Media. Pp. 139–190.

Kindig, D., and G. Stoddart. 2003. What is population health? *American Journal of Public Health* 93(3):380–383.

King, W. D., M. D. Wong, M. F. Shapiro, B. E. Landon, and W. E. Cunningham. 2004. Does racial concordance between HIV-positive patients and their physicians affect the time to receipt of protease inhibitors? *Journal of General Internal Medicine* 19(11):1146–1153.

Kirst, M. W., and A. Venezia. 2004. From high school to college: Improving opportunities for success in postsecondary education. San Francisco, CA: Jossey-Bass.

Kneebone, E., and N. Holmes. 2015. The growing distance between people and jobs in metropolitan America. Washington, DC: Metropolitan Policy Program at Brookings.

Kokua Kalihi Valley. n.d. Kokua Kalihi Valley. http://www.kkv.net (accessed December 2, 2016).

Krieger, J., and D. L. Higgins. 2002. Housing and health: Time again for public health action. *American Journal of Public Health* 92(5):758–768.

Krueger, P. M., M. K. Tran, R. A. Hummer, and V. W. Chang. 2015. Mortality attributable to low levels of education in the United States. *PLOS One* 10(7):e0131809.

Kulwicki, A., R. Khalifa, and G. Moore. 2008. The effects of September 11 on Arab American nurses in metropolitan Detroit. *Journal of Transcultural Nursing* 19(2):134–139.

Kwate, N. O. A. 2008. Fried chicken and fresh apples: Racial segregation as a fundamental cause of fast food density in black neighborhoods. *Health and Place* 14(1):32–44.

La Vigne, N. G., P. Lachman, S. Rao, and A. Matthews. 2014. Stop and frisk: Balancing crime control with community relations. Washington, DC: Office of Community Oriented Policing Services.

Landrine, H., and I. Corral. 2009. Separate and unequal: Residential segregation and black health disparities. *Ethnicity & Disease* 19(2):179–184.
Lauderdale, D. S. 2006. Birth outcomes for Arabic-named women in California before and after September 11. *Demography* 43(1):185–201.
LaVeist, T. A., and J. M. Wallace. 2000. Health risk and inequitable distribution of liquor stores in African American neighborhood. *Social Science and Medicine* 51:613–617.
Lee, I. M., E. J. Shiroma, F. Lobelo, P. Puska, S. N. Blair, and P. T. Katzmarzyk. 2012. Effect of physical inactivity on major non-communicable diseases worldwide: An analysis of burden of disease and life expectancy. *The Lancet* 380(9838):219–229.
Lehman, D., P. Fenza, and L. Hillinger-Smith. 2012. Diversity & cultural competency in health care settings. A Mather LifeWays orange paper. Racial and ethnic minority providers disparities cultural competence. https://www.matherlifewaysinstituteonaging.com/wp-content/uploads/2012/03/Diversity-and-Cultural-Competency-in-Health-Care-Settings.pdf (accessed December 2, 2016).
Levesque, C., and K. W. Brown. 2007. Mindfulness as a moderator of the effect of implicit motivational self-concept on day-to-day behavioral motivation. *Motivation and Emotion* 31(4):284–299.
Levy, D. K., J. Comey, and S. Padilla. 2006. In the face of gentrification: Case studies of local efforts to mitigate displacement. Washington, DC: Urban Institute.
Levy, D. J., J. A. Heissel, J. A. Richeson, and E. K. Adam. 2016. Psychological and biological responses to race-based social stress as pathways to disparities in educational outcomes. *American Psychologist* 71(6):455–473.
Like, R. C. 2011. Educating clinicians about cultural competence and disparities in health and health care. *Journal of Continuing Education in the Health Professions* 31(3):196–206.
Losen, D. J., C. L. Hodson, I. Keith, A. Michael, K. Morrison, and S. Belway. 2015. Are we closing the school discipline gap? The Center for Civil Rights Remedies at The Civil Rights Project, UCLA, February. https://www.civilrightsproject.ucla.edu/resources/projects/center-for-civil-rights-remedies/school-to-prison-folder/federal-reports/are-we-closing-the-school-discipline-gap/AreWeClosingTheSchoolDisciplineGap_FINAL221.pdf (accessed December 14, 2016).
Louie, V. 2007. Who makes the transition to college? Why we should care, what we know, and what we need to do. *Teachers College Record* 109(10):2222–2251.
Luber, G., K. Knowlton, J. Balbus, H. Frumkin, M. Hayden, J. Hess, M. McGeehin, N. Sheats, L. Backer, C. B. Beard, K. L. Ebi, E. Maibach, R. S. Ostfeld, C. Wiedinmyer, E. A. Zielinski-Gutiérrez, and L. Ziska. 2014. Chapter 9: Human health. In *Climate change impacts in the United States: The third national climate assessment*, edited by J. M. Melillo, T. C. Richmond, and G. W. Yohe. U.S. Global Change Research Program.
Lueke, A., and B. Gibson. 2014. Mindfulness meditation reduces implicit age and race bias: The role of reduced automaticity of responding. *Social Psychological and Personality Science* 6(3):284–291.
Lundborg, P., C. H. Lyttkens, and P. Nystedt. 2012. Human capital and longevity: Evidence from 50,000 twins. Health, Econometrics and Data Group (HEDG). The University of York. https://www.york.ac.uk/media/economics/documents/herc/wp/12_19.pdf (accessed December 12, 2016).
Lundborg, P., C. H. Lyttkens, and P. Nystedt. 2016. The effect of schooling on mortality: New evidence from 50,000 Swedish twins. *Demography* 53(4):1135–1168.
Lyons, C. J., and B. Pettit. 2011. Compounded disadvantage: Race, incarceration, and wage growth. *Social Problems* 58(2):257–280.
Malinowski, P. 2013. Neural mechanisms of attentional control in mindfulness meditation. *Frontiers in Neuroscience* 7(8).

Maqbool, N., J. Viveiros, and M. Ault. 2015. The impacts of affordable housing on health: A research summary. Washington, DC: Center for Housing Policy, National Housing Conference.

Margo, R. A. 1990. Race and schooling in the south, 1880–1950. Chicago, IL: The University of Chicago Press.

Marmot, M., J. Allen, P. Goldblatt, T. Boyce, D. McNeish, M. Grady, and I. Geddes. 2010. Fair society, healthy lives: Strategic review of health inequalities in England post 2010. London: University College London.

Marulis, L. M., and S. B. Neuman. 2010. The effects of vocabulary intervention on young children's world learning: A meta-analysis. *Review of Educational Research* 80(3):300–335.

Massetti, G. M., and A. M. Vivolo. 2010. Achieving public health impact in youth violence prevention through community-research partnerships. *Progress in Community Health Partnerships: Research, education, and action* 4(3):243–251.

Massey, D. S., and N. A. Denton. 1988. The dimensions of residential segregation. *Social Forces* 67(2):281–315.

Massey, D. S., and N. A. Denton. 1989. Hypersegregation in U.S. metropolitan areas: Black and Hispanic segregation along five dimensions. *Demography* 26(3):373–391.

Massie, V. M. 2016. To understand the Dakota Access Pipeline protests, you need to understand tribal sovereignty. Vox, October 28. http://www.vox.com/2016/9/9/12851168/dakota-access-pipeline-protest (accessed December 2, 2016).

Mathews, T. J., and M. F. MacDorman. 2007. Infant mortality statistics from the 2004 period linked birth/infant death data set. National Vital Statistics Reports. Hyattsville, MD: National Center for Health Statistics 55(15):1–32.

Mathews, T. J., M. F. MacDorman, and M. E. Thoma. 2015. Infant mortality statistics from the 2013 period linked birth/infant death data set. National Viral Statistics Reports. Hyattsville, MD: National Center for Health Statistics 64(9):1–30.

Mays, V. M., S. D. Cochran, and N. W. Barnes. 2007. Race, race-based discrimination, and health outcomes among African Americans. *Annual Review of Psychology* 58:201–225.

McConville, M. 2013. Creating equitable, healthy, and sustainable communities: Strategies for advancing smart growth, environment justice, and equitable development. U.S. Environmental Protection Agency. https://www.epa.gov/sites/production/files/2014-01/documents/equitable-development-report-508-011713b.pdf (accessed October 12, 2016).

McCormack, G. R., and A. Shiell. 2011. In search of causality: A systematic review of the relationship between the built environment and physical activity among young adults. *International Journal of Behavioral Nutrition and Physical Activity* 8(125).

McDougle, L., D. P. Way, W. K. Lee, J. A. Morfin, B. E. Mavis, D. Matthews, B. A. Latham-Sadler, and D. M. Clinchot. 2015. A national long-term outcomes evaluation of U.S. premedical postbaccalaureate programs designed to promote health care access and workforce diversity. *Journal of Health Care for the Poor and Underserved* 26(3):631–647.

McEwen, B. S. 2012. Brain on stress: How the social environment gets under the skin. *Proceedings of the National Academy of Sciences* 109(Suppl 2):17180–17185.

McGee, R. E., and N. J. Thompson. 2015. Unemployment and depression among emerging adults in 12 states, Behavioral Risk Factor Surveillance System. *Preventing Chronic Disease* 12(3):140451.

McGinnis, J. M. 2016. Income, life expectancy, and community health: Underscoring the opportunity. *JAMA* 315(16):1709–1710.

McGinnis, J. M., P. Williams-Russo, and J. R. Knickman. 2002. The case for more active policy attention to health promotion. *Health Affairs* 21(2):78–93.

McGuire, T. G., and J. Miranda. 2008. New evidence regarding racial and ethnic disparities in mental health: Policy implications. *Health Affairs* 27(2):393–403.

McKee-Ryan, F., Z. Song, C. R. Wanberg, and A. J. Kinicki. 2005. Psychological and physical well-being during unemployment: A meta-analytic study. *Journal of Applied Psychology* 90(1):53–76.

McKinnish, T., R. Walsh, and T. K. White. 2010. Who gentrifies low-income neighborhoods? *Journal of Urban Economics* 67(2):180–193.

McLeroy, K. R., D. Bibeau, A. Steckler, and K. Glanz. 1988. An ecological perspective on health promotion programs. *Health Education Quarterly* 15:351–377.

McNeill, L. H., M. W. Kreuter, and S. V. Subramanian. 2006. Social environment and physical activity: A review of concepts and evidence. *Social Science & Medicine* 63(4):1011–1022.

Meara, E., S. Richards, and D. Cutler. 2008. The gap gets bigger: Changes in mortality and life expectancy by education, 1981–2000. *Health Affairs* 27(2):350–360.

Miller, J. 2015. Community close up: Rolling Hills Apartments, St. Paul, Minnesota. http://buildhealthyplaces.org/whats-new/rolling-hills-apartments-st-paul-minnesota-2 (accessed October 19, 2016).

Minkler, M., A. P. Garcia, J. Williams, T. LoPresti, and J. Lilly. 2010. Si se puede: Using participatory research to promote environmental justice in a Latino community in San Diego, California. *Journal of Urban Health* 87(5):796–812.

Moiduddin, E., and D. S. Massey. 2008. Neighborhood disadvantage and birth weight: The role of perceived danger and substance abuse. *International Journal of Conflict and Violence* 2(1):113–129.

Montez, J. K., and L. F. Berkman. 2014. Trends in the educational gradient of mortality among US adults aged 45–84 years: Bringing the regional context into the explanation. *American Journal of Public Health* 104(1):e82–e90.

Mosavel, M., R. Ahmed, D. Daniels, and C. Simon. 2011. Community researchers conducting health disparities research: Ethical and other insights from fieldwork journaling. *Social Science & Medicine* 73(1):145–152.

Ms. Foundation for Women. 2015. A Ms. Foundation for Women survey: A fresh look at the public's view toward issues and solutions. https://d18t6orusej5w.cloudfront.net/wp-content/uploads/2015/10/Ms-National-Survey-Executive-Summary.pdf (accessed December 2, 2016).

Mueller, N., D. Rojas-Rueda, T. Cole-Hunter, A. de Nazelle, E. Dons, R. Gerike, T. Gotschi, L. Int Panis, S. Kahlmeier, and M. Nieuwenhuijsen. 2015. Health impact assessment of active transportation: A systematic review. *Preventive Medicine* 76:103–114.

NASEM (National Academies of Sciences, Engineering, and Medicine). 2015. *The growing gap in life expectancy by income: Implications for federal programs and policy responses*. Washington, DC: The National Academies Press.

NASEM. 2016. *Systems practices for the care of socially at-risk populations*. Washington, DC: The National Academies Press.

Nashville Area Metropolitan Planning Organization. n.d. Nashville Area Metropolitan Planning Organization. http://nashvillempo.org (accessed October 17, 2016).

National Initiative for Building Community Trust and Justice. 2015. Implicit bias. Community-oriented trust and justice briefs. Washington, DC: Office of Community Oriented Policing Services.

NCHS (National Center for Health Statistics). 2016. Health, United States, 2015: With special feature on racial and ethnic health disparities. Hyattsville, MD: U.S. Centers for Disease Control and Prevention.

Neal, D., and A. Rick. 2014. The prison boom and the lack of black progress after Smith and Welch. Working paper 20283. Cambridge, MA: National Bureau of Economic Research.

NEJAC (National Environmental Justice Advisory Council). 2009. Reducing air emissions associated with goods movement: Working towards environmental justice. Washington, DC: U.S. Environmental Protection Agency.

North Carolina Institute of Medicine Task Force on Prevention. 2009. Chapter 11: Socioeconomic determinants of Health. In *Prevention for the health of North Carolina: Prevention action plan*. Morrisville: North Carolina Institute of Medicine.

NRC (National Research Council). 2012. *Education for life and work: Developing transferable knowledge and skills for the 21st century*. Washington, DC: The National Academies Press.

NRC. 2014. *The growth of incarceration in the United States: Exploring causes and consequences*. Washington, DC: The National Academies Press.

NRC and IOM (National Research Council and Institute of Medicine). 2013. *U.S. health in international perspective: Shorter lives, poorer health*. Washington, DC: The National Academies Press.

OECD (Organisation for Economic Co-operation and Development). 2015. In it together: Why less inequality benefits all . . . in the United States. Organisation for Economic Cooperation and Development. https://www.oecd.org/unitedstates/OECD2015-In-It-Together-Highlights-UnitedStates-Embargo-21May11amPArisTime.pdf (accessed December 1, 2016).

Olshansky, S. J., T. Antonucci, L. Berkman, R. H. Binstock, A. Boersch-Supan, J. T. Cacioppo, B. A. Carnes, L. L. Carstensen, L. P. Fried, D. P. Goldman, J. Jackson, M. Kohli, J. Rother, Y. Zheng, and J. Rowe. 2012. Differences in life expectancy due to race and educational differences are widening, and many may not catch up. *Health Affairs* 31(8):1803–1813.

Olson, M. E., D. Diekema, B. A. Elliott, and C. M. Renier. 2010. Impact of income and income inequality on infant health outcomes in the United States. *Pediatrics* 126(6):1165–1173.

Otiniano Verissimo, A. D., C. E. Grella, H. Amaro, and G. C. Gee. 2014. Discrimination and substance use disorders among Latinos: The role of gender, nativity, and ethnicity. *American Journal of Public Health* 104(8):1421–1428.

Padela, A. I., and M. Heisler. 2010. The association of perceived abuse and discrimination after September 11, 2001, with psychological distress, level of happiness, and health status among Arab Americans. *American Journal of Public Health* 100(2):284–291.

Paez, K. A., J. K. Allen, M. C. Beach, K. A. Carson, and L. A. Cooper. 2009. Physician cultural competence and patient ratings of the patient-physician relationship. *Journal of General Internal Medicine* 24(4):495–498.

Pager, D., and H. Shepherd. 2008. The sociology of discrimination: Racial discrimination in employment, housing, credit, and consumer markets. *Annual Review of Sociology* 34(1):181–209.

Pampel, F. C., P. M. Krueger, and J. T. Denney. 2010. Socioeconomic disparities in health behaviors. *Annual Review of Sociology* 36:349–370.

Paradies, Y. 2006a. A systematic review of empirical research on self-reported racism and health. *International Journal of Epidemiology* 35(4):888–901.

Paradies, Y. 2006b. Defining, conceptualizing and characterizing racism in health research. *Critical Public Health* 16(2):143–157.

Pascoe, E. A., and L. Smart Richman. 2009. Perceived discrimination and health: A meta-analytic review. *Psychological Bulletin* 135(4):531–554.

Paul, K. I., and K. Moser. 2009. Unemployment impairs mental health: Meta-analyses. *Journal of Vocational Behavior* 74(3):264–282.

Pearce, N., and G. D. Smith. 2003. Is social capital the key to inequalities in health? *American Journal of Public Health* 93(1):122–129.

Pereiram, G., L. Wood, S. Foster, and F. Haggar. 2013. Access to alcohol outlets, alcohol consumption and mental health. *PLOS One* 8(1).

Perez, L., F. Lurmann, J. Wilson, M. Pastor, S. J. Brandt, N. Kunzli, and R. McConnell. 2012. Near-roadway pollution and childhood asthma: implications for developing "win-win" compact urban development and clean vehicle strategies. *Environmental Health Perspectives* 120(11):1619–1626.

Perkins, D. D., and R. T. Taylor. 1996. Ecological assessments of community disorder: Their relationship to fear of crime and theoretical implications. *American Journal of Community Psychology* 24(1):63–107.

Peterson, R. D., and L. J. Krivo. 2010. Divergent social worlds: Neighborhood crime and the racial-spatial divide. New York: Russell Sage Foundation.

Pew Research Center. 2016. On views of race and inequality, blacks and whites are worlds apart. Pew Research Center. June 27. http://www.pewsocialtrends.org/2016/06/27/on-views-of-race-and-inequality-blacks-and-whites-are-worlds-apart (accessed October 31, 2016).

Phillips, D., L. Flores, Jr., and J. Henderson. 2014. Development without displacement. Oakland, CA: Causa Justa.

Picard-Fritsche, S., and L. Cerniglia. 2013. Testing a public health approach to gun violence: An evaluation of Crown Heights Save Our Streets, a replication of the Cure Violence model. New York: Center for Court Innovation.

Picker, L. 2007. The effects of education on health. The NBER Digest. National Bureau of Economic Research. March. http://www.nber.org/digest/mar07/w12352.html (accessed October 31, 2016).

Pinderhughes, H., R. A. Davis, and M. Williams. 2015. Adverse community experiences and resilience: A framework for addressing and preventing community trauma. Oakland, CA: Prevention Institute.

Polednak, A. P. 1996. Segregation, discrimination and mortality in U.S. blacks. *Ethnicity & Disease* 6(1–2):99–108.

Pollack, C. E., C. Cubbin, A. Sania, M. Hayward, D. Vallone, B. Flaherty, and P. A. Braveman. 2013. Do wealth disparities contribute to health disparities within racial/ethnic groups? *Journal of Epidemiology & Community Health* 67(5):439–445.

Polling Report. n.d. LGBT. http://pollingreport.com/lgbt.htm (accessed December 2, 2016).

Powell, L. M., S. Slater, D. Mirtcheva, Y. Bao, and F. J. Chaloupka. 2007. Food store availability and neighborhood characteristics in the United States. *Preventive Medicine* 44(3):189–195.

Prevention Institute. 2011. Fact sheet: Links between violence and health equity. Oakland, CA: Prevention Institute.

Priest, N., Y. Paradies, B. Trenerry, M. Truong, S. Karlsen, and Y. Kelly. 2013. A systematic review of studies examining the relationship between reported racism and health and wellbeing for children and young people. *Social Science & Medicine* 95:115–127.

Pucher, J., R. Buehler, D. R. Bassett, and A. L. Dannenberg. 2010. Walking and cycling to health: A comparative analysis of city, state, and international data. *American Journal of Public Health* 100(10):1986–1992.

RAMP (Regional Asthma Management and Prevention). 2009. Asthma and diesel. Oakland, CA: Regional Asthma Management and Prevention.

Reardon, S. F., and K. Bischoff. 2016. The continuing increase in income segregation, 2007-2012. Stanford, CA: Stanford Center for Education Policy Analysis.

Reardon, S. F., R. A. Valentino, and K. A. Shores. 2012. Patterns of literacy among U.S. students. *Future of Children* 22(2):17–37.

Remington, P. L., B. B. Catlin, and K. P. Gennuso. 2015. The County Health Rankings: Rationale and methods. *Population Health Metrics* 13:11.

Richardson, L. S., and P. A. Goff. 2013. Implicit racial bias in public defender triage. *The Yale Law Journal* 122(8):2626–2649.

Richeson, J. A., and N. Shelton. 2003. When prejudice does not pay: Effects of interracial contact on executive function. *Psychological Science* 14(3):287–290.

Roberto, E. 2008. Commuting to opportunity: The working poor and commuting in the United States. Washington, DC: Brookings Institution, Metropolitan Policy Program.

Roberts, C. B., A. I. Vines, J. S. Kaufman, and S. A. James. 2008. Cross-sectional association between perceived discrimination and hypertension in African-American men and women: The Pitt County Study. *American Journal of Epidemiology* 167(5):624–632.

Rodriguez, J., A. Geronimus, J. Bound, and D. Dorling. 2015. Black lives matter: Differential mortality and the racial composition of the U.S. electorate, 1970–2004. *Social Science & Medicine* 136–137:193–199.

Rosenbaum, J. E., and A. E. Person. 2003. Beyond college for all: Policies and practices to improve transitions into college and jobs. *Professional School Counseling* 6(4):252–260.

Ross, A. 2016a. New data highlights vast and persistent racial inequities in who experiences poverty in America. National Equity Atlas. http://nationalequityatlas.org/data-in-action/racial-inequities-poverty-in-america (accessed August 30, 2016).

Ross, A. 2016b. An overview of America's working poor. National Equity Atlas. http://nationalequityatlas.org/data-in-action/overview-america-working-poor (accessed December 16, 2016).

Rostron, B. L., J. L. Boies, and E. Arias. 2010. Education reporting and classification on death certificates in the United States. National Center for Health Statistics. Vital and Health Statistics 151:1–21.

Rouse, C. E., and L. Barrow. 2006. U.S. elementary and secondary schools: Equalizing opportunity or replicating the status quo? *The Future of Children* 16(2):99–123.

Rudolph, L., S. Gould, and J. Berko. 2015. Climate change, health, and equity: Opportunities for action. Oakland, CA: Public Health Institute.

RWJF (Robert Wood Johnson Foundation). 2009. Beyond health care. Robert Wood Johnson Foundation Commission to Build a Healthier America.

RWJF. 2015a. Everett culture of health story. http://www.rwjf.org/en/library/articles-and-news/2015/10/coh-prize-everett-ma-story.html (accessed October 21, 2016).

RWJF. 2015b. From vision to action: A framework and measures to mobilize a culture of health. Robert Wood Johnson Foundation. http://www.rwjf.org/content/dam/COH/RWJ000_COH-Update_CoH_Report_1b.pdf (accessed February 7, 2016).

Ryan, C. L., and K. Bauman. 2016. Educational attainment in the United States: 2015. Current Population Reports. U.S. Census Bureau. http://www.census.gov/content/dam/Census/library/publications/2016/demo/p20-578.pdf (accessed October 31, 2016).

Sabin, J., B. A. Nosek, A. Greenwald, and F. P. Rivara. 2009. Physicians' implicit and explicit attitudes about race by MD race, ethnicity, and gender. *Journal of Health Care for the Poor and Underserved* 20(3):896–913.

Salway, S., P. Chowbey, E. Such, and B. Ferguson. 2015. Researching health inequalities with community researchers: Practical, methodological and ethical challenges of an "inclusive" research approach. *Research Involvement and Engagement* 1(1).

Schnittker, J., and K. Liang. 2006. The promise and limits of racial/ethnic concordance in physician-patient interaction. *Journal of Health Politics, Policy and Law* 31(4):811–838.

Schroeder, S. A. 2007. We can do better—Improving the health of the American people. *The New England Journal of Medicine* 357:1221–1228.

Schulman, K. A., J. A. Berlin, W. Harless, J. F. Kerner, S. Sistrunk, B. J. Gersh, R. Dubé, C. K. Taleghani, J. E. Burke, S. Williams, J. M. Eisenberg, and J. J. Escarce. 1999. The effect of race and sex on physicians' recommendations for cardiac catheterization. *The New England Journal of Medicine* 340(8):618–626.

Sedaghat, A. R., E. C. Matsui, S. N. Baxi, M. E. Bollinger, R. Miller, M. Perzanowski, and W. Phipatanakul. 2016. Mouse sensitivity is an independent risk factor for rhinitis in children with asthma. *Journal of Allergy and Clinical Immunology*: In Practice 4(1):82–88.

Shapiro, I., C. Murray, and B. Sard. 2015. Basic facts on concentrated poverty. Washington, DC: Center on Budget and Policy Priorities.

Shavers, V. L., P. Fagan, D. Jones, W. M. Klein, J. Boyington, C. Moten, and E. Rorie. 2012. The state of research on racial/ethnic discrimination in the receipt of health care. *American Journal of Public Health* 102(5):953–966.

Shepard, P. 2005/2006. Breathe at your own risk: Transit justice in West Harlem. *Race, Poverty, and the Environment* (Winter):51–53.

Shonkoff, J. P., and A. S. Garner. 2012. The lifelong effects of early childhood adversity and toxic stress. *Pediatrics* 129(1):e232–e246.

Sims, M., A. V. Diez-Roux, A. Dudley, S. Gebreab, S. B. Wyatt, M. A. Bruce, S. A. James, J. C. Robinson, D. R. Williams, and H. A. Taylor. 2012. Perceived discrimination and hypertension among African Americans in the Jackson Heart Study. *American Journal of Public Health* 102(Suppl 2):S258–S265.

Singh, G. K., and S. M. Yu. 1995. Infant mortality in the United States: Trends, differentials, and projections, 1950 through 2010. *American Journal of Public Health* 85(7):957–964.

Skiba, R. J., R. H. Horner, C.-G. Chung, M. K. Rausch, S. L. May, and T. Tobin. 2011. Race is not neutral: A national investigation of African American and Latino disproportionality in school discipline. *School Psychology Review* 40(1):85–107.

Smith, E. J., and S. R. Harper. 2015. Disproportionate impact of K-12 school suspension and expulsion on black students in southern states. Philadelphia: University of Pennsylvania, Center for the Study of Race and Equity in Education.

Smith, S. G., P. A. Nsiah-Kumi, P. R. Jones, and R. J. Pamies. 2009. Pipeline programs in the health professions, part 1: Preserving diversity and reducing health disparities. *Journal of the National Medical Association* 101(9):836–840, 845–851.

Staats, C., K. Capatosto, R. A. Wright, and V. W. Jackson. 2016. State of the science: Implicit bias review. Columbus, OH: Kirwan Institute for the Study of Race and Ethnicity.

Steptoe, A., and P. J. Feldman. 2001. Neighborhood problems as sources of chronic stress: Development of a measure of neighborhood problems, and associations with socioeconomic status and health. *Annals of Behavioral Medicine* 23(3):177–185.

Stiefel, M., and K. Nolan. 2012. A guide to measuring the Triple Aim: Population health, experience of care, and per capita cost. Cambridge, MA: Institute for Healthcare Improvement.

Strutz, K. L., V. K. Hogan, A. M. Siega-Riz, C. M. Suchindran, C. T. Halpern, and J. M. Hussey. 2014. Preconception stress, birth weight, and birth weight disparities among US women. *American Journal of Public Health* 104(8):125–132.

Sturm, R., and D. Cohen. 2014. Proximity to urban parks and mental health. *Journal of Mental Health Policy and Economics* 17(1):19–24.

Sturtevant, L. 2014. The new District of Columbia: What population growth and demographic change mean for the city. *Journal of Urban Affairs* 36(2):276–299.

Subramanyam, M. A., S. A. James, A. V. Diez-Roux, D. A. Hickson, D. Sarpong, M. Sims, H. A. Taylor, Jr., and S. B. Wyatt. 2013. Socioeconomic status, John Henryism and blood pressure among African-Americans in the Jackson Heart Study. *Social Science & Medicine* 93:139–146.

Sue, D. W., C. M. Capodilupo, G. C. Torino, J. M. Bucceri, A. M. Holder, K. L. Nadal, and M. Esquilin. 2007. Racial microaggressions in everyday life: Implications for clinical practice. *American Psychologist* 62(4):271–286.

Suglia, S. F., R. C. Shelton, A. Hsiao, Y. C. Wang, A. Rundle, and B. G. Link. 2016. Why the neighborhood social environment is critical in obesity prevention. *Journal of Urban Health* 93(1):206–212.

Sundeen, M. 2016. What's happening in Standing Rock? *Outside*, September 2. https://www.outsideonline.com/2111206/whats-happening-standing-rock (accessed December 2, 2016).

Taylor, D. E. 2014. Toxic communities: Environmental racism, industrial pollution, and residential mobility. New York: NYU Press.

Thornton, R. L., C. M. Glover, C. W. Cene, D. C. Glik, J. A. Henderson, and D. R. Williams. 2016. Evaluating strategies for reducing health disparities by addressing the social determinants of health. *Health Affairs* 35(8):1416–1423.

TRB and IOM (Transportation Research Board and Institute of Medicine). 2005. Does the built environment influence physical activity? Examining the evidence. TRB special report 282. Washington, DC: The National Academies Press.

UCR (Uniform Crime Report). 2015. Hate crime statistics, 2014. Washington, DC: U.S. Department of Justice, Federal Bureau of Investigation. https://ucr.fbi.gov/hate-crime/2014/topic-pages/victims_final.pdf (accessed October 28, 2016).

U.S. Census Bureau. 2015. QuickFacts: Fresno County, California. http://www.census.gov/quickfacts/table/PST045215/06019 (accessed December 12, 2016).

US DOT (U.S. Department of Transportation). 2015. Equity. https://www.transportation.gov/mission/health/equity (accessed September 20, 2016).

U.S. News & World Report. n.d. Reagan High School. http://www.usnews.com/education/best-high-schools/texas/districts/austin-independent-school-district/reagan-high-school-18613 (accessed December 12, 2016).

U.S. Task Force on Community Preventive Services. 2001. Increasing physical activity: A report on recommendations of the Task Force on Community Preventive Services. *Morbidity and Mortality Weekly Report* 50(RR18):1–16.

Valente, T. W., P. Gallaher, and M. Mouttapa. 2004. Using social networks to understand and prevent substance use: A transdisciplinary perspective. *Substance Use & Misuse* 39(10-12):1685–1712.

van Ryn, M., and J. Burke. 2000. The effect of patient race and socio-economic status on physicians' perceptions of patients. *Social Science & Medicine* 50:813–828.

van Ryn, M., and S. S. Fu. 2003. Paved with good intentions: Do public health and human service providers contribute to racial/ethnic disparities in health? *American Journal of Public Health* 93(2):248–255.

Velez, M. B., C. J. Lyons, and B. Boursaw. 2012. Neighborhood Housing Investments and Violent Crime in Seattle, 1981-2007. *Criminology* 50(4):1025–1056.

Villeneuve, P. J., M. Jerrett, J. G. Su, R. T. Burnett, H. Chen, A. J. Wheeler, and M. S. Goldberg. 2012. A cohort study relating urban green space with mortality in Ontario, Canada. *Environmental Research* 115:51–58.

Volandes, A. E., M. Paasche-Orlow, M. R. Gillick, E. F. Cook, S. Shaykevich, E. D. Abbo, and L. Lehmann. 2008. Health literacy not race predicts end-of-life care preferences. *Journal of Palliative Medicine* 11(5):754–762.

Wahowiak, L. 2015. Addressing stigma, disparities in minority mental health: Access to care among barriers. *The Nation's Health* 45(1). http://thenationshealth.aphapublications.org/content/45/1/1.3.full (accessed October 27, 2016).

Waldron, H. 2007. Trends in mortality differentials and life expectancy for male social security-covered workers, by socioeconomic status. *Social Security Bulletin* 67(3):1–28.

Wallace, R., and D. Wallace. 1997. Socioeconomic determinants of health: Community marginalisation and the diffusion of disease and disorder in the United States. *BMJ* 314(7090):1341–1345.

Wang, H., and R. Horton. 2015. Tackling climate change: The greatest opportunity for global health. *The Lancet* 386(10006):1798–1799.

Weiss, C. C., M. Purciel, M. Bader, J. W. Quinn, G. Lovasi, K. M. Neckerman, and A. G. Rundle. 2011. Reconsidering access: Park facilities and neighborhood disamenities in New York City. *Journal of Urban Health* 88(2):297–310.

WHO (World Health Organization). 2006. Report of the WHO technical meeting on quantifying disease from inadequate housing (November 28-30, 2005). Bonn, Germany: World Health Organization, European Centre for Environment and Health.

WHO. 2011. 10 facts on health inequities and their causes. http://www.who.int/features/factfiles/health_inequities/en (accessed December 2, 2016).

Wigle, D. T., T. E. Arbuckle, M. Walker, M. G. Wade, S. Liu, and D. Krewski. 2007. Environmental hazards: Evidence for effects on child health. *Journal of Toxicology and Environmental Health* 10(1–2):3–39.

Wildeman, C. 2012. Imprisonment and infant mortality. *Social Problems* 59(2):228–257.

Willett, W. C., J. P. Koplan, R. Nugent, C. Dusenbury, P. Puska, and T. A. Gaziano. 2006. Prevention of chronic disease by means of diet and lifestyle changes. In *Disease control priorities in developing countries*. New York: Oxford University Press.

Williams, D. R., and C. Collins. 2001. Racial residential segregation: A fundamental cause of racial disparities in health. *Public Health Reports* 116(September–October):404–416.

Williams, D. R., and S. A. Mohammed. 2009. Discrimination and racial disparities in health: Evidence and needed research. *Journal of Behavioral Medicine* 32(1):20–47.

Williams, D. R., and S. A. Mohammed. 2013. Racism and health II: A needed research agenda for effective interventions. *American Behavioral Scientist* 57(8).

Williams, D. R., H. W. Neighbors, and J. S. Jackson. 2003. Racial/ethnic discrimination and health: Findings from community studies. *American Journal of Public Health* 93(2):200–208.

Williams, D. R., S. A. Mohammed, J. Leavell, and C. Collins. 2010. Race, socioeconomic status, and health: Complexities, ongoing challenges, and research opportunities. *Annals of the New York Academy of Sciences* 1186:69–101.

Wilson, V. 2016. State unemployment rates by race and ethnicity at the end of 2015 show a plodding recovery. Washington, DC: Economic Policy Institute.

Witt, W. P., H. Park, L. E. Wisk, E. R. Cheng, K. Mandell, D. Chatterjee, and D. Zarak. 2015. Neighborhood disadvantage, preconception stressful life events, and infant birth weight. *American Journal of Public Health* 105(5):1044–1052.

Woolf, S. H., and J. Q. Purnell. 2016. The good life: Working together to promote opportunity and improve population health and well-being. *JAMA* 315(16):1706–1708.

Woolf, S. H., R. E. Johnson, R. L. Phillips, and M. Philipsen. 2007. Giving everyone the health of the educated: An examination of whether social change would save more lives than medicine. *American Journal of Public Health* 2007(97):4.

Woolf, S. H., L. Aron, L. Dubay, S. M. Simon, E. Zimmerman, and K. X. Luk. 2015. How are income and wealth linked to health and longevity? Washington, DC: Urban Institute and Virginia Commonwealth University.

Yonas, M. A., N. Jones, E. Eng, A. I. Vines, R. Aronson, D. M. Griffith, B. White, and M. DuBose. 2006. The art and science of integrating Undoing Racism with CBPR: Challenges of pursuing NIH funding to investigate cancer care and racial equity. *Journal of Urban Health* 83(6):1004–1012.

Zestcott, C. A., I. V. Blair, and J. Stone. 2016. Examining the presence, consequences, and reduction of implicit bias in health care: A narrative review. *Group Processes & Intergroup Relations* 19(4):528–542.

Zhang, S., and V. Bhavsar. 2013. Unemployment as a risk factor for mental illness: Combining social psychiatric literature. *Advances in Applied Sociology* 03(02):131–136.

Zimmerman, E., and S. H. Woolf. 2014. Understanding the relationship between education and health. Discussion paper. Washington, DC: Institute of Medicine.

Zimmerman, R., C. E. Restrepo, H. B. Kates, and R. Joseph. 2015. Final report: Suburban poverty, public transit, economic opportunities, and social mobility. New York: University Transportation Research Center.

Zonderman, A. B., N. A. Mode, N. Ejiogu, and M. K. Evans. 2016. Race and poverty status as a risk for overall mortality in community-dwelling middle-aged adults. *JAMA Internal Medicine* 176(9):1394–1395.

Zuk, M., A. H. Bierbaum, K. Chapple, K. Gorska, A. Loukaitou-Sideris, P. Ong, and T. Thomas. 2015. Gentrification, displacement, and role of public investment: A literature review. Federal Reserve Bank of San Francisco working paper no. 2015-05. Community Development Investment Center working paper series. http://www.frbsf.org/community-development/publications/working-papers/2015/august/gentrification-displacement-role-of-public-investment (accessed October 31, 2016).

4

The Role of Communities in Promoting Health Equity

The previous chapter provided evidence concerning the many social, economic, and environmental factors that shape health and contribute to health disparities, and indicating that successful community-level interventions to improve health equity need to target both people and places. (See Box 4-1 for definitions of community and community-based solution as used in this report.) These factors largely take place in communities but are also affected by larger forces such as state and federal policy (see Chapter 6 for more on the policy context). Community action plays a vital role in effecting sustainable change. This chapter will first discuss why communities and community-driven actions to promote health are essential components in promoting health equity. This is followed by a discussion of the evidence on community-based collaboration. Conditions to foster actions toward health equity are reviewed as are the evidence and data necessary to inform community-driven solutions.

Below, a first-person account of the Thunder Valley Community Development Corporation is provided as an example of the way in which one community organization is promoting health equity.

> **BOX 4-1**
> **Definitions**
>
> *Community* is any configuration of individuals, families, and groups whose values, characteristics, interests, geography, or social relations unite them in some way (adapted from Dreher, 2016[a]). However, the word is used to denote both the people living in a place, and the place itself. In this report the committee focuses on shared geography, i.e., place, as a key component of community—in other words, community is defined as the people living in a place, such as a neighborhood. Therefore a *community-based solution* to promote health equity is an action, policy, program, or law that is driven by the community (members), and that affects local factors that can influence health and has the potential to advance progress toward health equity.
>
> ---
>
> [a] Draft manuscript from Melanie C. Dreher, Rush University Medical Center, provided to staff on February 19, 2016, for the Committee on Community-Based Solutions to Promote Health Equity in the United States. Available by request from the National Academies of Sciences, Engineering, and Medicine's Public Access Records Office. For more information, email PARO@nas.edu.

Taking Community Action to Promote Health Equity: The Thunder Valley Community Development Corporation
Written by Nick Tilsen, Founder and Executive Director of the Thunder Valley Community Development Corporation[1]

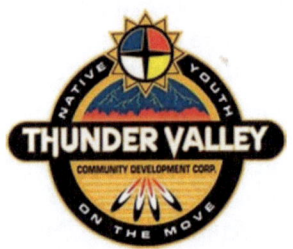

Thunder Valley Community Development Corporation[2] (CDC) is a Lakota-led, grassroots, community development organization located on the Pine Ridge Indian Reservation in southwest South Dakota. Thunder Valley CDC has

---

[1] Committee member Nick Tilsen is the founder and executive director of the Thunder Valley Community Development Corporation.
[2] See more at http://thundervalley.org and https://www.youtube.com/watch?v=-6aBQ09SjNI (both accessed December 5, 2016).

developed a comprehensive, innovative, and grassroots approach to collaborating with and empowering Lakota youth and families on the Pine Ridge Indian Reservation in order to improve the health, culture, and environment of our community in a way that heals and strengthens our identity. Our organization was founded by a group of young people who were reconnecting to Lakota spirituality and identity through ceremonies. They were presented with a challenge: "When are you going to make a way for your people, are you not warriors? It's time to stop talking and start doing." We recognized from that point that it would take systemic change to bring an ecosystem of opportunity to our community and solve the systemic and historic injustices we deal with daily.

The Pine Ridge Reservation is home to about 30,000 Oglala Lakota people. Eighty percent of the population is unemployed, and 50 percent lives below the federal poverty line. Life expectancy on the reservation is the lowest of anywhere in the Western Hemisphere besides Haiti, and the infant mortality rate is five times the national average. Fifty percent of the population is under the age of 18. To address these realities, we launched into deep community engagement with hundreds of hours of listening and visioning sessions with members of our community, including youth, elders, political leaders, and parents (see Figure 4-1 for the community theory of change). We challenged our community to think about what is possible and not just the challenges we face. We received a U.S. Department of Housing and Urban Development Sustainable Communities grant to facilitate this process and create a sustainable development plan for the region.

The community engagement process was at times very challenging—it is difficult to envision and dream about things that you have never seen before. This became evident in some intergenerational tensions. In one community engagement session, children were drawing what they believed was possible for the community on a white board. In the back of the room, there were a couple of elders grumbling that our community could never have these things, that we could not afford them. In that moment, the youth became angry that their hopes and dreams were being challenged. We were able to use that moment to create a mentality shift in the room by challenging the group and asking if it cost anything to dream, and what was the real cost if we did not? This mentality shift gave the elders a perspective in which to participate in the creation of what was possible. In going through this process, Thunder Valley CDC was able to create the Oyate Omniciye Oglala Regional Plan, which was adopted by the Oglala Sioux Tribe as the official Sustainable Regional Planning Document. Thunder Valley CDC has taken on a model community initiative through a 34-acre regenerative community development plan that provides the opportunity to begin to address the lack of physical, political, and economic infrastructure that exists and to create our own pathway out of poverty by building local skill and leadership capacity.

Along with our work to develop the regenerative community in a way that honors our cultural heritage and is adapted for the needs and vision of our local community, we are intentionally disrupting the status quo by creating models

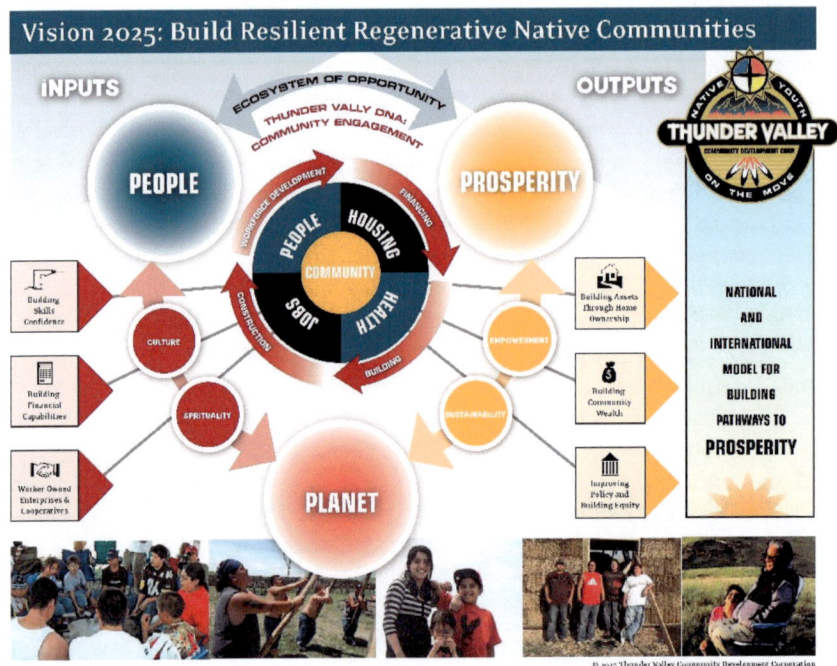

FIGURE 4-1 Thunder Valley Community Development Corporation's Theory of Change.
SOURCE: Thunder Valley CDC, 2016.

of change that will overcome intergenerational poverty and build momentum towards regional equity. These initiatives are focused on homeownership, food sovereignty, social enterprise, youth leadership development, regional equity, and the Lakota language.

Through our complex ecosystem of opportunity, the solutions we are creating will be able to address the root inequalities that negatively affect the social determinants of health.

Today, Thunder Valley CDC operates at about $4 million with support from multiple federal agencies, foundations, and individuals, including Northwest Area Foundation, Doris Duke Charitable Foundation, Surdna Foundation, Novo Foundation, W.K. Kellogg Foundation, Administration for Native Americans, and the U.S. Department of Agriculture. We are working to ensure the sustainability of our organization through building the capacity of our community to continue operating and growing the organization as well as ensuring sustainable funding. We also work diligently to try to diversify our funding streams and help shape trends in philanthropy.

To build the capacity of our organization we have been able to identify key people in our community who can be leaders in a specific area. This system builds power in our community by keeping our organization locally run. In addition, a core principle of our organization from the beginning is admitting what we do not know. This has allowed us to bring in consultants and experts from across the country to help build our knowledge of this work, especially in the areas of development and community design.

It is important to us that we are creating repeatable models—not a cookie cutter replica for other communities, but strategies that can be replicated in communities across the United States. To do this we have invested in the evaluation of our organization over the next five years, according to a sustainable triple bottom line, which holds people, planet, and prosperity in equal standing. For this evaluation we are measuring the impact of each of our initiatives and programs, the impact of the regenerative community, and the impact of our organization across the region. We also are measuring our community engagement. Ultimately, our work is aimed at improving health outcomes in our community by creating a healthy community and environment as a catalyst to decreasing health disparities across the reservation.

COMMUNITY ACTION: VITALLY NECESSARY

Community is any configuration of individuals, families, and groups whose values, characteristics, interests, geography, or social relations unite them in some way (adapted from Dreher, 2016[3]). However, the word is used to denote both the people living in a place, and the place itself. In this report the committee generally focuses on shared geography—in other words, community is defined as the people living in a place, such as a neighborhood. Therefore, a community-based solution is an action, policy, program, or law that is driven by the community (members), affects local factors that can influence health, and has the potential to promote health equity.

The potential of community-based solutions to advance health equity is a focus because the Robert Wood Johnson Foundation asked the Committee on Community-Based Solutions to Promote Health Equity in the United States to consider solutions that could be identified, developed, and implemented at the local or community level. However, the report focus should not be interpreted to suggest that community-based

---

[3] Draft manuscript from Melanie C. Dreher, Rush University Medical Center, provided to staff on February 19, 2016, for the Committee on Community-Based Solutions to Promote Health Equity in the United States. Available by request from the National Academies of Sciences, Engineering, and Medicine's Public Access Records Office. For more information, email PARO@nas.edu.

solutions represent the primary or sole strategy or the best opportunity to promote health equity. Communities exist in a milieu of national, state, and local level policies, forces, and programs that enable and support or interfere with and impede the ability of community residents and their partners to address the conditions that lead to health inequity. Therefore, the power of community actors is a necessary and an essential, but not a sufficient, ingredient in promoting health equity.

In addition to the support of high level policies, such as those that address structural inequities (e.g., residential segregation), community-based solutions described in this report also rely on multi-sectoral and multilevel collaborations and approaches: for example, engaging business and other nontraditional partners. It is a strength of multi-sectoral collaboration and efforts that are not primarily health focused that they, by definition, ensure diverse approaches to improving community health equity and well-being. Such diverse approaches also are a manifestation of the fact that not all communities start out observing the unfair differences in life expectancy between one side of town and another and thereafter seek to address those inequities. Some communities aim to improve high school graduation or expand affordable housing or create jobs. This report is for communities that believe improving health among their residents is important, but it is also for communities that believe better transit, more affordable housing, safer streets, and more small businesses are important. Whether health is the end or the means to an end, communities can benefit by understanding how health is connected to other goals important to them, and improving education, housing, or employment can also help improve health and mitigate health inequity.

As illustrated in the Thunder Valley CDC example, and detailed in Chapter 3, the community serves as the bedrock of health, a foundation for achieving other important goals, and key to building a productive society. Communities differ in the causes of health inequity they experience, from the availability of health care providers, the affordability and quality of housing, and employment opportunities, to schools, transportation systems, safety, the availability of parks and green space, and other aspects of the physical environment. Some of the challenges faced by vulnerable communities are unique, while others may be common among multiple communities and populations, or they may be present in every community.

Not only is each community unique in the degree and nature of its health inequities, but so too are the means to address those issues, in terms of such resources as locus of power and community values. What communities share, however, is that they are each experts on their local needs and assets and thus need to drive community-based solutions. The nine community examples provided in Chapter 5 illustrate the ability of local community organizations to directly address the determinants of health in order to improve health inequities. In each case, community action was supported, enabled, or facilitated by federal or state policies and programs because, as noted earlier in this report, community action is a necessary, but not sufficient, contributor to achieving health equity. Communities exist in a milieu of public- and private-sector policies, forces, and programs that enable and support or interfere with and impede the ability of community residents and their partners to address the conditions that lead to health inequity. Community action requires a supportive context, which may range from government policies and programs to the activities of an anchor institution[4] such as a university or business.

Many communities strive to achieve greater well being and economic vibrancy. Communities might aim to improve high school graduation rates, expand affordable housing, create more jobs, or improve their children's health. Whether health is a community's ultimate goal or the means to an end, communities can benefit by pursuing health equity. Examining health outcomes in the community can help communities understand how health is connected to other desired objectives, and improving education or housing or employment can also help improve health. Communities can see the potential for win-wins. Although it is possible that some communities will notice health disparities and target them as a priority, that is not always the case. When it is not, it may be helpful to encourage communities to consider health equity as a potential co-benefit and to open up additional avenues for measurement, evaluation, and planning. For example, introducing a community coalition working to expand employment opportunities to the concept of health equity could help expand the ways in which members view the value of their collaborative undertaking: that is, not only are they creating jobs and helping to train people for them, this can also have positive effects on health equity in the community. In other words, this report is for communities that believe promoting health equity among their residents is important, but it is also for communities that believe better transit, more affordable housing, complete streets, and more small businesses are essential to a thriving community.

THE EVIDENCE ON COMMUNITY-BASED EFFORTS

Communities might not all be successful at building the type of organizational and collaborative capacity needed to achieve the changes they

---

[4] Dubb et al. describe an anchor institution as a place-based institution that is tied to its location "by reason of mission, invested capital, or relationships to customers or employees and hence have a vested interest in improving the welfare of their surrounding communities" (Dubb et al., 2013, p. vii).

desire (e.g., improved educational attainment, a more widely accessible transit system) that can also improve health equity. What accounts for successful community interventions for promoting health equity? Why are some communities and organizations able to come together and effect change while others are not? The answers to these questions are complex and involve both the characteristics of the communities and organizations themselves and the broader aspects of the social, economic, environmental, and political context in which communities operate.

The evaluation of community efforts is extremely difficult and complex, both to identify the effects of community action on the determinants of health and to identify the effects on health and health equity (Fawcett et al., 2010). There are multiple barriers, including the complexity of webs of influence and causation and the existence of many confounding variables. Much of the existing research on community-based interventions and on the effectiveness of collaborative efforts to improve community health has been of limited usefulness.[5] Research findings have been mixed or negative on the effectiveness of partnerships, and insufficient duration may be one challenge (Shortell et al., 2002). Research also has primarily focused on the "low-hanging fruits" in this space such as individual-level interventions, single interventions,[6] and interventions implemented under highly controlled conditions not generalizable to socioculturally diverse communities (Trickett et al., 2011). Tobacco use is one case where the evidence of community-based interventions—along with the evidence on clinical interventions and integration of the two—is robust, as shown by the U.S. Preventive Services Task Force and the Community Task Force (Ockene et al., 2007). The evidence-based nonclinical interventions recommended by the Community Task Force included: smoking bans and restrictions, increasing the unit price for tobacco, and media campaigns.

In 2002, Shortell and colleagues conducted a study of 25 public–private community health partnerships (out of 283 partnerships in the Community Care Network that responded to a request for application from the Health Research and Educational Trust of the American Hospital Association. Between 1995 and 2000, the partnerships had grown from an average of 10 to an average of 22 member organizations, including "hospitals, health systems, managed care organizations, clinics, public health departments, physician organizations, nursing homes, schools and school districts, local government agencies, state health departments, citizen groups, chambers of commerce, social service agencies, and local businesses" (Shortell et al., 2002, p. 52). Based on both qualitative and

---

[5] A growing body of research, not discussed here, focuses specifically on coalition functioning (see, for example, Shapiro et al., 2015).

[6] See, for example, Holder et al., 1997.

quantitative analysis of the partnerships, researchers identified six characteristics shared by the five highest-performing partnerships and absent in the lowest-performing partnerships. These characteristics—"managing partnership size and diversity, developing multiple, approaches to leadership, maintaining focus, managing conflict, recognizing life cycles, and redeploying or patching resources are challenges faced by all community health coalitions in all types of environments"—they concluded (Shortell et al., 2002).

Fawcett and colleagues (2010) provide an overview of some of the factors that contribute to poor performance in achieving population health goals, including health equity, as established in Healthy People 2010, and some of the causes, including challenges in "engaging stakeholders at multiple ecologic levels in building collaborative partnerships for population health." The authors offer seven recommendations for strengthening collaborative partnerships for population health and health equity: measure progress, "develop and use action plans that assign responsibility," facilitate natural reinforcement for cross-sectoral collaboration, assure adequate base funding, provide training and technical support, establish participatory evaluation systems to document and review progress and make course corrections, and "arrange group contingencies to ensure accountability for progress and improvement" (Fawcett et al., 2010, p. 5).

A Cochrane Collaboration systematic review and meta-analysis by Hayes and colleagues (2012) examined 16 studies with a total of 28,212 participants "comparing local collaborative partnerships between health and government agencies with standard working arrangements" (Hayes et al., 2012, p. 2). Hayes et al. found only two good-quality studies: one showed no health improvement while the other showed modest benefit. The systematic review also included three studies that examined environmental changes, and two out of three showed some health benefit. In their recent study, Mays and colleagues (2016) examined 16 years worth of data from the National Longitudinal Survey of Public Health Systems based on a sample of 360 metropolitan communities and found decreased mortality from preventable causes in areas with a high level of comprehensive population health system capital. The researchers used a quasi-experimental research design and identified categories of system capital. Communities with comprehensive population health system capital had "a broad scope of population health activities supported through densely connected networks of contributing organizations" (Mays et al., 2016, p. 2007). The study authors noted that it is more challenging to develop comprehensive levels of system capital in rural, low-income, and minority communities, and they suggested that "efforts to build system capital in low-income, minority, and rural communities may go a long way toward reducing inequities in population health" (Mays et al., 2016, p. 2012).

Qualitative and practice-based studies have suggested that certain attributes—including leadership, a backbone or an integrator organization, an infrastructure for collaboration, a common vision, shared language, a strategy for diversifying funding—are required for communities to succeed in health improvement efforts (Community Tool Box, 2016; FSG, 2011, 2013; Hayes et al., 2012; Prybil et al., 2014; Verbitsky-Savitz et al., 2016), and many of these are likely to apply to community efforts to organize and mobilize for health equity as well. In addition to the three elements of health equity as a shared vision and value, collaboration, and capacity, findings suggest that the success of community organization and mobilization for health equity is a function of the following factors:

- the qualities of the community organization itself, such as committed, charismatic leaders, community support, and resources;
- the larger social, economic, environmental, and political conditions that set the stage for change.

These factors are briefly discussed in more detail below.

The characteristics of community organizations, such as having passionate and competent leadership (see, for example, the Delta Health Center and WE ACT for Environmental Justice community examples in Chapter 5), are important for successful interventions for health equity. However, as noted above, communities cannot always achieve sustainable change on their own. Successful community interventions are often not simply the product of extraordinary people doing extraordinary things. Research in sociology and political science indicates that the broader social, economic, environmental, or political context can influence whether organizations succeed, and it is likely that these contextual aspects can also affect the efforts of communities to bring about change (Hojnacki et al., 2012; Polletta, 2008). Evidence from the sociology of social movements may be useful in this context, given the centrality of community organizing to community-driven change efforts (Skocpol et al., 2000), the nearly three-decades-long Healthy Communities movement (Norris and Pittman, 2000), and the relationship between mobilization for political participation and shared membership in a voluntary organization (Campbell, 2013) such as a community health coalition. According to the predominant theories of political process, the political environment, often called the "political opportunity structure," strongly shapes whether social movement mobilization is successful, sustainable, and leads to substantive policy change (Meyer, 2004; Polletta, 2008). Furthermore, researchers have shown that the ability of communities to organize successfully depends, in part, on the receptivity of local political actors and structures to the communities' needs (McAdam, 1982).

Scholars measure the openness of political structures in a variety of ways, including the receptivity of elected officials to movement demands (Meyer and Minkoff, 2004), which may be greater if elected officials reflect the demographics of their communities (Browning et al., 1984); the extent to which policy makers have made policy decisions favorable to constituent needs (McAdam, 1982); the ability of minorities to have access to and influence over policy decisions (Eisinger, 1972); and the amenability of the audience, including the voting electorate, to movement issues (Santoro, 2008). These "opportunity structures" facilitate the ability of communities, even in the context of grave challenges, to come together to agree upon and solve problems, including those related to health equity.

For example, the greatest progress in reducing tobacco use in the United States came when local smoking-control ordinances were combined with state and federal efforts to increase tobacco taxes. The taxes not only made cigarettes more expensive, dampening demand; they also helped fund advertising campaigns warning people of the dangers of cigarettes and supported smoking quit lines. This multipronged effort to change policy, backed by a powerful communications and educational strategy, created a snowball of change that transformed norms and expectations around smoking (Prevention Institute, 2014). Ultimately, this changing policy environment sparked and facilitated effective community-led initiatives to reduce smoking-related illness.

Funding is another element of the larger policy context supporting community action. In the Thunder Valley CDC example described earlier, funding from the U.S. Department of Housing and Urban Development (HUD), the U.S. Department of Agriculture (USDA), and foundations allowed the community to create a sustainable development plan for the region. Both state and federal funding decisions can influence how collaboration and community participation unfold on the ground. Funding can also incentivize community participation. For example, the HUD Sustainable Communities Regional Planning Grant Program aims to support locally led collaborative efforts with partnerships that include a range of interests beyond traditional partners—such as arts and culture or recreation organizations, food systems, regional planning agencies, and public education entities—and which target such varied aims as housing and economic development in order to create jobs and regional economic activity (HUD, 2016).

In contrast, some policy environments can negatively affect community efforts to improve health equity. Certain areas suffer disproportionately from poor infrastructure that does not support healthy and walkable communities (e.g., a lack of sidewalks and fully accessible crosswalks). Although planning is a local issue, some states have policies in place to support complete streets policies (Smart Grow America, 2014) at the local level. When there is not a supportive policy framework at the regional, state, or national level, creating community-level change can be more challenging.

These factors and examples can be applied across all of the determinants of health from a regional, state, and federal policy perspective. To build on the land use and transportation example, the U.S. Department of Transportation's Transportation Investment Generating Economic Recovery (TIGER) discretionary grants program is helping jurisdictions such as Pittsburgh, Pennsylvania, build infrastructure that will, in Pittsburgh's case, "reconnect the Hill District to downtown Pittsburgh, more than 60 years after highway and arena construction razed a middle income African American community" through a project that will improve neighborhood streets, sidewalks, and crosswalks, add a bus stop, a bike-sharing station, and Americans with Disabilities Act–compliant walkways, and will create open space for transportation and recreation (DOT, 2016).

ELEMENTS OF SUCCESSFUL COMMUNITY EFFORTS

Communities working to promote health equity or to address social or environmental conditions in their neighborhoods may use different types of partnerships that include community-based organizations, local government agencies, and residents themselves. Such varied coalitions represent an important part of the opportunity structure for change. In the section that follows, the committee discusses in detail the three elements identified in its conceptual model introduced in Chapter 1 (see Figure 4-2), which were used to guide its review and selection of illustrative examples of community-based solutions detailed in Chapter 5:

1. Multi-sector collaboration
2. Health equity as a shared vision and value
3. Community capacity to shape outcomes

1. Multi-Sector Collaboration

First, successfully addressing health inequities, like other community interventions, requires the committed collaboration of organizations situated in and outside the health and health care sector (Hoying et al., 2012). The Robert Wood Johnson Foundation (RWJF) Culture of Health Action Framework's drivers for cross-sectoral collaboration are quality of partnerships, investment in collaboration, and policies that support collaboration (e.g., systems in place to encourage health as a mutual goal on an ongoing basis). Information on the roles of different sectors and

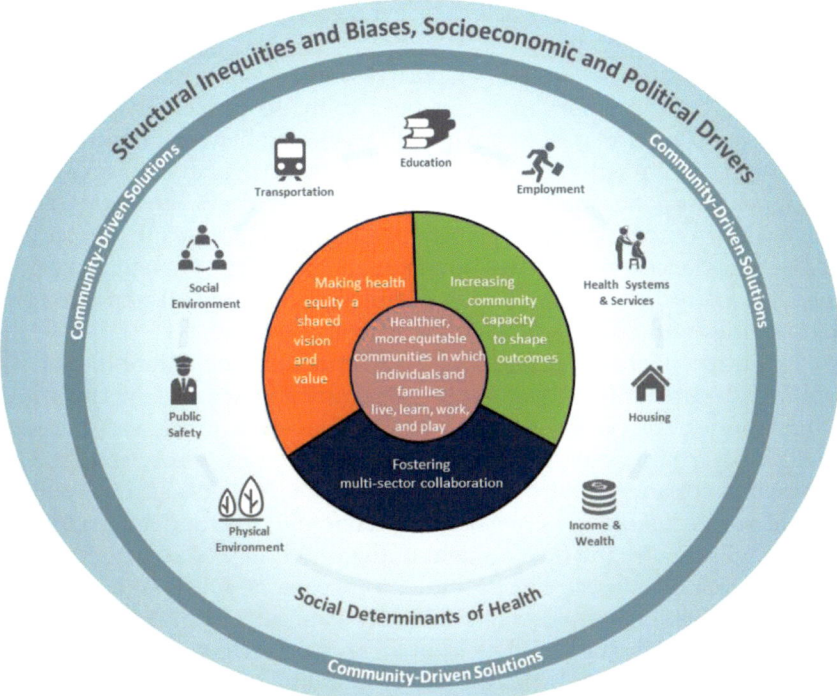

FIGURE 4-2 The three elements of community success in implementing community-driven solutions to promote health equity.

stakeholders is discussed in more detail in Chapter 7, including some examples of work on the horizon.

Many organizations have identified the fostering of cross-sector or multi-sector collaboration as a key ingredient for promoting health and health equity (Mattessich and Rausch, 2014; Prybil et al., 2014). Multi-sector collaboration—the partnership that results when government, nonprofit organizations, private entities, public organizations, community groups, and individual community members come together to solve problems that affect the whole community—has the potential to solve systemic problems that affect health outcomes. A multi-sector approach challenges the common silo approach to public health (and other fields), wherein advocates work only within their respective fields with little or no communication or alignment across fields. Although much can be learned from expertise in specific fields, the determinants of health do not reside in one sector alone, and no one sector, even health, holds the solution to improving health equity. Moreover, cross-sector collaboration may also enable community actors to leverage a wider range of supports for community-driven work.

Drawing on the resources, perspectives, and insights of multiple sectors to address a problem increases the likelihood of effective and systemic impact. In their assessment of the association between multi-sector population health activities and health outcomes over time, Mays and colleagues found that communities with *comprehensive system capital*—rich networks of organizations working together to effect health improvement—experienced significantly lower death rates from preventable conditions (e.g., cardiovascular disease, diabetes, and influenza) compared to communities without this capital (Mays et al., 2016).

Achieving health equity depends on addressing the determinants of health in the broader context in which they are situated (see Figure 4-2). Although there are policy strategies that can have a significant impact on all of the determinants of health, programmatic approaches depend on the community for successful planning, implementation, and sustainability. If there is a focus on any one social or economic determinant, an intervention will require the involvement of the multiple sectors that overlap with the area of interest. For example, transportation affects (access to) housing, education, employment: thus, only a multi-sector collaboration that brings together stakeholders from these other areas will succeed. The overarching milieu in which all these disparate sectors come and work together is the community itself.

One implication of this is that openness is an important characteristic of successful community organizations. Open contexts (to use a term drawn from the sociology literature) encourage constituencies of historically marginalized populations to mobilize and advocate for government responses to their concerns. For example, the Dudley Street Neighborhood Initiative, the Indianapolis Congregation for Action, and WE ACT for Environmental Justice (see Chapter 5 for more information on these community examples) engage and empower traditionally excluded communities through leadership development. Open contexts can engender trust in the political system among historically marginalized populations and thus encourage residents of minority neighborhoods to become civically engaged, develop a sense of attachment to and ownership of their neighborhoods, and mobilize on behalf of neighborhood concerns (Bobo and Gilliam, 1990; Williams, 1998). Open contexts can also provide resources and opportunities across a myriad of domains that enhance community capacity and viability (Lyons et al., 2013). In contrast, closed contexts are less receptive and responsive to the claims and needs of marginalized constituencies. In relatively closed contexts, even the most impassioned leadership can fail to produce sustained and successful interventions (Lyons et al., 2013).

2. Health Equity as a Shared Vision and Value

Effective community partnerships have a "well-articulated and shared vision" (Shortell et al., 2002; see also Mattesich and Rausch, 2014), and it is reasonable to expect that success in addressing health inequities also requires a shared vision and shared values. Holding health equity as a shared vision and value is an aspirational notion; in many community-based partnerships to address any number of community challenges, health equity may simply be an implicit vision and value.

Shared value refers to two relevant concepts. One dimension of shared value refers to social or cultural values. In this context, the set of beliefs and ideas held in common that allow collaborators to work together despite differences (e.g., in social status, sector, philosophy, race and ethnicity, and ability) in order to craft interventions that have the sufficient resources, cultural awareness, and inclusiveness as well as a path to sustainability for lasting change (RWJF, 2015[7]). The other dimension of shared value comes from the business literature—particularly the work of Porter and Kramer (2011)—and refers to "policies and operating practices that enhance the competitiveness of a company while simultaneously advancing the economic and social conditions in the communities in which it operates. Shared value creation focuses on identifying and expanding the connections between societal and economic progress" (Porter and Kramer, 2011). Combining the two meanings therefore means that a shared vision is the "glue" that holds multi-sector collaboration together, elevating the desired change above individual and organizational interests in order to improve the health and well-being of all those who are part of the community.

3. Community Capacity to Shape Outcomes

Third, increasing community capacity to shape outcomes is a recurring theme and need, as the committee found while reviewing community examples and the relevant literature (see, for example, Hargreaves et al., 2016; Hoying et al., 2012). Community capacity refers to the ability of communities to come together to identify common needs and to build

---

[7] The RWJF Culture of Health Action Framework identifies making health a shared value as one of its four action areas for realizing a culture of health in the United States. The drivers identified for making health a shared value include "mindsets and expectations" that promote health and well-being as a priority, civic engagement, and a sense of community (the social connections needed for a community to thrive). The description of the framework's first dimension states "Making Health a Shared Value emphasizes the importance of individuals, families, and communities in prioritizing and shaping a Culture of Health. Everyone should feel engaged with their community's decisions and believe that they have a voice in the process" (RWJF, 2015).

social and political capital by drawing on ties with actors both inside (including residents, local businesses, and elected officials) and outside of the community (Chaskin, 1999). Thus defined, the concept of community capacity parallels other concepts central to research on different dimensions of community well-being. Notions of power, community empowerment, social network ties, and social capital are also relevant to this discussion of community capacity. In the organizational behavior literature, power is defined as asymmetrical control over valued resources (Anderson and Brion, 2014), and scholarship in political science reflects on power relations and on the formation of social capital (Campbell, 2013; Jacobs and Soss, 2010). Robert Putnam's (2000) research identified and measured five broad dimensions of social capital: community organizational life, engagement in public affairs, community volunteerism, informal sociability, and social trust (see also NRC, 2014). In the sociology of community safety and crime, "collective efficacy" (Sampson et al., 1997) refers to the ability of residents of a given area to exert control over the behavior of individuals and groups and thereby create a safe and orderly environment. Collective efficacy, like community capacity, requires some degree of trust, cohesion, and shared norms of intervention for the common good of the community. Community members who come to know and trust their neighbors and have a sense of ownership and belonging in the place where they live are more likely to work collectively to solve common problems related to promoting health equity.

True community-led action is only possible insofar as communities have the capacity to organize for health equity. For a community to be able to change the conditions in which its members live, members need the capacity and ability to act—they need vision, leadership, voice, and power (see Box 4-2). Thus, building community capacity is the primary mechanism that ensures the democratization of decision making around health equity. Furthermore, community capacity (and community involvement more generally) is key for sustained change (Verbitsky-Savitz et al., 2016). For change to be long lasting, normative innovations need to be adopted into the very fabric of community social life. Communities with a greater capacity for social organization and collective efficacy are more adept at integrating change into community life because members of the community are themselves part of the intervention.

As discussed earlier, a community movement or action does not occur spontaneously. What Doran Schrantz from ISAIAH, a faith-based coalition, calls "invisible work" needs to be done first: "the work of organizers and organizations like ISAIAH or [the PICO Network] or countless other community organizations across this country. There are conversations at kitchen tables, in church basements, in little meeting rooms, [and] in your

> **BOX 4-2**
> **Power, Voice, Leadership, Collective Action**
>
> **Building power and voice to increase capacity** (Schrantz, 2016). In addition to a lack of economic resources, a lack of political power can contribute to poor community health. Empowering individuals through community organizing to exercise their collective political influence can create policy changes that improve health and well-being.
>
> **Building leaders** (Community Tool Box, 2016). In many cases, emerging community organization leaders are novices in the area of community action. Often, despite successful work experience, they have not acquired the unique knowledge and skills required to lead a successful community organization. According to *Community Organizing: Ground Rules for Grass Roots Organizers* (CIL Management Center, 2005), such knowledge and skills include making the case for change and assembling the data into actionable information to support the case, recruiting the support of anchor organizations, building a base of public support and political power, engaging the media, and securing dependable funding.
>
> **Acting collectively as a community.** This refers to constructing democratic, sustainable, and community-driven organizations that are multi-issue and can work on many different needs over time (FSG, 2011; Kania and Kramer, 2011). See Chapter 8 for an additional discussion of collective impact.

neighborhood in which people go through the experience of being trained and how to have the public skills to pull that off" (Schrantz, 2016).

Depending on the community challenges being addressed, the appropriate range of knowledge and experience will need to be assembled. For example, a kindergarten-through-12th-grade intervention would ideally have expertise not only in education but also in cognitive development, the social environment, public safety, transportation, and other sectors, and the intervention would need to engage parents, caregivers, and, when appropriate, students themselves. Individuals participating from different sectors bring to the table a wide range of knowledge and skills, and there may well be a need for capacity to work collaboratively, with attention given to differences in power and status, in order to attain authentic partnerships with members of the affected community. See, for example, the Magnolia Community Initiative in Chapter 5 for a collaborative community initiative with partners across government, nonprofits, private entities, and faith organizations. Just as a shared vision is important to unite a multi-sector collaboration, authentic partnership with representatives from all affected community segments is essential to help community interventions succeed.

The current state of community health inequities did not emerge overnight or in a vacuum. Policies that intentionally or unintentionally create structural inequities based on bias, whether conscious or unconscious, and discrimination, whether blatant or subtle, continue to shape communities; some are decades old, and others are recent or under consideration. Communities working on interventions to achieve health equity need to engage in dialogue about or directly address these structural challenges in order to pursue effective and successful programs.

Conclusion 4-1: Making health equity a shared vision and value, building community capacity, and fostering multi-stakeholder collaboration are vital in the development of community-driven solutions for promoting health equity.

Conclusion 4-2: It is essential for entities initiating efforts to promote health equity in communities (e.g., government agencies, foundations, and other funders) to require explicit strategies for achieving authentic community engagement and ownership at each stage of such efforts. Specifically, it is important for leaders of such efforts to document and describe on an ongoing basis the engagement of different parts of the community, particularly residents not usually at the table and those most affected by inequitable health conditions.

BUILDING EVIDENCE TO SUPPORT COMMUNITY ACTION

There are numerous examples of successful community-based solutions that promote health equity. However, the partners involved in working to promote community-level intervention have faced challenges to achieving success. Based on the literature concerning the elements that support successful community-level intervention, on examining case examples, and on evaluating current gaps, it is clear that increasing the right kinds of evidence base (see Box 4-3), training, and access to experience would support further advancements in community-level action.

Evidence Base for Community Solutions

A major barrier to the spread of effective community solutions is the mismatch between what may be the most promising solutions and the knowledge base that is available for communities to draw on (Schorr, 2016). The current knowledge base consists primarily of *programs or individualized interventions* that have been shown to work with the use of experimental methods of evaluation, especially randomized controlled

> **BOX 4-3**
> **Why Community-Level Evidence Is Needed**
>
> The Adverse Childhood Experiences (ACE) study (Felitti et al., 1998) captured attention because it documented the long-term effects of childhood trauma. The impact of trauma extends beyond the individuals who directly witness or experience violence. Its long-term damage can also be produced by structural violence, which prevents people and communities from meeting their basic needs. The result is both high levels of trauma across the population and a breakdown of social networks, social relationships, and positive social norms across the community—all of which could otherwise be protective against violence and other health outcomes. The predominant approach to dealing with trauma is medical: individual screening and treatment. Because much of the trauma experienced by young children and their families is present in the social-cultural environment, the physical and built environments, and the economic environment, medical responses should be supplemented with community-level interventions. An enhanced framework and an expansion of supportive literature will be necessary to guide communities in implementing community-level interventions.

trials. As with evidence-based public health practice and policy more broadly (Fielding and Briss, 2006), such traditional methods are a poor fit with the knowledge needed to design and implement cross-sector community solutions that will be effective in achieving health equity. Currently more is known about the *problems* of health inequities than about the *solutions*. Additionally, more is known about the *programs* that have worked in the past to marginally improve health equity than about the *strategies* and *broad, interactive, crosscutting interventions* that could bring greater and more widespread progress in the future.

Building an Evidence Infrastructure Toward Greater Impact

Efforts to design and implement cross-sector community solutions are hampered by the absence of an infrastructure to support knowledge development and dissemination, implementation, continuous improvement, and expanded data collection to inform this evidence base (see data discussions in Chapters 2 and 8 for more information). A strengthened infrastructure to guide community-level interventions will (1) identify the *essential elements* of successful interventions; (2) take account of the *power of systems* to determine results; and (3) assist all stakeholders to engage in *ongoing disciplined inquiry*.

1. Identify the *essential elements* of successful interventions.

An intervention's *essential elements*—or core components, active ingredients, or effectiveness factors—are the functions or principles and activities necessary to achieve successful outcomes, including the implementation and contextual conditions of the solution (e.g., political and regulatory context or funding). When these attributes can be described, communities can be much more rigorous and intentional about what can be and needs to be adapted and what needs to be held constant. The National Scientific Council on the Developing Child reviewed the evidence on commonalities among child care environments that promote healthy development and found that the critical elements are ensuring "that relationships in child care are nurturing, stimulating, and reliable, [leading to] an emphasis on the skills and personal attributes of the caregivers, and on improving the wages and benefits that affect staff turnover" (National Scientific Council on the Developing Child, 2004). This finding is at odds with policies that predominantly define "quality" in terms of more easily quantified but less meaningful metrics such as adult–child ratios, group size, and physical facilities (National Scientific Council on the Developing Child, 2004).

Once identified, these essential elements can be re-bundled to fit a new population and unique circumstances. They are portable, effective guides to action, and can have a multiplying effect because they are more transferable to a wider range of settings than model programs. As noted earlier in the chapter, Thunder Valley CDC has invested in long-term evaluation plans to identify the core elements of its programs and inform strategies in other communities.

To systematically extract these essential elements requires good data, rigorous analysis, and thoughtful judgment as well as the infrastructure and desire to create a better understanding of the core elements of programs, contexts, and systems change aimed at significant outcomes.

2. Take account of the *power of systems* to determine results.

Much of what makes interventions effective is often undermined by the systems in which they operate, especially when the intervention is expanded to reach large numbers. As Patrick McCarthy, president of The Annie E. Casey Foundation, has pointed out, if the road to scale is to reach ambitious goals, it needs to run through public systems (McCarthy, 2014). And decades of experience, McCarthy says, "tell us that a bad system will trump a good program—every time, all the time" (McCarthy, 2014). Whether a community-based collaboration is concerned with youth in the juvenile justice system, students in public schools, families in the child welfare system, the youngest children and their families, or the survivors of domestic violence, even the greatest program cannot succeed in a lasting way if it is housed in a dysfunctional system. It is illusory to think that an effective intervention can be scaled without full recognition of the power of the system that can determine program priorities, budget allocations, staffing levels, and eligibility criteria, and that can nurture or sabotage a culture of trust.

3. Assist all stakeholders to engage in *"ongoing disciplined inquiry."*

To achieve greater impact in the future will require applying evidence that is generated by ongoing disciplined inquiry among practitioners, policy makers, and researchers. This ongoing disciplined inquiry needs to be based on a deep understanding of the problem it seeks to solve, of the systems that produce the current outcomes, of the detailed practical knowledge necessary for good ideas to actually work, and a willingness to constantly reassess operations and make changes that evidence and experience suggest will lead to improvement.

Community College Pathways (CCP) is an example of ongoing, disciplined inquiry in action. The Carnegie Foundation for the Advancement of Teaching created CCP in response to the extraordinarily high failure rates among the half million community college students annually assigned to remedial math instruction as a prerequisite to taking college-level courses. CCP consists of a network of college faculty, administrators, researchers, program designers, and implementers working together to "achieve big results, reliably and at scale" (CSSP, 2016b) for community college students struggling with remedial math. When CCP began, 80 percent of the students enrolled in these courses did not complete or pass them. Through monthly meetings to learn from the real-world experience of network participants and by adapting research-based ideas from diverse domains, CCP networks changed the way that remedial math classes are conducted, introduced new e-curricula, changed students' own expectations about their ability to succeed at math, and developed support networks among students. Within 2 years, CCP tripled the success rates of remedial math students, who consistently outperformed comparison group students. CCP is now working in ever-wider circles to show how disciplined inquiry can develop effective responses to a problem previously perceived as intractable (Bryk et al., 2015).

In selecting interventions or elements of intervention to implement, communities attempting to draw from existing directories of effective programs find a severely limited knowledge base (Hayes et al., 2012; Schorr, 2016; Woulfe et al., 2010). Even when it comes to individual programmatic interventions that have been shown to have an impact in the contexts in which they have been tested, users cannot reliably conclude that the same intervention will produce similar results in their own system or community (CSSP, 2016a).

Communities determined to promote health equity by bridging the gaps among research, practice, and policy recognize the need to go beyond identifying and scaling up individual "evidence-based" programs. As they pursue broader change in the conditions for health, they find a dearth of systematic, organized information and guidance to help them set common goals and measures of success; select multifaceted and mutually reinforcing strategies, grounded in strong theory; align implementation efforts, and make the necessary system and community-level changes to adapt and continuously improve. A centralized resource for communities is needed, and several partially relevant models exist, some of which could potentially be modified to operate in an expanded capacity. These include the County Health Rankings (CHR) What Works for Health database, the CDC Community Health Improvement (CHI) Navigator, and also, perhaps, the Agency for Healthcare Research and Quality's (AHRQ's) Measures Clearinghouse and the National Library of Medicine (which serves as a knowledge curation resource through its special queries). The CHR What Works for Health database provides information for community health improvement organized by expected beneficial outcomes, potential beneficial outcomes, evidence of effectiveness, effect on disparities, implementation examples, implementation resources, and citations. The CHI Navigator[8] is intended for individuals and groups who lead or participate in community health improvement work

> within hospitals and health systems, public health agencies, and other community organizations. It is a one-stop shop that offers community stakeholders expert-vetted tools and resources for depicting visually the who, what, where, and how of improving community health; making the case for collaborative approaches to community health improvement; establishing and maintaining effective collaborations; and finding interventions that work for the greatest impact on health and well-being for all. (CDC, 2015)

Recommendation 4-1: A public–private consortium[9] should create a publicly available repository of evidence to inform and guide efforts to promote health equity at the community level. The consortium should also offer support to communities, including technical assistance.

---

[8] For more information, see http://www.cdc.gov/chinav (accessed December 5, 2016).

[9] This could be done through such mechanisms as a collaboration among CDC (home of the Community Health Improvement Navigator initiative), university-based centers (see the example of the University of Wisconsin Population Health Institute that operates the County Health Rankings [CHR] What Works for Health database), and one or more philanthropic organizations.

The repository could include databases that provide and integrate information from multiple relevant sectors (e.g., education, health, housing) at the national, state, and metropolitan levels as well as for smaller local geographies such as census tracts; and information on effective intervention approaches and the knowledge necessary to strengthen the capacity of communities to take action on such needs as educational attainment, job training and job creation, civil rights, decent and stable housing, and other determinants of health by race, ethnicity, gender, disability status, age, sexual identity/orientation, and other demographic characteristics. Providing relevant assistance, guidance, and support to local community leaders (e.g., identifying data sources, accessing funding available from federal agencies, and using civil rights law) could improve the chances of success for community organizations. Creating or building on existing resources that could become a repository of information and a source of technical assistance could also be complemented by efforts to build learning networks, thus allowing communities to share experiences with other local community leaders (see, for example, the possibilities suggested by Community Commons[10] and others).

REFERENCES

Anderson, C., and S. Brion. 2014. Perspectives on power in organizations. *Annual Review of Organizational Psychology and Organizational Behavior* 1(1):67–97.

Bobo, L., and F. D. Gilliam. 1990. Race, sociopolitical participation, and black empowerment. *American Political Science Review* 84(2):377–393.

Browning, R. P., D. R. Marshall, and D. H. Tabb. 1984. *Protest is not enough: The struggle of blacks and Hispanics for equality in urban politics.* Berkeley: University of California Press.

Bryk, A. S., L. M. Gomez, A. Grunow, and P. G. LeMahieu. 2015. *Learning to improve: How America's schools can get better at getting better.* Cambridge, MA: Harvard Education Press.

Campbell, D. 2013. Social networks and political participation. *Annual Review of Political Science* 16:33–48.

CDC (U.S. Centers for Disease Control and Prevention). 2015. *CDC community health improvement navigator.* https://www.cdc.gov/chinav (accessed December 5, 2016).

CIL Management Center. 2005. Community organizing: Ground rules for grass roots organizers. Chapter 10: Leadership development. 10.3: Leadership development skills. http://wnyil.org/community-organizing/chapter10_3.html (accessed October 18, 2016).

Chaskin, R. J. 1999. *Defining community capacity: A framework and implications from a comprehensive community initiative.* Chicago, IL: Chapin Hall Center for Children at the University of Chicago.

---

[10] For more information, see https://www.communitycommons.org (accessed December 5, 2016).

Community Tool Box. 2016. *Chapter 1. Section 7. Working together for healthier communities: A framework for collaboration among community partnership, support organizations, and funders.* http://ctb.ku.edu/en/table-of-contents/overview/model-for-community-change-and-improvement/framework-for-collaboration/main (accessed October 18, 2016).

CSSP (Center for the Study of Social Policy). 2016a. *Better evidence for decision-makers.* Washington, DC: Center for the Study of Social Policy.

CSSP. 2016b. *Carnegie math pathways: Case study.* http://www.cssp.org/policy/body/Carnegie-Math-Pathways.pdf (accessed October 26, 2016).

DOT (U.S. Department of Transportation). 2016. *Tiger discretionary grants.* https://www.transportation.gov/tiger (accessed October 13, 2016).

Dubb, S., S. McKinley, and T. Howard. 2013. *Achieving the anchor promise: Improving outcomes for low-income children, families and communities.* Takoma Park, MD: The Democracy Collaborative at the University of Maryland.

Eisinger, P. K. 1972. *The conditions of protest behavior in American cities.* Madison: University of Wisconsin.

Fawcett, S. B., J. Schultz, J. Watson-Thompson, M. Fox, and R. Bremby. 2010. Building multisectoral partnerships for population health and health equity. *Preventing Chronic Disease* 7(6):1–7.

Felitti, V. J., R. F. Anda, D. Nordenberg, D. F. Williamson, A. M. Spitz, V. Edwards, M. P. Koss, and J. S. Marks. 1998. Relationship of childhood abuse and household dysfunction to many of the leading causes of death in adults: The Adverse Childhood Experiences (ACE) study. *American Journal of Preventive Medicine* 14(4):245–258.

Fielding, J. E., and P. A. Briss. 2006. Promoting evidence-based public health policy: Can we have better evidence and more action? *Health Affairs (Millwood)* 25(4):969–978.

FSG (Foundation Strategy Group). 2011. *Collective impact.* http://www.fsg.org/ideas-in-action/collective-impact (accessed October 18, 2016).

FSG. 2013. *Using collective impact in a public health context: Introduction.* http://www.fsg.org/blog/using-collective-impact-public-health-context-introduction (accessed October 18, 2016).

Hargreaves, M. B., N. Verbitsky-Savitz, B. Coffee-Borden, L. Perreras, P. J. Pecora, C. Roller White, G. B. Morgan, T. Barila, A. Ervin, L. Case, R. Hunter, and K. Adams. 2016. *Advancing the measurement of collective capacity to address adverse childhood experiences and resilience.* Gaithersburg, MD: Community Science.

Hayes, S. L., M. K. Mann, F. M. Morgan, H. Kitcher, M. J. Kelly, and A. L. Weightman. 2012. Collaboration between local health and local government agencies for health improvement. *The Cochrane Database of Systematic Reviews* (10):Cd007825.

Hojnacki, M., D. C. Kimball, F. R. Baumgartner, J. M. Berry, and B. L. Leech. 2012. Studying organizational advocacy and influence: Reexamining interest group research. *Annual Review of Political Science* 15(1):379–399.

Holder, H. D., R. F. Saltz, J. W. Grube, R. B. Voas, P. J. Gruenewald, and A. J.Treno. 1997. A community prevention trial to reduce alcohol-involved accidental injury and death: Overview. *Addiction* 92 (Suppl 2):S155–S171.

Hoying, A., N. Sambourskiy, and B. Sanders. 2012. *A structured approach to effective partnering: Lessons learned from public and private sector leaders.* Atlanta, GA: U.S. Centers for Disease Control and Prevention.

HUD (U.S. Department of Housing and Urban Development). 2016. *Sustainable communities regional planning grants.* http://portal.hud.gov/hudportal/HUD?src=/program_offices/economic_resilience/sustainable_communities_regional_planning_grants (accessed October 18, 2016).

Jacobs, L. R., and J. Soss. 2010. The politics of inequality in America: A political economy framework. *Annual Review of Political Science* 13(1):341–364.

Kania, L., and M. Kramer. 2011. Collective impact. *Stanford Social Innovation Review* Winter:36-41. https://ssir.org/articles/entry/collective_impact (accessed October 18, 2016).

Lyons, C. J., M. B. Velez, and W. A. Santoro. 2013. Neighborhood immigration, violence, and city-level immigrant political opportunities. *American Sociological Review* 78(4):604–632.

Mattessich, P. W., and E. J. Rausch. 2014. Cross-sector collaboration to improve community health: A view of the current landscape. *Health Affairs* 33(11):1968–1974.

Mays, G. P., C. B. Mamaril, and L. R. Timsina. 2016. Preventable death rates fell where communities expanded population health activities through multisector networks. *Health Affairs (Millwood)* 35(11):2005–2013.

McAdam, D. 1982. *Political process and the development of black insurgency, 1930-1970*. Chicago, IL: University of Chicago Press.

McCarthy, P. T. 2014. The road to scale runs through public systems. *Stanford Social Innovation Review* Spring:12-13. https://ssir.org/articles/entry/the_road_to_scale_runs_through_public_systems (accessed October 18, 2016).

Meyer, D. S. 2004. Protest and political opportunities. *Annual Review of Sociology* 30:125.

Meyer, D. S., and D. C. Minkoff. 2004. Conceptualizing political opportunity. *Social Forces* 82(4):1457–1492.

National Scientific Council on the Developing Child. 2004. *Young children develop in an environment of relationships*. Cambridge, MA: Harvard University Center on the Developing Child.

Norris, T., and M. Pittman. 2000. The healthy communities movement and the coalition for healthier cities and communities. *Public Health Reports* 115(2/3):118–124.

NRC (National Research Council). 2014. *Civic engagement and social cohesion: Measuring dimensions of social capital to inform policy*. Washington, DC: The National Academies Press.

Ockene, J. K., E. A. Edgerton, S. M. Teutsch, L. N. Marion, T. Miller, J. L. Genevro, C. J. Loveland-Cherry, J. E. Fielding, and P. A. Briss. 2007. Integrating evidence-based clinical and community strategies to improve health. *American Journal of Preventive Medicine* 32:244–252.

Polletta, F. 2008. Culture and movements. *Annals of the American Academy of Political and Social Science* 619(1):78–96.

Porter, M. E., and M. R. Kramer. 2011. Creating shared value. *Harvard Business Review* 89(1-2 January-February 2011):62–77.

Prevention Institute. 2014. *Making connections for mental health and wellbeing among men and boys in the U.S.* Oakland, CA: Prevention Institute.

Prybil, L., F. D. Scutchfield, R. Killian, A. Kelly, G. Mays, A. Carman, S. Levey, A. McGeorge, and D. W. Fardo. 2014. Improving community health through hospital-public health collaboration: Insights and lessons learned from successful partnerships. In *Health management and policy faculty book gallery: Book 2*. Lexington, KY: Commonwealth Center for Governance Studies, Inc.

Putnam, R. D. 2000. *Bowling alone: The collapse and revival of American community*. New York: Simon and Schuster.

RWJF (Robert Wood Johnson Foundation). 2015. *From vision to action: A framework and measures to mobilize a culture of health*. Princeton, NJ: Robert Wood Johnson Foundation.

Sampson, R. J., S. W. Raudenbush, and F. Earls. 1997. Neighborhoods and violent crime: A multilevel study of collective efficacy. *Science* 277(5328):918–924.

Santoro, W. A. 2008. The civil rights movement and the right to vote: Black protest, segregationist violence and the audience. *Social Forces* 86(4):1391–1414.

Schorr, L. B. 2016. Reconsidering evidence: What it means and how we use it. *Stanford Social Innovation Review*. https://ssir.org/articles/entry/reconsidering_evidence_what_it_means_and_how_we_use_it (accessed October 18, 2016).

Schrantz, D. 2016. PowerPoint presentation to the Committee on Community-Based Solutions to Promote Health Equity in the United States in Washington, DC, April 27, 2016. http://www.nationalacademies.org/hmd/~/media/Files/Activity%20Files/PublicHealth/COH_Community%20Based%20Solutions/April%20Meeting/Schrantz%20D.pdf (accessed October 18, 2016).

Shapiro, V. B., J. D. Hawkins, and S. Oesterle. 2015. Building local infrastructure for community adoption of science-based prevention: The role of coalition functioning. *Prevention Science* 16(8):1136–1146.

Shortell, S. M., A. P. Zukoski, J. A. Alexander, G. J. Bazzoli, D. A. Conrad, R. Hasnain-Wynia, S. Sofaer, B. Y. Chan, E. Casey, and F. S. Margolin. 2002. Evaluating partnerships for community health improvement: Tracking the footprints. *Journal of Health Policy and Law* 27(1).

Skocpol, T., M. Ganz, and Z. Munson. 2000. A nation of organizers: The institutional origins of civic voluntarism in the United States. *The American Political Science Review* 94(3):527–546.

Smart Grow America. 2014. *State-level complete streets policies*. https://www.smartgrowthamerica.org/app/legacy/documents/cs/policy/cs-state-policies.pdf (accessed October 18, 2016).

Thunder Valley CDC (Community Development Corporation). 2016. *Theory of Change*. http://thundervalley.org/change/theory-change (accessed October 23, 2016).

Trickett, E. J., S. Beehler, C. Deutsch, L. W. Green, P. Hawe, K. McLeroy, R. L. Miller, B. D. Rapkin, J. J. Schensul, A. J. Schulz, and J. E. Trimble. 2011. Advancing the science of community-level interventions. *American Journal of Public Health* 101(8):1410–1419.

Verbitsky-Savitz, N., M. B. Hargreaves, S. Penoyer, N. Morales, B. Coffee-Borden, and E. Whitesell. 2016. *Preventing and mitigating the effects of aces by building community capacity and resilience: Appi cross-site evaluation findings*. Washington, DC: Mathematica Policy Research.

Williams, M. S. 1998. *Voice, trust, and memory: Marginalized groups and the failings of liberal representation*. Princeton, NJ: Princeton University Press.

Woulfe, J., T. R. Oliver, S. J. Zahner, and K. Q. Siemering. 2010. Multisector partnerships in population health improvement. *Preventing Chronic Disease* 7(6):A119. https://www.cdc.gov/pcd/issues/2010/nov/10_0104.htm (accessed October 23, 2016).

5

Examples of Communities Tackling Health Inequity

Communities across the United States are developing and putting into action strategies that can contribute to the reduction of health inequities. Too often these community efforts go unmentioned in the media while stories of blight, crime, or community unrest receive more attention. The committee was asked to identify and examine six or more examples of community-based solutions (see the report conceptual model in Figure 5-1) that address health inequities, drawing from interventions or activities that intentionally or indirectly promote equal opportunities for health. The examples identified in this chapter span health and non-health sectors and take into account the range of factors that contribute to health inequity in the United States, such as systems of employment, public safety, housing, transportation, education, and others. The committee provides a summary of each example to demonstrate both the innovative work conducted by communities and the challenges that they face. The committee also comments on a number of crosscutting essential elements that show promise for promoting health equity in communities. Finally, the committee summarizes a number of lessons learned from both the success and the failures of the strategies described.

PROCESS OF SELECTION

The committee engaged in a robust process, described in complete detail in the Chapter 5 Annex, to review a total of 105 examples gathered and select the 9 community examples that are outlined in this chapter.

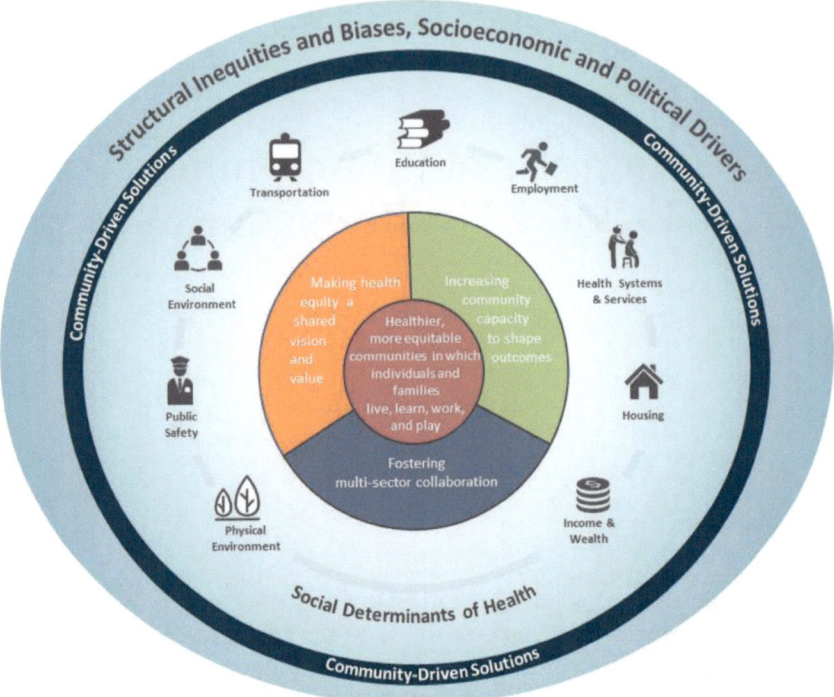

FIGURE 5-1 Report conceptual model for community solutions to promote health equity.
NOTE: The community-driven solutions are highlighted here to convey the focus of this chapter.

In brief, the committee queried local and state organizations, relevant philanthropic organizations, researchers and others; reviewed relevant reports and publications on the topic of community health; and undertook a literature review. It is important to note that the committee did not evaluate the overall effectiveness of these community efforts. Rather, the committee sought out community-driven solutions that target the social determinants of health with strong links to health outcomes, as evidenced by the literature. The committee developed three sets of criteria to guide the selection of the case studies:

1. **Core criteria:** All examples chosen for this chapter must
    - address at least one (preferably more) of the nine social determinants of health identified by the committee (education, employment, health systems and services, housing, income

and wealth, physical environment, public safety, social environment, and transportation) and be
   - community-driven
   - multi-sectoral
   - evidence-informed
2. **Aspirational criteria:** Examples were considered based on the convening organization's ability to engage nontraditional partners and to work in an interdisciplinary and multilevel manner and also on the documentation of plans to achieve outcomes and sustain the effort.
3. **Contextual criteria:** Examples were chosen to reflect a diversity of communities, populations, solutions, and demographic characteristics.

COMMUNITY EXAMPLES[1]

The following section summarizes the strategies of nine communities whose efforts focus on addressing the social determinants of health across a number of different geographic locations, environments, and community challenges (see Figure 5-2 for the geographic distribution). These summaries highlight the core and aspirational criteria that the committee developed and the approach that each community took toward making health equity a shared vision and value, increasing community capacity to shape outcomes and fostering multi-sector collaboration as well as showing how the strategies addressed the broader socioeconomic and political context to ultimately achieve healthier, more equitable communities. For easy reference, Table 5-1 lists the nine communities, the social (or environmental, or economic) determinants of health they address, and the key sectors with which each community partnered to implement its solutions. The community efforts described are not intended to reflect the full range of communities across the United States and of effective community-driven efforts to improve well-being and health equity. For example, the communities do not include an example from the lesbian, gay, bisexual, and transgender (LGBT) community or one that reflects individuals with disabilities or individuals with mental illness.[2]

---

[1] Community examples are provided in alphabetical order.
[2] For example, LGBT advocates, addressing the regulatory hurdles to timely and appropriate research for better AIDS treatments, protested and advocated for change and succeeded in substantially altering the way the National Institutes of Health reviews and conducts human subjects research across all domains. For other examples of successful efforts among these groups, see http://dralegal.org/cases (accessed July 17, 2016) for a list of lawsuits conducted by Disability Rights Advocates, the mental health parity work conducted by the National Alliance on Mental Illness (NAMI), or the Bithlo Transformation Effort (http://stakeholderhealth.org/transformative-partnership/case-study-bithlo [accessed August 28, 2016]).

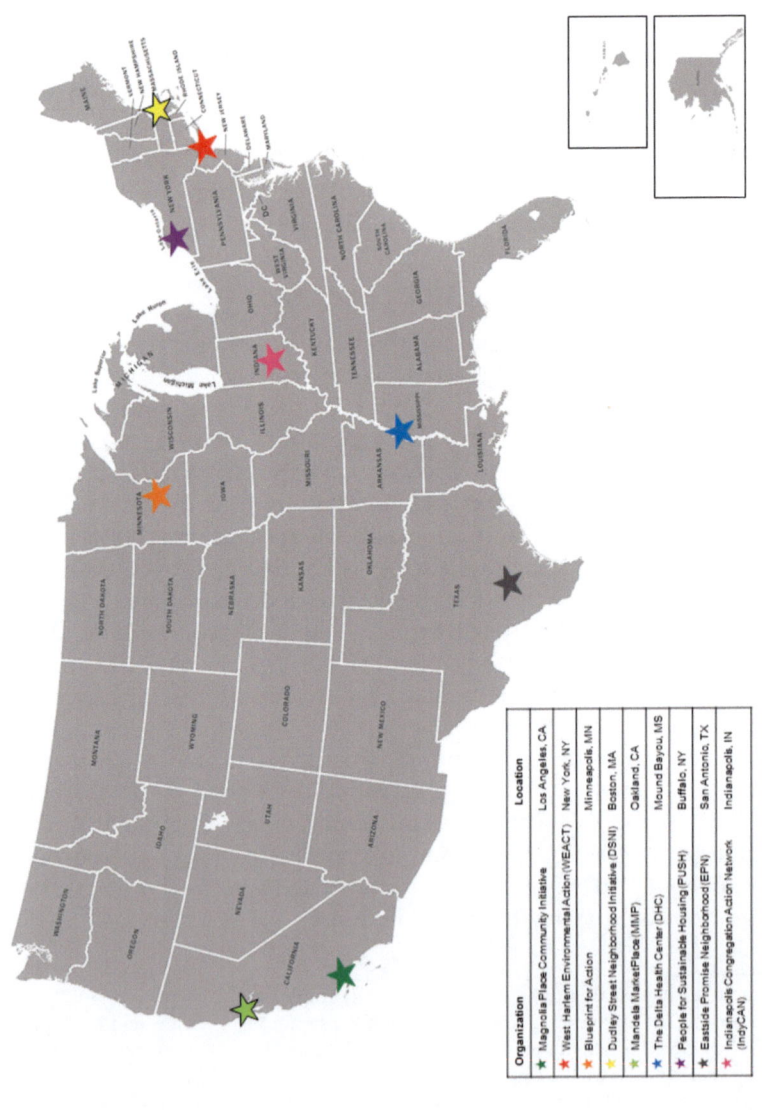

FIGURE 5-2 Geographic distribution of the nine community examples.

Each of the nine community initiatives is at a different phase of development: some have been around for more than 40 years, while others emerged in the past few years, and each has a unique approach. Because the examples went beyond traditional health or health care approaches, the outcomes are often tied to specific project goals rather than to the long-term health outcomes that emerge from these benefits. For example, a community whose focus is on housing might measure the number of low-income housing units that became available, and a community effort focused on education might measure improvement in third-grade reading levels or increased levels of high school graduation rates—all measures that are proxies for the long-term achievement of improved health. The committee also used these examples to identify some of the intangible qualities needed to initiate, maintain, and sustain community efforts.

The committee was inspired by the communities described in this chapter and is grateful to them for their willingness to share their history and accomplishments for this report. These examples serve as a proof of principle that communities can mobilize to promote effective change that addresses multiple determinants of health. These examples are not blueprints. Exact replicas of these communities' interventions might not work in other communities, but their lessons learned will prove valuable to many communities that hope to create positive change.

Minneapolis Blueprint for Action to Prevent Youth Violence[3]

Background and History

The Minneapolis Blueprint for Action to Prevent Youth Violence[4] is a community-driven, grassroots response to the issue of youth violence, originally developed in 2008. From 2002 to 2011, homicide was

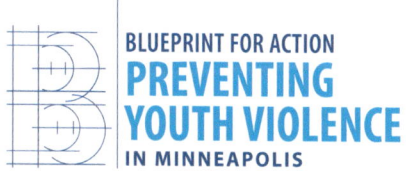

---

[3] This summary is an edited account that was prepared on the basis of templates completed by staff of each community initiative. Statements and opinions expressed are those of the community organization and have not been endorsed or verified by the National Academies of Sciences, Engineering, and Medicine.

[4] For more information, see http://www.minneapolismn.gov/health/youth/yvp/blueprint (accessed September 13, 2016).

TABLE 5-1 Nine Community Examples—Brief Information

	Blueprint for Action	Delta Health Center	Dudley Street Neighborhood Initiative	Eastside Promise Neighborhood
Location	Minneapolis, MN	Mississippi Delta	Boston, MA	San Antonio, TX
Social determinant of health				
Education	•	•		•*
Employment	•		•*	•
Health systems and services	•	•*		
Housing			•	
Income and wealth		•	•	
Physical environment	•	•	•*	•
Public safety	•*		•	•
Social environment	•	•		•
Transportation	•	•		
Key community partners	County and city departments, local school district, local youth agencies, faith-based organizations, local businesses	Community health associations, educational institutions, agricultural co-ops	Other community stakeholder organizations, educational institutions, nonprofit organizations	Local nonprofits, local school district, city agencies, faith-based organizations, educational institutions, health providers, local elected officials
Outcomes	From 2007–2015: • 62% reduction in youth gunshot victims • 34% reduction in youth victims of crime • 76% reduction in youth arrests with a gun	• Rate of low birth weight babies decreased from 20.7% in 2013 to 3.8% in 2015	From 2014–2015: • Percent of high school students at or above grade level according to state mathematics assessments increased from 36% to 63%	From 2015–2016, number of survey respondents who answered that: Child care is available to them when needed most of the time or sometimes increased from 80% to 100%

EXAMPLES OF COMMUNITIES TACKLING HEALTH INEQUITY   217

	Indianapolis Congregation Action Network	Magnolia Community Initiative	Mandela MarketPlace	People United for Sustainable Housing	WE ACT for Environmental Justice
	Indianapolis, IN	Los Angeles, CA	Oakland, CA	Buffalo, NY	West Harlem, NY
	• • • • •	• • •*	 • • •* •	 •* • •	 • •* • •
	Faith-based organizations, businesses, government, community leaders	More than 70 partner organizations, including government, nonprofit, for-profit, faith, and community group associations that connect programs and providers	Local businesses, educational institutions, youth development organizations, housing developers, government agencies, foundations	Government agencies (housing, energy, parks), local elected officials, nonprofits and NGOs, private-sector businesses	Academic institutions and CBPRers, housing groups, legal partners, energy and solar providers, government agencies, local elected officials
	• Average PICO member engages in 76% more civic duty than average resident • Reduction in incarceration in Marion County will be measured using data submitted to U.S. Annual Survey of Jails	• In 2016, 57.3 percent of children ages 0 to 5 had access to a place other than an emergency room when sick or in need of health-related services	• 641,000+ pounds of produce distributed in food insecure communities • 76% of shoppers reported increased consumption of fruits and vegetables	• Currently conducting regional mapping project (to be completed end of 2016) measuring number of redevelopers	• New policies and legislative reform on issues related to air quality monitoring and use of harmful compounds such as BPA and

continued

TABLE 5-1 Continued

	Blueprint for Action	Delta Health Center	Dudley Street Neighborhood Initiative	Eastside Promise Neighborhood
			• Four-year adjusted cohort graduation rate increased from 51% to 82% • Percent of students who enroll in a 2-year or 4-year college or university after graduation increased from 48% to 69%	They work with others to improve their neighborhood increased from 58% to 83% Their neighborhood has safe places for kids to play increased from 40% to 67%

NOTES: Outcomes as calculated and reported by each of the community initiatives. An asterisk (*) denotes the main social (or environmental or economic) determinant(s) of health on which the community focused. BPA = bisphenol A; CBPR = community-based participatory research; NGO = nongovernmental organization; PICO = People Improving Communities through Organization.

the leading cause of death among Minneapolis residents ages 15–24 years, accounting for 39 percent of deaths in this age group and disproportionately affecting youth of color (Blueprint for Action, 2013). Resident perceptions of safety differed across racial/ethnic groups as well. In 2006, a county survey revealed that gangs were considered a neighborhood problem by 40 percent of Hispanics, 35 percent of African Americans, 24 percent of Asians/Pacific Islanders, and 11 percent of whites (see Table 5-2 for data on Minneapolis demographics) (Blueprint for Action, 2013).

By 2008, the city of Minneapolis had already been expending its resources through various law enforcement strategies to address the staggering rates of youth violence, but the city was not seeing sufficient results from those efforts (Zanjani, 2011). A call for governmental action

Indianapolis Congregation Action Network	Magnolia Community Initiative	Mandela MarketPlace	People United for Sustainable Housing	WE ACT for Environmental Justice
• Increased access to jobs through expanded transit by using Indianapolis Metropolitan Planning Organization's geographic information system mapping data	• In 2015, 78.2 percent of students graduated from high school • In 2016, 45.7 percent of students enrolled in a two or four year college or university after graduation • From 2014 to 2015, 75.7 percent of students reported that they felt safe both at school and while traveling to and from school	• $5.5+ million in new revenue generated • 26+ job/ ownership opportunities generated	housing units, number of employed workers, amount of carbon emission reduction, and utility bill cost savings for low-income households	phthalates in consumer products, pesticides, and flame retardants

was put out by community members and stakeholders, including members of an advisory group comprised of youth-serving organizations and community leaders who were knowledgeable about the various cultural communities in Minneapolis.

The outcome was the first Blueprint for Action, which is a coordinated, strategic plan to apply the public health approach to violence prevention through evidence-based strategies and by engaging multiple partners and stakeholders. The mayor recommended a roster of stakeholders to engage and the city council adopted a motion that specifically identified partners to include in the process of development. Leaders who came together to develop the blueprint included representatives from law enforcement, juvenile supervision, public health, youth programs,

TABLE 5-2 City of Minneapolis Demographics

Total	~410,939 residents
Race/Ethnicity	63.8% White
	18.6% African American
	10.5% Latino or Hispanic
	5.6% Asian
	2.0% Native American/American Indian
Gender	49.7% female
Age	6.9% under 5 years
	20.2% under 18 years
	8.0 % 65 years and over
Education	89% completed high school
	16% received bachelor's degree or higher
Employment	3.3% unemployed
Income	$50,767 median income
	22.6% in poverty

NOTE: Percentages may not add up to 100 percent due to varied reporting, rounding, and missing data from source.
SOURCES: BLS, 2016; U.S. Census Bureau, 2015b.

education, social services, faith communities, neighborhoods, and city and county government. The goals of the current blueprint[5] are to

- foster violence-free social environments
- promote positive opportunities and connections to trusted adults for all youth
- intervene with youth and their families at first sign of risk
- restore youth who have gone down the wrong path
- protect children and youth from violence in the community

These goals provided a framework under which to align the many programs, services, and other efforts that were incorporated into the blueprint, some of which were already under implementation by community groups, nonprofits, and government agencies in Minneapolis.

When the call for action to respond to youth violence was received, a citywide collaborative effort, supported by the Minneapolis Foundation and the mayor, was undertaken. First, the Minneapolis City Council passed a resolution declaring youth violence a public health issue and it created a steering committee that led to the development of the Blueprint for Action. The Minneapolis health department and Minneapolis

---

[5] For more information on the 2013 Blueprint for Action, see http://www.minneapolismn.gov/www/groups/public/@health/documents/webcontent/wcms1p-114466.pdf (accessed September 13, 2016).

Foundation examined youth arrest and detention data and upstream risk and protective factors for youth violence. This evidence informed such blueprint program components as employment programs, an anonymous tip line, a gang prevention and healthy youth development curriculum, and a neighborhood clean sweep program.[6]

Across neighborhoods, disparities in economic conditions are apparent throughout the city of Minneapolis. For example, the annual household income is quite different in such low-income communities as Near North (median income $24,733) and Phillips (median income $25,125) than it is in communities such as Southwest (median income $94,667, a nearly fourfold difference) (Minnesota Compass, 2016). The blueprint was developed with the understanding that the communities suffering from concentrated poverty were also experiencing disproportionate amounts of youth violence. According to a county-level survey in 2010, more than half (57 percent) of the adults in the Camden and Near North communities and about one-third (33 percent) of the adults in the Central, Phillips, and Powderhorn communities cited gangs as a serious problem, compared with only 10 percent of adults who lived in other neighborhoods of Minneapolis (Blueprint for Action, 2013).

Initially, the program focused on youth ages 8–17 who resided in neighborhoods experiencing the highest rates of crime and violence. In 2009 the program expanded to 22 neighborhoods, and the target age range was extended to age 24, based on indicators that demonstrated a higher risk of youth violence in Minneapolis for this population. These indicators were based on data compiled by the local health department from sources across various sectors, including the U.S. Census, the Minneapolis Police Department, Minnesota Hospital Association, and the Minneapolis Park and Recreation Board. The blueprint also developed criteria factors for the target neighborhoods based on available data:

- rate of homicides
- rate of violent crime
- rate of firearm-related assault injuries
- population under 15 years of age
- percent of families in poverty with related children under 18
- access to a Minneapolis Park and Recreation center

According to the Minneapolis Health Department, "the ultimate success of the blueprint is reliant on the extent to which community

---

[6] For a list of the ongoing activities under the Blueprint for Action, see http://www.minneapolismn.gov/www/groups/public/@health/documents/webcontent/wcms1p-114466.pdf (accessed September 19, 2016).

stakeholders remain a part of the process" (Blueprint for Action, 2013). Community stakeholders include neighborhood associations, faith groups, schools, libraries, parks, local businesses, and block clubs. Furthermore, the blueprint connects with other communities facing similar challenges and applying a prevention approach to violence through networks such as the Prevention Institute's UNITY initiative, the National Forum on Youth Violence Prevention (see Figure 5-3 for alignment of goals with the National Forum), and Cities United.

Solutions to Address the Social Determinants of Health

The underlying causes and correlates of violence overlap substantially with those of health inequity (Prevention Institute, 2011). Therefore, a multidisciplinary public health approach to the issue of youth violence, such as the one taken by Blueprint for Action, can have a significant impact on the social determinants of health.

Public safety The primary goal of the blueprint is to reduce homicides and firearm-related injuries, in addition to improving juvenile interactions with the criminal justice system as needed. One program that seeks to do

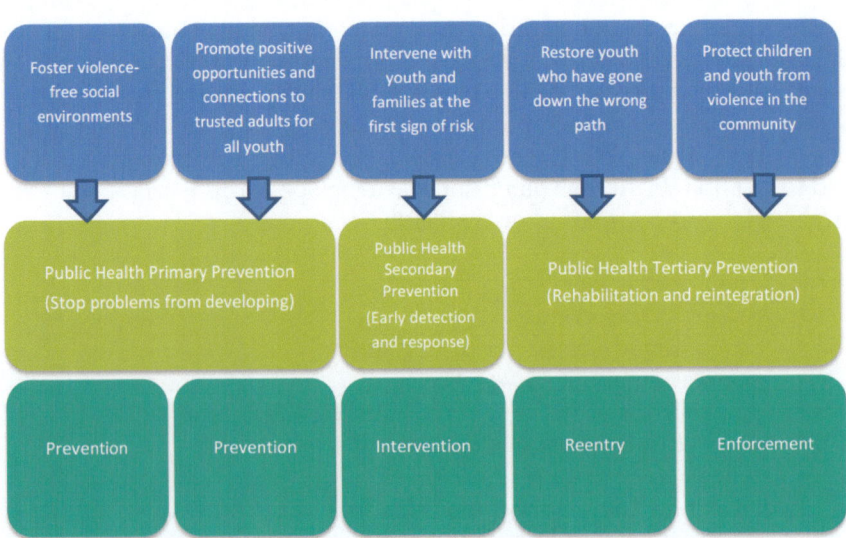

FIGURE 5-3 The alignment of the five Minneapolis blueprint goals with the National Forum to Prevent Youth Violence Strategies and the continuum of public health services.
SOURCE: Blueprint for Action, 2013. Used with permission.

this is the Speak Up tip line, a confidential tip line for youth to report a threat of weapons in the community. The idea for this tip line originated from feedback given by young men in a dialogue portion of a meeting to develop the blueprint. While Speak Up received about 10–12 calls per month, data show that usage of the tip line is highly correlated with the amount of funding allocated to public awareness campaigning in the community.[7] The blueprint also employs youth outreach teams in downtown Minneapolis and at high schools to facilitate the creation of an environment that redirects youth to positive activities.

For youth at risk of violent injury, the blueprint offers Inspiring Youth, a case management program, in addition to parental education and support for the youth's families. The program serves 60 youth per year, with plans to increase the number of youth served in 2017. Inspiring Youth has received $100,000 per year from the City of Minneapolis general fund and $45,000 in 2016 and again in 2017 from the Minnesota Department of Public Safety Office of Justice Programs in the form of a Youth Intervention Program grant.

> Inspiring Youth developed out of a repeated experience that the mayor had when he attended funerals of young people. He often heard 'I knew this would happen' from community members who knew the young person. The program was created to both identify youth at risk of being injured violently and to offer them support and services to help them avoid the risk of being involved in violence. —Gretchen Musicant, Commissioner of Health, City of Minneapolis Health Department, 2016

The blueprint implements BUILD, a gang prevention and healthy youth development curriculum for middle schoolers, and provides school resource officers who are evaluated based in part on the number of positive interactions they have with students. The BUILD curriculum provides youth with opportunities to learn about positive decision making, goal setting, and conflict resolution. Thus far, BUILD has been implemented at 10 sites, with the recent development of BUILD Leaders, a program focused on older youth, ages 18–24. Currently, there are two culturally specific groups applying this model in a Native American and an African American community.

Employment The blueprint provides employment and workforce development opportunities for youth as an alternative to engaging in delinquent or violent behavior. The North4 program is operated by Emerge, a place-based community development agency, and provides workforce and life skills training for youth who are gang-involved and who have

---

[7] Source available by request from the National Academies of Sciences, Engineering, and Medicine's Public Access Records Office (PARO@nas.edu).

had previous involvement with the juvenile justice system. This program works to remove barriers to employment that former offenders face when reintegrating into society. Another program designed to create employment opportunities for youth and reduce gang violence is BUILD Leaders, a program that employs older youth to teach an anti-gang curriculum to younger youth. Step Up is a summer employment program for youth (ages 16–21) in the private, nonprofit, and government sectors.

Physical environment The blueprint seeks to create and maintain a physical environment that is conducive to safe and peaceful activities in the community. For example, pop-up parks are part of a collaborative effort with the Minneapolis Park Board to bring activities to abandoned properties, under-programmed parks, and community events. This also entails an innovative graffiti prevention program which is designed to assist communities with projects for removing and preventing graffiti (see Figure 5-4). The Neighborhood Clean Sweep program partners with neighborhood associations to make neighborhoods cleaner.

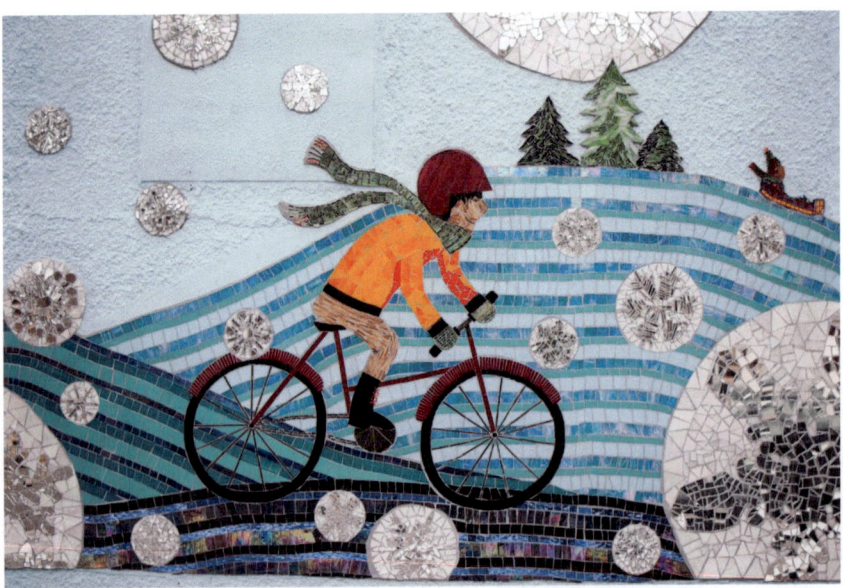

FIGURE 5-4 Bryant market mural, 2011, community mosaic project designed by mosaic artist Sharra Frank.
NOTE: Used with permission by the artist.

Social environment As listed in its core goals, the blueprint is intended to foster a culture of nonviolence and positive interactions between youth and adults. The city's participation in the national Youth Violence Prevention Week annually features community-based organizations that are fostering pro-social activities for youth and peacemaker awards for youth and adults. The awards result in a small financial grant to schools for additional peacemaking activities. Additionally, the blueprint has succeeded in expanding summer hours for out-of-school time, for youth to engage in structured, positive activities.

Health systems and services The blueprint has partnered with two local level I trauma center hospitals to improve health care services for victims of violence. Together, they developed a protocol for intervening and providing psychosocial assessments within 24 hours to every youth (ages 10–24) presenting with a violent injury to the emergency room. This protocol is active in one of the two hospitals, with plans to expand implementation to the other hospital. The blueprint's next step is to implement an emergency department-based program at a level I trauma center hospital that connects youth injured violently with a staff member who knows the community to facilitate access to post-discharge resources and case management. Also in the planning phase is Project Connect, a program that addresses adolescent dating violence at school-based clinics in local high schools. Project Connect is funded by a state grant from the U.S. Department of Justice's Office on Violence Against Women.

Education In addition to the above-mentioned activities in the school setting (e.g., school resource officers and Project Connect), the blueprint supports college scholarships for local students. The Power of You program provides tuition-free scholarships for community college which have been demonstrated to increase the number of students attending college and also retention rates (Minneapolis CPED, 2011). In fact, 80 percent of recipients report that the scholarship influenced their decision to go to college (Minneapolis CPED, 2011).

Transportation Because a lack of access to transportation can be a barrier to accessing important resources, especially in neighborhoods with high rates of violence, the blueprint seeks to increase access to safe transit for youth. Students in Minneapolis high schools are given free bus passes for transportation to and from school and to meet other transportation needs as well.

Data and Outcomes

The blueprint is intended to reduce outcomes that are measured systematically at the local level, such as number of firearm-related assault injuries, the number of youth homicides, the number of youth involved in violent crime, and other various outcomes related to the goals of the blueprint. Minneapolis collects data on performance measures and indicators for each goal across multiple sectors. Results Minneapolis[8] is a management tool the city uses to systematically track performance toward achieving its goals, with data coming from the Minneapolis Police Department, schools, the Minneapolis hospital association, Department of Community Planning and Economic Development, and more. A review panel of city and community leaders meets to track progress and discuss strategies on key performance measures. By regularly tracking performance data at these "progress conferences," city leaders identify areas where the city is excelling as well as opportunities for improvement. Following the implementation of the blueprint, Minneapolis saw an improvement in key outcomes. From 2007 to 2015, the number of youth gunshot victims decreased 62 percent, the number of youth victims of crime decreased by 34 percent, and the number of youth arrests with a gun decreased by 76 percent (City of Minneapolis, 2016).

Promoting Health Equity: Key Elements

The impetus for the blueprint originated from a shared vision for a unified city in which all youth are safe and able to thrive (Blueprint for Action, 2013). Achieving this vision will require a shift in norms and values throughout the community. Community members identified increased communication and outreach about blueprint efforts as well as the availability of safe spaces for youth as priorities for the blueprint in order to mobilize community members around the vision for a violence-free social environment (Blueprint for Action, 2013).

According to Sasha Cotton, the youth violence prevention coordinator at the Blueprint for Action, multi-sector collaboration has been essential to achieving outcomes in Minneapolis. Working closely with other city departments (e.g., juvenile corrections, police department), the county, the school district, local youth-serving agencies, faith-based organizations, local businesses, and other community stakeholders has given the effort a diversity of opinion and perspectives. The multi-sector partnerships required increased communication to reduce the redundancy of programs

---

[8] For more information, see http://www.ci.minneapolis.mn.us/coordinator/rm/index.htm (accessed September 19, 2016).

across agencies (Zanjani, 2011). Other elements that are key to sustained relationships across sectors include relationship building through identifying co-benefits, shared responsibility, and strong leadership. These partnerships allowed for the coordination of data collection from various sectors to inform the blueprint's objectives and priorities in addition to systematically tracking progress.

The blueprint has resulted in an increased capacity across multiple levels in Minneapolis, including the creation of a Youth Violence Prevention Executive Committee and a youth congress. The youth congress created a mechanism for youth to influence decisions and policies on education, housing, safety, employment, transportation, and health (Rybak, 2012). The youth congress has been able to shape important educational and employment programs such as The Power of You scholarship program.

The blueprint has also been able to leverage resources to support community-driven youth development initiatives. In the past 3 years, the Blueprint Approved Institute was created to build the organizational capacity of small community-based organizations serving youth. The institute provides a mechanism for grassroots organizations to gain insights into city government processes, in addition to providing opportunities for the city government to better meet the needs of the community it serves. One of the objectives of the Blueprint Approved Institute is to empower community-based organizations to have better success in competing for grant funding.

Challenges and Lessons Learned

One of the major barriers to sustaining the work of the blueprint, a plan that seeks to address community-level violence, is the transitional nature of the public's interests and of public administration. To begin with, the issue of violence is not uniform from one neighborhood to the next. Each community will have varying concerns, needs, and tailored approaches for achieving its goals, which are always evolving with respect to current events. Furthermore, interests and priorities can shift with the advent of new political administrations. The blueprint team cites strong leadership and deep connections to the community as elements that are critical to stabilizing a plan such as Blueprint for Action across neighborhoods and over time.

Sustaining Success

In 2009 the City of Minneapolis successfully lobbied for the passage of state legislation—the Youth Violence Prevention Act of 2009—which declared youth violence as a public health issue statewide and created three additional pilot sites in Minnesota. During the first year of the blueprint, the city budget adopted by the mayor included $175,000 to support implementation. Over the years, both ongoing and one-time funding from the city has been augmented by state and national grants as well as by some private philanthropic grants. As a result of the blueprint's success, blueprint recommendations continue to inform budget decisions made by the mayor and city council. In order to maintain the cross-sector relationships, biweekly multi-jurisdictional meetings are held to facilitate shared information, relationship building, and problem solving. Furthermore, the blueprint established a youth violence prevention coordinator position which is housed in the Minneapolis Health Department. The placement of this role in the city's health agency, rather than in an elected official's office, has been a critical component of the sustainability of the initiative.

Delta Health Center[9]

Background and History

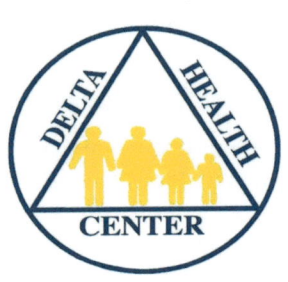

Delta Health Center, Inc. (DHC) had its origins in 1965 as the first neighborhood health center established under the auspices of the Office of Economic Opportunity (OEO). It ultimately became the first rural federally qualified health center (FQHC).[10] DHC provides primary medical and dental care services to individuals and families who reside in Bolivar, Sunflower, Washington, Issaquena, and Sharkey counties in the Mississippi Delta. Employing a community-oriented primary care (COPC) model, DHC develops and implements community development initiatives and projects, all coordinated through the clinic. DHC operates nine community health centers in Mound Bayou (the primary

---

[9] This summary is an edited account that was prepared on the basis of templates completed by staff of each community initiative. Statements and opinions expressed are those of the community organization and have not been endorsed or verified by the National Academies of Sciences, Engineering, and Medicine.

[10] For more information, see http://www.deltahealthcenter.org (accessed September 26, 2016).

site), Greenville (two sites), Indianola, Cleveland, Moorehead, Hollandale, Mayersville, and Rolling Fork.

Not long after the authorization of the Community Action program of the OEO in 1964, the staff began to explore whether it might be able to support some substantial changes in how health care for poor populations was organized. The challenge was to improve the health and well-being of low-income families—and, as public health official Alonzo Yerby put it at a 1965 White House conference, to assure that poor people would no longer be "forced to barter their dignity for their health" (Schorr, 1988).

Two developments moved these ideas from visions to real possibilities. First, the passage of Medicare and Medicaid legislation in 1965 meant that there would be a significant source of funding that could support newly designed service structures in disadvantaged communities. Second, a group of health care reformers, led by Jack Geiger[11] of Harvard University and Count Gibson of Tufts University, came to OEO with thoughtful plans for new entities they called neighborhood health centers. These would be established where the needs were greatest, with the Mississippi Delta as a prime example: an area of concentrated poverty where the infant mortality rate was 70 deaths per 1,000 live births (Longlett et al., 2001), the median family income was $900 per year, and the median level of education was 5 years (Geiger, 2002).

The first OEO health center grant was made in 1966 to create DHC in Mound Bayou, with the goal of demonstrating that it was possible to provide high-quality health care and related services and supports to many who had never benefited from the U.S. health care system and to do so in ways that would be cost-effective. Geiger was then appointed as project director for DHC.[12] The Mississippi Delta community continues to face barriers to health (see Table 5-3 for demographic data). DHC provides services to more than half of the population living below the federal poverty level in the Mississippi Delta. Mound Bayou, the town where DHC's main campus is located, is the oldest predominantly African American community in the country. The level of black-white residential segregation in Bolivar County measures at 61 out of a total 100[13] on the index of dissimilarity (County Health Rankings, 2016a).

---

[11] For an oral history interview with Jack Geiger conducted by John Dittmer in 2013, see https://www.loc.gov/item/afc2010039_crhp0076 (accessed September 26, 2016).

[12] For a short film (produced and directed by Judy Schader Rogers in 1970) that documents the origin of the Delta Health Center, see https://vimeo.com/6659667 (accessed October 17, 2016).

[13] The residential segregation index ranges from 0 (complete integration) to 100 (complete segregation).

TABLE 5-3 Demographics of the Delta Health Center Catchment Population

Total	~9,629 residents
Race/ethnicity	98% African American
	1.0% White
	<1.0% Latino or Hispanic
Health	27.8% uninsured
	35.6% Medicaid patients
	48.7% patients with asthma
	21.6% patients with diabetes
Age	27.7% under 18 years
	61.2% 18–64 years
	11.1% 65 years and over
Education	73.5% high school graduate in Bolivar County
Income	98.2% patients at or below federal poverty line

NOTE: Percentages may not add up to 100 percent due to varied reporting, rounding, and missing data from source.
SOURCES: HRSA, 2015; U.S. Census Bureau, 2015a.

Community-Oriented Primary Care Model

COPC is a systematic approach to health care derived from principles in the disciplines of epidemiology, primary care, preventive medicine, and health promotion which was first pioneered by Sidney and Emily Kark in a South African rural community (Geiger, 2002; Longlett et al., 2001). Geiger asserts that although community development and social change are not explicit goals of the COPC model, they are implicit in the model's emphasis on community organization and local participation with health professionals (Geiger, 2002). DHC employs this model using a multipronged approach that includes the development and implementation of community development projects that improve health, such as an agricultural cooperative, transportation company, and an integrated primary health care system. The integrated primary care system consists of multidisciplinary teams of physicians, nurses, and health educators. COPC also moves beyond the traditional integration of "community engagement" (e.g., a community advisory board). Rather than involving the community in COPC practice, it involves the practice in basic processes and structures within the community (IOM, 1983).

Solutions to Address the Social Determinants of Health

Although DHC is a health care service provider for the community, it targets more than just health care by using insights from the COPC model to act on multiple factors outside of the traditional health care setting that are pertinent to the community.

Health systems and services DHC provides comprehensive health care services at nine sites. Services include dental care; a diabetes clinic; family medical care; a laboratory; nutritional counseling from dieticians; pediatric care; a pharmacy; social services support from licensed social workers; women's health care services; obstetrics, neonatal, and gynecological care; and X-ray services. DHC also offers a smoking cessation program and provides referrals to local mental health centers for its patients. To better meet patients' needs, DHC offers a prescription assistance program for those without prescription coverage who meet income guidelines. Furthermore, the patients' ability to pay is determined using a sliding-scale self-pay tool, based on the 2015 poverty guidelines published by the U.S. Department of Health and Human Services.

Start Strong is a DHC outreach program that targets maternity patients with the goal of reducing barriers and providing incentives for patients to see a provider during their first trimester. Through group counseling and providing access to healthy produce and other essential goods, the program has been able to engage maternity patients who were not initially obtaining usual care during their pregnancies.

Education In the 1970s, DHC established an office of education which sought out aspiring high school and college graduates, assisting them with college and professional school applications as well as connecting them with scholarship information and university contacts (Geiger, 2002). At night DHC also offered high school and college preparatory courses for students. Some of the students who benefited from these educational services returned to work for DHC in various positions—as a clinical director, a staff pediatrician, and executive director (Geiger, 2002). There are plans to reinstate some classes at DHC—specifically, General Education Development (GED) test courses for community residents. Today, DHC partners with the tri-county school system to invite youth ages 14–18 who have an interest in medical careers to shadow providers and assist with local health fairs.

Social environment DHC improves social capital by creating ties to community-based institutions to address the race- and class-based isolation of poor and minority communities (Geiger, 2002). Among these institutions were 10 local community health associations, each of which had a community center and associated programs.

Physical environment DHC developed an agricultural co-op, the North Bolivar County Farm Co-op, with the assistance of a foundation grant from the Federation of Southern Cooperatives in 1968 (see Figure 5-5).

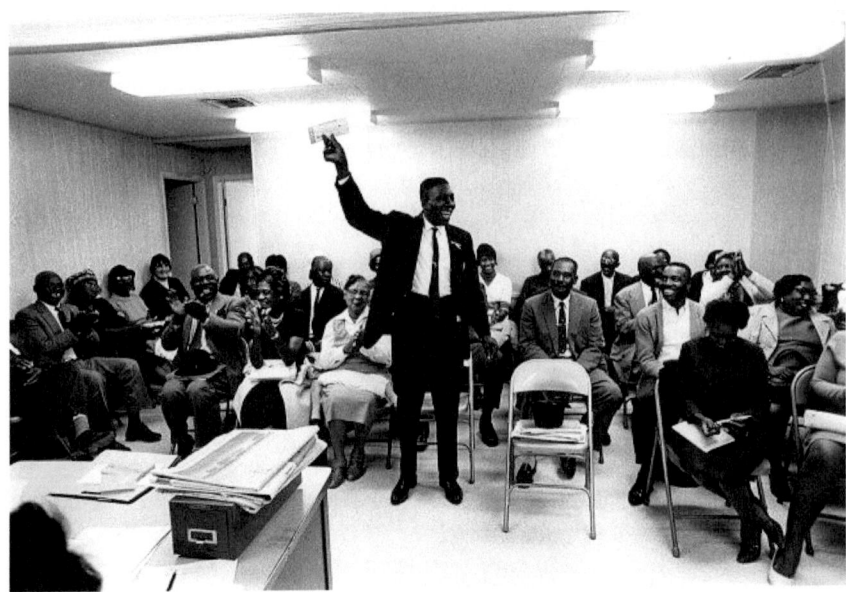

FIGURE 5-5 At a 1968 meeting of the North Bolivar County Health Council at the Delta Health Center, Mound Bayou, Mississippi, William Finch announces the arrival of a Ford Foundation check that will launch a farming cooperative to grow vegetables for a malnourished population.
SOURCE: Photo by Dan Bernstein. Used with permission.

This initiative brought together 1,000 families to harness their labor and operate a 600-acre vegetable farm, building on agricultural skills that were already present in the community. DHC still operates a farm on 6.8 acres of land, producing fruits and vegetables that are made available to its patient population. This work is done in collaboration with Delta Fresh Foods[14] Initiative, which provides funding, and Alcorn State University, which assists with farming services. In an effort to encourage healthy eating, the DHC diabetes clinic initiated a program, Ticket to Pick It, in which patients who visit the clinic receive a ticket that allows them to access fresh produce on the farm at no cost.

Income and wealth In the 1960s the health council of DHC sought to end local discriminatory banking practices. DHC leveraged its funding by proposing that it would deposit the council's funding and cash flow

---

[14] For more information on Delta Fresh Foods, see http://deltafreshfoods.org (accessed September 28, 2016).

with the first local bank that opened a branch in a predominately African American neighborhood, hired community residents as tellers, and engaged in fair employment and mortgage loan practices (Geiger, 2002).

Transportation DHC provides transportation services to and from the clinic sites for all patients in partnership with the Bolivar County Community Action Agency. This service is intended to mitigate the effects of a lack of access to transit as a barrier to receiving health care services. Specifically, maternity patients with children at home but no child care would be unable to visit the center. DHC ensures that transportation for multiple passengers is provided to patients for this reason. In addition, DHC operates a car seat initiative for maternity patients, in which mothers are trained to safely install and use car seats and car seats are provided to each participating family at no cost. In 2016, DHC donated more than 200 car seats to maternity patients.

Data and Outcomes

As a Health Resources and Services Administration health center program grantee, DHC is required to report on the center's performance using measures defined in the Uniform Data System (UDS) every year. UDS measures include patient characteristics (e.g., race/ethnicity, age, income status, insurance status, homelessness, and more), clinical data (e.g., rates of preventive screening services and chronic disease management), and cost data (e.g., grant expenditures and cost per patient). The adoption of electronic medical records and the availability of annual data facilitate data collection for trend analyses. For example, the rate of low-birthweight babies has decreased from 20.7 percent in 2013 to 3.8 percent in 2015 (HRSA, 2015). DHC staff attributes this in part to the increase in obstetrics and gynecology providers on-site over the past few years and also to the targeted programs for maternity patients.

Promoting Health Equity: Key Elements

DHC works across sectors and disciplines to serve the needs of the community in the Mississippi Delta. In 2015 the center partnered with educational institutions such as Emory University and Mississippi State University to engage student volunteers who worked on affordable housing and gardening projects (see Figure 5-6).

DHC illustrates the potential outcomes of capacity building in a community over a sustained period of time. For the past 40 years it has been owned and operated by the North Bolivar County Health and Civic

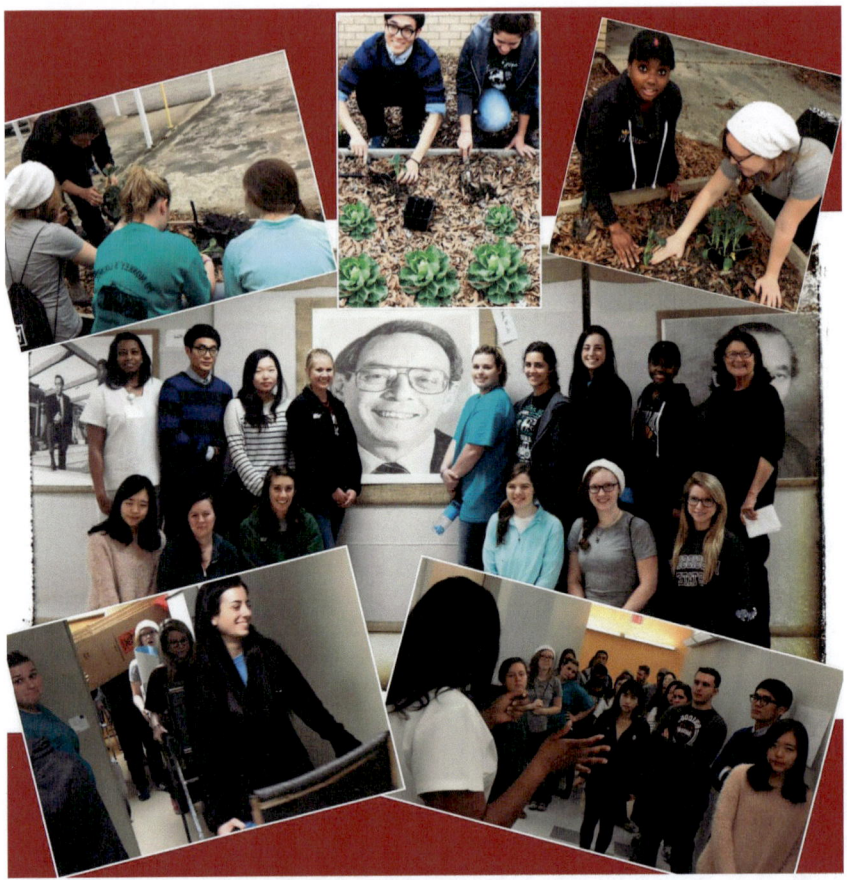

FIGURE 5-6 Mississippi State University students visit DHC and work on community garden with Delta Fresh Foods (2015).
SOURCE: DHC, 2015. Used with permission.

Improvement Association, an organization that the center played a role in creating with the community (Geiger, 2016).

Challenges and Lessons Learned

One of the challenges that DHC currently faces in serving its community is the significant number of residents who fall in the health insurance coverage gap, which amounts to 108,000 people in the state overall (Garfield and Damico, 2016). Among these residents, 52 percent are people of color, 54 percent are women, and 58 percent are in a working family

(Garfield and Damico, 2016). Mississippi is one of the states that opted not to expand Medicaid coverage through the provision of the Patient Protection and Affordable Care Act (ACA), an expansion that estimates indicate could have provided insurance coverage for an additional 181,000 residents in Mississippi (Garfield and Damico, 2016).

Overcoming the historical mistrust of medical institutions among underserved communities and the fear of privacy violations among patients has been a challenge for DHC staff. By remaining visible and active in community activities (e.g., festivals, health fairs, career day in schools), in addition to being transparent about adhering to Health Insurance Portability and Accountability Act privacy rules, DHC has worked to build trust among community residents. DHC also adapts to the literacy needs of its patient population, a high proportion of which have low literacy levels. DHC trains patient navigators to tailor services to a patient's level of literacy.

DHC, being a rural and community-based health center, has found it challenging to secure a network of providers. Many of the current programs and initiatives that DHC engages in are informed by provider interactions with patients, which instruct providers about the barriers patients face and contributing upstream factors that shape them (e.g., a lack of money for transportation, child care issues, and illiteracy). As a result, DHC also trains its providers to be advocates for their patients.

Geiger wrote in 2002 that there are two important lessons to be learned from DHC's history:

1. communities suffering from poverty are rich in potential and ingenuity; and
2. health services have the capacity to address the root causes of poor health through community development and the social change that it produces (Geiger, 2002).

Sustaining Success

As an FQHC, DHC receives funding from the federal government and abides by the requirements in Section 330 of the Public Health Service Act. It initially received funding in 1965 and is governed and overseen by a board of directors. Other sources of funding for DHC include the Mississippi Department of Health, W.K. Kellogg Foundation ($825,000 during 2014–2017), and Delta Fresh Foods. Furthermore, as an FQHC, 51 percent of the DHC board of directors must be drawn from current patients in the program. The success of DHC led to the establishment of 200-plus health centers in the United States by 1973 and approximately 1,200 by 2010 (Longlett et al., 2001).

According to DHC, the center prides itself in being a "one-stop shop" for community residents in a rural community where convenience is rare. DHC builds off of the legacy of the center's community-driven origins and has provided a centralized space where the community can access medical care, social services, insurance assistance, a pharmacy, and other important resources necessary to empower residents to lead healthy lives.

Dudley Street Neighborhood Initiative[15]

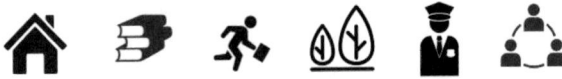

Background and History

The Dudley Street Neighborhood Initiative (DSNI) is a nonprofit, community-driven organization located in the Roxbury and North Dorchester neighborhoods of Boston, Massachusetts. Established in 1984, 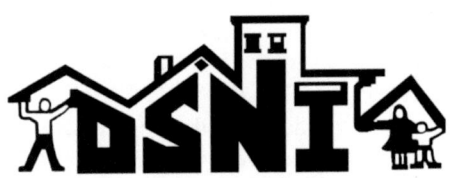 its mission is "to empower Dudley residents to organize, plan for, create, and control a vibrant, diverse, and high quality neighborhood in collaboration with community partners" (DSNI, 2016d). One of DSNI's distinguishing strengths is its focus on channeling individual concerns into a collective voice to achieve shared goals and facilitate community empowerment. DSNI originated from and continues to be shaped by residents' ability to leverage their collective power to influence and control the changes taking place in their community. In addition to its emphasis on community empowerment to carry out its mission, DSNI also focuses on sustainable economic development and youth opportunities and development. The organization's commitment to these values is a key factor in its successful implementation over the past three decades of various initiatives aimed at improving the health and well-being of the community it serves.

As a community organizing and planning group, DSNI's membership includes approximately 3,600 residents as well as community stakeholder

---

[15] This summary is an edited account that was prepared on the basis of templates completed by staff of each community initiative. Statements and opinions expressed are those of the community organization and have not been endorsed or verified by the National Academies of Sciences, Engineering, and Medicine.

TABLE 5-4 Dudley Village Campus Demographics

Total	~27,500 Residents
Race/ethnicity	57% African American
	28% Latino
	20% Cape Verdean
Gender	53% female
Age	26% of residents are under age 18
	62% of households with at least one child age 0–17
Education	81% completed high school
	11% of residents over age 25 have a bachelor's degree
Employment	17% unemployed
Income	Median household income is $34,000
	62% spend almost one-third of their monthly income on rent
Language	47% speak a language other than English at home

NOTE: Percentages may not add up to 100 percent due to varied reporting, rounding, and missing data from source.
SOURCES: DSNI, 2016a; 2014–2015 American Community Survey.

groups, such as other nonprofits, religious institutions, educational institutions, and local businesses. Participation from low-income residents is encouraged through low-cost, sliding-scale membership dues. The structure of DSNI's 35-member board of directors is designed to reflect the diversity of the community (see Table 5-4 for demographic information of the community DSNI serves, known as the Dudley Village Campus). Four board seats are reserved for African American residents, four for Cape Verdean residents, four for Latino residents, four for white residents, four for youth, seven seats for local health and human service nonprofits, two for community development corporations, two for small businesses, two for religious organizations, and two seats for residents appointed by the board (DSNI, 2016b).

DSNI's founding was in response to residents' concerns and frustrations over the deterioration of their community caused by arson fires and dumping (DSNI, 2016c). Broader socioeconomic issues such as disinvestment, poverty, and white flight had also negatively affected the neighborhoods of the community and led to further resident discontent. DSNI was founded with assistance from the Mabel Louise Riley Foundation, a foundation based in Boston that expressed interest in assisting the Dudley area after a site visit. In 1984 the Riley Foundation convened a group of community stakeholder groups, forming the Dudley Advisory Group. A neighborhood revitalization plan was proposed to residents but met with overwhelming dissatisfaction at the lack of resident representation on the governing board. By 1985 a revised plan was designed by a broadly

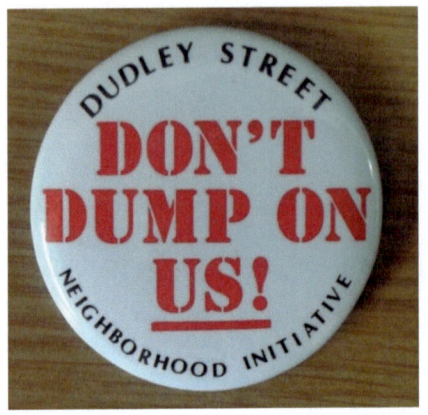

FIGURE 5-7 Button from Dudley Street Neighborhood Initiative's first neighborhood revitalization campaign.
SOURCE: Personal communication with DSNI staff. Available by request from the National Academies of Sciences, Engineering, and Medicine's Public Access Records Office (PARO@nas.edu). Used with permission.

representative group which established a resident majority on the board and firm community control of redevelopment.

In 1986 DSNI launched Don't Dump on Us (see Figure 5-7 for a button from this community revitalization campaign), its first neighborhood revitalization campaign, which cleaned vacant lots and shut down illegal trash transfer stations. During this time, a comprehensive neighborhood revitalization plan was also developed and officially adopted by the city of Boston in 1987.

Community Land Trust Model

One of DSNI's most notable accomplishments was its establishment of an urban community land trust (CLT).[16] CLTs have existed for more than 45 years in the United States, with more than 270 in various cities across the country (Cho et al., 2016), but the establishment of DSNI's CLT in 1988 was particularly noteworthy as it was the first time a community group sought out and won the power of eminent domain to acquire vacant land for resident-led development. Furthermore, it remains the second-largest CLT in the country. In the year of its founding, the organization purchased vacant lots in Boston to rebuild the land into affordable housing, urban agricultural and gardening sites, a town commons, parks and

---

[16] The National Community Land Trust Network describes community land trusts with the following description: "CLTs develop rural and urban agriculture projects, commercial spaces to serve local communities, affordable rental and cooperative housing projects, and conserve land or urban green spaces. However, the heart of their work is the creation of homes that remain permanently affordable, providing successful homeownership opportunities for generations of lower income families" (National Community Land Trust Network, 2016).

playgrounds, a charter school, community facilities, and spaces for new businesses. DSNI's CLT, known as Dudley Neighbors, Inc., owns more than 30 acres of land, providing 226 units of permanently affordable housing to low-income residents (Cho et al., 2016). An analysis of the CLT's stabilizing effects on neighborhoods shows lower vacancy and foreclosure rates and higher owner-occupancy rates (Dwyer, 2015). Dudley Neighbors also provides affordable land to urban farmers. Many urban agricultural and gardening activities have emerged from the establishment of the land trust, including several farms (some commercial and others operated by The Food Project, a local nonprofit), many community gardens, and a 10,000-square-foot greenhouse (Loh and Shear, 2015).

Boston Promise Initiative

The U.S. Department of Education awarded DSNI a Promise Neighborhood planning grant of $500,000 in 2010 and a $5,000,000 implementation grant in 2012, from which DSNI launched the Boston Promise Initiative. The initiative is intended to support families, schools, and neighborhoods in ensuring that every child in the community has "cradle to career" opportunities to succeed through access to quality education, social support systems, and safe environments. The Boston Promise Initiative has developed and implemented several initiatives that aim to achieve these outcomes, many of which emphasize teen involvement in youth education. The initiative also aims to build organizational capacity by leveraging information gained from social network analysis.

Solutions to Address the Social Determinants of Health

DSNI has developed and implemented a range of community initiatives to address the social determinants of health. Many of these initiatives are operated through partnerships with a range of other community stakeholder organizations. Several initiatives focus their efforts on specific, more vulnerable populations within the community.

Housing Dudley Neighbors, Inc., promotes the CLT model to provide affordable housing and encourage community control of land development (DSNI, 2016e; Dudley Neighbors, 2016). In partnership with the Dorchester Bay Economic Development Corporation and Nuestra Comunidad Development Corporation, Dudley Neighbors ensures affordable housing for low-income residents by selling homes built by these local development corporations to qualifying residents at affordable prices (Cho et al., 2016). This model provides a sustainable alternative to allowing the housing market to inflate prices and create unjust financial barriers for low-income residents seeking to become homeowners (Cho et al., 2016). DSNI also participates in the Greater Boston Community Land Trust Network in cooperation with other local organizations to further promote the development of affordable housing and open spaces through the community land trust model (DSNI, 2016e).

In addition to reducing barriers to affordable housing, another goal of DSNI is to reduce homelessness and provide services to support individuals and families at risk of becoming homeless. In partnership with Project Hope, a nonprofit based in Boston providing supportive housing services, DSNI established the No Child Goes Homeless initiative to support children and their families facing homelessness or possible eviction by providing services and other resources made available through a network of schools, city agencies, and other service providers (Boston Promise Initiative, 2016; DSNI, 2016e). In 2016, DSNI and Project Hope participated in a city-level conversation hosted by the Boston Department of Neighborhood Development, which also included the mayor's chief of education, the Boston Housing Authority, and leaders from Boston Public Schools. At this meeting, the No Child Goes Homeless initiative was highlighted as a promising practice. Project Hope and DSNI were asked to shape and potentially lead a pilot to demonstrate the effectiveness of cross-sector collaboration for replication across the city.

Education In conjunction with community empowerment and sustainable economic development, DSNI prioritizes youth leadership development and has launched a range of initiatives that provide opportunities and enable access to quality education for youth of all ages. Achieve Connect Thrive (ACT) is an evidence-based framework developed by DSNI to improve academic performance and facilitate successful career opportunities. The Learning Our Value in Education campaign holds educational events that are open to all community members to attend, and DSNI also supports a youth committee and an education committee to further facilitate educational opportunities for residents and community leaders. The Boston Promise Initiative also supports an early childhood education initiative called Dudley Children Thrive, which fosters a network of teachers and parents of children ages 5 and under. The initiative is intended to promote early childhood literacy and school readiness by encouraging parents to read to their children (Sandel et al., 2016). The School Readiness Roundtable brings early childhood educators and policy makers face-to-face with parents from the neighborhood, where they openly discuss strategies that work and those that do not to support young children.

DSNI's early learning work illustrates how neighborhood-level interventions can improve childhood opportunity and lift children out of poverty (Sandel et al., 2016). In 2015, 50 percent of families participating in the initiative had increased the number of times they read to their children, and 80 percent read to their children three or more times per week (DSNI, 2016c). DSNI also implements many other educational efforts to support youth and their families from early childhood through higher education, including parent advocacy and leadership programs, the Highland Street AmeriCorps mentoring program, a youth council, a college readiness program, and a young alumni network.

Employment DSNI works to increase employment opportunities for residents of racial and ethnic minority backgrounds, women, and women of racial and ethnic minority backgrounds through the Dudley Workforce Collaborative, which supports business developers to increase the number of construction work hours offered to residents in these marginalized groups. For construction related to the Boston Promise Initiative, the collaborative was successful in ensuring that 51 and 15 percent of the construction workforce consisted of racial and ethnic minorities and women, respectively (DSNI, 2016e). In 2013, DSNI helped secure 44 percent of total subcontract value on Choice Neighborhoods construction projects for minority-owned enterprises, totaling $16,438,519, with an additional 10 percent of subcontract value for women-owned enterprises, totaling $3,656,263 (DSNI, 2016c).

Physical environment DSNI supports food security by partnering with two other Boston-based nonprofits—the Food Project and Alternatives for Community & Environment—to increase residents' access to healthy and locally grown food options through the Dudley Real Food Hub and to provide loans for new and existing local food businesses. The collaborative effort also provides opportunities for residents, particularly youth, to participate in community gardening and educational activities to increase awareness and encourage consumption of healthy and locally sourced food options. As part of the Dudley Real Food Hub, Commonwealth Kitchen, an equipment-sharing incubator, has supported more than 50 community-based food businesses. Additionally, with DSNI's endorsement, a neighborhood grocery store, FT & Davey's Supermarket, successfully raised $5,000 from the community to purchase an industrial freezer, a key component in the local fresh produce distribution chain.

Public safety DSNI works to address public safety issues. In 2012, a series of shootings prompted the organization to convene a diverse group of community stakeholders, including local officers from the Boston Police Department, to support neighborhood watch groups. After the widely publicized closing of a state drug lab in 2012, following a scandal in which it was revealed that more than 24,000 drug cases from 2003 to 2012 were compromised, DSNI's advocacy efforts, in coordination with other community stakeholders, helped secure $5 million from the state to support community-based reentry services.

Social environment Another of DSNI's goals is to improve the community's cultural and artistic economy. The organization leads the Fairmont Cultural Corridor, an initiative begun in 2012 through which local artists, businesses, and arts and cultural organizations collaborate to implement activities such as art installations, public place-making, and outdoor markets (Fairmont Cultural Corridor, 2016). The arts create thriving public spaces for the neighborhood, and DSNI also engages residents in participatory action research to co-create knowledge about the neighborhood. Residents have been recruited and paid as researchers in neighborhood surveys for the Boston Promise Initiative and for studies commissioned by the Healthy Neighborhoods Equity Fund, a participatory action research initiative investigating the effects of real estate development on residents' health.

The arts and data merge in the form of interactive data visualizations at neighborhood events. In 2015, DSNI conducted a focus group with young people about their perceptions of future success. The transcript from the focus group was turned into a word cloud, and the words from the word cloud were burned onto wood blocks left over from an art installation. The blocks were then given to children to create their own found poems (see Figure 5-8). The activity provides a strong example of how the arts and data can work together to inform and inspire community residents.

Data and Outcomes

DSNI's initiatives aspire to achieve the following community change outcomes:

- strong and healthy families
- vibrant and thriving communities
- children entering school ready to succeed
- successful students and schools
- postsecondary completion and career readiness

DSNI has made progress in achieving these outcomes through its many initiatives. The Dudley Real Food Hub has facilitated a community-driven planning process to identify key strategies for helping families improve their food environment, and families have also strengthened

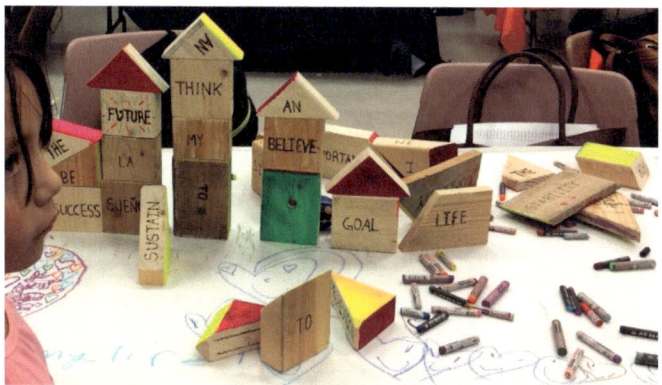

FIGURE 5-8 Wood block poems from a neighborhood event that merged data and arts to help inspire children to achieve success.
SOURCE: Personal communication with DSNI staff. Available by request from the National Academies of Sciences, Engineering, and Medicine's Public Access Records Office (PARO@nas.edu). Used with permission.

their financial literacy through enrollment in Fair Chance for Family Success. Cultural initiatives such as the Fairmont Cultural Corridor have contributed to more vibrant and thriving communities. Dudley Neighbors, Inc., has contributed to the creation of a Chinatown community land trust and, as a certified state community development corporation, secured $100,000 in community tax investment credits. To help children achieve greater school readiness, residents and community stakeholders have convened working groups to assist families with children ages 0 to 5. To increase opportunity for students to succeed in school, mentoring programs have matched 18 students with mentors of color who are primarily from the neighborhood. The No Child Goes Homeless program has also provided support services to students and their families at risk of eviction. Greater career readiness has also been accomplished, with 48 young people hired and efforts under way to engage youth 18 to 24 years old to develop educational and career pathways.

DSNI's peer-to-peer financial literacy and learning program, Fair Chance for Family Success, has enrolled 100 families and achieved significant outcomes since the initiative began in 2014. Table 5-5 displays some of Fair Chance's key outcomes and results.

As a Promise Neighborhood grantee, DSNI reports data collected for 15 Government Performance Results Act (GPRA) indicators, which are measures that quantify achievement of outcomes related to health care services, education, exercise, nutrition, exercise, and others. Table 5-6 provides some of the key results DSNI has measured from 2014 to 2015.

TABLE 5-5 Results of DSNI's Fair Chance for Family Success Program (2014–2016)

Outcome	Result (n = 74)
Average amount in savings accounts	Increased from $3.43 to $1,555.26
Average amount in checking accounts	Increased from $200.51 to $775.83
Average amount in total assets	Increased from $452.42 to $5,899.46
Average subsidy income	Reduced from $128.25 to $47.56

SOURCE: Personal communication from Andrew Seeder to National Academies staff on September 21, 2016. Available by request from the National Academies of Sciences, Engineering, and Medicine's Public Access Records Office (PARO@nas.edu).

TABLE 5-6 Results Related to GRPA Indicators

Outcome	2014	2015
Percent of kindergarteners who demonstrate at the beginning of the school year age-appropriate functioning across multiple domains of early learning (n = 116)	59%	65%
Percent of high school students at or above grade level according to state mathematics assessments (n = 64)	36%	63%
Four-year adjusted cohort graduation rate (n = 72)	51%	82%
Percent of students who enroll in a 2-year or 4-year college or university after graduation (n = 86)	48%	69%
Percent of children who participate in at least 60 minutes of vigorous physical activity daily (n = 142)	16%	22%
Percent of children who consume five or more servings of fruits and vegetables daily (n = 195)	27%	30%
Student mobility rate (n = 1,871 [total enrollment of schools])	61%	46%

SOURCE: Personal communication from Andrew Seeder to National Academies staff on September 21, 2016. Available by request from the National Academies of Sciences, Engineering, and Medicine's Public Access Records Office (PARO@nas.edu).

Promoting Health Equity: Key Elements

Since its early days up to the present, one of DSNI's main goals has been to empower the Dudley community by "changing residents' perceptions of their neighborhood and of their own power to change the conditions in which they live" (Schorr, 1997). In carrying out this goal, the organization has cultivated a shared vision among residents, families, local organizations, and local businesses to achieve a healthier and more vibrant community. DSNI has fostered increased community engagement and a greater sense of community within neighborhoods previously ravaged by unjust disinvestment and policies that led to poor health outcomes. The organization's many ongoing efforts emphasize access to basic needs such as housing and education as well as emphasizing economic opportunity and healthy behavior in driving a unified vision of health equity.

As evidenced by its diverse and growing membership of individuals and stakeholder groups, DSNI recognizes the need to foster multi-sector collaboration to achieve a more vibrant community of healthier residents. Its encouragement of and engagement in collaboration with various entities spanning many different sectors is one of its core strengths. Through efforts relating to its community land trust, the organization engages with development organizations and other nonprofits to improve housing and land use management. Through initiatives such as the Boston Promise Initiative, Dudley Real Food Hub, Dudley Workforce Collaborative, and Fairmont Cultural Corridor, the organization engages with businesses, local arts and cultural institutions, and other nonprofits to improve economic, agricultural, and cultural development. Partnerships with educational institutions are also well established through DSNI's range of youth education programs.

DSNI builds social capital and community leadership among residents to create a thriving community. The Boston Promise Initiative's Fair Chance for Family Success, a peer-to-peer financial learning support network funded by the Family Independence Initiative, has achieved significant quantifiable outcomes. Over the course of 2 years, from 2014 to 2016, families in Fair Chance saw average savings increase from $3.43 to $1,553.36, while average checking account balances increased from $200.51 to $775.83. On average, total assets increased from $452.42 to $5,899.46. The Fair Chance program is a model for how peer-to-peer social networks can drive social change.

DSNI's commitment to youth development has also built strong capacity among its younger residents to sustain and build on the work begun by the previous generation and create greater opportunities for future generations. Many of DSNI's educational initiatives specifically support the needs of children of low-income, impoverished, and homeless families, providing needed services and social support as well as pathways to educational and career success. These initiatives not only contribute to reducing health disparities but also facilitate the development of youth in the community into the next generation of community leaders who give back to the community that has supported them and their success. Building youth capacity has thus contributed to a cycle of residents helping residents, which has helped sustain DSNI's success over the past three decades since its founding.

DSNI is a values-first organization; it is a data-informed organization driven by values. In working with youth, for example, DSNI recognizes the power of the neighborhood's young people who want to be engaged and play a leadership role in the community. When youth are offered a supportive and challenging leadership environment that values their engagement, perspective, and growth, they are empowered to invest in their own and their community's development. This means that young people are at the table and actively providing their voices during decision-making processes. Additionally, DSNI organizes to ensure that anchor institutions make upstream investments in the social determinants of health in alignment with the ACA's changes to how hospitals and other health providers make investments in community health. DSNI and its partners are moving forward with a major campaign to reassert community voice in the determination of needs, community benefits agreements, and payments in lieu of taxes.

Challenges and Lessons Learned

One of DSNI's most significant challenges is convincing residents to prioritize long-term gains over short-term benefits. Many low-income residents prioritize day-to-day needs and emergency conditions, such as the risk of eviction, paying bills, and feeding and getting their kids to school. To help these families achieve healthier outcomes, DSNI is interested in strategies to mitigate the effects of these barriers and to shift residents' thinking from short to long term.

A critical component of DSNI's success has been its innovative and inclusive approach to governance through its board of directors. The board is guided by a vision of collective leadership, and its membership is representative of the community both through racial/ethnic composition and youth involvement. Additionally, the board's joint decision making with the City of Boston for development of community-owned land has led to the building of housing, open and green neighborhood spaces, and local businesses that meet the needs of community residents.

EXAMPLES OF COMMUNITIES TACKLING HEALTH INEQUITY

Sustaining Success

Youth development is a core component of DSNI's work which has helped to sustain its success. Investing in youth has helped to achieve long-term community change and yielded substantial long-term benefits, as some youth who participate in DSNI's work expand their participation, developing into leaders as full-time staff members (Bhatt and Dubb, 2015). DSNI also provides opportunities for residents to develop leadership skills through activities such as its Sustainable Economic Development Committee, through which residents gain valuable training and real-world experience in community organizing, planning, and development.

> Through organizing, residents get the chance to take leadership responsibility and apply some of what they've learned to the real world. Facilitating a meeting with a developer and hammering out a community benefits agreement is something you can take a workshop on, but it's different in the real world.
>
> —Harry Smith, Director of Sustainable Economic Development, Dudley Street Neighborhood Initiative

Eastside Promise Neighborhood[17]

Background and History

The Eastside Promise Neighborhood (EPN) was founded as an implementation site of the U.S. Department of Education (ED) Promise Neighborhood grant program, which provides funding to nonprofit organizations, educational institutions, and Indian tribes to support the revitalization of disadvantaged communities through investment in youth education and development (ED, 2016). The Promise Neighborhood goals are based on the 10 promises listed in Table 5-7.

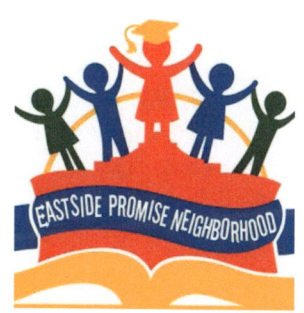

---

[17] This summary is an edited account that was prepared on the basis of templates completed by staff of each community initiative. Statements and opinions expressed are those of the community organization and have not been endorsed or verified by the National Academies of Sciences, Engineering, and Medicine.

TABLE 5-7 Eastside Promise Neighborhood 10 Promises

Educational Success	Family and Community Support
1. Children enter kindergarten ready to succeed in school.	6. Students are healthy and access aligned learning and enrichment activities.
2. Students improve academic performance and are proficient in core subjects.	7. Students feel safe in their school and community.
3. Students successfully transition from elementary to middle to high school.	8. Students live in stable communities.
4. Students graduate from high school.	9. Families and community members support learning in Promise Neighborhood schools.
5. Students earn a college degree or a job training certification.	10. Students have access to 21st century learning tools.

SOURCE: EPN, 2016a.

EPN emerged from a 2010 planning grant awarded to the United Way of San Antonio and Bexar County to continue the process of revitalizing the Eastside neighborhood of San Antonio, Texas, by identifying the factors that affect academic success and to design a plan to create a collection of solutions to improve educational outcomes in schools throughout the area. Using the $312,000 1-year planning grant to inform and develop a Promise Neighborhood proposal, a community stakeholder group of residents and local experts conducted a variety of information-gathering activities, including a needs assessment, focus groups, and forums for community discussion. The needs assessment identified problems in the local school system, including inadequate access to quality early education programs, low-performing schools, low graduation rates, poor student health outcomes, and insufficient or ineffective social support services. A proposal to address these community needs was developed and submitted, and in 2011, a 5-year $23.7 million (EPN, 2016b) implementation grant was awarded to launch EPN as a joint initiative of the United Way of San Antonio and Bexar County, the San Antonio Independent School District, the San Antonio Housing Authority, Family Services Association, the City of San Antonio, the P–16+ Council, Community Information Now, and SA2020.[18] The area is also home to a U.S. Department of Housing and Urban Development Choice Initiative, a U.S. Department of Labor Promise Zone Designation, and two Byrne Criminal Justice initiatives. The term "EastPoint" is used to describe the area of collective impact for all of the activity occurring as a result of this significant federal investment.

---

[18] SA2020 is "a community vision and movement born from a series of public forums in 2010 to develop goals for improving San Antonio by the year 2020." For more information, see http://www.sanantonio.gov/sustainability/SA2020.aspx (accessed December 5, 2016).

EPN's mission is to "[unite] institutional and resident stakeholders to leverage and strengthen the neighborhood's assets and resources so that children and families are inspired to stay, grow, graduate, and stay" (EPN, 2016c). Its 5-year goal was "to break down traditional government and non-profit silos" to develop and implement more collaborative solutions to address the complex barriers faced by students in disinvested neighborhoods (EPN, 2016b).

In the 1950s the Eastside neighborhood was a predominately African American community afflicted with segregation in housing, schools, and businesses. In addition to a 2.58 percent decrease in the population since 2000 (compared to a 16 percent overall increase in San Antonio), the race and ethnicity distribution of EPN's population has also changed over the past two decades. See Table 5-8 for a summary of EastPoint demographics. Although the community has a rich cultural history and includes more than 50 churches, 6 EPN-designated schools, almost 300 businesses, and an array of social service organizations, its residents face significant socioeconomic disadvantages that negatively affect their attainment of good health. The American Community Survey found that from 2005 to 2009 the neighborhood's annual median household income was $19,766, as compared with $43,087 for all of San Antonio (Drennon, 2011; PolicyLink, 2014). In the same time period, about 60.1 percent of children were living in poverty, almost three times the national child poverty rate of 21.9 percent (Drennon, 2011; PolicyLink, 2014). Many families in the community are younger than the average in San Antonio and experience higher rates of poverty (Drennon, 2011; PolicyLink, 2014). Educational outcomes are also worse than in San Antonio, as access to and quality of early childhood education, schools, and social support services are low (Drennon, 2011; PolicyLink, 2014).

TABLE 5-8 EastPoint Demographics

Total	~18,000 residents (2010)
Race/Ethnicity	~68% Hispanic
	~25% African American
	~7% white
Income	Annual median household income from 2005 to 2009: $19,766
	60.1% of children living in poverty

NOTE: Percentages may not add up to 100 percent due to varied reporting, rounding, and missing data from source.
SOURCES: Drennon, 2011; PolicyLink, 2014.

Solutions to Address the Social Determinants of Health

EPN focuses on improving educational outcomes through many programs that provide educational and growth opportunities for children and youth from early childhood through postsecondary education and career support.

Education EPN is committed to providing a sustainable pathway for youth to achieve educational success and be ready for college or the workforce. Its goal of establishing family and community stability reflects its recognition that environmental barriers must be addressed in order for children to achieve educational and employment success. EPN's vision is for students to graduate from high school ready for college, careers, and self-sufficiency with the support of a revitalized and thriving community. Its cradle-to-career pathway consists of the promises that the community strives to make to its youth in supporting their education and development. Figure 5-9 illustrates the types of community resources that are available to achieve each goal along the pathway.[19] Healthy and financially stable families who have access to social support and services are the foundation of the pathway. School readiness, access to quality education (including early childhood; science, technology, engineering, and mathematics [STEM]; post-secondary; and trade certification opportunities), meaningful engagement from parents and caregivers, and a safe environment are also emphasized as essential components of EPN's pathway to achieving academic success.

EPN partners with the San Antonio Independent School District (SAISD) to create a continuous, integrated pipeline to success for students attending the schools in the EPN, which include the Tynan Early Childhood Education center; three elementary schools (Bowden, Washington, and Pershing Elementary Schools); Wheatley Middle School, which serves as the District's site for a ED-funded Community School; and Sam Houston High School. SAISD redesigned its education plan to emphasize successful and sustainable STEM education for students. Other priorities in the redesigned plan include meeting state standards in all core subjects and strengthening teacher capacity through increased training. EPN's talent development strategy, led by Trinity University, has also been integrated into the district's new 5-year Blueprint for Excellence plan.

EPN provides funding and support for a number of programs that improve early childhood education and school readiness, including a number of Texas Rising Star–accredited early childhood centers and

---

[19] A video describing EPN's 10 promises is available at http://eastsidepromise.org/the-results (accessed December 5, 2016).

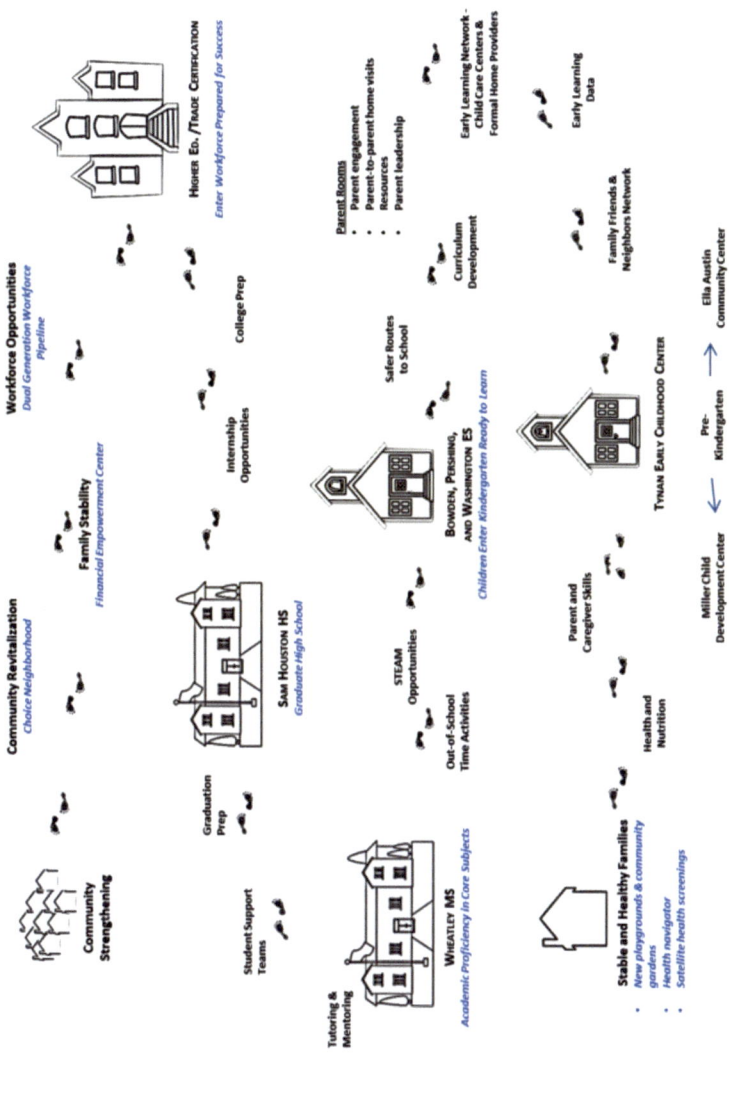

FIGURE 5-9 EPN's cradle-to-career pathway.
SOURCE: EPN, 2013. Used with permission.

summer camps; an online resource known as Ready Rosie to support kindergarten readiness; a Family, Friends, and Neighbors Network operated by the Family Service Association; a free Home Instruction for Parents of Preschool Youngsters program, managed by Catholic Charities, which encourages early reading; expert early childhood consultants to support quality improvements at the centers; and, thanks to a Chase Foundation grant, expanded opportunities for center staff to pursue a child development associate (CDA) certificate and associate of arts (AA) credentials. For the early childhood programs, 73 percent of licensed slots at the three child care centers in the area are currently utilized (244 out of 335). The target of 25 participants for the Family, Friends, and Neighbors Network has been exceeded, with 33 enrolled, and the available slots for CDA and AA participation were utilized at 100 percent.

EPN also implements a number of programs in collaboration with partners to promote educational success through secondary and postsecondary education. City Year, a nonprofit that partners with at-risk schools in impoverished communities to provide support to vulnerable students and teachers, partners with EPN to pair trained young adults (corps members) with students identified as most at risk from Wheatley Middle School and Sam Houston High School. Corps members support these vulnerable students to overcome attendance problems and achieve academic success.[20] EPN and its partners also provide students with resources to learn more about and enroll in colleges and universities. SAISD also receives funding from the ED's Gaining Early Awareness and Readiness for Undergraduate Programs to provide college readiness coaches, summer camps and programs, and other resources to prospective college applicants.

EPN-supported internship programs to develop leadership capacity and to provide career opportunities for talented youth were augmented by a Citibank grant to support a college match savings program for neighborhood students. Partnerships with several nonprofits (including the Boys and Girls Clubs of San Antonio, the Girl Scouts of Southwest Texas, HIS Bridgebuilders, and the YMCA of Greater San Antonio) provide after-school and summer programs that emphasize STEM education. Figure 5-10 summarizes EPN's cradle-to-career pipeline.

Meaningful parent and caregiver engagement is an essential aspect of EPN's educational programming. In partnership with the Family Service Association's Family–School–Community Partnership, United Way, SAISD, and City Year, EPN facilitates a range of services such as parent-led home visits, parent training, and school-based family activities

---

[20] For more information on City Year and its partnership with EPN, see http://eastsidepromise.org/city-year (accessed December 5, 2016).

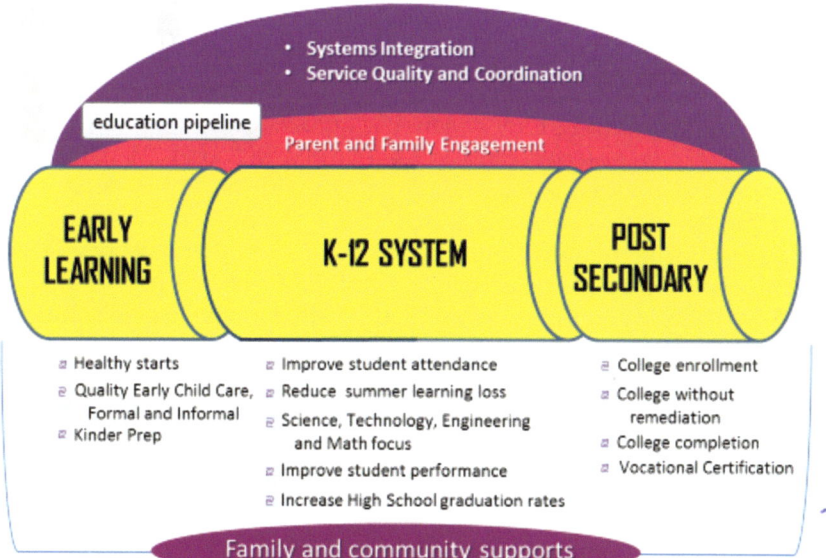

FIGURE 5-10 EPN's cradle-to-career pipeline to support success in education. SOURCE: EPN, n.d. Used with permission.

to deepen parent and caregiver involvement and empower families to resolve problems such as chronic absenteeism.

Physical environment In addition to educational success, EPN also works to improve the health of its community through investment in other social determinants of health. In addition to partnerships that have created children's playgrounds, community gardens, and farmer's markets, access to healthy food is also addressed through a partnership with the San Antonio Food Bank to provide families with fresh produce. Public safety for youth has also been addressed. The Byrne grant enabled EPN to contract with the San Antonio Police Department to provide additional patrols in the mornings and afternoons to ensure that the pathways to school were safe. In addition, a new initiative launched at one of EPN's elementary schools for the 2015 to 2016 school year is the Walking School Bus program, which involves adult supervision of children walking to and from school. The program addresses student safety concerns due to factors such as crime and unsafe construction as well as reducing tardiness, improving attendance, and improving students' health and well-being.

Data and Outcomes

United Way and its partners committed early in EPN's development to using data and community input to drive the initiative's decision-making process. During EPN's planning grant process, a review of longitudinal academic performance data revealed that only 31 percent of neighborhood children entered kindergarten with readiness skills. As a result, many of EPN's solutions related to early education were launched at the very beginning of the initiative. For programming developed during the implementation phase of the grant, EPN subcommittees participated in strategic planning sessions that resulted in identifying solutions which were ultimately sent to the advisory council for approval. The programs outlined above were either identified during the planning phase or developed during the implementation phase. Community input was prevalent throughout, either as a part of the numerous meetings held during the planning phase or as a part of work done at the subcommittee or advisory council level.

EPN's subcommittees spend time reviewing data associated with the funded programs, including usage rates and performance metrics. As part of its review, if a program is started that does not resonate with the community, the subcommittee evaluates the process for improvement before the next round of funding. For example, after the initial funding was provided for farmers markets, data revealed that a large number of customers were not from the footprint (the area being served). The committee changed the location of the markets to the community school and also provided funding for nutrition education and cooking classes to ensure that families understood the importance of utilizing fresh fruits and vegetables in their daily diets. Additionally, EPN and United Way staff review contracts on a bimonthly basis, including performance metrics, financials, and narrative reports submitted by funded agencies. This contract review process provides an opportunity for staff members to provide ongoing technical assistance for providers and consistent dialogue for program improvement. When EPN discovered that the out-of-school-time partners were not having the desired impact on academic achievement, a community of practice was created to give the partners the opportunity to collectively review the data and cross-pollinate best practices.

EPN's theory of change is guided by 21 neighborhood goals which include targets set by community members and stakeholders. The goals are developed based on the ED's Government Performance Results Act indicators, which are standard measurements for all Promise Neighborhood grant recipients. The target-setting process was conducted using the results-based accountability (RBA) framework and included 13 meetings with more than 200 residents, content experts, and partners and 10 small group meetings with over 50 individuals from specific workgroups (e.g., the Dual Generation Workforce Pipeline workgroup) or specific partnerships (e.g., Out of School Time providers, City Year, all SAISD campus principals and their teams). The RBA framework structures participation and dialogue by focusing on the end game and affords the opportunity for the necessary negotiations and debates which must be part of a community-owned agenda. Table 5-9 displays EPN's 10 promises as well as some of the key outcomes that the initiative has achieved in these areas.[21] Data to measure this progress have been collected on an annual basis through a neighborhood survey, a literacy assessment, an early development assessment, a census of child care enrollment, a collection of administrative data and annual graduation rates, and a school climate survey.

Promoting Health Equity: Key Elements

Through the role of committees in its governance process, EPN fosters a shared community vision for better educational and health outcomes. EPN supports four community committees comprised of residents, community stakeholders, content experts, and local partners who meet regularly to address issues related to early childhood learning, health and wellness, education, and school and neighborhood safety. The Promise and Choice Together (PaCT) Health and Wellness Committee, for example, has reviewed data collected from 6th- to 12th-grade students on fruit and vegetable consumption and participation in physical activity to develop several of its solutions. Furthermore, a health consultant funded by EPN has served on the committee and facilitated the committee's inclusion of Healthy People 2020 metrics related to health and wellness in order to develop interventions. EPN's committees have fostered shared accountability among resident participants and strengthened educational success and health equity as a shared vision.

EPN collaborates with organizations from many different sectors. Its key partners include the United Way of San Antonio and Bexar County, The Annie E. Casey Foundation, SAISD, the City of San Antonio, Ella Austin Community Center, Goodwill Industries, Alamo Colleges, St. Philip's College, San Antonio Growth on the Eastside, San Antonio Housing Authority, Workforce Solutions Alamo, Family Services Association, and the San Antonio Police Department. These core partnerships were formed during the planning phase of the process or the early implementation

---

[21] For more information on initiatives related to each of the 10 promises as well as outcomes data and targets for past years, see http://eastsidepromise.org/the-results (accessed December 5, 2016).

TABLE 5-9 EPN's 10 Promises and Key Outcome Measures

Promise 1	Children enter kindergarten ready to succeed in school.	• In 2016, 57.3 percent of children ages 0 to 5 had access to a place other than an emergency room when sick or in need of health-related services. • In 2015, 47.8 to 86.0 percent (depending on assessment) of children aged 3 and 41.0 percent of children in kindergarten demonstrated age-appropriate early learning functioning. • In 2016, 50.4 and 47.8 percent of children participated in formal and informal early learning programs, respectively.
Promise 2	Students improve academic performance and are proficient in core subjects.	• In fiscal year 2015–2016, 51.8 and 47.7 percent, respectively, of students in grades 3 through 8 were at or above grade level, according to state mathematics and language arts assessments.
Promise 3	Students successfully transition from elementary to middle to high school.	• Through the Family–School–Community Partnership of United Way and Family Service Associate, 1,126 parents from all 6 EPN schools were visited in 2015 by another parent to learn about and connect to available resources and services to support their children's success in school.
Promise 4	Students graduate from high school.	• In 2015, 81.3 percent of students graduated from high school (state graduation rate formula).
Promise 5	Students earn a college degree or a job training certification.	• In 2016, 45.7 percent of students enrolled in a 2- or 4-year college or university after graduation. • In 2011, 1.3 percent of students earned industry-recognized certifications.
Promise 6	Students are healthy, and their educational performance improves by accessing aligned learning and enrichment activities.	• In the 2015 to 2016 school year, 30.5 percent of students reported engaging in at least one hour of daily physical activity. • In the 2015 to 2016 school year, 36.7 percent of children reported consuming five or more daily servings of fruits and vegetables.
Promise 7	Students feel safe at school and in their community.	• From 2014 to 2015, 75.7 percent of students reported that they felt safe both at school and while traveling to and from school.
Promise 8	Students live in stable communities.	• After 2013 to 2014, EPN experienced a slight decrease in student mobility in 2014 to 2015.[a] Overall, little movement has been observed on mobility, with rates basically flat for the past four school-years with only minor overall fluctuation.[b]

TABLE 5-9 Continued

Promise 9	Families and community members support learning in Promise Neighborhood schools.	• From 2015 to 2016, 51.6 percent of families reported reading to their children three or more times a week, 70.5 percent of families reported encouraging their children to read books outside of school, and 83 percent of families reported talking to their children about post-high-school career opportunities.
Promise 10	Students have access to 21st-century learning tools.	• In 2015, 90 percent of students had access to [the] Internet at home and at school.

[a] The Wheatley Courts demolition and the relocation of families outside the footprint in early 2014 may have had an impact on the mobility of students at the target schools.
[b] Compared to the baseline year, Bowden and Wheatley have shown improvement, Sam Houston stayed virtually unchanged, and Pershing and Washington experienced increased mobility. Compared to the 2015 to 2016 target of 20 percent, only Bowden Elementary is close to meeting the target with a 23.6 percent mobility rate.
SOURCE: EPN, 2016a.

phase and are maintained through regularly scheduled meetings at the subcommittee, staff, and leadership levels. The mutual accountability structure for EastPoint has three levels of partnership and accountability. The structure includes periodic reports to the mayor and city council of San Antonio delivered by the anchor partners. These reports include an overview of the progress of each of the major initiatives occurring as a part of the EastPoint collective impact model.

Some of the other organizations that EPN has partnered with are public libraries, faith-based organizations, sororities and fraternities, the National Association for the Advancement of Colored People (NAACP), and the San Antonio Spurs. Its key partners in carrying out its health and wellness initiatives include the Martinez Street Women's Center, the San Antonio Food Bank, Methodist Health Care Ministries, the City of San Antonio, University Health Systems, CommuniCare, SAISD, University of the Incarnate Word Bowden Eye Care and Health Center, the San Antonio Metropolitan Health District, HIS Bridgebuilders, and the University of Texas Health Science Center.[22] Additionally, EPN engages with local politicians in its governance process. Representatives from the mayor's and city councilmen's offices have designated seats on EPN's advisory council. Staff members from the offices of local elected officials are also invited to serve as members of EPN subcommittees.

---

[22] For a full list of organizations who partner with EPN, see http://eastsidepromise.org/the-partners (accessed December 5, 2016).

EPN has built resident capacity through its process of holding subcommittee and advisory council meetings that include representation from neighborhood associations. These neighborhood associations are composed of residents and property owners who hold regular community meetings to discuss and advocate for causes raised by their membership. Each has its own governing rules with elected leadership and may collect voluntary dues. Currently, three exist in EPN: Dignowity Hills, Government Hill Alliance, and Harvard Place/East Lawn.

EPN has developed organizational capacity by taking advantage of a DOE investment in training in results-based accountability. RBA is "a management tool that can facilitate collaboration among human service agencies, as a method of decentralizing services, and as an innovative regulatory process" (Schilder, 1997). Several of EPN's staff members and community partners received RBA training in the initiative's early implementation phases. RBA continues to inform the work of EPN and its partners in ongoing development and implementation of its programs.

Challenges and Lessons Learned

An important element contributing to EPN's success has been its development and use of a process or framework to guide its governance process. EPN's subcommittees have used RBA to develop and implement a range of health and educational programming. Another important aspect of EPN's programmatic development has been the use of data to guide decision making, monitor progress over time, and make corrections and adjustments as necessary. EPN partners with a community data intermediary called CI:Now (Community Information Now), which has, over time, built a data warehouse and multiuser bridge underwritten by three funding sources and which enables the review of relevant student and family indicators to monitor progress across a range of programs (EPN, 2016b).

One of EPN's ongoing challenges is ensuring that informal and formal communication systems successfully facilitate knowledge of the variety of resources available to community residents, as many families face transportation and access barriers and may not be aware of the resources and events available to them. EPN includes three neighborhoods, each with its own distinct characteristics and communication challenges. Developing a multipronged approach to reach residents across the footprint is an area for continuous improvement. The preferred method of communication continues to be "word of mouth," as it generally comes from a vetted source that has a connection to the community. The Family–School–Community Partnership, which places Parent Rooms at each campus, and the school district's Parent Family Liaisons are the main distribution points, as they are highly connected to families in the footprint. EPN also created the position of family navigator to help connect families to available programs and events in the area. Finally, the Health and Wellness Committee recommended a solution that included hiring community connectors who visit homes to conduct an information and referral assessment to assist those with children ages 0 to 5 with accessing a medical home. These promotora-style peer home visitors also provide information about upcoming events and resources, including job fairs and career training opportunities in the neighborhood.

Over time, the implementation team has experienced some challenges that affected its problem-solving role and effectiveness. In recognition of this changing dynamic, plans are under way to ensure that the leadership of the implementation team is fortified to serve in its intended role and prepare for the transition to post-grant sustainability. The tri-chairs of the implementation team have agreed to participate in a self-assessment of the team's current structure to provide insight to help identify and determine areas that may need adjustments for continued success in implementing collective initiatives.

Sustaining Success

EPN displays a deep commitment of accountability to the neighborhood. Entering the final stage of the EPN grant, sustainability is a key discussion. Stakeholders—including residents, volunteers, and organizations indigenous to the footprint—have begun sustainability efforts with a focus on creating a long-term strategy that identifies successful solutions to increase service value and build capacity for the most promising practices to be financially sustained. A series of meetings will be held in 2016, including community information-sharing sessions; visits to local neighborhood association meetings coined as "EPN Road Shows"; and community subject matter convenings to identify sustainable solutions, partner agencies who are interested in carrying the work forward, and potential areas for capacity-building for those partner agencies and gaps in service if no partner can be identified. The information captured will be used to design an EPN-recommended long-term sustainability strategy that will be submitted to the advisory council for approval and shared with the coordinating council. This will serve as a recommendation from the EPN community regarding the community's voice for what its members feel is needed to stay on the course to success—a true reflection of the community-driven approach that initially launched EPN's work. The EPN plan should also serve as a template for the future sustainability work

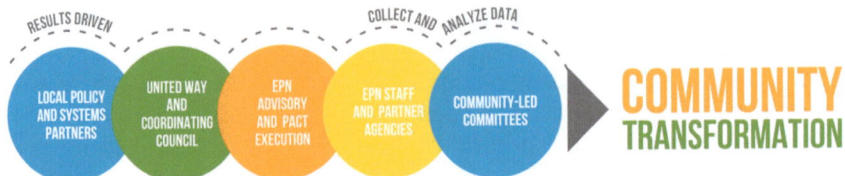

FIGURE 5-11 Eastside Promise Neighborhood's key community actors.
SOURCE: Personal communication with EPN staff. Available by request from the National Academies of Sciences, Engineering, and Medicine's Public Access Records Office (PARO@nas.edu). Used with permission.

of the coordinating council for EastPoint, the Eastside, and greater San Antonio. Figure 5-11 displays the key actors who drive EPN's community-driven approach.

The combined leadership of the EastPoint Coordinating Council also recognizes the importance of sustainability in its broadest sense. Initial collaborations and collective successes in the targeted EastPoint footprint have been a testament of how working together can achieve greater success and will be the foundation to the forthcoming initiatives for the City of San Antonio. Considering what has taken place thus far, the city council leadership has allocated funds for the coordinating council to develop a sustainability plan for continued EastPoint revitalization. Following a qualitative and quantitative evaluation of the various grant programs and initiatives, a sustainability plan for EastPoint efforts will be used to develop strategies and recommendations on which programs and initiatives should be replicated in other parts of the Promise Zone and other parts of the city as well as sustainability strategies for replication.

Indianapolis Congregation Action Network[23]

Background and History

The Indianapolis Congregation Action Network (IndyCAN) is a multiracial, multi-faith, nonpartisan organization in central Indiana that catalyzes marginalized people and faith communities to act collectively for racial and economic equity. Founded in 2012, the mission of IndyCAN is to "build the leadership capacity of low- and moderate-income people who live, work, and worship in central Indiana, empowering them to work alongside service providers, policymakers, and other stakeholders to increase collaboration, leverage resources, and improve the systems impacting their lives."[24] IndyCAN's expanding alliance reaches tens of thousands of people from Indiana's 17 largest denominations and the Catholic Archdiocese. IndyCAN is a member of the People Improving Communities through Organization (PICO) National Network,[25] a network of faith-based community organizations working to create innovative solutions to problems facing urban, suburban, and rural communities.

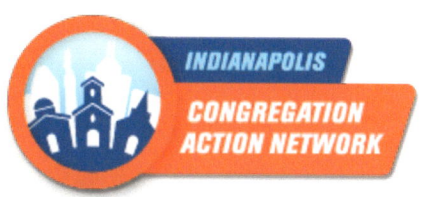

IndyCAN seeks to achieve its vision of "Opportunity for All" by building the power of traditionally excluded communities through leadership development, amplifying the prophetic voice, awakening the electorate, and creating strategic partnerships that reshape the environment to advance regional, state, and national policy campaigns (IndyCAN, 2014) (see Figure 5-12). When launched in 2012, IndyCAN had one major goal: to connect 10,000 families affected by economic hardship to employment by addressing the issues of mass incarceration and gun violence, economic dignity, and immigrant integration and inclusion in the community. This overarching goal brought together a large coalition of clergy, people of

---

[23] This summary is an edited account that was prepared on the basis of templates completed by staff of each community initiative. Statements and opinions expressed are those of the community organization and have not been endorsed or verified by the National Academies of Sciences, Engineering, and Medicine.

[24] For more information, see http://www.indycan.org/about (accessed September 13, 2016).

[25] For more information, see http://www.piconetwork.org (accessed September 13, 2016).

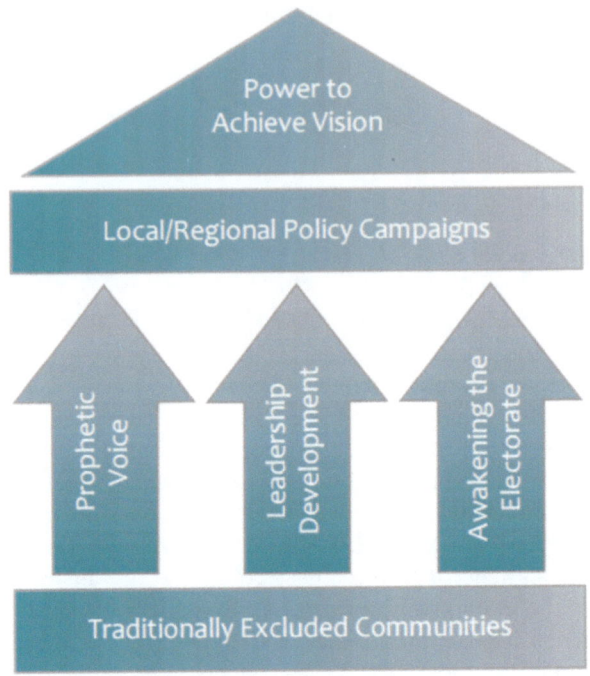

FIGURE 5-12 IndyCan's model to build the power of traditionally excluded communities to achieve its vision.
SOURCE: Indianapolis Congregation Action Network. 2014. Annual Strategic Report. Used with permission.

faith, and civic and business leaders. Today, IndyCAN's "Opportunity for All" Policy Platform has the following objectives:

- create career pathways to jobs of the future
- invest in equitable regional transit that gets people to work
- reduce mass incarceration and gun violence
- and pass a fair, direct, and inclusive pathway to citizenship for 11 million aspiring Americans (IndyCAN, 2014)

The Indianapolis metropolitan area faces many economic and social challenges (see Table 5-10 for the demographics of Marion County). The area has the eighth fastest-growing poverty rate in the nation, which also translates into a lack of economic opportunity (IndyCAN, 2014). The state of Indiana is ranked 49th in the country for economic mobility—that is, the likelihood that a poor child will transition out of poverty and into

TABLE 5-10 Marion County, Indiana, Demographics

Total	~934,243 residents
Race/Ethnicity	57.9% white
	27.1% African American
	9.8% Latino or Hispanic
	2.6% Asian
	0.5% Native American/American Indian
	0.1% Native Hawaiian/other Pacific Islander
Health	32% adult obesity
	19% adults report having poor or fair health
	19% uninsured
Violence	45% increase in murder rates (2010–2014)
	144 victims of homicide in 2015
Education	76% of students graduate from high school
Employment	6.5% unemployed
Income	82% increase in poverty over the last decade
	31% of children living in poverty

NOTE: Percentages may not add up to 100 percent due to varied reporting, rounding, and missing data from source.
SOURCES: County Health Rankings, 2016b; IndyCAN, 2014, 2016b.

the middle class (IndyCAN, 2014). The percentage of children in Marion County living in single-parent households is among the highest in the state, at 47 percent (County Health Rankings, 2016b). Between 1985 and 2014, the per capita jail population in Marion County doubled, with African Americans being 3.1 times as likely to be in jail than their white counterparts (IndyCAN, 2016b).

Marion County ranks 83rd out of 92 counties in Indiana for health outcomes, and based on measures of health behaviors, clinical care, social and economic factors, and the condition of the physical environment, it ranks last out of 92 counties for health factors (County Health Rankings, 2016b).

The IndyCAN model for action is adapted from the PICO Community Organizing Model as a faith-based, broad-based organizing model that makes shared values and social relationships the binding factors that hold organizations together, rather than specific issue-based organizing. This creates a sustainable vehicle for state wide organizing and building capacity. The organization is rooted in local organizing committees, which engage community members through dialogue, local and regional trainings, and research meetings to identify the priorities of the community. The 38 participating congregations[26] that make financial contributions,

---

[26] For a full list of participating congregations, see http://www.indycan.org/about/congregations (accessed December 5, 2016).

"missional members," receive training to build capacity among their clergy and laity teams.

IndyCAN has various community, regional, and state-level partners outside of the realm of health. The organization has an extensive legal network, including the American Civil Liberties Union (ACLU), to support its work to protect immigrant families and promote criminal justice reform. IndyCAN leadership holds meetings with local and state-level policy makers, thought leaders, policy experts, and public officials to develop strategies and inform their decisions. IndyCAN has partnered with Indiana University, the University of Minnesota, the University of Wisconsin, the Vera Institute, and others to support community-led research as well.

Integrated Voter Engagement

Integrated Voter Engagement (IVE) is a year-round program that connects voter engagement to issue-based organizing in order to build power, sustainability, and impact over multiple election cycles. IVE is a more sustainable model for voter engagement in contrast to traditional campaigning methods, which tend to be seasonal operations (Paschall, 2016). In preparation for the 2014 midterm elections, IndyCAN volunteers garnered more than 15,000 pledges to vote, including pledges from more than 5,000 unlikely voters who were predominately low-income and people of color (Paschall, 2016). In 2014, IndyCAN doubled the African American and Latino turnout in three pilot districts, and by 2015, IndyCAN voter contact grew to 11 percent of every person that cast a ballot in Marion County, Indiana (IndyCAN, 2016a). IndyCAN has been successful in leveraging the already existing social networks within congregations and clergy voice, seen as credible messengers, to strengthen its voter program. These social networks and relationships are integral to promoting civic engagement and ensuring that people who pledge to vote will follow through (Paschall, 2016).

Addressing the Social Determinants of Health

While at first glance IndyCAN may not appear to be directly targeting health outcomes, it is clear that the work of the organization seeks to improve many of the social and economic determinants of health to achieve its mission of racial and economic equity.

Employment Employment opportunities as a means to promote economic dignity are a critical issue within IndyCAN's mission, as it supports opening and expanding pathways to jobs with family-sustaining wages, developing career pipelines that align training with employer needs, and removing barriers to employment, good wages, and benefits. In an effort to expand entry points for low-income and entry-level workers to middle-class careers in high-growth industries, the organization works to align workforce development and educational programs directly to employer needs. Since its founding, IndyCAN has promoted policies that have contributed to 9,738 new jobs and 52,620 trained workers and have removed barriers to employment for 253,600 immigrants, formerly incarcerated "returning citizens," and excluded workers in the region. For example, IndyCAN advocated for the first local hire requirement implemented in the state, which requires 30 percent of jobs created through downtown development tax increment financing to be directed to local low-income residents and allocates $3.5 million in job training and micro loans for minority businesses, which has resulted in good jobs for residents facing economic hardship (IndyCAN, 2014). IndyCAN also convenes educational institutions, workforce development organizations, and community members to expand the career pipeline by putting best practices, such as on-the-job training, in place.

Public safety Faced with rising homicide and incarceration rates, in addition to the associated costs of violence, IndyCAN has prioritized public safety and incarceration on its agenda. Specifically, the organization strives to reduce violence by advocating for the implementation of the U.S. Department of Justice's top-rated, evidence-based, nationally recognized strategy, Ceasefire. The Ceasefire approach has cut homicides by 30 to 60 percent in cities across the nation[27] by linking those who are at the highest risk of engaging in violence to jobs and alternatives to street life, healing the broken relationship between law enforcement and communities of color, and better integrating immigrants and previously incarcerated individuals into the community. To address recidivism, IndyCAN also promotes strategies such as transitional jobs and housing for the formerly incarcerated. IndyCAN currently partners with the mayor and the county sheriff with the goal of reducing Marion County's incarceration rate by 20 percent in 2018. This plan includes diversion programs for people with mental illness, addiction, and for low-level nonviolent offenders.

When the city of Indianapolis announced its plans to build a new $1.75 billion criminal justice center in 2014, residents expressed concerns that it would perpetuate the cycle of mass incarceration for low-income communities of color. IndyCAN organized residents and put forth a campaign that "brought together an unparalleled coalition of business, government,

---

[27] For more information, see https://nnscommunities.org/impact/results (accessed October 18, 2016).

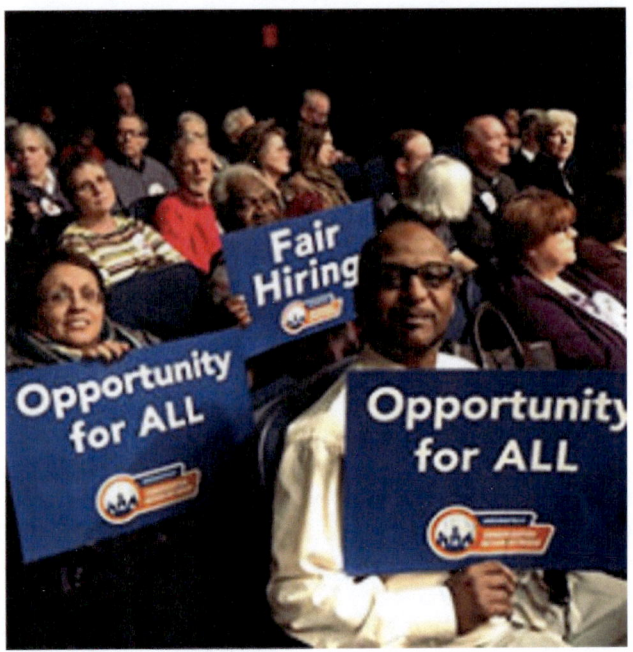

FIGURE 5-13 IndyCAN Ban the Box action, 2014.
SOURCE: Personal communication with Shoshanna Spector to National Academies staff on September 20, 2016. Available by request from the National Academies of Sciences, Engineering, and Medicine's Public Access Records Office (PARO@nas.edu). Used with permission.

and community leaders" that prompted the city council to halt the project and commit to restorative criminal justice reform strategies (Paschall, 2016). IndyCAN's current Jobs Not Jails initiative is informed by the body of evidence that suggests the disproportionate burden of incarceration on low-income communities of color as well as the importance of employment opportunities in reducing violence and recidivism. Jobs Not Jails outlines concrete steps[28] for the city to take to ensure that a new criminal justice center reduces violence and keeps people out of jail. In 2014, IndyCAN successfully campaigned to "ban the box," leading to the passage of an ordinance that prohibits city or county agencies and vendors from inquiring into an applicant's conviction history until after the first interview (see Figure 5-13). It should also be noted that the organizing

---

[28] For more information, see http://www.indycan.org/issues/mass-incarceration (accessed September 14, 2016).

efforts of IndyCAN laid the groundwork for the Indiana Supreme Court decision in September 2016 to end money bail practices for all low-level nonviolent, offenders.

Transportation IndyCAN works to achieve its vision of an equitable public transit system through its Ticket to Opportunity initiative.[29] The initiative was developed after the organization commissioned a study that revealed a broad base of support for new investment in mass transit, in addition to the effect that inadequate transit has as a barrier to employment opportunities and other important resources (IndyCAN, 2016a). IndyCAN is organizing to pass a regional transit expansion referendum in November 2016 that will triple bus service in Indianapolis. This expansion is projected to fuel economic development and increase job access for low-income communities threefold (IndyCAN, 2016a). The Ticket to Opportunity field program is initiating dialogue with 80,000 marginalized voters of color through large-scale integrated voter engagement to build sustained capacity for achieving transit equity. Thus far, more than 2,000 community members have communicated with their legislators in town hall sessions, in-person meetings, statehouse visits, calls, letters, and media events in efforts to convince them to support the passage of this bill (IndyCAN, 2014).

Education IndyCAN advocates for increased access to higher education and works to increase the accessibility of higher education to all immigrant students. The organization's priorities include providing equal access to in-state tuition for all students who graduate from high schools in Indiana and working to pass the DREAM Act in Indiana. IndyCAN is also organizing to expand quality prekindergarten education in the state of Indiana.

Social environment Efforts to improve the social environment are integrated throughout the work of IndyCAN. For example, IndyCAN provides civic gathering places at member congregations in various neighborhoods, many of which do not have other stable venues for civic gathering purposes. Furthermore, IndyCAN develops leaders who become involved in civic engagement, often for the first time. In 2015, IndyCAN trained 874 people who engaged 4,945 participants in its campaigns through personal visits, congregational events, town halls, vigils, research actions, and voter outreach, in addition to shaping IndyCAN's Jobs Not Jails platform. IndyCAN clergy, staff, and leaders conducted 108 trainings, including

---

[29] For more information, see http://www.indycan.org/transit/the-ticket-to-opportunity-platform (accessed September 14, 2016).

two leadership assemblies, four strategy team meetings, 96 trainings in congregations, and 12 clergy councils.

Finally, IndyCAN builds relationships and social networks across racial and ethnic differences to strengthen the social fabric of communities and to develop residents' sense of purpose and self-worth, all of which contribute to social and emotional health.

Data and Outcomes

As a member of the PICO network, many measures of progress that IndyCAN tracks are measures of civic engagement and community organizing. This includes estimates of the numbers of participants at trainings, conferences, and other organizing activities; the number of trainings given; the number of votes secured for particular ballot measures; the size of the voter contact network; and the levels of empowerment. Speer and colleagues found that the average PICO member engages in 76 percent more civic activities than the average resident (Speer et al., 2010) (see Figure 5-14).

IndyCAN also relies on data sources across various sectors to inform and support their platforms on issues such as public safety and transit expansion. For instance, IndyCAN's goal to reduce incarceration in Marion County will be measured using data submitted to the U.S. Annual

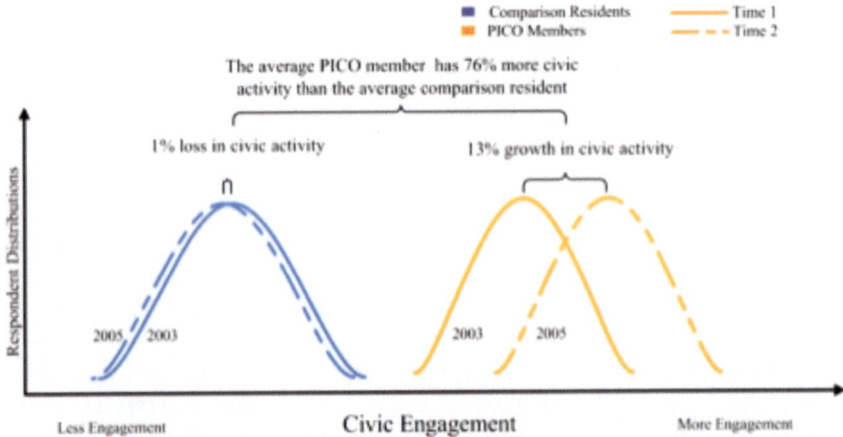

FIGURE 5-14 Changes in levels of civic engagement from 2003 to 2005 among PICO members and non-PICO members.
NOTE: This figure is drawn from an unpublished dataset. A subset of these data is presented in Speer et al., 2010.
SOURCE: Speer et al., 2010. Used with permission.

Survey of Jails. IndyCAN aims to build commitment from the U.S. Department of Justice to track and make accessible data to better identify racial disparities and assess outcomes. Additionally, IndyCAN measures access to jobs through expanded transit by using the Indianapolis Metropolitan Planning Organization's geographic information system mapping data.

Promoting Health Equity: Key Elements

IndyCAN's main platform, "Opportunity for All," is based on the premise that every person should have equal opportunity to access the conditions and resources necessary for the region to achieve racial and economic equity. This shared vision of opportunity for all is central to achieving community health, economic growth, and, ultimately, health equity. IndyCAN uses its extensive network of congregations to harness and uplift the collective voice of its communities and, in particular, marginalized populations. IndyCAN also recognizes and uses the power of faith-based leaders to create a shared vision and value among congregants. Religious leaders are a trusted source of guidance in Indiana, which is the 16th "most churched state in the nation" and where one in three voters is Catholic and 84 percent of African Americans say that religion is important to their decision making (IndyCAN, 2016a). IndyCAN works to equip faith-based leaders with the tools to teach and act on the imperative for achieving equity in transit, justice, and economic dignity.

A key element of IndyCAN's work is the formation of strategic partnerships across sectors to enable the community to act collectively as a region and to leverage collaboration to achieve its shared goals. IndyCAN has been able to create a strong coalition of business, government, and community leaders across sectors to mobilize around issues that are important to residents. Since its founding in 2012, the organization has launched three coalition partner tables covering the areas of transit expansion, immigrant integration, career pathways, and criminal justice reform, with participation from elected officials, policy makers, and several other partners. Collaboration with policy makers and public officials has proven to be vital to achieving long-term, measurable systemic outcomes. Data collection is one of many important activities of IndyCAN that has required partnerships across sectors, including such partners as the Metropolitan Planning Organization, EmployIndy, and the Bureau of Justice Statistics.

IndyCAN builds leadership and community capacity from the grassroots level, empowering individuals into a collaborative, organized movement of people with shared values and power. Through the facilitation of civic gatherings and providing leadership training that teaches residents to use the tools of democracy to improve their communities, IndyCAN is creating sustained community capacity. Low-income leaders—including people of color, immigrants, and returning citizens—continue to guide all aspects of decision making in the organization. Campaign decisions are initiated by local congregations and then ratified through local organizing committees (LOCs). Low-income LOC leaders maintain an ongoing dialogue with hundreds of low-income families through regular one-on-one conversations, check-in calls, and congregation-wide assemblies to ensure accountability and invite participation in decisions. At least two delegates, elected by each member congregation, vote at six Council of Representative (COR) meetings per year and shape countywide issue campaigns and strategy, set organizational direction, and review the annual budget. COR meetings also provide an entry point for new low-income leaders to participate in the broader organization.

IndyCAN also produces tool kits and other resources[30] for communities seeking to initiate dialogue and organize their congregations.

Sustaining Success

In order to sustain its work, IndyCAN raises funds from partners, individual donors, corporations, and foundations. While the primary source of funding is external donors, 25 percent of resources come from fundraising from internal resources.

IndyCAN's work is building a vehicle for statewide community organizing. The organization has recently begun initial efforts to create a chapter in northeastern Indiana, with plans to scale up across the state over the next 5 years. The organizing infrastructure that IndyCAN has built across an extensive network of local congregations allows for sustained relationships, and the training programs build a sustained capacity to shape outcomes. For example, in 2015 IndyCAN's training program focused on deepening its capacity to identify and challenge structural racism, race privilege, and implicit bias in all of its policy change campaigns. The training program is often the only place in the area where people gather and build relationships across race, class, and religion to understand the intersections of IndyCAN's work and build a shared commitment to the work of racial and economic justice.

---

[30] For more information, see http://www.indycan.org/tools (accessed September 14, 2016).

Magnolia Community Initiative[31]

Background and History

The Magnolia Community Initiative (MCI) originated from a strategic planning process within the Children's Bureau of Southern California,[32] a private, nonprofit agency, in 2001. By asking, "How can we prevent many of the social ills that rob vulnerable children of their future?" and "How can this be done in an environment where government and philanthropic resources are limited?" the Children's Bureau identified the key areas that research had shown to be necessary for creating safe and supportive environments in which children achieve the best results and live free of abuse and neglect.

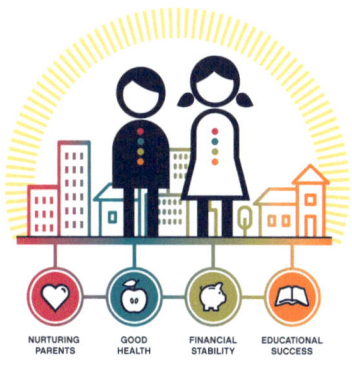

Based on this, the Children's Bureau then became the catalyst for what is now MCI.[33] Officially launched in late 2008, MCI's mission was to "unite the county, city, and community to strengthen individual, family, and neighborhood protective factors by increasing social connectedness, community mobilization, and access to needed supports and services." Today, more than 70 partners are involved in MCI's work to transform an entire community by uniting the residents and public and private organizations to change how both residents and organizations think and act as well as how parents behave. The main goal is to improve outcomes for those living in a metro Los Angeles community that is plagued with economic and social barriers. MCI's approach is a shift from using individual

---

[31] This summary is an edited account that was prepared on the basis of templates completed by staff of each community initiative. Statements and opinions expressed are those of the community organization and have not been endorsed or verified by the National Academies of Sciences, Engineering, and Medicine.

[32] For more information, see https://www.all4kids.org (accessed December 5, 2016).

[33] For an overview presentation on the MCI, see https://www.youtube.com/watch?v=tc2drcfNHPM (accessed December 5, 2016).

or program-level outcomes to promoting collective responsibility for improving outcomes for children by positively influencing family conditions, neighborhood conditions, protective factors, and positive parenting routines.

MCI's primary approach is to

- support a learning system that helps partners align their activities toward the mission and strategies of MCI and promote collective actions;
- support a holistic approach characterized by empathy and an understanding that positive neighborhood and family factors need to exist and interact in order to produce health and well-being outcomes;
- focus on a linkage system to effectively connect families with appropriate supports;
- promote changes in practice that help organizational partners cope with new demands as they incorporate change and support residents' positive actions in their own sphere of influence; and
- provide actionable data to inform partners' efforts and galvanize residents to make changes and achieve improved health and developmental outcomes.

The West Adams, Pico Union, and North Figueroa Corridor neighborhoods served by MCI have 35,000 youth, of which almost one-third are under 5 years of age. (See Table 5-11 for more demographics.) High rates of child abuse, child neglect, and spousal abuse are also present within this community. These neighborhoods are vulnerable, high-need, and

TABLE 5-11 Demographics of MCI Catchment Area in West Adams, Pico Union, and North Figeroa Corridor Neighborhoods

Total	~35,000 youth residents
Race/ethnicity	75% Latino
	11% Asian
	8% White
	5% African American
Health	35% of children are obese
Education	40% of children enter kindergarten unprepared
	73% of children are not proficient in reading by third grade
	40% of students will not graduate from high school on time
Income	65% of children live in poverty

NOTE: Percentages may not add up to 100 percent due to varied reporting, rounding, and missing data from source.
SOURCE: Bowie, 2011.

EXAMPLES OF COMMUNITIES TACKLING HEALTH INEQUITY

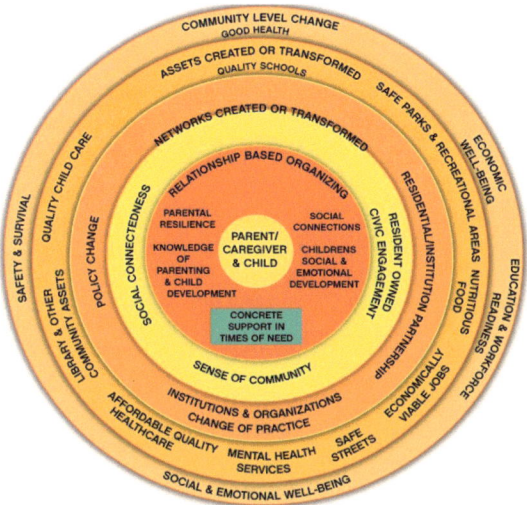

FIGURE 5-15 Magnolia Community Initiative community change model.
SOURCE: Bowie, 2011. Used with permission.

low-resource areas with multiple threats, as evidenced by the presence of low-performing schools and low student achievement, high poverty, low employment rates, a high incidence of diabetes and asthma, and high rates of involvement with the child welfare system (Bowie, 2011).

Community Level Change Model

The Magnolia Community Initiative Partners, along with the Children's Council of Los Angeles and First 5 LA, developed a Community Level Change Model. This model highlights the logic behind building resilience at the individual, family, and societal levels and the community-level changes sought. It is a graphic representation of a theory of change built upon research, some key assumptions, and years of implementing and learning from community-based prevention strategies (see Figure 5-15).

Within the model, the foundation for achieving individual-family and community-level change is increasing the protective factors for and mitigating the risk factors of family and community members. Informed by the Asset Building Community Development Model of John McKnight, resident groups are formed, and by virtue of members coming together to deepen their connections with one another, be each other's support systems, and learn and grow as individuals, the groups then become more aware of and involved in improving their neighborhoods (Kretzmann and McKnight, 1993).

Residents participating in neighborhood groups make social connections, increase their resilience for coping with stress, gain knowledge of parenting techniques and the stages of child development, foster their children's social and emotional growth, and create mutually supportive relationships that provide concrete support in times of need. From these protective factors come a greater sense of community and connectedness plus a move toward civic engagement that is truly resident-owned and resident-led. Resident-owned and -led actions result in partnerships that change institutional policies and practices, transforming and creating neighborhood assets such as high-quality schools and child care, economically viable jobs, good affordable health care and mental health services, safe and affordable housing, safe streets and parks, and other community elements such as libraries, banks, stores, and transportation options. Ultimately, these neighborhood-level assets contribute to the health and well-being of those living within them by contributing to the community-level outcomes of good health, safety and survival, economic well-being, social and emotional well-being, and education and workforce readiness.

Diverse Network of Partners

The Magnolia Community Initiative network includes an array of partners across various sectors. These include multiple partners operated by the Los Angeles County Chief Executive Office, including social services, child support, and child protection; regional organizations responsible for populations of children (e.g., the Los Angeles County Unified School District, Women Infants and Children Nutrition Program, and child care resource and referral); and private and nonprofit community-based organizations providing health care, early care and education, including Head Start and Early Head Start, family support, and banking and economic development services and supports.

The initiative began with a small group of cross-sector organizations recruited by the Children's Bureau. This core group established the overall approach with which to engage others. Individuals from these organizations coalesced around the shared goal of looking beyond one's programmatic achievements and embracing the collective goal of improving outcome for the full population of residents within the community, with improved outcomes for young children as the demonstrated marker of this success. Currently, MCI uses an open Web-based platform for communication. There is an orientation process for individuals and agencies asking to join the initiative. However, there are no barriers to entry or exit within MCI. All partners participate voluntarily, contributing what they can to the collective endeavor. Partners collaborate to align their work and function as a system, shifting from solely delivering individual services to a preventive and holistic approach for each person served (Inkelas and Bowie, 2014).

MCI also created a learning system for partners which consists of meetings, working groups, and improvement projects that build relationships and which aligns actions among agencies and with community residents, improves staff practices, builds agency capacity to better use data to understand the effects of one's practice, and introduces improvement science approaches to improve change processes. Through their involvement, partners are able to improve their individual practice and staff capacities, reflect with others on how to function as a "system" to improve conditions for children and families, and, ultimately, improve outcomes for their community. It is the voluntary nature of MCI that supports its sustainability, as partners serve without shared funding.

Solutions to Address the Social Determinants of Health

MCI's approach supports and is in alignment with cross-sector efforts, as each organization provides services within the sector of its competency. MCI then works on processes that enable different sectors across the social determinants of health to function more fully as a system to achieve positive results.

Social environment At the same time, MCI staff facilitates Belong Neighbor Circles, which are structured discussions of residents that introduce the concepts of protective factors, empathy, and belonging, with the goal of motivating residents into action. These discussions are intended to increase personal connections among the participants; expand the relationships of participants within their neighborhood; expand and strengthen participants' connections to community resources, supports, and information; and empower residents to acknowledge when they have a concern about the well-being of a neighbor or family member and act on those concerns to improve the well-being of individual families and therefore the community at large. Pre- and post-survey data reveal an increase in positive attitudes in the community around available resources, social cohesion, and perceptions of safety (see Figure 5-16).

Data and Outcomes

To collect data to measure community-level outcomes, MCI first created a community profile from publicly available datasets. In addition, MCI used the Early Development Index (EDI), a validated population

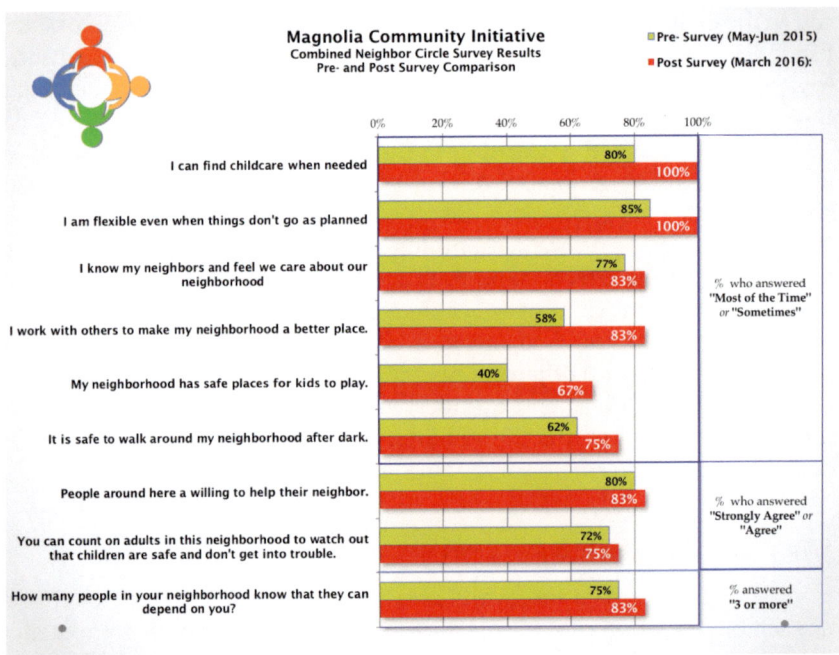

FIGURE 5-16 Magnolia Community Initiative Combined Neighbor Circle survey results: Pre- and post-survey comparison.
SOURCE: Personal Communication with Ron Brown to National Academies staff on November 18, 2016. Available by request from the National Academies of Sciences, Engineering, and Medicine's Public Access Records Office (PARO@nas.edu). Used with permission.

measure of children's well-being. EDI measures child development in 5-year-olds based on their kindergarten teacher's assessment across the following developmental domains: (1) physical health and well-being, (2) social competence, (3) emotional maturity, (4) language and cognitive skills, and (5) communication skills and general knowledge (Bowie, 2011). The results based on this index can be geographically mapped to neighborhoods (see Figure 5-17).

MCI created a Protective Factor and Community Belonging Survey by drawing items from multiple validated surveys and administered it biannually to individuals living in the catchment area beginning in 2009, with 2015 the most recent year it has been administered. The survey asks about wellness behaviors, protective factors, family conditions, access to services and supports, and contact with network partners.

MCI has also developed a dashboard that displays monthly and quarterly progress on actions related to family behaviors and their experiences

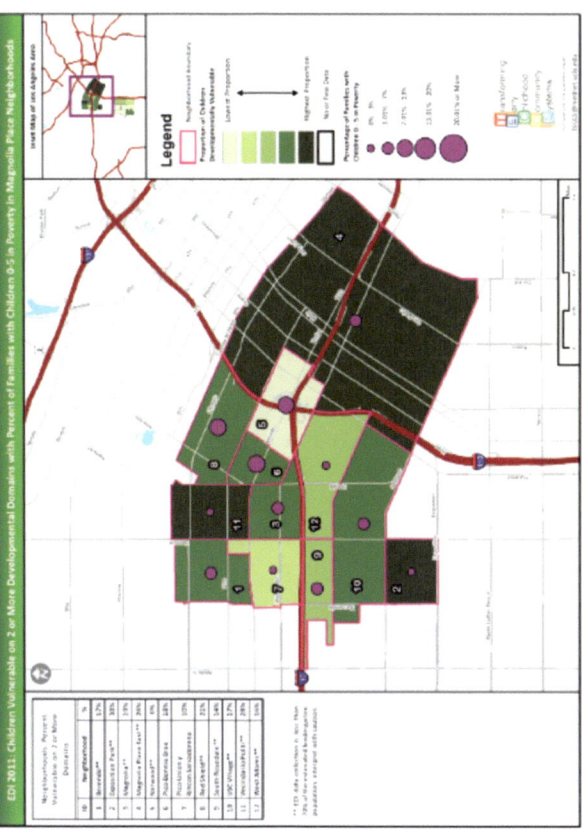

FIGURE 5-17 EDI results mapped by the proportion of children vulnerable on two or more developmental domains with percent of families with children 0–5 in poverty in Magnolia Place Neighborhoods.
NOTE: The UCLA Center for Healthier Children, Families, and Communities, under license from McMaster University, is implementing the Early Development Instrument with its sublicenses in the United States. The EDI is the copyright of McMaster University and must not be copied, distributed, or used in any way without the prior consent of UCLA or McMaster. @McMaster University, The Offord Centre for Child Studies. Used with permission.
SOURCE: Personal communication with Ron Brown to National Academies staff on November 18, 2016. Available by request from the National Academies of Sciences, Engineering, and Medicine's Public Access Records Office (PARO@nas.edu).

with organizational partners. The MCI dashboard includes feedback from residents regarding their experiences while engaged with partner organizations, linkage and referrals made using its MCI CareLinQ system, Innovation group progress, and the latest MCI Community Survey outcomes (2015).

Promoting Health Equity: Key Elements

A shared vision for improved outcomes among children and families is what binds together the network of more than 70 government and private-sector partner organizations that make up MCI. The initiative also works toward a vision for a socially connected community by enhancing the linkages and partnerships within its network. This translates to shared accountability and a fostering of relationships among network partners (i.e., enhancing familiarity with each other, linking clients to one another) to strengthen their impact on the community as a whole (Inkelas and Bowie, 2014).

Engaging residents has been a key component of MCI from its inception. The initiative recognizes that community members and residents need to play an active role not only in working to improve neighborhood and family conditions but also in the stages of providing input on what kind of changes they would like to see. MCI is predicated on the belief that residents who engage with each other within the construct of the initiative will increase community capacity, which is necessary to sustain improvements in child safety, health, and nurturing. To that end, the Belong Campaign[34] effort to engage and mobilize residents focuses on strategies to build social connections, develop ties with neighbors, and create leaders (neighborhood ambassadors) who can help connect residents to the resources available in the community. (See Figure 5-18 for a photograph of Belong participants.) By building their network of support, neighbors will have greater opportunities to increase each other's potential to be a positive force in their families and in their neighborhoods.

MCI also has strategies to improve organizational capacity for using data and cross-systems approaches to improve collective action. The strategies range from innovation groups that are using and teaching improved approaches—which include iterative testing and the use of data and charts for assessing change coupled with an improvement coach—to larger group collective action projects such as prototyping and testing the Web-based linkage and referral platform (CareLinQ). MCI has also developed a fellowship program. Currently in its fourth year, the fellowship

---

[34] For more information, see https://www.youtube.com/watch?v=CUEtCD_I9iU (accessed December 5, 2016).

EXAMPLES OF COMMUNITIES TACKLING HEALTH INEQUITY

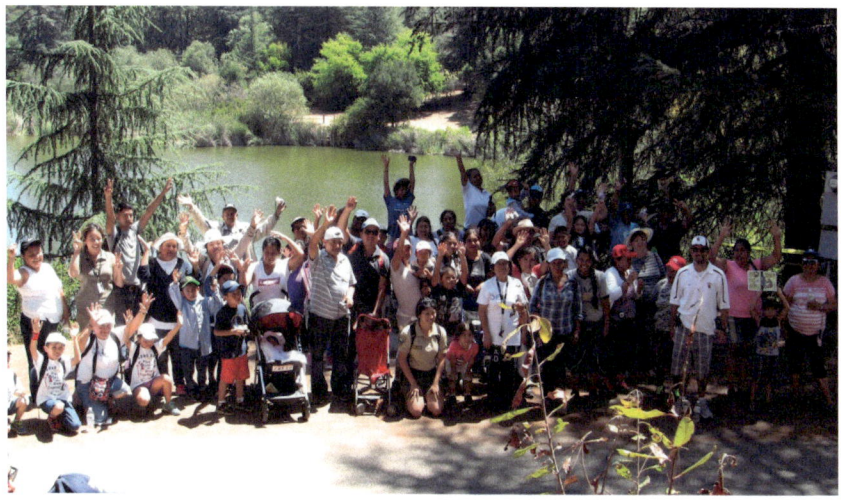

FIGURE 5-18 Participants in the Belong Campaign activities.
SOURCE: Personal communication with Patricia Bowie to National Academies staff on October 12, 2016. Available by request from the National Academies of Sciences, Engineering, and Medicine's Public Access Records Office (PARO@nas.edu). Used with permission.

supports mid-level and emerging agency leaders in building their professional capacity to adopt and support the data, improvement and other approaches that MCI has adopted for itself and its agency and at the same time to continue to deepen and foster cross-sector relationships among the MCI partners.

An especially noteworthy aspect of MCI is its ability to foster and maintain a culture of collaboration with many partners across a variety of sectors and disciplines. The initial recruitment strategy for partners was led by the Children's Bureau. A factor in the selection of partners that was crucial to facilitating a culture of collaboration was capturing a diverse group committed to the overarching goals of MCI and willing to lead through collaboration and not simply competition. This is especially challenging, because community groups and organizations are constantly shifting between cooperation and competing for limited resources to meet their organizational needs (Bowie, 2011). In MCI, collaborative groups are developed based on interest and are led by those partners with the time, resources, and expertise to advance a project. Leadership within the initiative is informal and not prescriptive, and there is no monetary compensation for participation.

Challenges and Lessons Learned

The challenges to taking on this level of work and desired outcome are seemingly endless. For example, maintaining involvement and participation, fostering cooperation over competition, sustaining one's own agency or family and having enough time and resources to contribute to a collective good or goal, having sufficient resources to achieve the necessary scale for large-scale change, and tracking progress in ways that are meaningful to a diverse group of key stakeholders, each with varying interests and ways of viewing success.

MCI has embraced a collective response in order to both address the interrelatedness and complexity of today's problems and to enable equitable access to the opportunities needed to thrive given today's possibilities. The initiative also recognizes that these collective endeavors require new ways of working, which includes new structures, social processes, and practices from the individuals, organizations, and the larger systems of which they are a part.

Yet there remains very little in the way of sharing the exploration and "testing" of what new structures, processes, and practices might better ensure equitable access and opportunity to thrive in the realities of today's economy. Maintaining sufficient momentum and sufficient engagement to change culture and practice to achieve better results within any one sector is well documented, and adapting these processes continues to be an ongoing exploration across many fields. However, applying this learning to achieve societal goals and address community-specific challenges remains an ongoing process of exploration, testing, learning, adapting, and resilience to all other things happening at the same time. Maintaining this as the focus is likely to be MCI's greatest challenge.

Sustaining Success

MCI was not designed as a 5- or 10-year plan, but rather as an approach that will expand over time and over generations within the community and organizations serving the community. For the first 2 years, the MCI director was the only staff member of the initiative. In more recent years, MCI has brought in other staff members to assist in strengthening some of the core support functions for the network. These include a data manager, an improvement coach, the MCI Belong organizing team, and a staff member focused on providing project management support of cross-agency projects. While recognizing that moving to managing a staff team requires a fair amount of time and energy, MCI decided at this time that having a stronger staff infrastructure will ensure success in sustaining MCI's approach to community change.

The MCI fellowship is a built-in sustainability mechanism which nurtures the next generation of leaders, grounding them in the MCI philosophy and practice. With each alumni group of mid-level managers, MCI ensures that its principles and practices are well integrated back into a partner organization. There is intended focus on passing on the vision, creating shared leadership so that the initiative continues to produce meaningful impacts on population community well-being and achieving the outcomes at a neighborhood level. Importantly, the building of data points over time to demonstrate change in the outcomes for children and families is a vital part of the sustainability strategy in order to ultimately attract ongoing investment and support from government and the philanthropic community. Recently, MCI received a $2 million collaborative gift from the Doris Duke Charitable Foundation and the Tikun Olam Foundation to assist with the data capture and communication strategy for sharing overall progress and lessons learned.

Mandela MarketPlace[35]

Background and History

Mandela MarketPlace creates sustained community economic development through investments and programming in local solutions to food system challenges in historically marginalized communities. To achieve this, Mandela implements community-informed 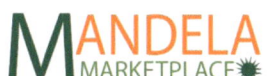 programming to increase food access and build economic opportunity—addressing issues of economic disinvestment, food insecurity, and health inequity by building on local assets. These programs span the breadth of the food chain, including producer support to increase market share, healthy food accessibility in urban markets, nutrition education and demand stimulation, and food retail business incubation.

Incorporated as a nonprofit in 2004 and based in West Oakland, Mandela MarketPlace's mission is "to work in partnership with local residents, family farmers, and community-based businesses to improve

---

[35] This summary is an edited account that was prepared on the basis of templates completed by staff of each community initiative. Statements and opinions expressed are those of the community organization and have not been endorsed or verified by the National Academies of Sciences, Engineering, and Medicine.

health, create wealth, and build assets through cooperative food enterprises in low-income communities" (Mandela MarketPlace, 2013). Recognizing that food-based strategies can provide an avenue for sustainable economic development, Mandela's model emphasizes investment in local communities to reverse the effects of long-term disinvestment and systemic racism.

Located in Alameda County, West Oakland is a historically African American neighborhood in the northwest region of Oakland that is home to about 36,000 people (City-Data.com, 2016b). Mandela MarketPlace's work has taken place primarily in a subarea of West Oakland with a population of about 25,000 people who have suffered severely from economic disinvestment and environmental injustices.[36] In 2010, West Oakland's population was 64 percent African American, 16 percent Latino, 9 percent Asian/Pacific Islander, and 7 percent white (City-Data.com, 2016b). Between 2000 and 2010, West Oakland's African American population declined 20 percent, while the number of Asian/Pacific Islander and white residents increased by 39 percent and 135 percent, respectively (Alameda County Public Health Department, 2015). West Oakland has the highest rates of poverty and unemployment in the county, with 45 percent of households earning an annual income of less than $25,000 (Healthy Food Access Portal, 2016). Additionally, only 23 percent of Oakland residents who are eligible for assistance from the Supplemental Nutrition Assistance Program (SNAP) actually receive benefits (FRAC, 2005; Unger and Wooten, 2006). West Oakland also has the highest rates in the county of certain diet-related chronic diseases, including diabetes rates that are three times greater than in the rest of the county (Alameda County Public Health Department, 2008). Approximately 48 percent of adults suffer from obesity (Healthy Food Access Portal, 2016), with persistent disparities by race and ethnicity. The prevalence of obesity by race and ethnicity is 28.9 percent for African Americans, 26.6 percent for Hispanics, and 5.5 percent for Asians/Pacific Islanders (Alameda County Public Health Department, 2014). As the neighborhood is surrounded by two freeways and adjacent to the Port of Oakland, residents of West Oakland suffer from greater exposure to environmental pollution and exposure-related health conditions. Compared to residents of the Bay Area, residents of West Oakland are exposed to three times more diesel pollution (Alameda County Public Health Department, 2014). West Oakland residents are also two and a half times more likely to develop cancer in their lifetime and have the highest rates of asthma hospitalization in the county (Alameda County Public

---

[36] Personal communication with Mandela MarketPlace staff. Available by request from the National Academies of Sciences, Engineering, and Medicine's Public Access Records Office (PARO@nas.edu).

TABLE 5-12 West Oakland Demographics

Total	~36,000 residents
Race/Ethnicity (2010)	64% African American
	9% Asian/Pacific Islander
	16% Latino
	7% white
Education	7.9% completed high school
	7.3% received an associate's degree
	14.1% received a bachelor's degree
Income	Median household income in 2013: $38,480
	33.9% below poverty level

NOTE: Percentages may not add up to 100 percent due to varied reporting, rounding, and missing data from source.
SOURCES: City-Data.com, 2016b; U.S. Census Bureau, 2010.

Health Department, 2014). See Table 5-12 for a summary of demographic information of West Oakland's population.

Throughout the early to mid-1990s, West Oakland was a prosperous working-class neighborhood of cultural activity, economic growth, and social activism. Host to a vibrant jazz and blues community in the 1940s and 1950s and the birthplace of the Black Panther Party in the 1960s, West Oakland was the last stop of the Transcontinental Railroad and thus also served as an economic and transportation hub (The Planning History of Oakland, n.d.). The neighborhood experienced devastating economic and cultural decline with the waning of the war economy, the onset of discriminatory housing and redlining policies, and the displacement of African American residents and the destruction of their homes and businesses due to urban renewal (Soliman, n.d.). Disinvestment and discriminatory social policies have had lasting destructive effects on the neighborhood.

> For far too long, communities like West Oakland have suffered intentional and sanctioned disinvestment—stripping people of financial assets, social cohesion, and human dignity. The primary challenges [facing West Oakland] are those of a community that is not only unequal but also inequitable. To bridge this equity gap, targeted investment in people and community builds a foundation for community re-investment—a foundation composed of engaged and honored community voices, resources directed specifically to empower those voices, and core values that honor community-owned solutions and economies for community benefit, grounded in a demand for health and a respect for culture.
>
> —Dana Harvey, Executive Director, Mandela MarketPlace

Residents of West Oakland have been rebuilding their community and fighting socioeconomic and environmental injustices that have lingered from the period of urban renewal. The founding of Mandela MarketPlace stemmed from these ongoing collective efforts, specifically the efforts of residents of color who had become increasingly concerned about the lack of access to affordable healthy food in their neighborhood. Through grassroots organizing efforts, residents established a comprehensive community planning process that recognized the need to provide economic opportunity to low-income residents of color and support under-resourced local farmers and local business owners in creating a sustainable community-owned food system.

In 1998 the University of California Cooperative Extension initiated a food and health needs assessment with the Environmental Justice Institute (EJI) and community residents. The results of the assessment affirmed residents' recognition of their community's need for food security and economic opportunity. EJI organized a series of community meetings, town halls, church events, nutrition workshops, and focus groups for residents, from which the West Oakland Food Collaborative was created in 2000 to provide a grassroots platform and community voting process through which residents developed a plan of community ownership and local employment and business expansion. In 2003 the U.S. Department of Agriculture (USDA) awarded a 3-year, $225,000 Community Food Projects grant that helped create the Mandela Farmers Market and the Healthy Neighborhood Store Alliance. In 2004 Mandela MarketPlace was incorporated as a 501(c)(3) nonprofit in order to support the opening and incubation of the Mandela Foods Cooperative. In 2009 Mandela Foods Cooperative opened and remains the only full-service grocery store serving West Oakland, operating as a worker cooperative owned by community members. It was incorporated by community members in 2004 as a worker-owned cooperative with grant and loan support from several sources, including the Walter and Elise Haas Fund, the West Oakland Project Advisory Community, a city council member, and the Oakland Business Development Center.

Solutions to Address the Social Determinants of Health

Mandela MarketPlace has launched a number of programs that increase food security, expand local employment opportunities, build individual and community wealth, provide health and nutrition education, improve the built environment, and strengthen outcomes through integration with the health care sector.

Employment and income Mandela has improved local workforce development by hiring and training local residents and supporting local farmers with a greater distribution network. Residents, farmers, business owners, and entrepreneurs of the community have also built wealth through opportunities to earn family-sustaining incomes, participate in business and entrepreneurial training, expand their customer bases, and receive microfinance loans.

An example of these opportunities put into action is Mandela Foods Cooperative, a 2,200-square-foot grocery store that stocks fresh produce, 50 percent of which is sourced from local farmers of color who grow their produce sustainably and are members of the Mandela Foods Distribution network, a venture of Mandela MarketPlace. Mandela Foods Cooperative does not sell alcohol, tobacco, or products with high fructose corn syrup. It is collectively owned by worker-owners who are all local residents of color. Currently the store is run by four worker-owners and employs two full-time employees and hopes to expand to eight worker-owners and three full-time employees in the near future. The store serves more than 250 customers daily and since opening has generated sales revenue of more than $4 million ($1 million in 2014 alone), which has benefited its worker-owners as well as members of the Mandela Foods Distribution network. Supported by a 2006 grant from The California Endowment and a 2011 grant from the California Department of Food and Agriculture, the network includes under-resourced farmers of color who operate within 200 miles of the Bay Area and who have access to flexible, no-interest loans that can be repaid with produce through Mandela MarketPlace's Harvest to Market loan program.[37]

Physical and social environment Mandela MarketPlace also provides a range of educational programming related to health and nutrition. Its programs include nutrition education workshops, cooking classes, and community outreach events. In partnership with Highland Hospital, Alameda County's safety net hospital, Mandela provides classes taught by dieticians to high-use patients. As of 2015, Mandela's educational programs had trained 26 peer educators, 10 youth, and 30 community residents on nutrition and food access. Community control of programmatic planning and allocation of resources has improved the social environment by building social capital among residents and community stakeholders. Mandela partners with local health clinics, hospitals, and senior centers to increase access to affordable healthy foods and provide education about the importance of healthy food consumption. Mandela has provided support to Oakland Based Urban Gardens to create Oakland's first land trust, a community garden near a local high school, and a park located in a residential neighborhood. Mandela has also supported Planting Justice,

---

[37] For more information on the Harvest to Market loan program, see http://media.wix.com/ugd/c3e56b_32738ccf66cf47ef9e967f295bcfd280.pdf (accessed December 5, 2016).

an Oakland-based food justice nonprofit, to undertake gardening projects at schools in East Oakland.

Data and Outcomes

Mandela's current data collection efforts[38] include obtaining monthly totals of produce sales through Mandela Foods Distribution; customer tallies at produce stands; randomized tallies of the number of fruit and vegetable customers at corner stores in its Healthy Retail Network; quarterly intercept surveying of fruit and vegetable customers at all retail sites (including corner stores, produce stands, and Mandela Foods Cooperative); customer receipt data from Mandela Foods Cooperative; and bi-weekly inventory records of produce distribution at each corner store. Figure 5-19 illustrates Mandela's community-owned food system model and some of the key overall outcomes Mandela has achieved.

Promoting Health Equity: Key Elements

Since its founding, Mandela has encouraged shared responsibility among community members and stakeholders in developing programs to achieve better health and socioeconomic outcomes. Meaningful resident and stakeholder engagement has been essential in the organization's

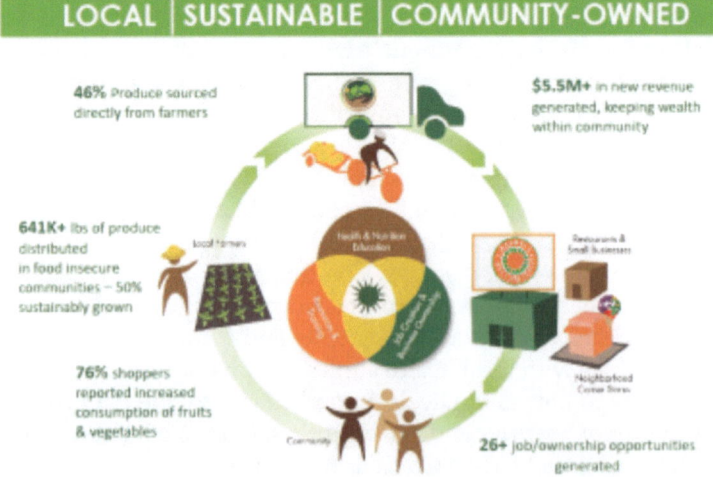

FIGURE 5-19 Mandela MarketPlace's model for a community-owned food system and outcomes data.
SOURCE: Mandela MarketPlace, 2013. Used with permission.

---

[38] Data collection is ongoing, and collected data have not yet been analyzed.

efforts to rebuild and reinvest in communities. Mandela has built a range of partnerships across different sectors to develop collaborative solutions to build healthier and more equitable communities and local food economies.

> The integration of economics and health forge natural partnerships among otherwise seemingly different sectors—we do business together, we support improved community health through education and food access, and we promote community ownership of the food system and the economies that develop within and around that system.
>
> —Dana Harvey, Executive Director, Mandela MarketPlace

Mandela's partnerships have involved businesses, educational institutions, youth development organizations, housing developers, government agencies (at the city, state, and federal levels), foundations, and others. Specific partners have included the University of California, Davis; Nutrition Policy Institute; Alameda Health Systems; Alameda County Public Health Department; East Bay Community Law Center; Sustainable Economies Law Center; PolicyLink; Centro Community Partners; Oakland Housing Authority; Resources for Community Development; Self-Help Credit Union; California FreshWorks Fund; FarmLink; Alameda County's Community Development Agency; City of Oakland's Community Action Partnership program; Mercury LLC (an advertising and marketing firm); California Wellness Foundation; Violet World Foundation; and Y & H Soda Foundation. Mandela has also received essential funding support from USDA, specifically from its Agricultural Marketing Service agency, Food Insecurity Nutrition Incentive program, Risk Management Agency, National Institute of Food and Agriculture, and Healthy Food Financing Initiative.[39]

Mandela's commitment to achieving better health and socioeconomic outcomes is also evident in its support of building capacity of local enterprises through business start-up support and loans. In 2013 Mandela received a $400,000 grant from the Healthy Food Financing Initiative to establish a $115,000 revolving fund to support local food enterprises and create 20 jobs. The fund has provided support for Mandela Foods Cooperative, Zella's Soulful Kitchen (a cafe located inside Mandela Foods Cooperative that is owned by a local entrepreneur), and Mandela Foods Distribution as well as three local food enterprises that sell at Mandela Foods Cooperative and other retail outlets. Mandela Foods Cooperative has supported employee and leadership

---

[39] The Healthy Food Financing Initiative is operated jointly by the U.S. Department of Agriculture, the U.S. Department of Health and Human Services, and the U.S. Department of the Treasury.

development by providing pathways from employment to ownership and training for its worker-owners and employees. Mandela also invests in youth development. From 2007 to 2013, Mandela supported the West Oakland Youth Standing Empowered program, which provided opportunities for local youth to engage in projects related to a range of community issues, including obesity prevention, improvement of walkable infrastructure and transportation, and neighborhood park improvement.

Challenges and Lessons Learned

Meaningful and sustained community engagement has been an essential component of Mandela MarketPlace from its early organizing efforts to the implementation of its many initiatives. The success of Mandela's programs has also depended on capable and committed leadership within the organization and from the community, including engagement from stakeholders to align community goals and recruit other areas of expertise when needed. During its early organizing phase, community organizers recognized a need for technical expertise in grocery retail and hired external consultants to provide assistance for developing a business model.

Mandela is regularly expanding its efforts to secure continuous sources of funding. Since its incorporation in 2004 as a 501(c)(3) nonprofit, Mandela has been able to leverage multiple funding sources from various foundations and government grant programs to expand and sustain its work. It has successfully secured funding from multiple sources by demonstrating a return on investment (see Figure 5-19) through important outcomes across different areas, including economic benefits from training employees and expanding businesses as well as community benefits from meeting the need for access to affordable healthy foods.[40]

Sustaining Success

Mandela has implemented several initiatives with community-based partners to sustain its community-owned food and local economies system model. A case study in Mandela's sustained relationships in community change can be seen in the organization's longtime work with James Berk, one of Mandela Foods Cooperative's co-owners. When Berk first walked into Mandela's office to participate in the CX3 community survey project, in partnership with Alameda County Public Health Department (ACPHD) and the California Department of Public Health (CDPH), he

---

[40] Personal communication with Mandela MarketPlace staff. Available by request from the National Academies of Sciences, Engineering, and Medicine's Public Access Records Office (PARO@nas.edu).

was 15 years old and attending a continuation school in West Oakland. Over the next 6 weeks, Berk and four other teams of adults and youth conducted surveys throughout West Oakland to assess the community for food access and walkability, including surveying corner markets, analyzing advertisements within 1,000 feet of schools, and documenting the condition of sidewalks and signage visible as students and families walked throughout the neighborhood.

Berk, along with and six other youth who were part of the summer program, charged themselves with using the data to identify and act on built environment improvements. With continued support from ACPHD and CDPH, Mandela MarketPlace and the youth team were able to make important changes in their community, building self-efficacy along with a series of projects aimed at improving their community, increasing healthy food access, and launching the Healthy Neighborhood Store Alliance program in West Oakland. Along the way, Berk matured as a leader in the team and in West Oakland. His work was recognized by the Ashoka Foundation, and the team was included in the Ashoka Youth Ventures program, receiving professional support, making presentations to investors, and traveling to other countries to connect with youth activists around the world. Berk was eventually recognized by Robert Redford's Art of Activism award in 2010 (Henry, 2011). When Mandela Foods Cooperative offered entrepreneurship training classes in an effort to identify new co-owners, Berk was a key participant. He became the youngest worker-owner, at 18 years old, and has remained an integral part of the Mandela family in the 7 years since.[41] See Figure 5-20 for a photo of Berk and other employees of Mandela Foods Cooperative.

Recent examples of successful community-driven partnerships include a public awareness campaign to increase health and nutrition knowledge and a multi-sectoral partnership to increase fruit and vegetable consumption for SNAP-eligible hospital patients. To increase awareness of healthy food availability and importance, Mandela partnered with a design firm and the California State Outdoor Advertising Association to develop and implement a strategic public awareness campaign that included twenty billboards placed throughout the county as well as posters and other materials displayed in local businesses. With 169 million views over 3 months, the billboards publicized the importance of healthy food systems to achieve positive health and socioeconomic outcomes and highlighted

---

[41] To read more about James Berk's work with Mandela and his achievements, see http://civileats.com/2011/05/06/james-berk-of-mandela-foods-brings-produce-to-his-people-video; http://blog.sfgate.com/inoakland/2010/06/10/local-teen-shines-while-receiving-art-in-activism-award; and http://www.homelessprenatal.org/news/founder-executive-director-martha-ryan-honored-at-redford-center-event (all accessed December 5, 2016).

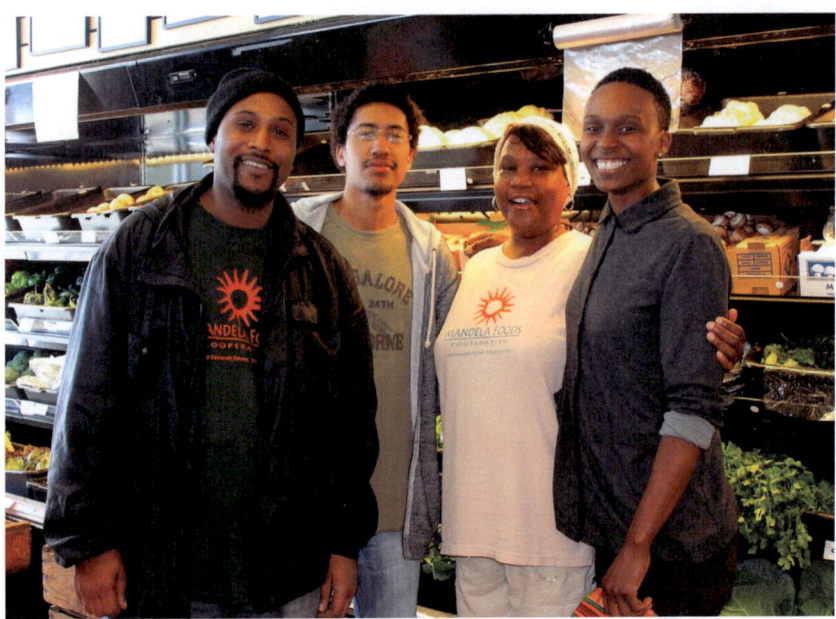

FIGURE 5-20 James Berk (left) with employees of Mandela Foods Cooperative.
SOURCE: Mandela MarketPlace, 2016. Used with permission.

the availability of affordable healthy foods through Mandela's network of stores and produce stands (Chakrabarti, 2016b). Building on Mandela's existing work with Highland Hospital, Mandela MarketPlace has launched its Fresh Creds program with support from a 3-year $422,500 grant from the Food Insecurity Nutrition Incentive program.[42] Mandela stores and produce stands in West, East, and North Oakland provide a 50 percent credit for each dollar spent on fruits and vegetables to low-income hospital patients who receive SNAP, known locally as CalFresh, benefits. Additionally, clinicians from the hospital assist low-income residents to enroll in CalFresh and provide health and nutrition education at Mandela stores. As demand for healthy foods grows, Mandela and its partners are sustaining engagement with partners across different sectors to ensure affordable access to healthy foods for low-income residents, in an area where points of access to receive CalFresh benefits are scarce (Chakrabarti, 2016a).

---

[42] For more information on the Fresh Creds program, see http://www.mandelamarketplace.org/freshcreds (accessed December 5, 2016).

The organization's commitment to developing solutions based on the needs and concerns of community residents has also been a critical success factor for sustainability. Mandela MarketPlace plays a key role in resourcing social, physical, and financial equity gaps that historically marginalized people and communities face. The reinvestment in communities and residents, with the ultimate goal that communities own the solutions, drives Mandela's work toward creating generational sustainability, uplifting cultural diversity, and increasing equal access to resources that cultivate thriving communities.

People United for Sustainable Housing[43]

Background and History

People United for Sustainable Housing (PUSH) is a nonprofit with a membership base of community residents that focuses on securing sustainable affordable housing for residents of the West Side neighborhood of Buffalo, New York. Its mission is "to mobilize residents to create strong neighborhoods with quality, affordable housing, expand local hiring opportunities, and to advance economic justice" (PUSH, 2012a). The organization's main activities are in the areas of ensuring affordable housing and living wage jobs, providing needed community services, and advocating for community members' needs through political activism. PUSH implements all of its many initiatives with a commitment to sustainable economic development.

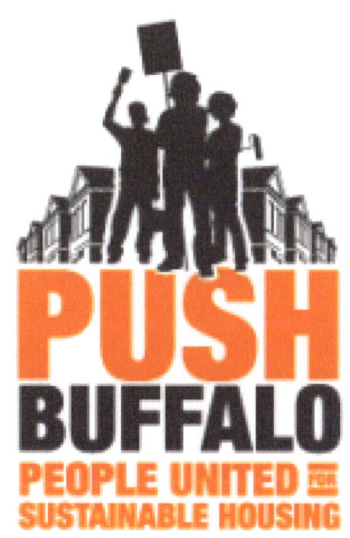

---

[43] This summary is an edited account that was prepared on the basis of templates completed by staff of each community initiative. Statements and opinions expressed are those of the community organization and have not been endorsed or verified by the National Academies of Sciences, Engineering, and Medicine.

TABLE 5-13 Demographics of Community Served by PUSH

Total	~25,000 residents
Race/Ethnicity	~25% African American
	~25% Puerto Rican
	~10% Asian
Income	Annual median household income in 2015: ~$26,000
	~40% of residents earned below the federal poverty line

SOURCE: Bhatt and Dubb, 2015.

The community served by PUSH is primarily low-income, and a majority of the community's residents live in poor-quality housing. See Table 5-13 for a demographic summary of the community served by PUSH.

The organization was founded in 2005 by Aaron Bartley and Eric Walker, who began their work with a 6-month canvassing effort surveying residents of the West Side. The door-to-door interviews conducted during the Block by Block campaign revealed that residents were concerned about the many hazardous vacant properties in their neighborhoods. PUSH discovered that a subagency of the New York State Housing Finance Agency owned 1,500 vacant, tax-delinquent lots in Buffalo (200 of which were in the West Side), which were then sold to the State of New York Municipal Bond Bank Agency. After that the properties were bundled and sold at a highly inflated price to the investment bank Bear Stearns (which later failed and was sold in the 2007 to 2008 financial crisis). The lots were not rehabilitated and remained vacant. PUSH petitioned for the release of the properties, and when its efforts were unsuccessful, it attempted to publicize the fraudulence through direct action campaigns that took aim at the governor at the time, whose successor eventually dismantled the bond and relinquished the properties back to the city of Buffalo. The lots could then be transferred to and redeveloped by PUSH or any of its partners, and an $8 million fund was established to assist in redevelopment.

Following these events in 2007, PUSH convened a community planning meeting to create a development plan for a 25-square-block area of the West Side where the annual per capita income was $9,000 (PUSH, 2012a). Annual community planning meetings followed, from which the Green Development Zone emerged in 2008. Many of PUSH's efforts as well as initiatives undertaken in collaboration with other partners take place within this zone of economic development. By 2013 more than 19 residential properties in the development zone had been completed, and a state grant was awarded to redevelop an additional 46 affordable housing units (PUSH, 2012b). The plan for the development zone includes not only the creation of affordable and energy-efficient housing but also the development of living-wage jobs that encourage a sustainable and community-driven urban economy (Boyer, 2013; PUSH, 2015). Figure 5-21 shows Buffalo residents rallying for energy sustainability.

Solutions to Address the Social Determinants of Health

PUSH operates several suborganizations whose efforts address disparities specific to housing, employment, and the physical and social environments.

Housing and employment The organization's main activity is reclaiming community control of vacant lots and redeveloping abandoned properties into sustainable, affordable housing for low-income residents. The Buffalo Neighborhood Stabilization Company is a nonprofit subsidiary corporation founded by PUSH that builds affordable housing in the Green Development Zone by operating a land bank in the Massachusetts Avenue Corridor of the West Side. Since 2014 the company has rebuilt more than

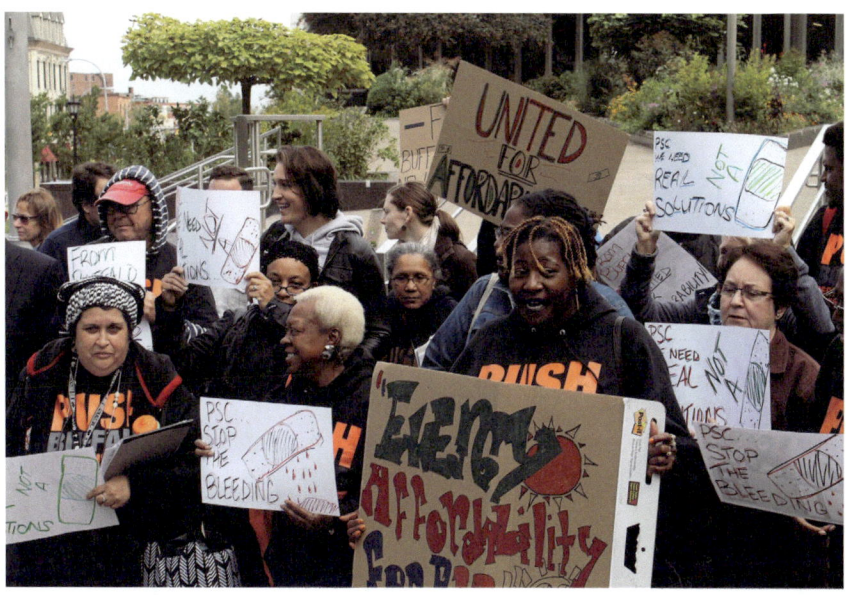

FIGURE 5-21 Buffalo residents rallying for energy sustainability.
SOURCE: Personal communication with PUSH staff. Available by request from the National Academies of Sciences, Engineering, and Medicine's Public Access Records Office (PARO@nas.edu). Used with permission.

25 vacant lots into affordable apartment units, in total creating about 500 energy-efficient homes for low-income residents.

Another housing initiative founded by PUSH is the Sustainable Neighborhoods Program, drafted in partnership with the state's housing agencies and signed in 2009. The program provides funding for housing redevelopment projects across the state that are community-driven and emphasize sustainability (PUSH, 2012e).

As part of the development plan for the Green Development Zone, PUSH also emphasizes energy-efficient housing improvement practices and sustainable jobs. PUSH helped to draft Green Jobs–Green New York, which was passed in 2009 with support from a broad-based multi-stakeholder coalition, including members from the labor community and environmentalists. The legislation encourages homeowners to retrofit their homes with energy-efficient upgrades and encourages contractors to hire more workers from marginalized groups. Through its first contract with the New York State Energy and Research Development Authority (NYSERDA) in 2010, PUSH Green was launched to provide weatherization and other house improvement services that promote energy efficiency to homes in western New York. Since 2011 PUSH Green has partnered with NYSERDA installation contractors to retrofit 500 homes. The initiative also focuses on reducing harm caused by indoor pollutants such as lead paint, asbestos, and mold (PUSH, 2012b). Through another NYSERDA grant in 2015, PUSH Green connected low- to moderate-income households to on-site solar photovoltaic incentives and financing offered by New York State.

In 2015 PUSH established PUSH Hiring Hall, a construction company with more than 20 full-time employees from marginalized groups who receive training and earn living wages (see Figure 5-22). Through a partnership with Solar Liberty, the largest solar panel installer in the area, the initiative trains a number of these workers in solar panel installation and provides these services at discount to residents. Over the next 3 years, the partnership will also provide 12 full-time, living-wage jobs in the private sector. PUSH Hiring Hall has also partnered with large developers, including Savarino Companies and Sinatra Development, to place workers in living wage jobs as skilled construction laborers. These development companies are recipients of public subsidies for market rate housing development in the city of Buffalo. Beginning in late 2016 PUSH will also undertake a new project to redevelop a vacant school in the West Side into 32 units of affordable housing specifically for elderly residents and a community hub with a recreational gym, community theater, and office space for local organizations.

PUSH has also expanded its work into other areas of environmental sustainability. PUSH Blue, which focuses on storm water interventions,

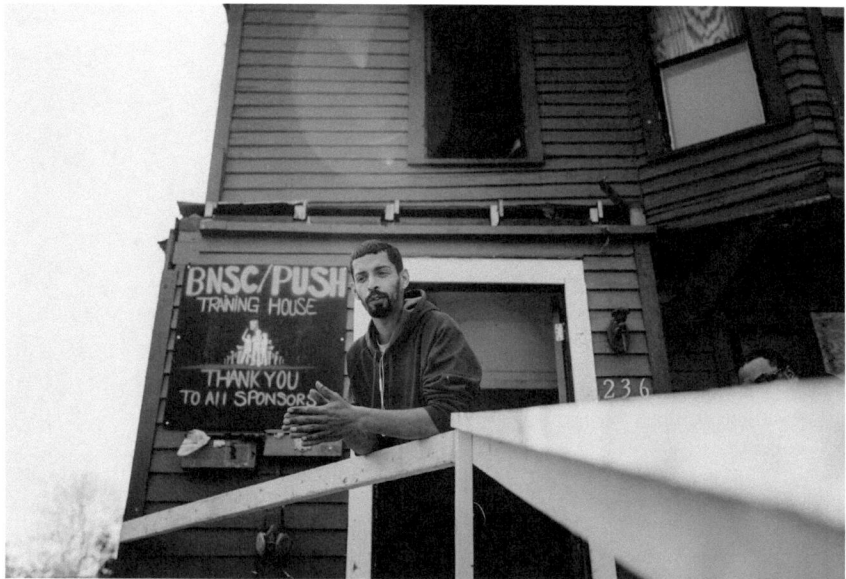

FIGURE 5-22 A member, Daniel Colon, of PUSH Buffalo's Hiring Hall/construction crew.
SOURCE: Personal communication with PUSH staff. Available by request from the National Academies of Sciences, Engineering, and Medicine's Public Access Records Office (PARO@nas.edu). Used with permission.

has created more than 10 new living-wage jobs and performed more than 30 projects in the Green Development Zone to help reduce the amount of raw sewage that flows into local water sources.

Partners of PUSH Blue include the Cleveland Botanical Garden, the Buffalo Sewer Authority, and the City of Rochester. As part of the Buffalo Sewer Authority's implementation of a citywide plan to control combined sewer overflow, PUSH Blue installed 75 bioretention systems on vacant lots owned by the city in 2015 and installed 69 more in 2016 (PUSH, 2015). PUSH also established a subsidiary business[44] called PUSH Gro, which markets and sells verniculture compost in partnership with cooperative businesses, including Lexington Cooperative Market and Urban Roots. Figure 5-23 shows a numbr of PUSH volunteers at a green infrastructure installation.

---

[44] PUSH Gro was established as a benefit corporation. Benefit corporations, or b corps, are "for-profit companies certified by the nonprofit B Lab to meet rigorous standards of social and environmental performance, accountability, and transparency" (B Lab, n.d.).

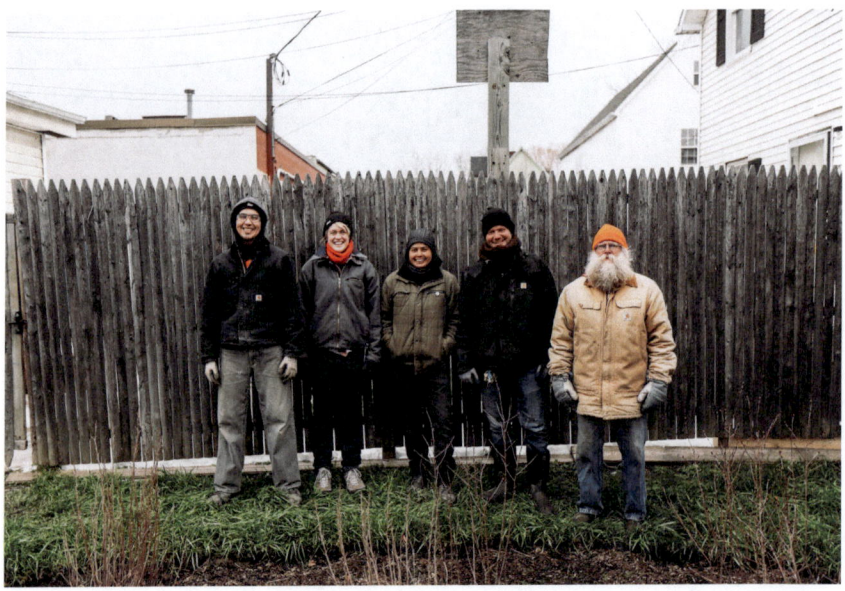

FIGURE 5-23 PUSH volunteers at a redevelopment site.
SOURCE: Personal communication with PUSH staff. Available by request from the National Academies of Sciences, Engineering, and Medicine's Public Access Records Office (PARO@nas.edu). Used with permission.

Physical environment PUSH has also worked to improve the West Side community's built environment. In 2011 the Massachusetts Avenue Park campaign successfully lobbied for $350,000 of funding to rehabilitate the largest park in the community (PUSH, 2012c). The organization has also created community gardens and urban agriculture plots in previously vacant lots in the Green Development Zone. It has also encouraged urban agriculture through collaboration with the Massachusetts Avenue Project, a nonprofit that operates a large urban farm on 13 previously vacant lots in the West Side (Massachusetts Avenue Project, 2016). PUSH works to create a more socially supportive environment through its operation of the Grant Street Neighborhood Center, a drop-in community center that provides programs and resources for West Side youth of all ages. Founded in 2009, the center supports an average of 60 youth each day, providing homework help, computers, movies, board games, a dance studio, and arts programs, including a new addition of a West Side Studios stop-frame animation course in partnership with Squeaky Wheel and Ujima Theatre Co., with intended tracks for higher education and workforce in the technology sector. In addition to providing day-to-day academic and social support, the center aims to provide "a safe, open, and productive space" and to promote youth development and leadership (PUSH, 2015).

Data and Outcomes

PUSH collects data on a number of different measures and is currently conducting a regional mapping project that will map data collected over time to elucidate progress and identify areas where further work is still needed. The measured outcomes include the number of redeveloped housing units, the number of employed workers, the amount of carbon emission reductions, and utility bill cost savings for low-income households. The organization plans to complete the mapping project by the end of 2016.

Promoting Health Equity: Key Elements

From its initial grassroots campaigns to the present day, PUSH's efforts have consistently reflected the concerns and needs expressed by residents of the community. Seventy-five percent of members of the organization's board of directors are community residents directly residing in PUSH's target zone—the Green Development Zone—and the organization convenes a community development committee monthly to determine resident needs and develop solutions to address these needs. The organization also convenes annual community planning congresses and invites professional planners to speak with residents to help identify and address resident concerns. Through these mechanisms, community input on housing, economic, and environmental issues has persisted as the driver of much of PUSH's work. The partnership between residents and PUSH (and its various suborganizations) ensures that the goals to improve the community are jointly shared.

PUSH has collaborated with many organizations and agencies, increasing stakeholder engagement in achieving its goals and fostering extensive multi-sector partnerships. In addition to partnerships with housing, energy, and parks departments, PUSH has also collaborated with more than 20 nongovernmental organizations, ranging from national organizations and foundations (including the Local Initiatives Support Corporation, People's Action Institute, Green for All, the First Niagara Foundation, the Center for Community Change, and the Center for Working Families) to other local nonprofits (including the Massachusetts Avenue Project, the Coalition for Economic Justice, the Partnership for the Public Good, VOICE-Buffalo, Open Buffalo, and West Side Housing). PUSH partners with private-sector companies, including a green architecture firm, a network of local contractors, and large banks such as Citizens, M&T, and HSBC, which have contributed financial donations for projects in the Green Development Zone (Bartley, 2016). The organization advocates for national policy change through its membership in the People's Action Institute (formerly National People's Action [NPA]), a network of grassroots organizations rallying around issues related to economic and social justice, and Green for All, a nonprofit that builds participation from minority communities in the green economy and climate change movements. PUSH and the NPA have spoken with the U.S. Department of Housing and Urban Development to encourage its assistance for community redevelopment efforts from federal programs (PUSH, 2012c). Additionally, PUSH held a public forum in 2009 with the Federal Reserve to encourage greater investment in sustainable development from the Community Reinvestment Act and reform lender oversight through the Home Mortgage Disclosure Act (PUSH, 2009).

PUSH's model of creating a sustainable urban economy through community-based redevelopment and organizing has built community capacity by prioritizing residents' concerns and encouraging neighborhood leaders to create and implement solutions. Extensive partnership building has helped strengthen the organization's capacity. Furthermore, many elements of its work could be scalable and transferrable to other low-income communities. For example, the organization's NetZero House, the first house in the region whose energy consumption is matched by its energy production, has garnered national recognition from media outlets and policy makers (PUSH, 2012d). Additionally, the organization often invites individuals from other organizations to tour the Green Development Zone and gain insights that can be taken back to their own communities.

Challenges and Lessons Learned

The barriers that PUSH has faced in carrying out its work have primarily related to the financing for housing redevelopment and workforce development and training. Premium and maintenance costs for energy-efficient and sustainable construction practices are often higher than for traditional housing redevelopment construction, and covering the premiums with state housing funding programs can be difficult. PUSH has advocated for the state's funding criteria to be more inclusive of sustainable construction in an effort to overcome this barrier. PUSH also faces challenges in sustaining employment opportunities for workers who receive training from the organization. Building connections with private-sector employers, such as PUSH Hiring Hall's partnership with Solar Liberty, will continue to be important for overcoming this barrier.

Another barrier is the growing real estate market and early gentrification in the West Side area that has complicated the Buffalo Neighborhood

Stabilization Company's efforts to acquire land and develop affordable housing. PUSH Hiring Hall has also faced challenges related to the employment-at-will doctrine, which has often been tied to discriminatory and racially motivated hiring, firing, and disciplinary practices.

> We've tried to position PUSH as a labor-management intermediary in order to protect and advance the interests of otherwise vulnerable contingent construction laborers, most of whom are men of color. We've worked to embed protections in our labor contracts, e.g., the right for PUSH to engage the host employer prior to adverse disciplinary action being taken against workers; a progressive disciplinary policy that takes seriously consideration of mitigating circumstances.
>
> —Clarke Gocker, Director of Policy and Initiatives, PUSH Buffalo

WE ACT for Environmental Justice[45]

Background and History

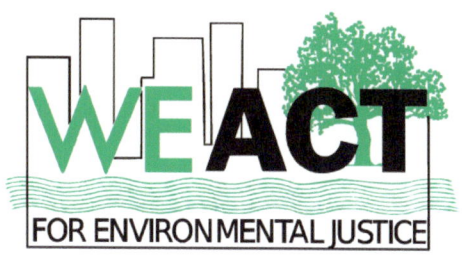

WE ACT for Environmental Justice (WE ACT), formally known as West Harlem Environmental Action, Inc., is a nonprofit, membership organization that engages in community organizing, community-based participatory research, and advocacy to fight environmental injustices faced by residents of color in West, Central, and East Harlem and Washington Heights/Inwood, marginalized neighborhoods located in northern Manhattan in New York City. WE ACT's mission is "to build healthy communities by ensuring that people of color and/or low income participate meaningfully in the creation of sound and fair environmental health and protection policies and practices" (WE ACT, 2016a). The organization focuses on improving environmental health and protection through community organizing, policy and legal advocacy, public awareness campaigns, community-based participatory

---

[45] This summary is an edited account that was prepared on the basis of templates completed by staff of each community initiative. Statements and opinions expressed are those of the community organization and have not been endorsed or verified by the National Academies of Sciences, Engineering, and Medicine.

research, civic engagement, and initiatives that influence local, state, and federal environmental health and protection policy and laws. WE ACT also promotes greater inclusion of marginalized communities in environmental reform and decision making by training and educating residents to become informed, empowered voters. See Table 5-14 for demographic information of the community WE ACT serves.

Founded in 1988 by three activists (see Figure 5-24) from West Harlem, WE ACT was the first environmental justice organization in New York City. The organization's creation was catalyzed by residents' protests of the North River Sewage Treatment Plant on the Hudson River, which had opened in 1986 and was releasing high levels of toxic emissions and odors. WE ACT cofounders Peggy Shepard, Chuck Sutton, and Vernice Miller-Travis mobilized the community for a civil disobedience protest on January 15, Martin Luther King, Jr. Day, in 1988 (see Figure 5-25). In conjunction with residents protesting across the road from the treatment plant, a small group of community activists and elected officials known as the "The Sewage Seven" rallied directly in front of the plant on the West Side Highway and were arrested for stopping traffic. Over the next few years, WE ACT gained support from local and state elected officials and recruited an environmentalist to research the plant's operations. In 1992, WE ACT served as the lead plaintiff with the Hamilton Grange Day Care Center and others in a nuisance lawsuit brought against the New York City Department of Environmental Protection (DEP), with pro bono attorneys from the Natural Resources Defense Council (NRDC) and Paul, Weiss, Rifkind, and Wharton. WE ACT cited that racial and class discrimination had motivated the decision to locate the plant in West Harlem rather than in a primarily white neighborhood in the Upper West Side that had originally been chosen for the plant's location. In late 1993, the parties reached a settlement that mandated a $55 million effort by the city to fix

TABLE 5-14 Harlem Demographics

Total	~125,528 residents
Race/Ethnicity	65.0% African American
	17.3% Hispanic
	11.7% white
	3.2% Asian
Education	40.4% completed high school
	41.1% completed post-secondary education
Employment	7.7% of population aged 25 to 64 unemployed
Income	Median household income in 2013: $36,395

NOTE: Percentages may not add up to 100 percent due to varied reporting, rounding, and missing data from source.
SOURCES: U.S. Census Bureau and American Community Survey data via (statisticalatlas.com, 2016) and (City-Data.com, 2016a).

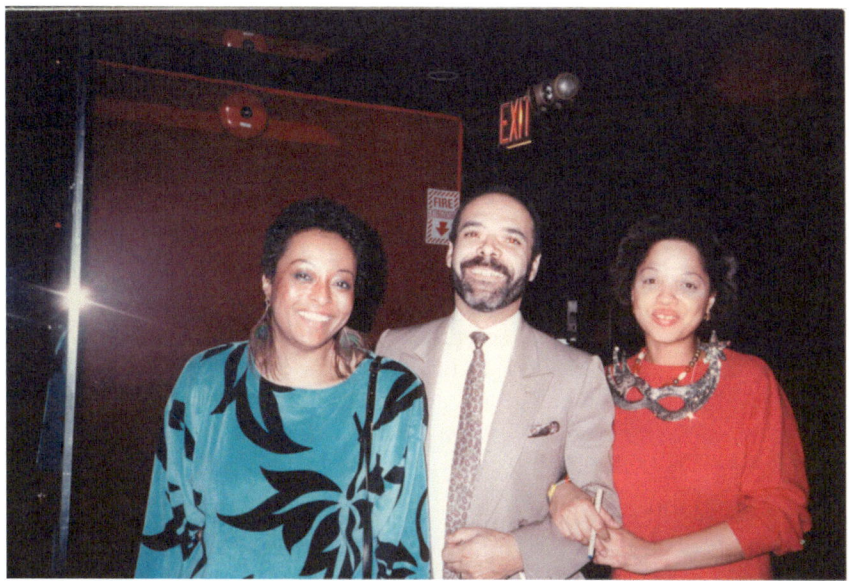

FIGURE 5-24 WE ACT cofounders Peggy Shepard, Chuck Sutton, and Vernice Miller-Travis.
SOURCE: Personal communication with WE ACT staff. Available by request from the National Academies of Sciences, Engineering, and Medicine's Public Access Records Office (PARO@nas.edu). Used with permission.

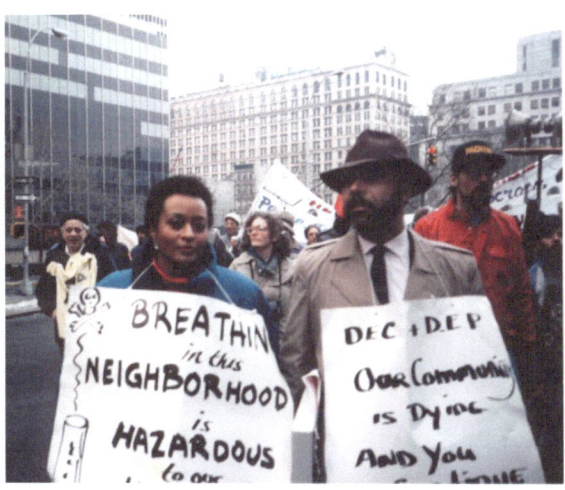

FIGURE 5-25 Two of WE ACT's supporters rallying in 1988 to protest the North River Sewage Treatment Plant.
SOURCE: WE ACT, 2016c. Used with permission.

the plant and established WE ACT and NRDC as monitors to oversee the court-ordered improvements to the plant, including hiring an engineering consultant to ensure that retrofit efforts were completed satisfactorily. The settlement also established a $1.1 million settlement fund to address the environmental concerns of the community, from which WE ACT acquired funds to hire its first three paid staff members in 1994. The settlement also established a $1.1 million Community Environmental Benefits Fund from penalties levied on the New York City DEP by the New York State Department of Environmental Conservation. WE ACT has since grown from a grassroots organizing effort led by a small group of West Harlem activists to a nationally recognized institution that supports and empowers residents to advocate for and achieve more environmentally healthy communities. The organization's annual budget is about $2 million, with about 85 percent provided by foundations, and it currently has 16 staff members (WE ACT, 2016c).

Civil Rights Law

WE ACT's origins and present-day efforts are grounded in using civil rights analysis and law to create policy changes that benefit residents and improve the health of communities. In addition to the environmental racism claims in the North River Sewage Treatment Plant case, the second of WE ACT's earliest activities also used civil rights law to create policy change.

In 1988, WE ACT filed an injunction in the state supreme court calling for an environmental impact statement by the Metropolitan Transit Authority (MTA) over its proposal to build a sixth diesel bus depot uptown in West Harlem, which was already disproportionately burdened by pollution-producing facilities. The northern Manhattan neighborhoods of East, West, and Central Harlem and Washington Heights/Inwood were hosting five of the six Manhattan bus depots. In 2000 WE ACT filed a Title VI[46] administrative complaint with the U.S. Department of Transportation against the MTA when it sold a bus depot in the South Bronx and sent 200 buses to over-capacity depots in northern Manhattan where the buses sat—often idling—near homes, schools, and parks. The MTA cited a "business necessity" for its actions at a time when studies were documenting that the Harlem community was experiencing asthma at alarmingly

---

[46] Title VI of the Civil Rights Act of 1964 (42 U.S.C. § 2000d to 2000d-7): "No person in the United States shall, on the ground of race, color, or national origin, be excluded from participation in, be denied the benefits of, or be subjected to discrimination under any program or activity receiving Federal financial assistance" (GPO, 2010).

higher rates (Corburn et al., 2006; Nicholas et al., 2005), as much as six times the rate of other Manhattan neighborhoods (Wakin, 2001).

From 1991 to 1992, WE ACT, as a member of the Coalition to Save St. Luke's Hospital, worked with the NAACP Legal Defense Fund, which filed a Title VI complaint with the U.S. Department of Health and Human Services for unjustly transferring maternity and neonatal beds in an uptown hospital to a downtown hospital affiliate.[47] The St. Luke's catchment area includes two large public housing projects that depend on the hospital for health services. In 2004 WE ACT and the NRDC filed a lawsuit against the U.S. Environmental Protection Agency (EPA) for its rat poison standards, which had failed to protect the health of children (WE ACT, 2016d). In 2016 WE ACT and other advocates from across the country partnered with Earthjustice and filed a lawsuit against the EPA for failing to update standards that protect families and their children against neurotoxic lead-based paint and lead dust, which many studies have shown can irreparably hinder children's learning ability and reduce their IQ (Bellinger, 2008; Needleman et al., 1990).

Solutions to Address the Social Determinants of Health

WE ACT works to build healthier communities by prioritizing identified healthy community indicators: air quality; open and green space; food justice; climate justice; toxic-free products; transportation; waste, pests, and pesticides; land use; and healthy indoor environments. The organization uses community organizing and training, community-based participatory research (CBPR), advocacy, and an empowered grassroots membership base to achieve its goals.

Physical environment WE ACT's work to improve the physical environmental focuses on improving the built environment, advocating for climate justice, and promoting toxic-free products.

Built environment WE ACT helped to create the West Harlem Piers Park (see Figure 5-26), which transformed a former 69,000-square-foot parking lot into a 105,526-square-foot park, redeveloping the Harlem waterfront to increase options for active living for uptown families. The park opened in 2009 after a decade of community organizing and planning that produced a community-driven plan developed by WE ACT and Manhattan Community Board 9 in partnership with more than 200

---

[47] Personal communication with WE ACT staff. Available by request from the National Academies of Sciences, Engineering, and Medicine's Public Access Records Office (PARO@nas.edu).

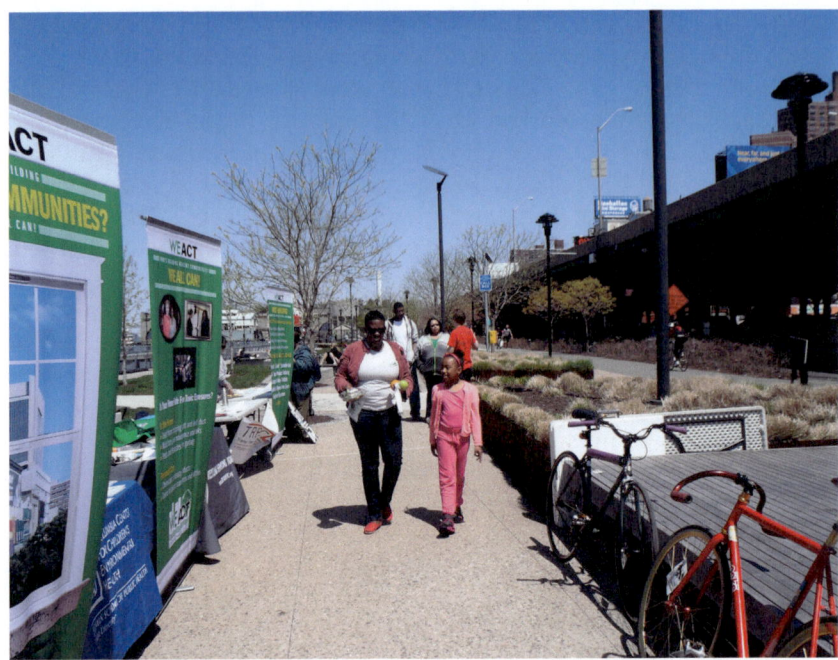

FIGURE 5-26 Harlem Piers Park.
SOURCE: Personal communication with WE ACT staff. Available by request from the National Academies of Sciences, Engineering, and Medicine's Public Access Records Office (PARO@nas.edu). Used with permission.

residents, representatives from the New York City Department of Parks and Recreation, and local elected officials. In 1999 the community-driven plan was submitted to the New York City Economic Development Corporation, which set aside a variety of commercial development proposals in favor of advancing the community-driven plan to a master plan for the waterfront park and the surrounding neighborhood.

Building on the success of the community-planning process for the Harlem Piers waterfront park, which encourages active living, WE ACT organized a 40-group Northern Manhattan Environmental Justice Coalition in a campaign known as Fair Share, not Lion's Share. The campaign achieved the decommissioning of the 135th Street marine transfer station (MTS), which resulted in an MTS being rebuilt in the affluent upper eastside of Manhattan. Under former Mayor Bloomberg's solid waste plan, each borough needed to be self-sufficient and provide for its own waste in order to reduce truck trips through overburdened communities of color and low income in Brooklyn and the South Bronx, where waste transfer stations proliferate. Mayor Bloomberg agreed in 2007 that WE ACT and Community Board 9 could organize community stakeholders to develop a community-driven plan for redeveloping the former MTS located on the Hudson River next to the new Harlem Piers waterfront park. These efforts created the From Trash to Treasure campaign, which has engaged residents to collaboratively develop a plan for the redevelopment of the 28,000-square-foot MTS. The closure of the MTS eliminated 200 to 300 trucks driving through the community to the MTS, which was operating 24 hours daily.

In response to Columbia University's plan to develop a satellite campus in the Manhattanville section of West Harlem, between 2005 and 2012 WE ACT and the West Harlem community, acting with Community Board 9, coalesced to hold the university accountable for its land use process that threatened to restrict community access and spur gentrification and displacement. WE ACT developed environmental recommendations to ensure that construction trucks used diesel retrofits and that buildings would be constructed to comply with Leadership in Energy and Environmental Design (LEED) standards. WE ACT partnered with Fordham Law School's Community Development Law Clinic, which produced legal research on land use and zoning and assisted community residents in developing their testimony for hearings on the environmental impact statement and the city's Uniform Land Use Review Process, which required city council approval. WE ACT's Deputy Director Cecil Corbin-Mark was a lead community negotiator acting to hold the university accountable for providing a community benefits agreement (CBA) of $150 million, with another $150 million provided by the city to relocate two buildings of tenants and to preserve affordable housing. The West Harlem Development Corporation administers the CBA and grants funds to West Harlem groups for projects that improve community health, job training, small business, and arts and culture.

Climate justice With a $100,000 grant from the Kresge Foundation, WE ACT engaged its members and 400 residents from four neighborhoods across northern Manhattan in a series of public workshops in 2015 and developed the Northern Manhattan Climate Action Plan. The plan focuses on energy security, emergency preparedness, and social hubs and emphasizes coordination by community members through bimonthly working groups which advance policy initiatives such as development of microgrids and solar installations for affordable multifamily housing. Other stakeholders who contributed to the development of the plan include academic partners at Columbia University's Mailman School of Public Health and the Icahn School of Medicine at Mount Sinai, the New York City Mayor's Office of Resilience and Recovery, elected officials, and consultant Dr. Michael McDonald of the Global Health Response and Resilience Alliance. The implementation strategy identified policy initiatives necessary to achieve the plan with a 3-year Kresge Foundation grant of $660,000.

In 2008 WE ACT organized the Environmental Justice Leadership Forum on Climate Change, a national coalition of 42 environmental justice organizations across 20 states. The forum publishes a Clean Power Plan Tool Kit,[48] which provides guidance for state agencies and stakeholders to conduct civil rights and environmental justice analyses and meaningful engagement with vulnerable communities in planning for and implementing the federal Clean Power Plan rule. Incorporating equity, health, data, and meaningful engagement are key elements of the planning process. The tool kit report published by the forum summarizes the environmental justice analysis under Title VI of the 1964 Civil Rights Act in this way:

- Describe what you plan to do.
- Consider the benefits and burdens for all communities.
- Consider the alternatives.
- Include people of color and low income in the decision-making process.
- Implement a plan to distribute benefits and burdens equitably and avoid discrimination.[49]

Currently, the forum is working with a consultant to develop an environmental justice analysis for states to guide their development of their state implementation plans.

Nontoxic products In response to growing evidence of the human health effects of harmful chemicals and pesticides, WE ACT worked with the New York Public Interest Research Group (NYPIRG) in 2005 to encourage the New York City Council to pass two bills that were aimed at reducing exposures to toxic chemicals contained in pesticides. Armed with findings from a collaborative 18-year research project of the Columbia Center for Children's Environmental Health (CCCEH) that has documented the exposure to banned pesticides of 720 mothers and newborns in northern Manhattan and the South Bronx, WE ACT and NYPIRG worked with members of the New York City Council to introduce bills requiring notification of neighbors when pesticides are applied and requiring a

---

[48] The Clean Power Plan Tool Kit is available at http://www.ejleadershipforum.org/clean-power-plan-tool-kit (accessed December 5, 2016).

[49] See page 28 of the Forum's *Environmental Justice State Guidance: How to Incorporate Equity & Justice into Your State Clean Power Planning Approach*, available at http://www.ejleadershipforum.org/wp-content/uploads/2016/01/EJ-State-Guidance-updated-March-7.pdf (accessed December 5, 2016).

reduction and elimination in the use of the worst toxic pesticides in New York City's stockpile. Both bills were passed by the council and signed into law in 2005.

Beginning in 2006 and continuing to the present, WE ACT and Clean and Healthy New York have served as coleaders of the Just Green Partnership, a statewide coalition of environmental, environmental justice, public health, health-affected, labor, and sustainable business advocates who have led the fight in New York to protect children and families from harmful toxic chemicals in many products used daily. In 2010 the U.S. Food and Drug Administration ruled that it could no longer declare that bisphenol A (BPA) was safe. WE ACT and Clean and Healthy New York worked with allies in the Just Green Partnership to implement a ban on BPA in children's products—including pacifiers, unfilled bottles, and sippy cups—and allowed for BPA-free products to be labeled as such. WE ACT engaged residents of northern Manhattan in signing petitions and postcards urging leaders of the New York State Assembly, Senate, and governor to protect New York's children from the harmful effects of BPA. In 2010 New York passed a ban on BPA in products used by children ages 3 and younger. In 2012 WE ACT and Clean and Healthy New York worked as the leaders of the Just Green Partnership to ban TCEP, a toxic flame retardant chemical, in children's products. Using findings from research conducted by CCCEH, WE ACT again engaged its members and northern Manhattan residents in pushing for a change in the law that would better protect their children. At the end of the legislative session in 2012 and with bipartisan support, Governor Cuomo signed into law a bill requiring that TCEP be banned in children's products in New York.

In 2015, in partnership with the Just Transition Alliance and the Connecticut Coalition for Environmental Justice, WE ACT created a public awareness and education campaign to gain support from the congressional Black and Hispanic caucuses, subcommittees, and other agencies and offices to back the Safer Chemicals, Healthy Families campaign. The campaign advocated for the reform of the Toxic Substances Control Act of 1976, an outdated national law regulating chemical safety that had allowed approximately 82,000 potentially unsafe chemicals to remain in use in the United States. The act was amended in 2016 by the Frank R. Lautenberg Chemical Safety for the 21st Century Act, which mandates safety reviews of chemicals currently in use as well as new chemicals not yet on the market and includes some protections for vulnerable communities.

Transportation In 1997 WE ACT launched its Dump Dirty Diesel campaign to promote public awareness among community residents of the high levels of pollution in many neighborhoods of northern Manhattan due to the toxic diesel exhaust fumes being released by MTA buses and the elevated risks of respiratory problems, chronic disease, premature mortality, and negative effects on birth outcomes caused by this pollution. The goal of the campaign was to encourage the MTA to renovate its diesel bus depots and invest in buses running on clean sources of energy. In 2000 WE ACT filed a Title VI complaint against the MTA for continuing to invest in diesel buses. As a result of the complaint, the U.S. Department of Transportation mandated that the MTA uphold civil rights law and take environmental concerns into consideration in its future decision making. In 2008 WE ACT, along with the MTA and a community task force, began holding community planning sessions to transform the Mother Clara Hale bus depot to comply with LEED standards. Since then, WE ACT has been successful in pushing the MTA to transform its entire city bus fleet to hybrids and compressed natural gas buses.

In 2011 WE ACT partnered with UPROSE (a Brooklyn-based nonprofit that promotes healthy and resilient communities through environmental, climate, and youth justice), Empire State Future (a coalition of organizations in upstate New York that encourages sustainable and equitable economic growth), and the Tri-State Transportation Campaign (a nonprofit working to reduce dependency on cars in New York, New Jersey, and Connecticut) to create the New York State Transportation Equity Alliance (NYSTEA), a statewide coalition of more than 50 organizations. The coalition's goal was to help build a more affordable and equitable transportation system in New York, providing improved public transportation options to residents without cars and addressing negative environmental health effects. As a result of the advocacy of NYSTEA and others, the 2014–2015 New York State budget included the first increases for public transit both upstate and downstate in many years. In 2014 WE ACT also established a Transit Riders Action Committee (TRAC) which has organized residents to campaign against unjust transit fare increases and closings of public transit options and to advocate for civil rights protection in transportation policy making (WE ACT, 2016b). The efforts of WE ACT's TRAC resulted in bus rapid transit service across 125th Street, a congested east-west commercial corridor, and faster bus service for hundreds of Harlem residents to access the job center that is LaGuardia Airport located in the borough of Queens.

Housing In 2014 WE ACT began implementing its Healthy Homes Campaign with the goal of improving health, safety, and quality of life among residents of color and low income in New York City. The project has three objectives: (1) mobilize and build a campaign power base, consisting of members, environment and housing advocates, scientists, policy advocates, government agencies, community-based organizations, and people with health conditions related to poor indoor environmental conditions, in order to identify and marshal efforts to close gaps in housing policies and codes that violate the warranty of habitability[50] and expose vulnerable tenants to environmental toxins and hazards; (2) develop campaign communication strategies that effectively position the campaign for high public visibility and legislative attention and action; and (3) advance effective New York City housing policies that address current housing, building code, and enforcement gaps; protect public health; and reduce harmful indoor environmental exposures. Since launching the campaign, WE ACT has worked to secure citywide healthy housing legislative and regulatory policies aimed at improving health outcomes in multifamily affordable housing by partnering with allies from a broad cross-section of social justice advocacy, housing, government, research, and green building sectors in a collaborative campaign that uses mobilization, convening, and communications strategies to educate city officials to support the Asthma-Free Homes bill pending at the New York City Council—a bill that would require landlords to fix housing violations that affect asthmatic tenants.

Health systems and services WE ACT currently works to improve the methods and practices by which three Harlem-based hospitals engage vulnerable communities in their catchment areas to achieve community health needs assessments and community benefits processes under the Patient Protection and Affordable Care Act. WE ACT aims to identify specific ways that the hospitals can engage with populations in their catchment area, identify community health needs, and determine the exact scope and type of community benefits they could provide in response to community health needs. WE ACT will produce a report that serves as a resource for advocates, policy makers, and hospital leaders seeking to strengthen the impact that hospitals have on the health and well-being of the populations they serve by providing in-depth analyses of the existing community benefits processes and deliverables as well as specific recommendations for improving existing community services based on robust local engagement with a broad cross-section of stakeholders.

Data and Outcomes

WE ACT's theory of change, including key short-term, intermediate, and long-term outcomes that the organization hopes to achieve, is illustrated in Figure 5-27.

---

[50] "Most jurisdictions read residential leases to include an *implied warranty of habitability*. This warranty requires landlords to keep their property 'habitable,' even if the lease does specifically require them to make repairs. Furthermore, the warranty conditions a tenant's duty to pay rent on the landlord's duty to maintain a habitable living space" (LII, n.d.).

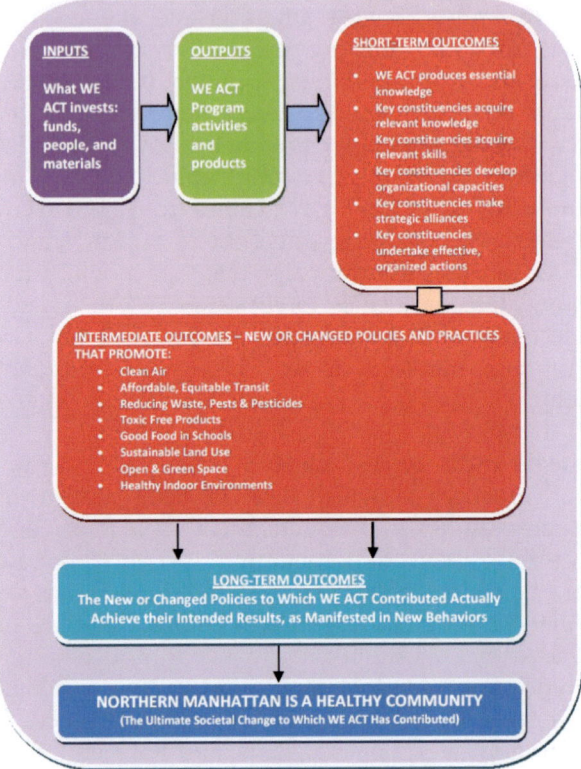

FIGURE 5-27 WE ACT's theory of change to create healthier communities in northern Manhattan.
SOURCE: WE ACT, n.d. Used with permission.

WE ACT partners with academic institutions to conduct CBPR and uses data as evidence to drive its campaigns. To demonstrate the effects of air pollutants, harmful chemicals, and pesticides on children's health and birth outcomes and to advocate for policy changes to improve these outcomes, WE ACT has collected data on air quality by producing maps showing sources of pollution overlaid with health and income data. WE ACT's data-driven advocacy efforts have led to new policies and legislative reform on issues related to air quality monitoring and the use of harmful compounds such as BPA and phthalates in consumer products, pesticides, and flame retardants.

Promoting Health Equity: Key Elements

WE ACT's work is based on the concerns of residents and members and driven by community efforts, including community organizing, community planning sessions, town halls, and public meetings between residents and elected officials. All steps in the development and implementation process for each of its initiatives are undertaken with meaningful community engagement, ensuring that the concerns and priorities of residents are the drivers of WE ACT's work. WE ACT engages partners from a range of sectors, including environmental health, land use and management, transportation, public health, energy, environmental health scientists and practitioners, and the legal system. Partners have included academic institutions, housing groups, law schools, solar energy providers, government agencies, and community-based participatory researchers.

WE ACT has partnered extensively with educational institutions to conduct research and collect data for its advocacy work. Its North River Sewage Treatment Plant complaint was submitted after conducting a CBPR project to determine whether high levels of pollution were to blame for the high rates of asthma among the community's children, a majority of whom were African American or Latino. With funding from the National Institute of Environmental Health Sciences (NIEHS), WE ACT and CCCEH collaborated to train 17 WE ACT interns to collect data on air quality in the uptown area. The collaborative research effort found unsafe levels of diesel particulates, results that were similar to those of the EPA's subsequent data collection (Minkler, 2010). WE ACT currently partners with the NIEHS Center for Environmental Health in Northern Manhattan (CEHNM)—which conducts research on the role that environmental pollution plays in the development of neurodegenerative diseases, respiratory diseases, and cancers with environmental risk factors—and CCCEH, both of them located at Columbia University's Mailman School of Public Health. As cochair of CEHNM's Community Outreach and Translation Core and a coprincipal investigator of CCCEH's Community Outreach Education Core, WE ACT disseminates the centers' research findings to community residents and organizations, health care providers, policy makers, and public interest groups. It organizes community conferences and policy briefings among its researchers, community residents and partners, and policy makers to inform and advocate for safer environmental health policies to protect and improve the health of low-income residents of color. For the past 18 years, WE ACT has had subcontracts with both research centers to carry out this work. CEHNM also provides $25,000 pilot grants to researchers and community partners to study air quality and other neighborhood concerns that affect environmental health. Partners at the research centers have also cooperated to apply for National

Institutes of Health grants (when WE ACT is ineligible to do so) that serve community concerns, such as understanding the impact of social cohesion on outcomes of public housing tenants affected by Hurricane Sandy. WE ACT has partnered with the University of Pittsburgh School of Public Health to study the cumulative effects of stress and air pollution on asthma throughout the five boroughs of New York City; with Montefiore Hospital to research effective methods for training parents on reducing exposure to indoor sources of lead; and with the Icahn School of Medicine at Mount Sinai to study the effects of climate change on children in northern Manhattan.

WE ACT has worked with elected officials and policy makers at the local, state, and national levels. Through its Kellogg Foundation–funded project, Establishing Health Resilience for Vulnerable Asthmatic Children, WE ACT works with partners in Louisiana, Michigan, Mississippi, and New York to strengthen the efficacy of federal strategies to reduce asthma disparities among vulnerable children by assessing the performance of strategies and mobilizing communities to advocate for needed reform. Specifically, the project seeks to understand how the four strategies identified in the Coordinated Federal Action Plan to Reduce Racial and Ethnic Asthma Disparities[51] have performed with regard to disparities among children in these communities between the ages of 0 and 8, given how critical these years are in a child's development. In 2017 WE ACT will disseminate a report on its findings and recommendations for how to improve these strategies. WE ACT has also hosted forums for candidates to speak on environmental justice issues and has trained residents to testify at city council hearings. It has mobilized residents to lobby with state legislators and, through its office in Washington, DC, galvanized residents to advocate for national policy change and legislative reform. WE ACT has also built support for national and global environmental justice movements and has taken on a leadership role in convening environmental justice organizations on climate issues.

WE ACT builds capacity by providing residents with opportunities to develop their leadership skills. In keeping with its theory of change (see Figure 5-27), the organization provides leadership training to community members through its Environmental Health and Justice Leadership Training (EHJLT) program, an 11-week course that educates participants about the issues confronting their northern Manhattan neighborhoods. Upon graduating, the class participants understand the impact of a range of environmental health issues and are ready to address them by taking a leadership role in organizing WE ACT's membership on related

---

[51] Available at https://www.epa.gov/asthma/coordinated-federal-action-plan-reduce-racial-and-ethnic-asthma-disparities (accessed October 27, 2016).

campaigns. The EHJLT training program has been adapted to train 60 high school students over 1 week in the predominately Latino Washington Heights Expeditionary Learning School. WE ACT is adapting its leadership training model with community-based organizations and high school students through a partnership with the University of North Carolina's Center for Environmental Health, Columbia University's Community Outreach and Engagement Core, and Harvard University's School of Public Health. The Climate Change and Health Fellows program will foster climate literacy among health professionals as well as high school students.

Challenges and Lessons Learned

As with many other environmental justice organizations, WE ACT has faced challenges in securing funding for its operations. These challenges have served as important opportunities for learning and growth. Funding for community organizing is often difficult to secure, as funders may not fully understand the costs associated with building a base of support for developing and implementing policy initiatives and mobilizing residents to vote, educate, and hold their elected officials accountable. A number of studies, including one by Dr. Daniel Faber at Northeastern University, document that environmental justice organizations receive half of 1 percent of all environmental funding nationally (Faber, 2001). Philanthropy has reported that environmental justice organizations comprise only 2 of the top 20 organizations receiving the small amount of environmental justice funding available (Environmental Grantmakers Association, 2015). Other philanthropy associations report that organizations led by directors of color receive even less funding from foundations (The Greenling Institute, 2006).

Strong grantsmanship has been essential for obtaining multiyear funding. Much of WE ACT's funding comes from larger foundations and federal grants. Securing funding from individual donors has proven to be particularly challenging, which can be problematic because donors often provide significant funding for general operations, including rent, administrative and fundraising staff, accounting, technological upgrades, and other elements that are critical to an organization's long-term success. Strong communications and public messaging that bolster the successes of an organization are critical to securing long-term sources of funding. Effective evaluation is also critical. WE ACT includes funding for evaluation consultants in proposals whenever possible and ensures that its staff members receive training in assessing outcomes and project effectiveness.

WE ACT designs its projects through a logic model process to help ensure that positive outcomes are achieved and objectives are met.

Sustaining Success

Vision, strategic planning, and developing a theory of change have been critical to planning the organization's future direction and identifying the methods and resources necessary to achieve WE ACT's objectives. Examples include the development of a federal policy office in Washington, DC, strategizing to develop a state legislative presence and exploring development as a 501(c)(4) organization. WE ACT has also sustained its success through strong membership development. Funding for a membership and organizing director took at least 5 years to secure, but in 2 years WE ACT's organizing team strategically recruited about 400 members who have been engaged in and provide leadership to the organization's campaigns. An emphasis on community-based planning has also helped to sustain success, engaging residents in visible and viable land use projects that improve community sustainability and public health. Community-based planning has improved social cohesion and created community consensus around projects that would be controversial if handled by city officials without resident input. Partnerships with academic institutions have provided critical data and findings for WE ACT's evidence-based campaigns and helped to increase the organization's visibility and credibility among policy makers and the media. Effective staff members are also essential for sustaining success by boosting confidence in the organization from policy makers and philanthropy and creating goodwill in the community.

Key elements that have facilitated WE ACT's success are its achievement of trust and a shared vision with the northern Manhattan neighborhoods plus a strong engagement with environmental justice organizations around the country. With strong partnerships with other nonprofits and academic institutions with similar goals, the organization has consistently sought outcomes that are beneficial for all stakeholders. WE ACT's activities have been informed by principles of collaboration developed by academic partners who engage in community efforts as well as formal processes such as the protocol for assessing community excellence developed by the National Association of County and City Health Officials. WE ACT has incorporated these principles and protocols in its work, but it has most successfully sustained its ties to the community through a commitment to resident solidarity over its decades of work. WE ACT has built high levels of trust that have sustained partnerships even after grant periods have ended and thus has created opportunities for ongoing collaboration.

SUMMARY OF CHALLENGES

As evidenced by the case examples discussed in this chapter, the barriers that organizations face in promoting health equity vary from larger contextual issues to more specific programmatic issues. For example, DHC struggles to overcome the challenges of patients who are left in the insurance coverage gap, and EPN works to keep communication systems effective to ensure that residents are aware of the resources made available to them. Also outside of the control of the community organizations highlighted in the chapter are the inevitable changes in political administrations, which can have implications for funding and political will. Another barrier that emerged from the community examples was the challenge of getting community residents to invest their time and energy into upstream factors and more long-term benefits, as compared to immediate needs. DSNI struggles with this, as many of the community residents are preoccupied with satisfying basic needs, such as shelter and food. Just as communities will require individualized approaches to solutions, responses to overcoming barriers should also be tailored to the strengths and needs of the community. The next section discusses how some of the challenges faced by the communities were addressed and other key components that made these communities successful.

SUMMARY OF KEY ELEMENTS, LEVERS, POLICIES, AND STAKEHOLDERS

Chapter 4 discusses the need to build the structures necessary to strengthen community solutions by undertaking systematic efforts to learn from both the successes and the failures in the strategies, initiatives, and other efforts currently under way and being developed. Although reviewing just nine examples does not constitute a systematic review, the communities described in this chapter make it clear that it is possible to act effectively at the community level to modify social determinants of health that may, in turn, reduce health disparities and promote health equity.

All of the nine community examples highlight the three key elements of effective community change from the committee's central figure: equity as a shared vision and value, increased community capacity, and enhanced multi-sectoral collaboration. Below, the committee addresses some of the ways these nine communities relied on the three key elements and applied a variety of elements, levers, and policies to achieve their desired outcomes.

Changing the Narrative

The most important, and perhaps least tangible, ingredient in all nine examples is the capacity to create a community vision in which residents will feel compelled to invest their time and energy. In a community where resources are scarce, jobs are few, money is tight, and parents cannot afford babysitters, getting started on community action for change may require great sacrifices and courage. Unless there is a belief that change is possible and that it might actually lead to a better quality of life, there will be no motivation for action. Creating a shared vision is the first and most essential task of leaders—a community needs to believe that people can change and that their circumstances can change. Without that willingness to hope for the possibility of change, nothing will get started. Dr. Jack Geiger, one of the early leaders of DHC, has argued that communities suffering from poverty, which are "all too often described only in terms of pathology, are in fact rich in potential and amply supplied with bright and creative people" (Geiger, 2002). This positive message is an example of how to inspire and engage.

Building Trust and Agency

A core element to changing the narrative and engaging the community in action is building trust and reciprocity among community residents and institutions. For many communities that face health inequity, divestment, land use and zoning policies, medical institutions, and other structural drivers have been a source of historical trauma and mistrust, and rightfully so. For DHC, overcoming historical mistrust has been achieved through ultimate transparency and a strong presence in community activities. In addition, over half of the board of directors must consist of current patients of the program. In the neighborhood of the DSNI, divestment had destructive effects on the social and economic environment. When the Riley Foundation first proposed its neighborhood revitalization plan to residents, it was met with discontent due to the lack of community representation. When the advisory group shifted power and ownership to the Dudley community members with a board that was majority residents, a community-driven agenda was established. This type of community power dynamic is reflected in many of the community examples and facilitates the building of trust between community institutions and residents. Trust among residents and other community stakeholders, in addition to the belief that change is possible, is essential for community actors to be empowered and develop agency. Interventions at the community level are uniquely positioned to empower community residents to seek change and galvanize communities to act.

Leadership

The Role of Leaders

In some, but not all, of the case examples, charismatic individuals united or mobilized a community and significant partners around a specific goal. Charismatic leaders can be extremely important in galvanizing change, but not every community may have such a person, at least initially. In some examples, leadership came from outside the community and helped build capacity within the community. This is the case with DHC. When DHC got started in the 1960s, many residents had not yet succeeded in overcoming infamous local barriers to voting. Local leaders took great risk in supporting the initiative, while local government and police were barriers, rather than supporters, of success. Today, DHC is community-owned, and its new generation of leadership and staff has strong community ties and effective partnerships with local government and other institutions. In this and other examples, an outside leader or leaders were successful because of a true partnership with a community, focusing on building capacity and empowerment.

The leaders in the nine examples differed widely in various ways, but they shared the ability to get the community working for change. By embarking on plans for change, leaders were sometimes able to secure relatively early victories, which led to more optimism and engagement. For example, an early protest march by leaders of WE ACT resulted in their arrest while blocking traffic. This arrest increased the visibility of the group and demonstrated its seriousness of purpose, which built community support and led to the group's successful partnership to sue New York City for greater environmental justice.

Leaders need not only to create hope but also to unite the community in working toward common goals. For IndyCAN, leaders belong to a faith-based network. This is not the only type of partnership that can produce change, but it has significant advantages in working with those who are already closely knit together into coherent congregations and who unite around the importance of large social and spiritual goals. Across the United States, numerous PICO organizations have effectively mobilized faith-based groups for social change.

Leadership Development

For DSNI, a foundation approached a community with a fully formed plan for change, and the community rejected it as ill-suited to its needs. Both the philanthropy and the community were flexible and insightful enough to keep working together and for the community to build the leadership capacity that would make it possible to create its own successful plan for change with the financial and other resources of the philanthropy in support. The responsivity and commitment of both parties, shown in the effort to continue working on the collaboration despite a setback, was vital to their success. MCI specifically set out through its Belong Campaign to build social connections, develop ties among neighbors, and create leaders. MCI fellowship is a built-in mechanism to develop the next generation of leaders. A few of the examples, including DHC, DSNI, and WE ACT, have persisted for decades. One factor that most likely contributed to the sustainability of these programs was that all focused explicitly on developing the next generation of leaders. DSNI created a Resident Development Institute. DHC set up educational programs for youth and assistance for those applying to college.

Building Diverse Network of Partners

All of these examples demonstrate the power of building an effective network, not just within the community but also with crucial additional partners who can support the community's goals. The number of partners is less important than the ability to unite a group of partners who may have disparate skills and domains of expertise but who maintain a shared vision. Many of these examples show collaborative interventions across many sectors; these broad partnerships were crucial in affecting change within challenging domains, ranging from youth violence to local poverty and unemployment.

The Minneapolis Blueprint for Action to Prevent Youth Violence is a striking example of multi-sectoral collaboration to address youth violence. Leaders, including the mayor, city council, and local philanthropy, along with the community, addressed multiple contributing factors ranging from lack of education, lack of job training, little follow-up with youth who presented to local hospitals with violent injuries, and the failure to reintegrate youth who had experienced legal difficulties into the community. The initiative built platforms for youth success, including college scholarships and youth leadership opportunities. WE ACT has served as a model for many other environmental organizations by forging partnerships among groups that had not previously worked together or thought to do so. These partners include academic institutions, housing groups, clean energy providers, community-based participatory researchers, nonprofits from other domains, and government agencies.

Relationship Building and Mutual Accountability

In creating a network of diverse partners, the communities in the examples created a shared commitment to their goals among partners.

One challenge that arises from collaborative work across sectors and disciplines is the competing interests of the partners. The partnerships within EPN, Blueprint, and MCI are forged with the understanding that if collaboration is effective, co-benefits can be realized. This also creates a mechanism for mutual accountability for resources and outcomes.

Governance Processes

All of the example communities had very specific governing practices and structures that were tailored to the needs and makeup of the community being engaged. Among the communities that had a leadership board, substantial and accurate representation of the community residents was vital. Generally, the communities in the examples employ structured, bottom-up approaches to decision making. IndyCAN employs the local organizing committee leaders to facilitate dialogues with community members, and elected delegates vote on important issues of strategy, budget, and more. EPN also uses committees, which are specialized. MCI uses a more informal and less prescriptive leadership model, which allows partners within the network to take initiative on issues based on interest and on the amount of resources available at the time.

Fostering Creativity

Creativity is another common feature of these initiatives. EPN realized multiple benefits in the domains of exercise, student safety, and community cohesiveness without great expenditure by mobilizing the Walking School Bus. When children at DHC showed clear signs of malnourishment, health professionals actually wrote prescriptions for food and organized a community garden for 1,000 member families, bringing in sustainable and improved nutrition for the community. The DSNI managed to obtain the power of eminent domain over abandoned properties in order to acquire land for resident-led development. This creative strategy opened up vast resources for community projects.

Planning for Sustainability

Leveraging Resources

Sustainability, whether financial or management sustainability, is a major consideration for any community-based solution. DSNI enhanced its sustainability by leveraging its success over 30 years to obtain a Promise Neighborhood grant. Mandela MarketPlace has addressed a different aspect of sustainability, looking to job creation, enhancement of the market for healthy food, and keeping wealth in the community. PUSH has also focused on creating jobs and job training, looking to maintain the initiative's benefits over time.

Training and Technical Expertise

Another factor that shapes a community initiative's sustainability, which many of the case examples capitalized on, is technical expertise and training. Educational institutions have emerged from the case examples as a valuable partner in this respect. WE ACT and IndyCAN partnered with education institutions for data collection and research, and DHC engaged students at local educational institutions to assist with the center's community projects. In the case of Mandela MarketPlace, when community organizers recognized a need for technical expertise, they commissioned external consultants to provide assistance developing a business model. Others of the example organizations trained within the community to develop the expertise needed. The Blueprint Approved Institute serves this purpose, providing a platform for grassroots organizations to learn about government processes and have the capacity to compete for funds. Training residents in community tools for action and mobilization was another common element of the case examples (EPN, IndyCAN, and WE ACT).

CONCLUSION

These nine examples are markedly diverse, yet as a group they provide common positive features that can inspire other communities to embark on or improve their own programs for change. They also share the capacity to raise the hope that communities, including those faced with daunting issues, can unite to produce real and lasting benefits in health outcomes and numerous related factors. None of these initiatives is a blueprint that can be simply copied and implemented anew in a different community with different residents, different history, and different challenges. Yet these widely varying communities illustrate that there are many different pathways to success.

The three key elements in the conceptual model for this report call attention to building in three domains: shared vision and values, community capacity, and multi-sector collaboration. In each of the nine initiatives described above, innovative and far-reaching efforts in these three domains created change for the better, recognizing and enhancing the potential for improved lives in these vibrant neighborhoods. These initiatives looked at their community challenges from widely varying perspectives. Some sought to link partners through spiritual bonds, while others focused on tackling poverty through job programs and education.

All were savvy in building effective and powerful partnerships. Key community partners—including community groups; local, state, and federal governments; philanthropies; educational institutions; and key local employers—played a vital role in collaborating to develop, implement, and sustain effective community solutions.

With the exception of a few, the communities featured in this chapter did not approach the design and implementation of their solutions with the frame of improving health. Instead, their ultimate goals were safe and affordable housing, economic development and dignity, safety, social cohesion, educational achievement among youth, neighborhood revitalization, or environmental justice—all of which are ingredients for a healthy community and foundational to health equity. The committee acknowledges that underserved communities that are struggling with poverty, violence, or divestment are not likely to have health as a priority on their agendas for improvement. However, the experiences and lessons learned from these nine communities reveal an opportunity for communities to address the social, economic, and environmental factors that contribute to a thriving community as well as improving health. Applying a health equity lens to community-driven solutions allows for the interdisciplinary, collaborative approaches with access to diversified funding sources that the nine communities were able to adopt. This also facilitates the realization of co-benefits (i.e., win-wins) for actors across sectors within the community, and especially for community residents, who can reap the benefits across multiple domains.

All were prudent in seeking diversified funding and carefully allocating resources. Furthermore, all nine communities built capacity among residents to identify key issues and to participate in devising strategies to meet their needs and build on their assets while recognizing the power of systems and other forces outside the community to enhance or undermine the effectiveness of their efforts. Long-lasting initiatives demonstrate wisdom in adapting their strategies and seeking new funding as times change, and in buffering themselves from the inevitable changes in political administrations over time. Box 5-1 outlines some guiding principles that emerged from the committee's review of the community examples and the existing literature on processes for community action to promote health equity.

> **BOX 5-1**
> **Some Guiding Principles for Community Consideration**
>
> As described above, community-based efforts to promote health equity require the following three key elements: (1) health equity as a shared vision and value, (2) community capacity to shape outcomes, and (3) multi-sector collaboration. Although no recipe for successful collaboration to promote health equity exists, some additional approaches emerging from the literature and community-based practices include
>
> - Leverage existing efforts whenever possible.
> - Adopt explicit strategies for authentic community engagement, ownership, involvement, and input throughout all stages of such efforts.
> - Nurture the next generation of leadership.
> - Foster flexibility, creativity, and resilience where possible.
> - Seriously consider potential community partners, including non-traditional ones.
> - Commit to results, systematic learning, cross-boundary collaboration, capacity-building, and sustainability.
> - Partner with public health agencies no matter the focus of the effort.
>
> SOURCES: Community Tool Box, 2016; FSG, 2011, 2013; Prybil et al., 2014; Verbitsky-Savitz et al., 2016.

Chapter 5 Annex

SELECTION PROCESS FOR COMMUNITY EXAMPLES

Identification

The committee identified potential examples through several avenues. Queries were sent to public health organizations such as the Association of State and Territorial Health Officials and the National Association and County and City Health Officials, philanthropies such as The California Endowment, and nonprofits, including Grantmakers in Health and the Prevention Institute. The committee also heard from many experts at its open meetings (see Appendix C for the meeting agendas) who presented many examples of community efforts to improve health and health equity in a range of sectors. Existing reviews of community efforts, reports on health disparities, healthy community websites, and other related publications were searched for relevant examples. Committee members also submitted examples from their respective fields. Finally, a literature review was undertaken.

Criteria

To guide the selection of the case examples for this report, the committee developed three sets of criteria (see Box 5-2 for a listing of all selection criteria). These criteria were informed by research and practice-based evidence as well as by the expertise of the committee. The first set consists of four core criteria, which must be met by all case examples. These core criteria assure that the examples chosen are substantively significant.

The first core criterion requires that the solution in the example addresses at least one (preferably more) of the nine social determinants of health identified by the committee: education, employment, health systems and services, housing, income and wealth, the physical environment, public safety, the social environment, and transportation. This criterion was informed by the wealth of literature suggesting the importance of targeting the social and economic conditions that affect health, especially at the community level (Bradley et al., 2016; Galea et al., 2011; Heiman and Artiga, 2015; Hood et al., 2016; Wenger, 2012). Furthermore, this criterion is basic to the committee's charge, which posits that the social determinants of health must be addressed to reduce health inequities.

The second core criterion states that each case example must be community driven. This requires that the solution is initiated by a community member, group, or local government or that prior engagement with the community is evident and subsequently incorporated into the solution.

BOX 5-2
Community Example Selection Criteria

Set 1: Core Criteria[a]

1. Solution addresses at least one, preferably more, of the nine social determinants of health identified by the Robert Wood Johnson Foundation (RWJF)/committee (health systems and services, education, employment, the physical environment, the social environment, housing, income and wealth, public safety, and transportation) and affects a local population that is affected by health inequities
2. Community-driven:
    a. engagement with the community is evident pre-intervention and incorporated in the solution, or
    b. the solution is initiated by the community/a community group/ or local government
3. Multi-sectoral
4. There is an assessment of evidence, including data or best available information, to
    a. Identify a problem
    b. Develop a solution that has a measurable outcome

Set 2: Aspirational Criteria[b]

5. Includes non-traditional partners and/or non-health domains
   Note: This is meant to be inclusive of non-traditional partners for communities to engage that may not necessarily be sectors (i.e., community organizers, PTA groups, etc.).
6. Interdisciplinary, multifactor
    a. The solution draws on multiple sources, including practice-based experience and research from multiple disciplines
7. Multilevel—the intervention has multiple levels of influence, such as individual, family, organizational/institutional, or governmental.
   Note: This does not mean that a solution must target each of these levels
8. The solution documents what it is trying to achieve, why that is important, and how it plans to achieve the desired outcome
9. Includes a plan for sustainability, including consideration of
    a. Long-term strategy and structure
    b. Funding, operating costs, resources, etc.
    c. Efficient use of resources
    d. Potential cost savings realized or return on investment
    e. Increased community capacity to shape outcomes
    f. Building the next generation of leaders
10. The solution has transferable key elements[c] that could practically be applied or adapted to similar contexts in order to scale impact
11. Evidence required of proposed intervention(s):
    a. Addresses a significant health disparity(or disparities), based on data of a documented need or problem and data showing impact on at least one proximal or distal measure of a health disparity

b. The actual or projected health benefits are substantial/meaningful to the vulnerable population(s) and community as a whole (not just statistically significant)
   c. Ongoing data collection of processes and outcomes (flexibility in terms of what type of data is generated and applied)
   Note: This includes health outcomes in a broad sense, related to social determinants (e.g., high school completion rates) that are strongly linked to health outcomes.
12. Implementation process is well documented, including
    a. The key elements and subtleties of how the solution is contributing to success (not referring to legal documents/individual health data)
    b. Particular practice (training, supervisory)
    c. Funding
    d. Regulatory context
    e. Political context
13. The solution is freely available to the community and not a proprietary resource

Set 3: Contextual Criteria[d]

14. Address a range of the nine determinants of health identified by RWJF/committee (health systems and services, education, employment, the physical environment, the social environment, housing, income and wealth, public safety, and transportation)
15. Varying community sizes
16. Rural and urban communities
17. Diversity in several of the following population characteristics:
    a. Race
    b. Ethnicity
    c. Age
    d. Gender identity
    e. Sexual orientation status
    f. Socioeconomic status
    g. Disability status
    h. Other statuses
18. Integration of civil rights concerns, including civil rights law into the solution
19. Solutions that require changes in the systems or policies within which the solution was implemented AND did not require changes in systems or policies to be effective
20. Various levels of political engagement

---

[a] To be included for consideration, the examples needed to meet each of the four core criteria.
[b] The examples need to meet at least one, and preferably more, of the aspirational criteria.
[c] Key elements are the functions or principles and activities of the solution that are necessary to achieve similar outcomes.
[d] These criteria were applied to the examples that met the four core criteria and a number of the aspirational criteria to ensure that the sample cases were diverse in terms of communities/populations, approaches to solutions, and other characteristics.

The community-driven element is significant because it highlights the distinction between solutions that are enacted on behalf of communities and *placed* in communities versus solutions in which the community is the driving force behind them (IOM, 2012). It is also important to note that the populations affected by health inequity are historically marginalized and underserved groups (Dicent Taillepierre et al., 2016). Community-driven solutions build the capacity and power for these marginalized groups to play a role in shaping their outcomes, which is especially noteworthy for groups that may be distrustful of governmental or medical institutions.

The third core criterion states that the solution must be multi-sectoral, meaning that it engages one or more sectors in addition to a traditional health sector (e.g., public health, health care, etc.). This criterion was drawn from the body of literature citing multi-sector collaboration as a powerful lever for addressing the social determinants of health and building a culture of health (APHA, 2015; Danaher, 2011; Davis et al., 2016; Kottke et al., 2016; Mattessich and Rausch, 2014). Multi-sector collaboration also has implications for the sustainability of the community-driven solutions, which traditionally have been under-resourced. Engaging stakeholders across multiple sectors provides the opportunity for innovative and cost-effective methods to sustain solutions at the community level.

The fourth core criterion requires the solution to be evidence-informed. This entails an assessment of evidence or the best available information to identify a problem and develop a solution that has a measurable outcome. Here, there is considerable flexibility in terms of the type of evidence that will qualify. This flexibility is based on the understanding that low-resource communities that suffer from health inequities often do not have the infrastructure, personnel, or financial resources to provide the highest standard of evidence.

The second set of criteria reflects the elements, processes, and outcomes of community-driven solutions that the committee identified as valuable for promoting health equity. These are not core criteria, in which case an example would be excluded if it did not meet one of them. Rather, they make up a set of aspirational criteria to inform the committee's selection of the cases. This set of criteria highlights important features of community-driven solutions, such as nontraditional partners or non-health domains (e.g., community organizers, public libraries, PTA groups, etc.) and interdisciplinary or multifactor in nature. This comes from the committee's understanding that engaging community stakeholders outside of the traditional health disciplines will facilitate cross-sector collaboration in addition to maximizing the impact on the social determinants of health. Such partnerships can increase reach and capacity by drawing on different backgrounds, skill sets, and knowledge bases (HHS, 2014).

For the examples to serve as a vehicle for sharing successful community-driven solutions with other communities affected by health inequities, the committee determined that there should be transferable key elements. All of the examples will be context dependent, and therefore they will not be replicable per se—that is, implemented in identical form. That being said, the key elements are the functions, principles, and activities of the solution that are necessary to achieve similar outcomes. They could practically be applied or adapted to similar contexts in order to scale impact (Schorr, 2016).

The criteria require that solutions illustrated in the examples will have documented their objectives, why those objectives are important, and how the solutions are expected to achieve the desired outcomes. Ideally they will have also thoroughly documented the implementation process so as to identify the key elements and subtleties of how the solutions contribute to success. This includes other significant contextual information such as the particular practice (training and supervisory), funding, regulatory context, and political context of the solutions. Furthermore, a plan for sustainability is outlined as a criterion for the community examples. To ensure sustained impact, the solutions should consider: long-term strategy and structure; funding, operating costs, and other resources; efficient use of resources; potential cost-savings or return on investment; and increased community capacity to shape outcomes.

The third set of criteria was developed to increase the likelihood that the examples will reflect a diversity of communities, populations, solutions, and other demographic characteristics representative of the United States, in addition to the characteristics of the solution itself. As a group the sample of examples should provide some variety in geographic regions and urban–rural classification. The committee also searched for examples that differ across the following population characteristics: race, ethnicity, age, gender identity, sexual orientation status, socioeconomic status, disability status, and other statuses applicable to health inequities. Finally, this set of criteria ensures the inclusion of solutions that integrate civil rights concerns; require changes in the systems, policies, or laws within which the solution was implemented; have various levels of political engagement (e.g., local, state, national); and result in a range of capacities developed within the community.

REFERENCES

Alameda County Public Health Department. 2008. Life and death from unnatural causes: Health and social inequity in Alameda County. *Alameda County Public Health Department Community Assessment, Planning, and Evaluation (CAPE) Unit.* http://www.acphd.org/data-reports/reports-by-topic/social-and-health-equity/life-and-death-from-unnatural-causes.aspx (accessed October 6, 2016).

Alameda County Public Health Department. 2014. *Alameda County health data profile, 2014: Community health status assessment for public health accreditation.* Alameda County Public Health Department Community Assessment, Planning, and Education (CAPE) Unit and Division of Communicable Disease Control and Prevention.

Alameda County Public Health Department. 2015 (unpublished). *West Oakland race and ethnicity 1940-2015 summary.*

APHA (American Public Health Association). 2015. *Opportunities for health collaboration: Leveraging community development investments to improve health in low-income neighborhoods.* Washington, DC: American Public Health Association.

B Lab. n.d. *What are B Corps?* https://www.bcorporation.net/what-are-b-corps (accessed October 27, 2016).

Bartley, A. 2016. *Green Development Zone.* https://www.changemakers.com/sustainableurbanhousing/entries/green-development-zone (accessed September 26, 2016).

Bellinger, D. C. 2008. Very low lead exposures and children's neurodevelopment. *Current Opinion in Pediatrics* 20(2):172–177.

Bhatt, K., and S. Dubb. 2015. *Educate and empower: Tools for building community wealth.* Democracy Collaborative.

BLS (U.S. Bureau of Labor Statistics). 2016. *Local area unemployment statistics.* http://www.bls.gov/web/metro/laulrgma.htm (accessed November 23, 2016).

Blueprint for Action. 2013. *Minneapolis Blueprint for Action to Prevent Youth Violence.* Minneapolis, MN: City of Minneapolis Health Department.

Boston Promise Initiative. 2016. *No Child Goes Homeless.* http://www.promiseboston.org/no-child-goes-homeless.html (accessed September 26, 2016).

Bowie, P. 2011. *Getting to scale: The elusive goal.* Seattle, WA: Casey Family Programs.

Boyer, M. A. 2013. Green housing: In Buffalo, it's not just for rich people anymore. *Yes! Magazine,* February 15.

Bradley, E. H., M. Canavan, E. Rogan, K. Talbert-Slagle, C. Ndumele, L. Taylor, and L. A. Curry. 2016. Variation in health outcomes: The role of spending on social services, public health, and health care, 2000-09. *Health Affairs* 35(5):760–768.

Chakrabarti, T. 2016a. *Growing resources for healthy economies in Alameda County, California.* http://nccd.cdc.gov/dchsuccessstories (accessed September 20, 2016).

Chakrabarti, T. 2016b. *A high profile for healthy economies.* http://nccd.cdc.gov/dchsuccessstories (accessed September 20, 2016).

Cho, S., K. Li, and T. Salzman. 2016. *Building a livable Boston: The case for community land trusts.* Medford, MA: Tufts University.

City-Data.com. 2016a. *Harlem neighborhood in New York, New York (NY), 10030, 10039, 10027, 10026, 10029, 10035, 10037 detailed profile.* http://www.city-data.com/neighborhood/Harlem-New-York-NY.html (accessed October 17, 2016).

City-Data.com. 2016b. *West Oakland neighborhood in Oakland, California (CA), 94607, 94608 detailed profile.* http://www.city-data.com/neighborhood/West-Oakland-Oakland-CA.html (accessed September 26, 2016).

City of Minneapolis. 2016. *Results Minneapolis (forthcoming).* Minneapolis, MN.

Community Tool Box. 2016. *Chapter 1. Section 7. Working together for healthier communities: A framework for collaboration among community partnership, support organizations, and funders.* http://ctb.ku.edu/en/table-of-contents/overview/model-for-community-change-and-improvement/framework-for-collaboration/main (accessed October 18, 2016).

Corburn, J., J. Osleeb, and M. Porter. 2006. Urban asthma and the neighbourhood environment in New York City. *Health & Place* 12(2):167–179.

County Health Rankings. 2016a. *Bolivar County snapshot.* http://www.countyhealthrankings.org/app/mississippi/2016/rankings/bolivar/county/outcomes/1/snapshot (accessed October 12, 2016).

County Health Rankings. 2016b. *Marion County snapshot.* http://www.countyhealthrankings.org/app/indiana/2016/rankings/marion/county/outcomes/overall/snapshot (accessed September 14, 2016).

Danaher, A. 2011. Reducing health inequities: Enablers and barriers to inter-sectoral collaboration. *Wellesley Institute* 3.

Davis, R., S. Savannah, M. Harding, A. Macaysa, and L. F. Parks. 2016. *Countering the production of inequities: An emerging systems framework to achieve an equitable culture of health.* Oakland, CA: Prevention Institute.

DHC (Delta Health Center). 2015. *2015 Mississippi Delta alternative spring break, Mississippi State University.* http://www.deltahealthcenter.org/2015-mississippi-delta-alternative-break-mississippi-state-university (accessed September 19, 2016).

Dicent Taillepierre, J. C., L. Liburd, A. O'Connor, J. Valentine, K. Bouye, D. H. McCree, T. Chapel, and R. Hahn. 2016. Toward achieving health equity: Emerging evidence and program practice. *Journal of Public Health Management and Practice* 22 (Suppl 1):S43–S49.

Drennon, C. 2011. *San Antonio's Eastside Proimise Zone: A neighborhood profile.* Trinity University Urban Studies Program.

DSNI (Dudley Street Neighborhood Initiative). 2016a. *About the neighborhood.* http://www.dsni.org/about-the-neighborhood (accessed September 26, 2016).

DSNI. 2016b. *Board of directors.* http://www.dsni.org/new-page (accessed September 26, 2016).

DSNI. 2016c. *History.* http://www.dsni.org/dsni-historic-timeline (accessed September 26, 2016).

DSNI. 2016d. *Home.* http://www.dsni.org (accessed September 26, 2016).

DSNI. 2016e. *Sustainable economic development.* http://www.dsni.org/sustainable-economic-development (accessed September 22, 2016).

Dudley Neighbors, Inc. 2016. *Dudley Neighbors Incorporated: The community land trust.* http://www.dudleyneighbors.org (accessed September 26, 2016).

Dwyer, L. A. 2015. Mapping impact: An analysis of the dudley street neighborhood initiative land trust. Cambridge, MA: MIT Department of Urban Studies & Planning.

ED (U.S. Department of Education). 2016. *Promise neighborhoods.* http://www2.ed.gov/programs/promiseneighborhoods/index.html (accessed September 26, 2016).

Environmental Grantmakers Association. 2015. *Tracking the field: Volume 5: Analyzing trends in environmental grantmaking.*

EPN (Eastside Promise Neighborhood). 2013. *Cradle-to-career pathway.* http://eastsidepromise.org/wp-content/uploads/2013/03/Cradle-to-Career-Pathway-e1363974021347.png (accessed September 19, 2016).

EPN. 2016a. The 10 promises. http://eastsidepromise.org/the-results (accessed September 22, 2016).

EPN. 2016b. *EPN schools.* http://eastsidepromise.org/epn-schools (accessed September 22, 2016).

EPN. 2016c. *Mission statement.* http://eastsidepromise.org/mission-statement (accessed September 26, 2016).

EPN. n.d. *Success in education from cradle to career.* http://eastsidepromise.org/k-12-pipeline (accessed September 19, 2016).

Faber, D. R. 2001. *Green of another color: Building effective partnerships between foundations and the environmental justice movement.* Northeastern University Philanthropy and Environmental Justice Research Project.

Fairmont Cultural Corridor. 2016. *Fairmont Cultural Corridor: Creating vibrant communities with arts and artists at the center.* http://www.fairmountculturalcorridor.org/history (accessed September 26, 2016).

FRAC (Food Research and Action Center). 2005. Food stamp access in urban America: A city-by-city snapshot. *Food Research and Action Center*. http://frac.org/wp-content/uploads/2009/09/cities2005.pdf (accessed October 6, 2016).

FSG (Foundation Strategy Group). 2011. *Collective impact*. http://www.fsg.org/ideas-in-action/collective-impact (accessed October 18, 2016).

FSG. 2013. *Using collective impact in a public health context: Introduction*. http://www.fsg.org/blog/using-collective-impact-public-health-context-introduction (accessed October 18, 2016).

Galea, S., M. Tracy, K. J. Hoggat, C. DiMaggio, and A. Karpati. 2011. Estimated deaths attributable to social factors in the United States. *American Journal of Public Health* 101(8):1456–1465.

Garfield, R., and A. Damico. 2016. *The coverage gap: Uninsured poor adults in states that do not expand Medicaid—an update*. Menlo Park, CA: The Henry J. Kaiser Family Foundation

Geiger, H. J. 2002. Community-oriented primary care: A path to community development. *American Journal of Public Health* 92(11):1713–1716.

Geiger, H. J. 2016. The first community health center in Mississippi: Communities empowering themselves. *American Journal of Public Health* 106(10):1738–1740.

GPO (U.S. Government Publishing Office). 2010. *42 U.S.C. §2000d to 2000d-7*. https://www.gpo.gov/fdsys/pkg/USCODE-2010-title42/pdf/USCODE-2010-title42-chap21-subchapV.pdf (accessed September 22, 2016).

The Greenling Institute. 2006. Legislative hearing before the California State Legislative Black Caucus, California Latino Legislative Caucus, and Asian Pacific Islander Legislative Caucus Paper on Foundation Giving to Minority-Led Nonprofits, April 24, 2016, Sacramento, CA.

Healthy Food Access Portal. 2016. *Profile: Mandela MarketPlace*. http://healthyfoodaccess.org/sites/default/files/HFA%20Portal%20Profile_Mandela%20Marketplace_FINAL2.pdf (accessed September 16, 2016).

Heiman, H. J., and S. Artiga. 2015. *Beyond health care: The role of social determinants in promoting health and health equity*. Menlo Park, CA: The Henry J. Kaiser Family Foundation.

Henry, S. 2011. *James Berk of Mandela Foods brings produce to the people (video)*. http://civileats.com/2011/05/06/james-berk-of-mandela-foods-brings-produce-to-his-people-video (accessed October 27, 2016).

HHS (U.S. Department of Health and Human Services). 2014. *Building sustainable programs: The framework*. Rockville, MD: U.S. Department of Health and Human Services.

Hood, C. M., K. P. Gennuso, G. R. Swain, and B. B. Catlin. 2016. County health rankings: Relationships between determinant factors and health outcomes. *American Journal of Preventive Medicine* 50(2):129–135.

HRSA (Health Resources and Service Administration). 2015. *2015 health center profile*. http://bphc.hrsa.gov/uds/datacenter.aspx?q=d&bid=040780&state=MS (accessed September 20, 2016).

IndyCAN (Indianapolis Congregation Action Network). 2014. *Indianapolis Congregation Action Network annual strategic report 2012–2014*. Indianapolis, IN: IndyCAN.

IndyCAN. 2016a. *Indycan "ticket to opportunity" campaign strategy*. Indianapolis, IN: IndyCAN.

IndyCAN. 2016b. *The people's agenda for ending mass incarceration and mass criminalization in Marion County*. Indianapolis, IN: IndyCAN.

Inkelas, M., and P. Bowie. 2014. The Magnolia Community Initiative: The importance of measurement in improving community well-being. *Community Investments* 26(1):18–24.

IOM (Institute of Medicine). 1983. *Community oriented primary care: New directions for health services delivery*. Washington, DC: National Academy Press.

IOM. 2012. *An integrated framework for assessing the value of community-based prevention*. Washington, DC: The National Academies Press.

Kottke, T. E., M. Stiefel, and N. P. Pronk. 2016. "Well-being in all policies": Promoting cross-sectoral collaboration to improve people's lives. http://nam.edu/wp-content/uploads/2016/04/Well-Being-in-All-Policies-Promoting-Cross-Sectoral-Collaboration-to-Improve-Peoples-Lives.pdf (accessed February 22, 2016).

Kretzmann, J. P., and J. L. McKnight. 1993. *Building communities from the inside out: A path toward finding and mobilizing a community's assets.* Evanston, IL: Institute for Policy Research.

LII (Legal Information Institute). n.d. *Implied warranty of habitability.* https://www.law.cornell.edu/wex/implied_warranty_of_habitability (accessed October 27, 2016).

Loh, P., and B. Shear. 2015. Solidarity economy and community development: Emerging cases in three Massachusetts cities. *Community Development* 46(3):244–260.

Longlett, S. K., J. E. Kruse, and R. M. Wesley. 2001. Community-oriented primary care: Historical perspective. *Journal of the American Board of Family Medicine* 14(1):54–63.

Mandela MarketPlace. 2013. *About us.* http://www.mandelamarketplace.org/about_us (accessed September 26, 2016).

Mandela MarketPlace. 2016. *Mandela MarketPlace: Building a community-based food system.* https://equityis.exposure.co/mandela-marketplace (accessed October 27, 2016).

Massachusetts Avenue Project. 2016. *About.* http://mass-ave.org/about (accessed September 26, 2016).

Mattessich, P. W., and E. J. Rausch. 2014. Cross-sector collaboration to improve community health: A view of the current landscape. *Health Affairs* 33(11):1968–1974.

Minkler, M. 2010. Linking science and policy through community-based participatory research to study and address health disparities. *American Journal of Public Health* 100(Suppl 1):S81–S87.

Minneapolis CPED (Community Planning and Economic Development). 2011. *The Minneapolis promise: A campaign for the most prepared workforce in the nation.* Minneapolis Department of Community Planning and Economic Development.

Minnesota Compass. 2016. *Profiles: Minneapolis-Saint Paul neighborhoods.* http://www.mncompass.org/profiles/neighborhoods/minneapolis-saint-paul#!community-areas (accessed September 19, 2016).

National Community Land Trust Network. 2016. *FAQ.* http://cltnetwork.org/faq (accessed September 22, 2016).

Needleman, H. L., A. Schell, D. Bellinger, A. Leviton, and E. N. Allred. 1990. The long-term effects of exposure to low doses of lead in childhood: An 11-year follow-up report. *New England Journal of Medicine* 322(2):83–88.

Nicholas, S. W., B. Jean-Louis, B. Ortiz, M. Northridge, K. Shoemaker, R. Vaughan, M. Rome, G. Canada, and V. Hutchinson. 2005. Addressing the childhood asthma crisis in Harlem: The Harlem Children's Zone asthma initiative. *American Journal of Public Health* 95(2):245–249.

Paschall, K. 2016. How integrated voter engagement builds power and changes policy. *Responsive Philanthropy*(1):3–6.

The Planning History of Oakland. n.d. http://oaklandplanninghistory.weebly.com. n.d. *The changing face of Oakland: 1945-1990.* http://oaklandplanninghistory.weebly.com/the-changing-face-of-oakland.html (accessed October 26, 2016).

PolicyLink. 2014. *Eastside Promise Neighborhood.* http://www.promiseneighborhoodsinstitute.org/sites/default/files/documents/pni/PNI_san%20antonio_091914_a_0.pdf (accessed September 16, 2016).

Prevention Institute. 2011. *Fact sheet: Links between violence and health equity.* Oakland, CA: Prevention Institute.

Prybil, L., F. D. Scutchfield, R. Killian, A. Kelly, G. Mays, A. Carman, S. Levey, A. McGeorge, and D. W. Fardo. 2014. Improving community health through hospital-public health collaboration: Insights and lessons learned from successful partnerships. In *Health management and policy faculty book gallery: Book 2*. Lexington, KY: Commonwealth Center for Governance Studies, Inc.

PUSH (People United for Sustainable Housing). 2009. *PUSH wins commitments from the fed!* http://pushbuffalo.org/push-wins-commitments-from-the-fed (accessed September 26, 2016).

PUSH. 2012a. *About us*. http://pushbuffalo.org/about-us (accessed September 26, 2016).

PUSH. 2012b. *Building green & affordable housing*. http://greendevelopmentzone.org/housing (accessed September 26, 2016).

PUSH. 2012c. *National campaigns*. http://greendevelopmentzone.org/campaigns/national-campaigns (accessed September 26, 2016).

PUSH. 2012d. *NetZero house*. http://pushbuffalo.org/netzero-house (accessed September 26, 2016).

PUSH. 2012e. *Sustainable neighborhoods*. http://greendevelopmentzone.org/campaigns/sustainable-neighborhoods (accessed September 26, 2016).

PUSH. 2015. *2015 annual report*. People United for Sustainable Housing.

Rybak, R. T. 2012. *City voices and perspectives: R.T. Rybak, mayor of Minneapolis*. Urban Networks to Increase Thriving Youth through Violence Prevention, Prevention Institute.

Sandel, M., E. Faugno, A. Mingo, J. Cannon, K. Byrd, D. A. Garcia, S. Collier, E. McClure, and R. B. Jarrett. 2016. Neighborhood-level interventions to improve childhood opportunity and lift children out of poverty. *Academic Pediatrics* 16(3 Suppl):S128–S135.

Schilder, D. 1997. *Overview of results-based accountability: Components of RBA*. http://www.hfrp.org/publications-resources/browse-our-publications/overview-of-results-based-accountability-components-of-rba (accessed October 27, 2016).

Schorr, L. 1988. *Within our reach: Breaking the cycle of disadvantage*. New York: Anchor Books.

Schorr, L. B. 1997. *Common purpose: Strengthening families and neighborhoods to rebuild America*. New York: Anchor Books.

Schorr, L. B. 2016. Evidence, replication and scaling up. Presented at ASPE HHS Roundtable on building evidence for domestic violence services and interventions, April 26, 2016, Washington, DC.

Soliman, J. n.d. *The rise and fall of seventh street in Oakland*. http://www.foundsf.org/index.php?title=The_Rise_and_Fall_of_Seventh_Street_in_Oakland (accessed October 26, 2016).

Speer, P. W., A. Peterson, A. Zippay, and B. Christens. 2010. Participation in congregation-based organizing: A mixed-method study of civic engagement. In *Using evidence to inform practice for community and organizational change*. Chicago, IL: Lyceum Books. Pp. 200–217.

statisticalatlas.com. 2016. *Overview of Harlem, New York, New York (neighborhood)*. http://statisticalatlas.com/neighborhood/New-York/New-York/Harlem/Overview (accessed October 27, 2016).

Unger, S., and H. Wooten. 2006. A food systems assessment for Oakland, CA: Toward a sustainable food plan. *Oakland Mayor's Office of Sustainability and University of California, Berkelely, Department of City and Regional Planning*. http://www.eukn.eu/e-library/project/bericht/eventDetail/a-food-systems-assessment-for-oakland-california-toward-a-sustainable-food-plan-2006 (accessed October 22, 2016).

U.S. Census Bureau. 2015a. *Education attainment: 2011-2015 American Community Survey 5-year estimates*. http://factfinder.census.gov/faces/tableservices/jsf/pages/productview.xhtml?src=CF (accessed October 17, 2016).

U.S. Census Bureau. 2015b. *Quickfacts: Minneapolis City, Minnesota*. http://www.census.gov/quickfacts/table/PST045215/2743000 (accessed November 23, 2016).

Verbitsky-Savitz, N., M. B. Hargreaves, S. Penoyer, N. Morales, B. Coffee-Borden, and E. Whitesell. 2016. *Preventing and mitigating the effects of ACEs by building community capacity and resilience: APPI cross-site evaluation findings.* Washington, DC: Mathematica Policy Research.

Wakin, D. J. 2001. Breathless. *The New York Times*, May 13. http://www.nytimes.com/2001/05/13/nyregion/breathless.html?_r=0 (accessed October 17, 2016).

WE ACT. 2016a. *Mission: Achieving environmental justice by building healthy communities since 1988.* http://www.weact.org/mission (accessed September 22, 2016).

WE ACT. 2016b. *NYSTEA.* http://www.weact.org/transportationequityalliance (accessed September 22, 2016).

WE ACT. 2016c. *History.* http://www.weact.org/history (accessed September 22, 2016).

WE ACT. 2016d. *Timeline.* http://www.weact.org/timeline (accessed September 22, 2016).

WE ACT. n.d. *Theory of change.* http://www.weact.org/theoryofchange (accessed September 22, 2016).

Wenger, M. 2012. *Place matters: Ensuring opportunities for good health for all.* Washington, DC: Joint Center for Political and Economic Studies.

Zanjani, B. 2011. *City voices and perspectives: Blueprint for Action—preventing violence in Minneapolis.* Urban Networks to Increase Thriving Youth through Violence Prevention, Prevention Institute.

6

Policies to Support Community Solutions

Communities operate in the context of federal and state policies that can affect local government decisions relevant to health through laws and regulations, through the allocation of resources, and by shaping political will on issues and approaches. Among the more widely recognized policies are those that fund or regulate health care delivery services. But policies in a variety of areas, ranging from education to land use and housing, the environment, and criminal justice, can be relevant to health disparities. Policies can vary significantly across geographic areas and over time in establishing priorities, providing funding, or encouraging collaboration. They can provide important opportunities or constitute barriers to promoting health equity. The policy context shapes the levers that are available to communities to address change.

It seems reasonable to assume that the better informed communities are about the implications of federal and state policy and policy changes, the greater their ability will be to respond effectively to address health disparities and help achieve change in the determinants of health. And, conversely, the more the needs of communities are considered in decision making at the federal and state levels, the more effective those policies will be. In other words, policy makers have the opportunity to lay the groundwork for community success. This policy context (i.e., socioeconomic and political drivers) is highlighted in the report's conceptual model in Figure 6-1.

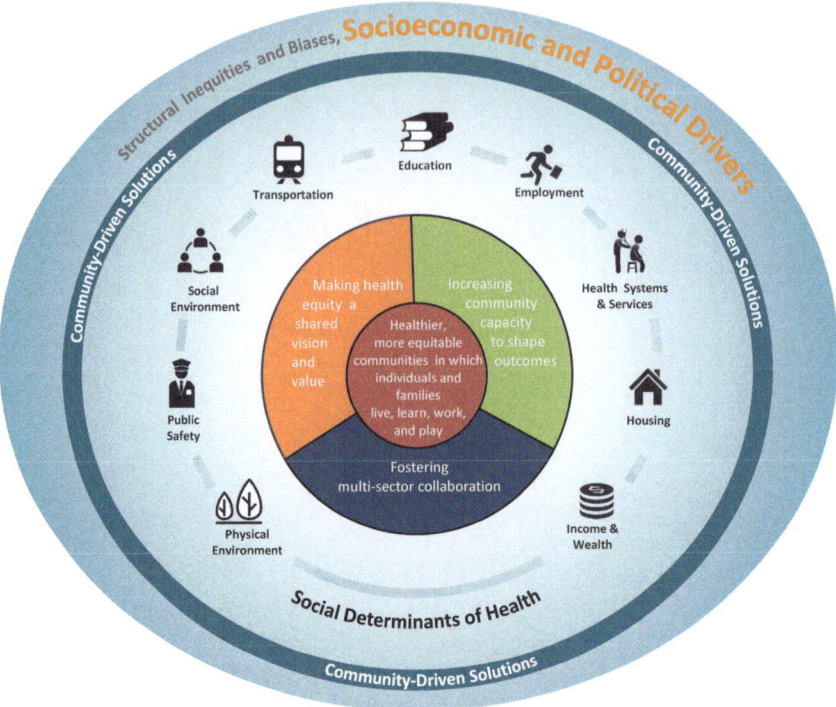

FIGURE 6-1 Report conceptual model for community solutions to promote health equity.
NOTE: The policy context is highlighted here to convey the focus of this chapter.

Frequently, community health initiatives, including collaborative activities, sometimes limit their vision and advocacy to policy changes related to health care and perhaps social services (Whittington et al., 2015). Communities—and the federal and state agencies that support them in their efforts to address health disparities—have multiple examples to follow in expanding their focus beyond health care and social services and examining opportunities in economic development, land use and housing, education, and criminal justice, areas which have not traditionally been the focus of health improvement efforts. Nevertheless, potential partners in those sectors are already working to improve outcomes, save money, and achieve other objectives that influence health. Examples include community development, justice reinvestment, and clean energy financing (Andrews et al., 2012; CSG, 2016; International Energy Agency, 2015). There are also policy changes that could be made at the federal and state level across non-health domains that would remove barriers or create opportunities for communities to promote health equity. The committee asserts that to attain health equity in the long term, policies that create structural barriers need to be addressed—addressing the root cause of the problem, not only treating the inequities that result. In this chapter, specific policies in six areas are discussed for their high relevance to community-based solutions that advance health equity: taxation and income inequality, housing and urban planning, education, civil rights, health, and criminal justice policy.

TAXATION AND INCOME INEQUALITY

As discussed in Chapter 3, income has been identified as one of many drivers of population health and health inequity over the life course, along with factors that are closely related to income such as education, occupation, and place of residence (Adler and Rehkopf, 2008; Chow et al., 2006; Cutler and Lleras-Muney, 2006).

The distribution of income is shaped by general economic conditions and by federal and state policies: most notably, taxes and government transfer programs such as Social Security, Supplemental Security Income (SSI), unemployment insurance, veterans' benefits, food stamps, the Supplemental Nutrition Assistance Program (SNAP), and the free and reduced-price school meal program. Thus, an individual's or a household's income results from a combination of reinforcing factors, including market conditions, government transfers, and taxes. A longitudinal analysis by the Congressional Budget Office (CBO) (2016) reviews changes in income inequality over time and notes that there has been increasing inequality along several measures: market income, "before-tax" income, and "after-tax" income. Market income (e.g., wages, salaries, business income, investment income, retirement pensions, and other money income), which excludes government transfers, rose over a 35-year period from 1979 to 2013 but grew 188 percent for households in the top 1 percent and only 18 percent for the bottom four income quintiles.

The CBO also examined before-tax income, which adds government transfers to market income. Government transfers reduce income inequality. Because government transfers largely benefit those at lower income levels, taking into account government transfers attenuates the income gap somewhat. So-called before-tax incomes rose between 32 and 39 percent in the lowest four quintiles, compared to 18 percent when government transfers are excluded. Because the highest quintile does not receive a significant amount of government transfers, its before-tax income grew at a similar rate as market income.

Finally, the CBO measured after-tax income, which takes into account both government transfers and taxes. Most federal revenues come from individual income taxes ($1.6 trillion) and payroll taxes ($1.1 trillion), with corporate income taxes ($300 billion) and other taxes playing smaller roles ($309 billion) (CBO, 2016). Over 35 years, households in the top 1 percent of the income distribution experienced an average 3 percent annual growth in inflation-adjusted, after-tax income compared with 1 percent for households in the bottom quintile. Thus, over 35 years, incomes at the top increased by 192 percent compared with an increase of 46 percent at the bottom. Half of tax offsets, including exclusions, deductions, preferential rates, and credits, go to those in the highest fifth of incomes (CBO, 2016). In 2013 average federal tax rates were below the 35-year average for most households, despite recent changes in tax law. Thus, across all three measures examined by the CBO, income inequality has grown substantially. These analyses also demonstrate the important role of government transfers and tax policy, as well as general economic conditions, in shaping income inequality.

The steady upward trend of income inequality in the United States has been documented and examined in a range of scholarship, including political science. Jacobs and Soss (2010) offer a typology of frameworks for analyzing how "economic inequalities result from and influence politics in the United States," one of which explores power relations, including how the state can create possibilities for agency (p. 345). A recent study underscores the stark relationship between income inequality and health and how this manifests locally. In the largest study of its kind, Chetty et al. (2016) examined more than 1 billion income tax and Social security records to report the association between income level and life expectancy from 1999 through 2014. Consistent with previous findings, they found that higher income is related to higher life expectancy and that lower income is related to lower life expectancy (NASEM, 2015; NRC and IOM, 2013; Waldron, 2007). The relationship found by Chetty et al. (2016) is dramatic: the gap in life expectancy for the richest and poorest 1 percent of the population was 14.6 years for men and 10.1 years for women. The relationship holds through the highest income percentiles, although the magnitude of the effect diminishes higher on the income distribution. Other studies have found that the income gradient also exists across racial and ethnic groups and that the relationship between income and health is stronger than between race and health (Woolf et al., 2015).

Chetty et al. (2016) examined the income-longevity relationship across time and across local areas. In certain local areas, the effect of being at the bottom of the income gradient is more pronounced than in others, with four- to fivefold differences. Trends in life expectancy also varied geographically, with some areas experiencing improvements and others declines.

There are a number of mechanisms through which income differences might drive local health patterns. Health behaviors, such as obesity and smoking, have been identified (Chetty et al., 2016; Mathur et al., 2013), as has pollution (Mohai et al., 2009) and access to healthy foods (Kyureghian et al., 2013). Low-income families that are food-insecure have also been found to choose high-calorie, nutrient-poor foods, contributing to worse health outcomes (Burke et al., 2016).

Federal means-tested programs are based on income and, whether through cash or in-kind benefits, can have a significant impact on health outcomes and thereby redress health inequity. The largest of these programs is Medicaid, which is discussed later in the chapter. The second largest program by expenditures is the earned income tax credit (EITC), which provides a tax credit to low-income families and individuals, followed by SSI, which provides benefits to low-income individuals with disabilities. Other programs include subsidized housing of various forms; SNAP, which supports food expenditures for low-income families and individuals; and Temporary Assistance for Needy Families, a cash benefit program that has contracted in size and is currently less than one-quarter the size of the EITC in aggregate (GAO, 2015). Finally, there are school food programs, Early Education, and the Special Supplemental Nutrition Program for Women, Infants, and Children, the latter of which provides vouchers for nutritional foods, counseling, health screening, and referrals for low-income infants, young children, and pregnant and postpartum women.

The programs vary significantly in the size of their benefits and in the number of people they reach. Over time, their growth rates have changed with economic conditions and changes in program rules. The recent Great Recession led to increases in most of these programs' spending between 2007 and 2011 and underscores the important role that these programs play in mitigating poverty (Bitler and Hoynes, 2013; Bitler et al., 2016). Program rules further shape the distribution of benefits among the low-income population: a study by Ben-Shalom et al. found that from 1984 to 2004, benefits to single mother households and non-employed[1] families declined by 19 and 21 percent, respectively, while benefits going to employed families, the elderly, and the disabled grew by 61 percent, 12 percent, and 15 percent, respectively (Ben-Shalom et al., 2011).

In many states a federal program is augmented through benefits or eligibility expansions. States have expanded the EITC, SSI, and SNAP beyond federal provisions (Bartilow, 2016), creating less inequity within the state but greater inequity across states. Thus, local community conditions can vary significantly over time and across regions.

The evidence base concerning the health effects of these means-tested programs varies. SNAP plays a crucial role in reducing poverty and

---

[1] Defined as families without a member over age 15 who worked in all 4 months prior to the interview.

food insecurity, particularly for children, and has also helped to reduce rates of obesity among its beneficiaries (Executive Office of the President, 2015). The U.S. Department of Agriculture (USDA), in collaboration with other organizations, released an obesity prevention tool kit, SNAP-Ed,[2] for states to promote this goal. Programs and policies such as SNAP have the potential to reduce childhood and adulthood obesity and provide substantial economic returns on investment, and their effects could potentially be amplified by local sugar-sweetened beverage or "soda tax" policies. Soda taxes have shown promise in Philadelphia (CHOICES, 2016) and could significantly benefit other areas, including the Bay Area and Boulder (Goldberg, 2016), as shown by research conducted by the Childhood Obesity Intervention Cost Effectiveness Study[3] initiative at the Harvard T.H. Chan School of Public Health.

In 2016 the federal EITC benefit, the largest means-tested federal program after Medicaid, provided cash transfers to 26 million people who work, primarily those with children (IRS, 2016). Studies have found that EITC benefits lead to improvements in a variety of health and mental health conditions for adults and children, as well as to reductions in smoking and other behaviors detrimental to health, improved parenting, and better school outcomes (Dahl and Lochner, 2005; Evans and Garthwaite, 2014; Hamad and Rehkopf, 2015, 2016; Strully et al., 2010). Twelve states play an important role in improving income and health equity by augmenting the EITC through state tax law. New York, for example, extends benefits to noncustodial parents, which has been found to increase employment and child support payments (Nichols and Rothstein, 2016). Because the EITC targets low- and middle-income workers, its expansion reduces income inequality and improves health equity.

In addition to the tax code and government transfers, federal and state laws shape incomes through minimum wage provisions. The federal government increased the minimum wage to $7.25 in 2009. In 21 states, the minimum wage is set higher than the federal level (Tax Policy Center, 2014). Given that minimum wages vary significantly due to state and local policies, such policies are another driver of health inequity at the community level. Declines in real minimum wages have been found to contribute to income inequality, particularly for women, between 1979 and 2012 (Autor et al., 2016). Studies of minimum wage and health have found that declining real minimum wage rates have contributed to increasing obesity rates in the United States (Meltzer and Chen, 2011) and that minimum wage policies are associated with lower maternal smoking and

---

[2] Tool kit is available at https://snaped.fns.usda.gov/snap/SNAPEdStrategiesAndInterventionsToolkitForStates.pdf (accessed December 19, 2016).

[3] For more information, see http://choicesproject.org (accessed December 19, 2016).

better birth outcomes (Wehby et al., 2016). A potential downside of minimum wage policies is their potential to decrease employment; research indicates that minimum wages can cause at least some unemployment, particularly for very low-skilled workers, including teenagers (Neumark et al., 2014).

HOUSING AND URBAN PLANNING POLICIES

Housing affordability has become a significant policy concern. From 2000 to 2012 the average rent burden for all renters grew from 26 percent of income to 29 percent of income, but for low-income families the burden has grown considerably more: renters in the bottom fifth of the income distribution spent about 63 percent of their income on rent in 2012, compared with 55 percent in 2000 (Collinson et al., 2015). In 2012, 49 percent of all renters and 89 percent of low-income renters spent more than 30 percent of their income on rent, an approximate 25 percentage point increase since 1960. This increase arose partly from improvements in housing and partly from stagnant incomes.

The federal government supports housing affordability through in-kind, means-tested programs and through the tax code. Roughly $42 billion is put toward numerous forms of means-tested housing assistance, such as vouchers to low-income families, subsidized rent in public housing projects, privately owned subsidized housing, and support for the construction of low-income housing. Two-thirds of federal subsidy recipients are either low-income elderly or people with disabilities. Significantly more support, roughly $228 billion, is given through tax deductions, such as mortgage interest deductions (OMB, 2016), the vast majority of which go to nonpoor households.

Among the earliest forms of housing assistance, public housing has faced numerous challenges. Historically, public housing developments were placed in disproportionately poor areas, distinct from their surrounding neighborhoods, which led to greater concentrations of poverty and racial segregation (Schill and Wachter, 1995). Today, funding for public housing is on the decline, and there are fewer than 1.1 million public housing units, down from 1.4 million units in the early 1990s, after an active effort to scale back public housing. The U.S. Department of Housing and Urban Development (HUD) HOPE VI program promoted demolition of public housing and sought to replace distressed public housing developments with lower-density, mixed-income developments (Schwartz, 2014); however, just over half of the demolished units have been replaced. Public housing units continue to be located in poorer neighborhoods than in other HUD programs (HUD, 2016b).

A number of other HUD-subsidized programs have supported privately owned, low-income housing by lowering construction costs or by providing rental subsidies to tenants. The Housing Choice Voucher (formerly Section 8) program awards vouchers to low-income families so that they can rent apartments on the private market. The program supports 2.4 million units for low-income households (HUD, 2016b). The remainder of the 5.3 million HUD-subsidized units is supported by project-based funding and other smaller programs. A significant policy issue is the low participation in housing assistance programs; only one in four eligible households currently receives a housing subsidy, and many areas report long waiting lists that combined are estimated to exceed 6.5 million households (Collinson et al., 2015). Finally, the Low Income Housing Tax Credit (LIHTC), begun in 1986, is now the largest federal housing program for the poor and has contributed to 2.78 million housing units becoming available from 1987 to 2014 (HUD, 2016a). The LIHTC program is administered by state entities that determine funding priorities within a federal framework.

A number of housing policies contribute to the economic status and welfare of low-income families. These include the overall size of federal housing assistance, which currently supports only one-quarter of eligible poor families; housing allocation processes; eligibility rules; and requirements on the quality of housing itself. At the same time, research findings on the impacts of housing policy on health equity are mixed. A recent review (Collinson et al., 2015) finds some evidence that families and children enjoy better health and overall well-being when living in more advantaged neighborhoods; however, housing subsidies do not necessarily move families to better neighborhoods. In particular, the public housing program appears to concentrate families in more economically and racially isolated neighborhoods than they would otherwise live in. In contrast, families receiving tenant-based subsidies like housing vouchers do not typically use them to move to neighborhoods that are substantially different from where they were previously living, although some research indicates that families receiving vouchers who have school-age children will move if housing is available near higher-performing schools (Ellen et al., 2016; Sanbonmatsu et al., 2011). Other research finds that although public housing is associated with reduced grade retention (i.e., repeating a grade) for African American students (but not for other students) (Currie and Yelowitz, 2000), housing vouchers were not found to improve educational attainment, crime, or health care use measured through Medicaid claims (Jacob et al., 2015). The HUD Moving to Opportunity experiment related to public housing found that children, mostly girls, benefited from moving out of public housing projects into a housing voucher program (Kessler et al., 2014; Sanbonmatsu et al., 2011). Relatively little research exists examining the effect of the LIHTC on recipients' living situations or health status.

Urban Planning Policies

Housing affordability and federal HUD policies are part of a larger dialogue concerning housing that also includes land use, residential and commercial development, natural resource use, transportation, and, even more broadly, changing neighborhoods and concerns over potential residential disruption. Urban planning policies shape the physical environment along with many other social determinants of health. Within federal and state initiatives, community actions can support local policy and implementation so that they benefit vulnerable populations.

Urban planning, while traditionally relying on geographic analytic tools, has the potential to influence health in a variety of ways, including access to health care services; disease outbreaks; physical activity among local residents; injuries related to motor vehicle, bicycle, and pedestrian traffic; air quality; crime; and employment (Kochtitzky et al., 2006). Increasingly, those involved in public health are being encouraged to include an urban planning lens, while those in urban planning are being encouraged to include a public health lens at the national level and in some states (Ricklin and Kushner, 2014).

One dimension of urban planning that can greatly influence health equity relates to so-called greening policies and programs. Two studies conducted in Philadelphia, including a randomized trial, found that programs to "green" and maintain vacant urban land—for example, through cleaning and plantings—led to lower rates of gun crime and vandalism; in addition, residents reported feeling safer, feeling less stress, and getting more exercise (Branas et al., 2011; Garvin et al., 2013; Huynh and Maroko, 2014). Because vacant lots are disproportionately situated in low-income areas, greening programs have the potential to promote health equity.

One of many urban planning challenges is around the larger issues of economic, job, and workforce development (Freeman, 2005; Newman and Wyly, 2006). Local economic development can revitalize blighted neighborhoods and create more jobs, but it can also lead to the displacement of low-income residents. In local areas where the housing supply is tight or where investment is improving the quality and amenities of the local housing stock, development can affect housing affordability, particularly for low-income residents, leading to displacement (Finch et al., 2016; PolicyLink, 2016b).

Displacement can exacerbate health inequities by limiting access to affordable housing, healthy food options, transportation, quality schools, bicycle and walking paths, exercise facilities, and social networks and also by increasing financial hardship (CDC, 2009). The disruption of social ties and networks can affect mental and physical well-being, especially for households that have lived in their original neighborhood for a long period of time (Phillips et al., 2014). A recent study in Philadelphia found that residents in a gentrified area of Philadelphia who stayed in that area experienced improvements in their financial well-being, as measured by credit scores. However, vulnerable residents who moved from that area tended to move to lower-income neighborhoods and experienced a worsening in financial well-being (Ding and Hwang, 2016; Ding et al., 2015). Despite concerns around the negative impacts of potential displacement, research attempting to quantify the scale and nature of residential displacement is limited and existing studies have relatively limited time horizons (Zuk et al., 2015).

The changing landscape of a number of cities in the United States suggests increasing income and racial segregation. Wyly and Hammel mapped the effects of housing market and policy changes in the 1990s in 23 large U.S. cities (Wyly and Hammel, 2004). Along with a resurgence in capital investment in the urban core, the authors found increased racial and class segregation in addition to intensified discrimination and exclusion in gentrified neighborhoods (Wyly and Hammel, 2004). This has implications for health inequity, as evidenced by the body of literature that suggests the negative health impacts of segregation and discrimination on people of color. At the same time, a number of equitable development and housing policy tools have been developed that can assist communities to balance opportunities across local groups so that more can benefit from development efforts (PolicyLink, 2016a; Wilson et al., 2008). Local communities and governments across the country have started to integrate processes and policies to advance health equity within the urban planning and land use context. For example, Multnomah County, Oregon, applies an "equity and empowerment lens" to local policy (Multnomah County, 2014a, b, n.d.), and Seattle–King County implemented an "equity in all policies" approach to all decision making and annually reports on what it terms "the determinants of equity" in the county (Beatty and Foster, 2015).

In a 2011 Institute of Medicine (IOM) report, the authoring committee recommended that "states and the federal government develop and employ a 'health in all policies' (HIAP) approach to consider the health effects—both positive and negative—of major legislation, regulations, and other policies that could potentially have a meaningful impact on the public's health" (IOM, 2011). The committee further recommended that "state and federal governments evaluate the health effects and costs of major legislation, regulations, and policies that could have a meaningful impact on health. This evaluation should occur before and after enactment." The recommendation below is made with an acknowledgment of the ongoing cross-sectoral work in many jurisdictions around the country and of the previous IOM recommendations.

> **Recommendation 6-1:** All government agencies that support or conduct planning related to land use, housing, transportation, and other areas that affect populations at high risk of health inequity should:
> - Add specific requirements to outreach processes to ensure robust and authentic community participation in policy development.
> - Collaborate with public health agencies and others to ensure a broad consideration of unintended consequences for health and well-being, including whether the benefits and burdens will be equitably distributed.[4]
> - Highlight the co-benefits of—or shared "wins" that could be achieved by—considering health equity in the development of comprehensive plans[5] (e.g., improving public transit in transit-poor areas supports physical activity, promotes health equity, and creates more sustainable communities).
> - Prioritize affordable housing, implement strategies to mitigate and avoid displacement (and its serious health effects), and document outcomes.

Strategies to expand affordable housing could include regulating the private housing market; establishing nonprofit-owned affordable housing; creating affordable home ownership opportunities; offering resident-controlled, limited-equity ownership; leveraging market rate development; and preserving publicly assisted affordable housing. Other policy tools to promote equitable development include the use of land trusts, legal covenants that protect and increase rent stabilization, inclusionary zoning, rent control, the use of Section 8 housing provisions, housing code enforcements, just-cause eviction controls, requirements for sufficient low-income housing to avoid displacement, and policies and tools that assist low-income residents in homeownership (ChangeLab Solutions, 2015). See Box 6-1 for an example of a community-driven neighborhood plan designed to make some of these changes.

---

[4] See Recommendation 7 in *For the Public's Health: Revitalizing Law and Policy to Meet New Challenges* (IOM, 2011).

[5] See, for example, ChangeLab Solutions' "Model Comprehensive Plan Language on Complete Streets" (ChangeLab Solutions, 2016).

> **BOX 6-1**
> **East Harlem Neighborhood Plan**
>
> When East Harlem was announced as a neighborhood for a possible rezoning, with the goal of creating new affordable housing, community stakeholders and leaders, including the Office of City Council Speaker Melissa Mark-Viverito, Manhattan Community Board 11, Community Voices Heard, and the Manhattan Borough President Gale A. Brewer, collectively sprang into action to inform the community about the rezoning proposal and catalyze a robust, community-driven neighborhood planning process. The East Harlem Neighborhood Plan Steering Committee was formed and convened local stakeholders in a community engagement process to create the East Harlem Neighborhood Plan. The goals of the neighborhood plan encompassed community organizing, political activism, social planning, and capacity building efforts targeted at multiple determinants of health in the context of New York City's increasing income inequality:
>
> - Collect and organize community concerns and ideas in order to influence city agencies' planning processes and rezoning efforts.
> - Create a needs assessment that takes into account East Harlem's current and future community.
> - Develop implementable recommendations that reflect community input.
> - Develop approaches to preserve existing affordable and public housing and generate new, permanently affordable housing.
> - Develop new tools for the preservation of culture, economy, and neighborhood character.
> - Provide a model for other communities and neighborhood planning efforts.
> - Create a human capital development plan that focuses on the advancement of East Harlem residents.
> - Build a base of engaged residents ready to advocate collectively for community needs.
>
> The East Harlem Neighborhood Plan evolved through 8 large (average of almost 180 individuals per session) public meetings, approximately 40 meetings to develop the objectives and recommendations around the 12 key themes, several informal meetings to gather more feedback and to provide more information on the ideas being discussed, community-based surveys, online comments, and meetings with agencies to test and gather feedback on the objectives and recommendations. Priorities were identified using a combination of online survey responses and voting via tokens at the final community forum on January 27, 2016. The two objectives per subgroup that received the most votes were selected. The resulting priorities and objectives were: arts and culture; open space and recreation; schools and education; pre-K, daycare and afterschool; housing authority developments; housing preservation; small business development; workforce and economic development; affordable housing development, zoning and land use; transportation, environment, and energy; safety; health; and seniors (WXY and Hester Street Collaborative, 2016).

EDUCATION POLICIES

The powerful role that education plays in producing—or reducing—inequitable health outcomes was discussed in Chapter 3. Educational attainment predicts life expectancy and such health status indicators as obesity and morbidity from acute and chronic diseases (see, for example, Woolf et al., 2007). The educational level of adults, particularly maternal educational achievement, is linked to their children's health and well-being. In all regions of the United States (Montez and Berkman, 2014), the gradient in health outcomes by educational attainment has steepened over the last four decades (Goldman and Smith, 2011; Olshansky et al., 2012), producing a larger gap in health status between Americans with high and low education levels. Thus, policies and practices to increase academic achievement and reduce education disparities make a critical contribution to reducing health inequities.

An important insight emerges from looking broadly across the array of education-related policies and practices. Desired improvements in education and health outcomes are unlikely to be achieved by one-dimensional interventions. Both the community examples that the committee has examined and other information the committee has gathered suggest that achieving greater equity in health outcomes will require collaboration and collective action across sectors and new forms of community engagement and partnership. At the community level, there may be unique opportunities to work in a coordinated manner. Part of the committee's charge was assessing and prioritizing these possibilities for more effective community-based efforts to improve health outcomes. In the context of education, there are a number of possibilities, including, notably, the opportunity to improve education outcomes themselves.

The current policy landscape in health and especially in education warrants serious consideration of policy as a key factor in shaping local action. New federal legislation, the Every Student Succeeds Act (ESSA),[6] makes an important contribution to any effort to promote community-based strategies for reducing health inequities by recognizing the need for schools to improve educational achievement and to embrace and support "whole child" strategies. (See the Chapter 7 section on education for more details on ESSA and how communities can leverage it.) The act makes this contribution by specifically acknowledging the importance of promoting physical and mental health and wellness as essential to reducing inequities in academic achievement. Within this broad vision are numerous components of the law that represent opportunities to strengthen the linkages between education and health, thereby creating the local conditions to reduce health inequities through education.

---

[6] S.1177 Every Student Succeeds Act. Public Law 114-95 (December 10, 2015), 114th Cong.

First, ESSA calls for the identification of evidence-based interventions. This is a significant development in education, a field that has been slow to make broad use of research as a basis for improving practice (West, 2016). The law sets forward specific tiers of evidence, ranging from randomized trials to correlational studies. There are current opportunities to expand significantly the evidence available to schools by making connections to the health community and scholars with interest in promoting educational equity.

School improvement plans represent another key feature of the new federal education legislation. Under Title I of ESSA, school districts, in partnership with stakeholders, must develop and implement plans that include evidence-based interventions. Their plans under Title IV, where Student Support and Academic Enrichment Grants (SSAEG) are awarded—a key local source of revenue for making more effective connections between education and health—must also be evidence-based. Furthermore, both Title I school improvement plans and Title IV plans must be informed by comprehensive needs assessments. Creating examples of needs assessments that effectively incorporate health and wellness will be of real value over the next 3 to 5 years as school districts work with community stakeholders in crafting these plans.

Finally, one of the most important components of ESSA pertains to its state and local accountability provisions. Historically these provisions have been preoccupied with testing and assessment in the hope that such data would ensure that more children were in fact doing well in school. States and localities are being given great latitude (without guidance) about how they should satisfy the ESSA accountability provisions going forward. The new education law provides an opportunity for communities to reframe how they think more broadly about student opportunity and student success in ways that embrace health and wellness. It is an opportunity, in this regard, to use additional types of data and use data in different ways. The law also reinforces the idea of thinking more broadly about who has a stake in student well-being. Because ESSA is clear that educators must work in partnership with their communities on behalf of children and youth, this is a chance for communities to seize these opportunities in ways that help them foster a genuine culture of health, which will improve education outcomes.

The Individuals with Disabilities Education Act (IDEA), first passed in 1975, is another federal law that promotes greater equity through the protection of rights for students with disabilities. A U.S. Department of Education (ED) analysis found that students of color are being identified as having a disability at increasingly more frequent rates and receive harsher discipline than their white peers (ED, 2016b). In early 2016, ED and the My Brother's Keeper Task Force established in 2014 by President Barack Obama proposed the Equity in IDEA rule to address these inequities by requiring standard approaches for identifying, disciplining, and supporting students with disabilities, particularly students of color with disabilities (ED, 2016c). Other efforts have been established to reduce inequity through early childhood intervention, including the Birth to Three Developmental Center[7] in Washington State that serves infants and toddlers who qualify for services under IDEA through various programs to support these children and their families.

To aid in its enforcement and oversight of federal civil rights laws, ED collects data from school districts about student characteristics, academic offerings, and disciplinary actions. It compiles these data into a publicly available, national data set called the Civil Rights Data Collection so that researchers, states, and school districts can conduct their own analyses. Importantly, in 2000–2001, and again in 2011–2012 and 2012–2013, ED included all K–12 schools in its data collection rather than taking a sample. Maintaining the comprehensive, national data collection through education opens an important opportunity for communities to improve education and address disparities. In addition to data within the education sector, schools can benefit from partnering with others in the community to identify needs and plan and implement solutions. Examples have been highlighted in the work of the National Collaborative on Education and Health (Healthy Schools Campaign, 2016). Also, a joint initiative between ED and the U.S. Department of Health and Human Services (HHS) identifies "build[ing] local partnerships and participat[ing] in hospital community health needs assessments" as one of five high-impact opportunities. The *Healthy Students, Promising Futures* tool kit states

> The community health needs assessments (CHNAs) that nonprofit hospitals are required to undertake include consultations with community members and public health experts, which can help launch productive partnerships between hospitals and schools. Schools and school districts can also partner with many other kinds of community-based organizations and institutions to enrich the health services available to students. (ED, 2016a)

Conducting community health needs assessments has long been an activity and role of local and state public health agencies. Public health accreditation, which a growing number of health departments undergo, requires that health departments conduct or participate in a collaborative process of comprehensive health needs assessment in their communities (PHAB, 2011).

An additional way to think about promoting community-based strategies for reducing education and health disparities is to consider the

---

[7] For more information, see http://www.birthtothree.org/programs (accessed September 21, 2016).

existing infrastructure of policies and programs within the education sector with an eye toward how this infrastructure might be strengthened, modified, or expanded in the interest of improving health outcomes. Schools can take actions to improve the immediate health and well-being of their students. For example, there are a number of policies and practices that exist at the community level pertaining to air quality and environmental standards in educational settings. Policies exist widely that are related to physical activity and wellness. In what education administrators might think of as student services, policies and procedures exist concerning screening for health conditions as well as for counseling and mental health services. In the context of intergovernmental coordination and cooperation, many local education agencies (e.g., school districts) have established advisory councils, established school-based clinics, and employed school health coordinators. In the context of curriculum and instruction, there is a broad array of programs that connect education and health, to include asthma awareness education; emotional, social, and mental health education; nutrition education; and, of course, physical education.

Recommendation 6-2: State departments of education should provide guidance to schools on how to conduct assessments of student health needs and of the school health and wellness environment. This guidance should outline a process by which schools can identify model needs assessments, including those with a focus on student health and wellness.

Recommendation 6-3: To support schools in collecting data on student and community health, tax-exempt hospitals and health systems and state and local public health agencies should:
- **Make schools aware of existing health needs assessments to help them leverage current data collection and analyses.[8]**
- **Assist schools and school districts in identifying and accessing data on key health indicators that should inform school needs assessments and any related school improvement plans.**

Furthermore, ED could consider leveraging the needs assessment mandate of ESSA and require that schools and school systems collect such information on student and community health. One important factor to take into consideration would be the disproportionate burden that such

---

[8] See, for example, the *Healthy Students, Promising Futures* tool kit from ED and HHS (ED, 2016a).

a requirement may place on schools already facing economic and infrastructure challenges.

CIVIL RIGHTS LAW AND POLICY

Civil rights, health, and environmental justice laws and policies provide a framework to promote equal access to publicly funded resources and prohibit discrimination based on race, color, national origin, income, gender, disability, and other factors. This crosscutting approach can be applied across different areas such as health, park access, education, housing, transportation, and others. Using the approach to support community-driven solutions draws on lessons from the civil rights movement and others such as the women's movement. The civil rights movement includes community stakeholders; social science experts; attorneys working in and out of court; grassroots organizing; legislation by Congress; executive action by the president; implementation by administrative agencies; popular support through the right to vote; and philanthropic support (Ackerman, 2014; Rodriguez et al., 2014).

Resting upon a number of federal and state laws, including the Civil Rights Act of 1964, the Fair Housing Act of 1968, the Americans with Disabilities Act of 1990, the Patient Protection and Affordable Care Act (ACA) of 2010, related regulations, and executive orders, a civil rights approach can lead to changes in structural inequities, policies, and practices that perpetuate racial, ethnic, and other disparities. In their implementation, these laws and associated regulations require that agencies collect data, measure compliance, assess complaints, and allow for midcourse corrections. Data also need to be available to communities for holding officials accountable and advocating for change. A civil rights approach to alleviating health disparities is not synonymous with litigation. Voluntary compliance with and enforcement of equal justice laws and policies can be preferable to court action as a means to achieve equal justice goals, including health equity. A comprehensive civil rights approach to ensuring health equity relies on planning, data collection and analysis, media, negotiation, policy advocacy, and coalition building—all as part of a larger problem-solving strategy (Rodriguez et al., 2014). Civil rights attorneys may work with community allies, clients, social scientists and academics, experts, and broader coalitions to seek racial and ethnic equity and overcome discrimination and structural barriers to a more equitable society.

Through a civil rights lens, health equity involves the fair distribution of both the benefits and the burdens of programs and activities. Equal justice means more than freedom from unhealthy, environmentally degraded communities. Applying civil rights law to health equity includes a positive vision to meet the needs of communities at risk for health inequity by reducing discriminatory burdens, removing barriers to participation in decision making, and increasing access to health and environmental benefits that help make all communities safe, vibrant, and healthy (USDA, 2012).

Federal Laws and Civil Rights

Numerous federal and state laws and policies support a civil rights approach to health equity. For example, Title VI of the Civil Rights Act of 1964 and corresponding regulations prohibit discrimination based on race, color, or national origin and promote equity in programs and activities by recipients of federal financial assistance.[9] The Fair Housing Act of 1968 prohibits discrimination and promotes equal opportunity in housing.[10] The ACA includes a provision, Section 1557, against health discrimination in federally funded or supported health programs or activities. Section 1557 and corresponding regulations prohibit discrimination based on race, color, national origin, limited English proficiency, gender, physical and mental ability, and age (HHS, 2016). The Americans with Disabilities Act affords similar protections against discrimination based on ability.[11] The National Environmental Policy Act also provides protections that can be used to buttress equal justice laws.[12] In addition, the President's Executive Order 12898 on environmental justice and health requires federal agencies to address the effects of programs, policies, and activities on minority and low-income populations.[13] Some states such as California have parallel laws that will become increasingly important to promote health equity,

---

[9] 42 U.S.C. § 2000d et seq.; 28 C.F.R. § 42.101 et seq. (U.S. Department of Justice regulations).
[10] 42 U.S.C. § 3601 et seq.
[11] 42 U.S.C. § 12101 et seq.
[12] 42 U.S.C. § 4321 et seq.
[13] See Exec. Order No. 12898, 59 Fed. Reg. 32 (Feb. 16, 1994), Section 1-101, https://www.archives.gov/files/federal-register/executive-orders/pdf/12898.pdf (accessed June 24, 2016); White House Memo re: Executive Order on Federal Actions to Address Environmental Justice in Minority Populations and Low-Income Populations (February 11, 1994), www.epa.gov/sites/production/files/2015-02/documents/clinton_memo_12898.pdf (accessed June 24, 2016); Memorandum of Understanding on Environmental Justice and Executive Order 12898 (2011), www.epa.gov/sites/production/files/2015-02/documents/ej-mou-2011-08.pdf (accessed June 24, 2016); and U.S. Department of Justice Guidance Concerning Environmental Justice (December 3, 2014), www.justice.gov/sites/default/files/ej/pages/attachments/2014/12/19/doj_guidance_concerning_ej.pdf (accessed June 24, 2016). See generally U.S. Department of Justice, Civil Rights Division, Title VI Legal Manual at pages 58–65 (January 11, 2001). Available at https://www.justice.gov/sites/default/files/crt/legacy/2011/06/23/vimanual.pdf (accessed June 24, 2016).

civil rights, and environmental justice and health with changes in federal enforcement and the political landscape in the years to come.[14]

The U.S. Commission on Civil Rights in 2016 issued a report emphasizing the need for the U.S. Environmental Protection Agency (EPA) to comply with and enforce civil rights and environmental justice laws.[15] Similarly, civil rights and environmental justice practitioners widely and strongly criticize EPA for being derelict in pursuing enforcement actions. Government enforcement is particularly important to guard against discriminatory impact because there is no private cause of action for individuals and organizations to seek justice through the courts under the discriminatory impact standard, according to the U.S. Supreme Court ("the *Sandoval* problem").[16] This is widely held to be a major problem in rights enforcement, as it can be more difficult to show intentional discrimination. These concerns are supported by publicly available information regarding EPA's failure to pursue filed administrative complaints, for example.[17] EPA released its *EJ 2020 Action Agenda* in 2016 as a strategic plan to promote civil rights, environmental justice, and health. Its imple-

---

[14] For example, California Government Code 11135 et seq. and corresponding regulations promote equal justice and prohibit discrimination by state agencies and state-funded programs and activities for specified classes, parallel to federal civil rights laws such as Title VI. Section 11135 was recently amended to strengthen compliance and enforcement. See, e.g., California Equal Justice Amendments Strengthen Law under 11135, http://www.cityprojectca.org/blog/archives/43834; and John Auyong et al., Opportunities for Environmental Justice in California Agency by Agency (Public Law Research Institute U.C. Hastings College of Law 2003), http://gov.uchastings.edu/public-law/docs/PLRI_Agency-by-Agency_03.pdf (accessed June 24, 2016).

[15] U.S. Commission on Civil Rights, *Environmental Justice: Examining the Environmental Protection Agency's Compliance and Enforcement of Title VI and Executive Order 12898* (September 2016). Available at http://www.usccr.gov/pubs/Statutory_Enforcement_Report2016.pdf (accessed June 24, 2016).

[16] According to the Court in *Alexander v. Sandoval*, 532 U.S. 275 (2001), the Title VI statute prohibits only intentional discrimination, and private individuals and organizations can enforce the statute in court. Congress did not intend to create a private cause of action to enforce the discriminatory impact regulations in court.

[17] See, for example, *Rosemere Neighborhood Association v. U.S. Environmental Protection Agency*, 581 F.3d 1169 (9th Cir. 2009) (EPA failed to process a single complaint from 2006 or 2007 in accordance with its regulatory deadlines); Lawyer: EPA Has Failed Civil Rights Law: Attorney Marianne Engelman Lado argues that the Environmental Protection Agency should enforce civil rights law in the low-income communities of color that she says carry the burden of pollution, NBC News (August 2, 2015). Available at http://www.nbcnews.com/video/nbcnews.com/57693524#58380209 (accessed June 24, 2016). Kristen Lombardi, Talia Buford, Ronnie Greene, Environmental Justice, Denied: Environmental racism persists, and the EPA is one reason why (Center for Public Integrity September 4, 2015) (EPA has not made a formal finding of discrimination in 22 years, despite having received hundreds of complaints, some exhaustively documented). Available at https://www.publicintegrity.org/2015/08/03/17668/environmental-racism-persists-and-epa-one-reason-why (accessed June 24, 2016).

mentation remains to be evaluated.[18] The recommendations and principles in the U.S. Commission on Civil Rights apply to other federal, state, and local agencies in addition to EPA. These and other examples demonstrate that environmental and civil rights laws can be used together, with the strengths in one body of policy and law shoring up challenges in the other.

A Planning Process

The following planning process is a policy and legal tool from the domain of civil rights and environmental justice—designed for use by federal, state, and local agencies and their grantees—that can be adapted to support community-based solutions to promote health equity. The process includes five major elements and can be used by community-based groups to assess both current policies and practices and those under consideration. This framework by public health, civil rights, and environmental justice experts is based on Title VI, Executive Order 12898, case law, and best practices by federal agencies[19] (Environmental Justice Leadership Forum on Climate Change, 2016b; The City Project, 2016b):

1. Describe what is planned in terms that are understandable to communities (for example, diversifying and broadening access to and support for healthy active living in parks and recreation areas).
2. Analyze the benefits and burdens on all people.
   a. The analysis can include numerical disparities (in park access, for example), statistical evidence, anecdotal evidence, empirical studies and surveys, demographic data, geographical information system mapping, and financial analysis. Who benefits, and who is left behind? To do this, data needs to be collected and made publicly available for independent

---

[18] See U.S. EPA, *EJ 2020 Action Agenda* (2016). Available at https://www.epa.gov/environmentaljustice/ej-2020-action-agenda-epas-environmental-justice-strategy; and Robert García and Marianne Engelman Lado, *EPA Environmental Justice Action Agenda: Major Steps Forward, and Opportunities for More* (NRPA Open Space Blog Nov. 4 2016), http://www.nrpa.org/blog/epa-environmental-justice-action-agenda-major-steps-forward-and-opportunities-for-more (accessed June 24, 2016).

[19] See, for example, Rodriguez et al., 2014, at pages 13–20 and authorities cited; Environmental Justice Leadership Forum on Climate Change, 2016b; and U.S. Department of Housing and Urban Development, *Affirmatively Furthering Fair Housing, Final Rule*, 24 C.F.R. Parts 5, 91, 92, et al., 80 Fed. Reg. 42272 (2015), https://www.gpo.gov/fdsys/pkg/FR-2015-07-16/pdf/2015-17032.pdf (accessed June 24, 2016).

analyses. Standards need to be defined to measure progress, allow for midcourse corrections, and hold officials accountable.
   b. The range of values at stake to be analyzed includes, for example, physical, mental, and social health; economic vitality, jobs, and displacement; climate and conservation; culture, history, art, and spiritual values; and equal justice and democratic participation.[20]
3. Analyze alternatives to what is being considered.
4. Include people of color, low-income people, and other stakeholders in every step in the decision-making process.
5. Develop an implementation plan to distribute benefits and burdens fairly and avoid discrimination.

An implementation plan through monitoring, compliance, and enforcement helps promote health equity and avoids unjustified discriminatory impacts regardless of intent, as well as intentional discrimination and implicit bias (DOT, 2012a; The City Project, 2016b).

Planning for health equity needs to take place early enough in the process to meaningfully guide the decision-making process and outcomes. The following sections will expand on this process, with each step premised on the participation of diverse stakeholders.

Planning, Data, Standards, Implementation, and Stakeholders

The application of the civil rights approach depends on outlining explicit priorities in planning, data, standards, implementation, and participation. The need for public participation based on full and fair information needs to be addressed in the process and cannot be assumed (Christensen, 2016; Garcia et al., 2016). The experience with the investment of park bond funds in California illustrates why specific priorities matter. California voters have passed billions of dollars in statewide resource, park, and water bonds for almost 20 years. Yet people of color and low-income people throughout California disproportionately lack access to parks, beaches, and recreation areas. To address these concerns, in 2006 voters passed Proposition 84, a bond measure authorizing $5.4 billion in public investments to improve water, parks, coastal protection, and natural resources. Proposition 84 and Assembly Bill (AB) 31—implementing legislation for the proposition—defined "park poor" and "income

---

[20] On the values at stake, see, for example, NPS, *Healthy Parks, Healthy People Community Engagement eGuide* at page 15 (2014). Available at www.nps.gov/public_health/hp/hphp/press/HealthyParksHealthyPeople_eGuide.pdf (accessed June 24, 2016).

poor" standards to prioritize the investment of $1.3 billion in local impact funds for park, water, and coastal projects (Garcia et al., 2016).[21] Fully 88 percent of the $400 million in funds invested under the AB 31 standards were invested in communities that are disproportionately of color and low-income. In contrast, 69 percent of the remaining $1 billion that were *not* invested using those standards were disproportionately invested in communities that tend to be park-rich, wealthy, and white. Not taking equity and disparities into account through planning, standards, data, and implementation can result in policy failure. Good intentions and vague commitments to "equity" or "local parks and urban greening" alone can exacerbate rather than alleviate disparities.

Discriminatory Impacts and Data Analysis

An important starting point for promoting health equity is the analysis of disparities that bear more heavily on one group of people than another. This includes, for example, numerical disparities for people of color or women based on statistical studies or anecdotal evidence.[22] Two recent cases by the U.S. Supreme Court emphasize the need to address civil rights compliance, enforcement, and data analysis by public agencies.[23] Federal entities such as the U.S. Department of Justice address the need for data collection and analysis in their regulations and guidance documents.[24]

---

[21] AB 31 is the Statewide Park Development and Community Revitalization Act of 2008, Pub. Res. Code §§ 5640 et seq. Prop 84 is the Safe Drinking Water, Water Quality and Supply, Flood Control, River and Coastal Protection Bond Act of 2006, Pub. Res. Code §§ 75001 et seq.

[22] See, for example, *Fisher v. University of Texas at Austin*, 579—U.S.—, slip opinion at pages 13–15 (2016); *Village of Arlington Heights v. Metropolitan Housing Dev. Corp.*, 429 U.S. 252, 265 (1977); *Griggs v. Duke Power Co.*, 401 U.S. 424 (1971); U.S. Department of Justice, Civil Rights Division, *Title VI Legal Manual* at pages 42–58 and cases cited (2001), available at https://www.justice.gov/sites/default/files/crt/legacy/2011/06/23/vimanual.pdf (accessed June 24, 2016); and Robert García and Erica Flores Baltodano, *Free the Beach! Public Access, Equal Justice, and the California Coast*, 2 Stanford Journal of Civil Rights and Civil Liberties 143, 187–190 and authorities cited (2005), available at goo.gl/RVgbJ.

[23] See *Fisher v. University of Texas at Austin*, 579—U.S.—(2016); *Texas Department of Housing and Community Affairs v. Inclusive Communities Project*, 576 U.S.–(2015); U.S. Department of Housing and Urban Development, *Implementation of the Fair Housing Act's Discriminatory Effects Standard*, 24 C.F.R. Part 100, 78 Fed. Reg. 11460 (February 15, 2013). Available at https://portal.hud.gov/hudportal/documents/huddoc?id=discriminatoryeffectrule.pdf (accessed June 15, 2016).

[24] The U.S. Department of Justice directs agencies to provide for "collection of data and information from applicants for and recipients of federal assistance sufficient to permit effective enforcement of Title VI." 28 C.F.R. § 42.406(a). This includes, for example, "(1) The manner in which services are or will be provided by the program in question, and related data necessary for determining whether any persons are or will be denied such services on

The U.S. Supreme Court in *Texas Department of Housing and Community Affairs v. Inclusive Communities Project* held that the prohibition against unjustified discriminatory impacts plays an important role in moving the nation toward overcoming a legacy of residential segregation and promoting equal opportunity for all. Proof of intentional discrimination is not required. The disparate impact standard allows people to counteract disguised animus, unconscious prejudices, and implicit bias that may escape easy classification as intentional discrimination. "A thoughtless policy can be as unfair as, and functionally equivalent to, intentional discrimination" (Rodriguez et al., 2014). The prohibition against unjustified discriminatory impacts promotes equal opportunity for all in access to health, housing, parks, beaches, transportation, jobs, contracts for diverse business enterprises, and other infrastructure and ecosystem services.[25] Overlapping evidence is relevant to prove discriminatory impact[26] and intent.[27]

---

the basis of prohibited discrimination; (2) The population eligible to be served by race, color, and national origin; . . . (4) [R]elated information adequate for determining whether the [program] has or will have the effect of unnecessarily denying access to any person on the basis of prohibited discrimination." 28 C.F.R. at § 42.406(b)(1), (2), (4). Similarly, FTA regulations address racial and ethnic data, demographic mapping, comparing benefits and burdens, public engagement, and planning. Federal Transit Administration, *Title VI Requirements and Guidelines for Federal Transit Administration Recipients, Circular FTA C 4702.1B*, pages IV -7, V-1 (Oct. 1, 2012); FTA, *Environmental Justice Policy Guidance for Federal Transit Administration Recipients, Circular (FTA C 4703.1)*, pages 6, 8, 11 (August 15, 2012). *Accord*, Executive Order 12898 on Environmental Justice, Sec. 3-3 (research, data collection, and analysis).

[25] See *Texas Department of Housing and Community Affairs v. Inclusive Communities Project*, 576 U.S.—2015. While the facts in that case involved the Fair Housing Act of 1968, the discriminatory impact standard is analogous under Title VI regulations and Affordable Care Act section 1557. See U.S. Department of Housing and Urban Development, *Implementation of the Fair Housing Act's Discriminatory Effects Standard*, 24 C.F.R. Part 100, 78 Federal Register. 11460 (2013). Available at https://portal.hud.gov/hudportal/documents/huddoc?id=discriminatoryeffectrule.pdf (accessed June 15, 2016).

[26] There are three prongs to the discriminatory impact inquiry: (1) Whether an action impacts one group more than another—numerical disparities based on race, ethnicity, or national origin shown through statistical studies or anecdotal evidence, for example. (2) If so, the funding recipient bears the burden of proving that an action is justified by business necessity—or by an analogous public policy in the case of a government agency. (3) Even if there is evidence of business necessity, the disparities are prohibited if there are less discriminatory alternatives to achieve similar objectives. See, for example, *Inclusive Communities* slip opinion at page 10.

[27] To evaluate an intentional discrimination claim, circumstantial evidence includes (1) whether an action impacts one group more than another, including numerical disparities shown through statistical studies and anecdotal evidence; (2) a history of discrimination; (3) departures from substantive norms; (4) departures from procedural norms; (5) a pattern of discrimination; and (6) the decision maker knows the harm a decision will cause. See, for example, *Village of Arlington Heights v. Metropolitan Housing Dev. Corp.*, 429 U.S. 252, 264–268 (1977); *Adarand Constructors, Inc. v. Peña*, 515 U.S. 200 (1995); and U.S. Department of Justice, Civil Rights Division, *Title VI Legal Manual* at pages 42–58 (2001). Available at https://

The U.S. Supreme Court in *Fisher v. University of Texas at Austin* in 2016 recognized the value of diversity in ways that support community-based solutions to promote health equity. Valuing diversity promotes cross-racial understanding, ending stereotypes, preparing for an increasingly diverse society and workforce, and cultivating leaders with legitimacy in the eyes of the public. The court emphasized the need to gather, analyze, and publish data based on race, color, and national origin in order to ensure that public benefits and burdens are distributed equally and to promote racial justice, human dignity, and diversity.[28]

Examples of the Planning Process in Action

Specific actions by several federal and local agencies illustrate how civil rights can be promoted to promote health equity through the planning process described above. The National Park Service (NPS) and the U.S. Army Corps of Engineers (the Corps) have used the systematic data-driven planning framework to analyze green access in the Los Angeles region. NPS and the Corps concluded as follows in the context of health and park access:

- There are disparities in green access based on race, color, or national origin;
- This contributes to health disparities based on those factors; and
- Environmental justice and civil rights laws require agencies to promote equity, compliance, and enforcement and alleviate these disparities.

These plans include the NPS plan to expand the Santa Monica Mountains National Recreation Area ("Rim of the Valley") (NPS, 2015; The City Project, 2016a), the NPS plan to create the San Gabriel Mountains National Recreation Area (NPS, 2013; The City Project, 2014b), and the Corps' plan to revitalize the Los Angeles River (The City Project, 2016c; U.S. Army Corps of Engineers, LA District, and Tetra Tech Inc., 2015).[29] HUD provides another example of the planning framework in action. HUD

---

www.justice.gov/sites/default/files/crt/legacy/2011/06/23/vimanual.pdf (accessed June 24, 2016).

[28] *Fisher v. University of Texas at Austin*, 579—U.S.—, slip opinion at pages 11, 14–15 (2016). While the facts of the case involved narrowly tailored race conscious admissions to promote the compelling state interest of diversity in a university, the value of diversity and the need for data are analogous in promoting health equity.

[29] The Corps has agreed to conduct a similar analysis of the benefits and burdens of, and alternatives to, the Dakota Access Pipeline, in consultation with the Standing Rock Sioux and with full public input before issuing any permits (Darcy, 2016). This is parallel to the Corps's analysis for revitalization of the Los Angeles River. The decision was made in large part in response to community organizing by the Sioux and its supporters.

withheld federal subsidies for a proposed warehouse project in response to significant local community action, pending a full study under the civil rights and environmental justice laws to consider a park alternative and the impact on people of color and low-income people. This community initiation and decision by HUD contributed to the creation of the L.A. State Historic Park and the greening of the Los Angeles River (Garcia, 2013; The City Project, 2014a).[30]

With these laws, equal access to publicly funded resources, such as parks and recreation for healthy active living, can be viewed as core civil rights issues. In *Brown v. Board of Education*, the U.S. Supreme Court struck down segregation in schools when it held that schools separated on the basis of race are inherently unequal, in violation of the Equal Protection Clause.[31] In *Watson v. City of Memphis* in 1963, the Supreme Court upheld equal access to public parks and recreation on equal justice grounds under *Brown*.[32]

The civil rights and equity framework is not limited to work in a single geographic area, such as Southern California, or to a specific substantive topic, such as health and park disparities (NPS, 2014). Echoing work by NPS and the Corps and recognizing the need for systematic data and analyses, EPA has released its online mapping and analysis tool called EJSCREEN. This tool includes nationwide data on health vulnerabilities, exposure to toxic chemicals and pollution, park access, and demographics, including race, color, national origin, income, and other variables and is described in more detail in Chapter 8 (EPA, 2016; The City Project, 2016d). WE ACT, a community example featured in Chapter 5, organized a coalition with 41 partners nationwide to address climate justice and health using the framework under Title VI of the 1964 Civil Rights Act (Environmental Justice Leadership Forum on Climate Change, 2016a,b).[33]

---

[30] Community advocates settled a related lawsuit under state law. The state then bought the land and created the park.

[31] *Brown v. Board of Education*, 347 U.S. 483 (1954). Discrimination is not just a black and white issue. Also in 1954, the Supreme Court held the Equal Protection Clause protects against discrimination based on race, color, national origin, ancestry, or descent in *Hernandez v. Texas*, 347 U.S. 475 (1954).

[32] *Watson v. City of Memphis*, 373 U.S. 526 (1963).

[33] A recent policy report explores the causes of such strong Latino support for environmental protection and government action to control climate change. Sam García, *Latinos and Climate Change: Opinions, Impacts, and Responses* (GreenLatinos and The City Project 2016), available at www.cityprojectca.org/blog/archives/43303 (accessed June 24, 2016). The communities that have shown the most consistent support for climate change, people of color, are generally marginalized or absent from the discussion by mainstream environmental organizations, academics, and government in carbon pricing schemes, including cap and trade, cap and dividend, and regulatory measures. The environmental justice movement has demonstrated that racially and ethnically identifiable communities are at a greater risk

> **BOX 6-2**
> **Economic Analysis of Improved Health Outcomes Using the Civil Rights Act of 1964 and Medicare Funding**
>
> One analysis of the effectiveness of using legal and policy advocacy using a rights-based framework to promote community-based solutions that result in improved health equity outcomes is by Stanford economic historian Gavin Wright. Wright analyzed improved health outcomes that resulted from desegregated health care services and facilities in the South as a result of the civil rights movement in his study, *Sharing the Prize: The Economics of the Civil Rights Revolution in the American South* (2013). This analysis is timely as the civil rights movement, civil rights legislation, legal advocacy, and the role of government in providing a social safety net are increasingly challenged.
>
> Health care and services were segregated, and this segregation resulted in health disparities in the pre-Civil Rights South. The health care community and civil rights attorneys worked together to achieve reform that had moral as well as material outcomes that benefited both people of color and non-Hispanic white people. The National Medical Association and NAACP Legal Defense Fund attorneys worked together, with the U.S. Department of Justice, to challenge the "separate but equal" provision under the Hill-Burton Act that funded segregated health care services through the early 1960s. In 1963, a federal court of appeals struck down "separate but equal" under the Act in *Simkins v. Moses H. Cone Memorial Hospital*. The court ruled in favor of a class that included African American physicians, dentists, and patients who were excluded from private non-Hispanic white hospitals that received federal funding. The following year, Congress passed Title VI of the Civil Rights Act of 1964 in response to the March on Washington led by Dr. Martin Luther King, Jr. President Lyndon Johnson, a southerner, persuaded southern senators to break the longest filibuster in the history of the nation to pass the legislation. Federal agencies enacted regulations to implement the Title VI statute. Congress passed the Medicare Act in 1965, which provided funding for medical services, as part of the War on Poverty. Medicare funding, coupled with the Title VI prohibition against discrimination by recipients of federal funding, resulted in improved outcomes in health equity and health outcomes for people of color and non-Hispanic white people.
>
> "The campaign to desegregate southern hospitals was a genuine part of the Civil Rights Movement." Medicare offered "a positive incentive to take patients they would formally have rejected, while at the same time giving the federal government a powerful financial threat to force compliance with Title VI." Wright asks: "The larger issue is whether hospital desegregation actually improved health outcomes." An analysis of post-neonatal infant mortality rates by race in the South and North between 1955 and 1975 and county-level data suggests that gains in health outcomes for people of color and non-Hispanic white people "were the direct result of desegregation and the Civil Rights Movement," concludes Wright on pages 236–240.
>
> Wright's analysis illustrates the myriad strategies of the Civil Rights Movement in action: civil rights attorneys in and out of court, courageous courts, organizing in the streets, legislation, executive action, administrative enforcement, and the power of the people who defeated the call to repeal civil rights laws.
>
> SOURCE: Wright, 2013.

The Federal Transit Administration addresses the framework in its civil rights and environmental justice guidance documents and has applied the framework to withhold federal funding in the transit context in Northern California (DOT, 2012a,b; The City Project, 2015). Box 6-2 describes an economic analysis of a policy intervention that advanced health equity.

Using Civil Rights Law

The following guidance can help civil rights attorneys, public health professionals, community groups, public agencies, recipients of public funding, foundations, and other stakeholders promote community-based solutions to promote health equity using civil rights tools and reinforce a culture of health (Rodriguez et al., 2014):

- Communities and other stakeholders can work together on compliance and equity plans for programs or activities by recipients of public funding that use the civil rights framework by describing what is to be done, analyzing the impact on all communities, analyzing alternatives, including full and fair participation by diverse communities, and promoting health equity.
- Compliance and equity plans can be used to guard against unjustified and unnecessary discriminatory impacts, as well as against intentional discrimination, in health and wellness programs and activities.
- Communities, when appropriate, can work with civil rights attorneys to use problem-solving strategies, including coalition building, planning, data collection and analysis, media, negotiation, policy and legal advocacy out of court, and access to justice through the courts.
- Communities can work with attorneys and public health experts together to promote a better understanding of the civil rights dimension of the challenge of health disparities and to show how to address these civil rights concerns for their communities to ensure that civil rights laws against discrimination in health and other publicly funded programs and activities are strengthened and not rolled back.

---

of environmental harms, disproportionately lack environmental benefits, pay a larger cost, and carry a heavier environmental burden than other communities regardless of class. Once these costs are considered the distribution of benefits must necessarily be structured to pay down that debt. Gerald Torres and Robert García, *Impact of Pricing Schemes on Environmental Justice Communities* (The City Project Policy Report 2016), available at www.cityprojectca.org/blog/archives/43641 (accessed June 24, 2016).

Conclusion 6-1: In the committee's judgment, civil rights approaches have helped mitigate the negative impacts of many forms of social and health discrimination. Continuing this work is needed to overcome discrimination and the structural barriers that affect health.

Conclusion 6-2: The committee concludes that using civil rights approaches in devising and implementing community solutions to promote health equity can guard against unjustified and unnecessary discriminatory impacts, as well as against intentional discrimination in programs that affect health. For example, those implementing community solutions can employ methods and data in ways that include full and fair participation by diverse communities.

See Chapter 8 for additional discussion on how civil rights law can support community-based solutions.

HEALTH POLICY

The Patient Protection and Affordable Care Act

The ACA has changed the financing, organization, and delivery of U.S. health care services in a number of important ways. It not only expands private and public health insurance but also reforms how Medicare and Medicaid services are delivered and revises the tax code in important ways that encourage nonprofit hospitals to invest in their local communities in new ways. The following section briefly reviews selected features of the ACA and discusses both how these features affect communities and how federal policy could be changed to affect health equity at the community level.

The ACA has expanded access to Medicaid coverage and private insurance to millions of individuals. Nationally, since 2010, rates of uninsured have dropped from 16.0 percent in 2010 to 9.2 percent in 2015 (Cohen and Martinez, 2015). Significantly, in part because 32 states expanded their Medicaid programs and 19 did not, the rates of uninsured among the non-elderly population varies significantly from a low of 5 percent in Massachusetts to a high of 19 percent in Texas (Kaiser Family Foundation, 2015, 2016). State decisions regarding Medicaid expansion were controversial and highly politicized in many states (Jacobs and Callaghan, 2013). Yet, these state decisions have important implications for communities. The variation in uninsured rates is more dramatic across metropolitan areas; among the 25 largest metropolitan areas the rates range from 4 to 19 percent (U.S. Census Bureau, 2015). On average, urban and rural counties have higher rates of the uninsured than suburban counties. Moreover, geographically uninsured whites are more likely to live in areas with high poverty census tracts, whereas minorities are more likely to be uninsured wherever they live (REACH Healthcare Foundation, 2016).

State policy around health insurance, particularly through Medicaid decision making, has serious implications for health and other disparities. On the one hand, the impact of health insurance on health outcomes has been found to be mixed, at least in the short run. For instance, while biometric measures of health were not found to improve in a study of the Oregon Medicaid expansion, self-reported health was found to improve. Other studies have also found improvements in self-reported health (Sommers et al., 2012), but not consistently (Wherry and Miller, 2016). On the other hand, health insurance is seen as a potential mechanism for increasing use of preventive and other medical care services. Although health insurance lowers the cost of care to individuals, other factors may also be important and counter lower costs, such as wait times for appointments, distances to services, and the perceived discomfort of the care itself. The empirical literature has found overwhelmingly that insurance expansions improve access to medical care (Finkelstein et al., 2012; Miller, 2012; Van Der Wees et al., 2013). Additionally, greater health insurance plays an important financial role by shielding individuals from out-of-pocket medical costs and improving their overall financial status (Hu et al., 2016). The annual cost of inpatient care for a person between the ages of 18 and 64 who was hospitalized in 2012 was approximately $15,000, and the annual cost of all types of care for that person in the same year was $25,000 (Hu et al., 2016). Individuals without health insurance often have difficulty paying medical expenses and may need to borrow money or forego other necessities such as food, heat, or rent. They are more likely to be contacted by collection agencies and are more likely to declare bankruptcy (Cunningham, 2008; Dobkin et al., 2016; Doty et al., 2008; Finkelstein et al., 2012). Thus, medical bills play a large role in individuals' overall financial picture, including their ability to save and make other investments. The expansions of Medicaid, including expansions under the ACA, have been found to substantially reduce the financial burden of medical care on low-income individuals and to increase their financial well-being (Baicker et al., 2013; Gross and Notowidigdo, 2011; Hu et al., 2016).

The health insurance provisions of the ACA have important implications for local communities. Although communities individually may have little influence over state and federal policy change, they can leverage existing policies to their advantage. Thus, communities can actively promote health insurance enrollment activities and help increase the number of individuals with health insurance in their communities, leading to greater financial well-being.

Hospital Community Benefit

Another important provision of the ACA for communities relates to charitable or nonprofit hospitals (in 2014, 78 percent of approximately 5,000 U.S. hospitals were nonprofit, exempt from most federal, state, and local taxes [Berwick et al., 2008; James, 2016]). In particular, the ACA changed the Internal Revenue Code such that all charitable hospitals must conduct community health needs assessments (CHNAs) and adopt an implementation strategy that addresses the needs identified in that assessment. Furthermore, the process must include "persons who represent the broad interests of the community served by the hospital facility, including those with special knowledge of or expertise in public health." Moreover, regulations issued in 2014 specify that the CHNA should include "the need to address financial and other barriers to accessing care, to prevent illness, to ensure adequate nutrition, or to address social, behavioral, and environmental factors that influence health in the community" (C.F.R. 501(r)3(4)), and it was later clarified in an executive update that this includes some forms of housing improvements. Nonetheless, federal reporting forms and instructions have caused some confusion related to community benefit, investments in improving the social determinants of health, and CHNAs. As health insurance coverage has expanded, the level of uncompensated care provided by hospitals has declined, leaving hospitals to consider other areas and ways to invest community benefit dollars. Some hospitals have shown greater interest in community-wide health investments and the underlying factors that affect population health rather than maintaining the more narrow focus on health care services and funding offsets (Rosenbaum and Choucair, 2016). In the report *Can Hospitals Heal America's Communities?* Howard and Norris wrote that by "addressing these social determinants of health through their business and non-clinical practices (for example, through purchasing, hiring, and investments), hospitals and health systems can produce increased measurably beneficial impacts on population and community health" (Howard and Norris, 2015, pp. 1–2). Examples of efforts that have used community benefit investments to build, hire, and invest in the local community include Kaiser Permanente in California and elsewhere and Promedica in Cleveland (NASEM, 2016d).

> **Recommendation 6-4: Through multi-sectoral partnerships, hospitals and health care systems should focus their community benefit dollars to pursue long-term strategies (including changes in law, policies, and systems) to build healthier neighborhoods, expand access to housing, drive economic development, and advance other upstream initiatives aimed at eradicating the root causes of poor health, especially in low-income**

communities. Hospital and health systems should also advocate for the expansion of efficient and effective services responding to health-related social needs[34] for vulnerable populations and people living in poverty.

This work should include meaningful participation by members of low-income and minority populations in the community. In addition to leveraging federal tax provisions around community health benefit in order to improve the social determinants of health and health equity, work by the Institute for Healthcare Improvement has shown that hospitals effectively tackle health equity not only in the community but also within their own institutions (Wyatt et al., 2016). Box 6-3 features an example of policy-driven work to reduce disparities in Maryland.

Triple Aim

Another component of the ACA is an emphasis on improving care, improving population health, and reducing the per capita cost of care. This notion of the "Triple Aim" is a term coined by the Institute for Healthcare Improvement and incorporated in ACA implementation, becoming part of the U.S. national strategy for tackling health care issues (AHRQ, 2016a; Berwick et al., 2008; Whittington et al., 2015). States, such as Massachusetts, also focus on Triple Aim outcomes: for example, through the Massachusetts Quality and Cost Council (AHRQ, 2016b; Holahan and Blumberg, 2006).

In its original conception, the Triple Aim seeks to improve the individual experience of care, improve the health of populations, and reduce the per capita costs of care for populations (Berwick et al., 2008). The Triple Aim is notably silent on health disparities. Perhaps this perspective stems from an initial focus on the private actors in the United States carrying out the Triple Aim, by selecting populations of interest, improving quality, and lowering costs. In fact, the architects of the Triple Aim approach cautioned that equity could be sacrificed in pursuit of the Triple Aim: the health of one population could be achieved at the expense of another. More recently, others have called for a "triple aim for health equity" that broadens the focus and embeds health care in a community-based

---

[34] Alley et al. describe services addressing health-related social needs, including transportation and housing (Alley et al., 2016). Others define services addressing such needs as "wraparound services," referring to linkages or services health care providers can offer to ensure, for example, that patients have transportation to routine health care appointments, have adequate food in their homes, and obtain legal (e.g., for tenant-landlord disputes about environmental exposure to asthma triggers) or social service assistance. See, for example, Bell and Cohen (2009).

> **BOX 6-3**
> **Maryland Health Enterprise Zones**
>
> In 2012 Maryland passed the Maryland Health Improvement and Disparities Reduction Act. One component includes a joint initiative between the Maryland Community Health Resources Commission and the Maryland Department of Health and Mental Hygiene initiative around "health enterprise zones" (HEZ). Under this 4-year pilot program, communities identified areas with measurable and documented economic disadvantage and poor health outcomes and proposed collaborative plans to address health outcomes and disparities. The HEZ statute provides financial incentives to recruit and retain health care providers to HEZs, including loan repayment assistance and income tax credits for newly hired practitioners, hiring tax credits for the employers of new HEZ practitioners, grant funding, and technical assistance. The HEZ pilot program is still under way and will be formally evaluated.
>
> The state statute also requires the Maryland Health Care Commission to establish and incorporate a standard set of measures regarding racial and ethnic variations in quality and outcomes and to track health insurance carriers' and hospitals' efforts to combat disparities. In addition, state institutions of higher education that train health care professionals will be required to report to the Governor and General Assembly on their actions aimed at reducing health care disparities. The latter is not slated to be formally evaluated. Nonetheless, the increased transparency around disparity-reduction activities can help tracking by agencies and outside researchers and help to shape future policy.

framework (Ehlinger, 2015). At issue is that the pursuit of the Triple Aim could perpetuate and even worsen disparities unless the concept is expanded to incorporate a health equity focus. A continued focus on rewarding health outcomes at the mean, without rewarding a compression in the variations in health, is likely to encourage interventions that target healthier, and socially less disadvantaged, populations in order to demonstrate improvements. Under such a reward system gaps in health between advantaged and disadvantaged populations may grow even wider.

Frequently, the pursuit of the Triple Aim is combined with an emphasis on care integration and bundled payment for services across settings in order to encourage efficiency and cost control (Berwick et al., 2008). The challenge from a health disparities standpoint is the skewed nature of health expenditures, with 1 percent of the population accounting for approximately 21.4 percent of health care expenditures, with average per-person annual expenditures of $87,570 (Cohen and Uberoi, 2013). Thus, there is a strong incentive for integrated health systems and those receiving bundled payment to avoid the 1 percent of patients who present the highest costs. This subgroup also is disproportionately socially disadvantaged. Some evidence indicates the existence of potential challenges with respect to disadvantaged groups for programs such as the accountable care organizations that arose from the Triple Aim approach. In particular, a recent study found that commercial and Medicare accountable care organization networks were relatively less likely to include physicians in areas where a higher percentage of the population was African American, living in poverty, uninsured, disabled, or had a rate of high school education less than in other areas (Yasaitis et al., 2016). Even where variation in health outcomes is used as a performance metric, a strategy of encouraging the enrollment of those at low risk and avoiding those at high risk can artificially inflate performance measures. The implication is that high-powered financial incentives, such as capitation and bundled payment, may elicit unintended responses from delivery systems and perpetuate health inequities.

> **Recommendation 6-5: Government and nongovernment payers and providers should expand policies aiming to improve the quality of care, improve population health, and control health care costs[35] to include a specific focus on improving population health for the most vulnerable and underserved. As one strategy to support a focus on health disparities, the Centers for Medicare & Medicaid Services could undertake research on payment reforms that could spur accounting for social risk factors in the value-based payment programs it oversees.**

The National Academies Committee on Accounting for Socioeconomic Status in Medicare Payment Programs has shown in its reports (NASEM, 2016a,b,c,e) that value-based payment systems that do not account for social risk factors can have unintended adverse consequences, including providers and health plans avoiding low-income patients and underpayment to providers disproportionately serving socially at-risk populations (such as safety net providers). These unintended consequences could in turn lead to deterioration in the quality of health care for socially at-risk populations and widening health disparities. That committee has stated that reducing disparities in access, quality, and outcomes is one of four policy goals in accounting for social risk factors (NASEM, 2016a,b,c,e), and its reports suggest that reforms to value-based payment programs that compensate providers fairly and increase fairness and accuracy in

---

[35] Better care, better population health, and lower cost are often described as the Triple Aim (Berwick et al., 2008).

public reporting can help achieve goals to reduce disparities and improve quality and efficiency of care for all patients.

CRIMINAL JUSTICE POLICY

The criminal justice system plays an important role in shaping health equity through multiple mechanisms. The first, which is conceptually straightforward, includes the health care screening and treatment services that the system provides to adult and juvenile prisoners and probationers. The second is more complex and far-ranging and includes the set of policies that determine if an individual becomes involved in the justice system, for how long, whether or not alternative sanctions will be offered, and how individuals will reenter the community after incarceration. These policies have long-term implications for education completion, employment, and income—all of which in turn affect health. Because the justice-involved population is disproportionately people of color and disproportionately comprises other vulnerable populations such as persons with mental illness, criminal justice policies have important implications for health equity.

The United States today has the highest rate of incarceration in the world, with a cost to states and the federal government of $80 billion in 2010 alone (DOJ, 2013). This remarkably high rate of incarceration stems from policies adopted by federal and state governments starting in the early 1980s, particularly around mandatory sentencing, "three strikes and you're out," and increasing drug-related incarceration (Blumstein and Beck, 1999; Mauer, 2001).

The current era of mass incarceration can be understood as a powerful policy intervention in the lives of the poor and people of color (Pettit and Western, 2004). Indeed, criminal justice policy and practice disproportionately affect minorities in a number of ways, and there is a large racial disproportionality at most stages of the criminal justice system for both adults and juveniles (Harris et al., 2009).

Policies related to the "war on drugs" since the 1980s have played an especially pivotal role in institutionalizing disproportionate minority contact with the criminal justice system. Many scholars have remarked that federal drug policies have targeted racial and ethnic minorities and especially African Americans and their communities. The differences in mandatory minimum sentencing guidelines for crack cocaine, which has been associated with poor and minority users, versus powder cocaine, whose users tend to be white (Palamar et al., 2015), is a case in point. Although the two substances are virtually identical on a molecular level, the Anti-Drug Abuse Act of 1986 stipulated a 100:1 weight ratio for powder versus crack cocaine when determining mandatory minimum sentences for possession (Palamar et al., 2015). In practice, this meant that 5 grams of crack, for example, mandated the same sentence (5 years in prison) as 500 grams of cocaine. Although the disparity was recently revised to an 18:1 ratio by the 2010 Fair Sentencing Act, scholars and community advocates have long argued that any disparity targets crack and, by extension, poor and minority users (Palamar et al., 2015). As a result, federal drug policies that sanction crack more than powder cocaine have exacerbated a widescale racial inequity that characterizes criminal justice sanctions for drug use and possession.

Blumstein highlights several other mechanisms by which racial and socioeconomic disproportionality can compound itself in the criminal justice system (Blumstein, 2009). Because more serious crimes occur in poor neighborhoods, police patrol them more densely. This also leads individuals in these areas to be more likely to be arrested (Blumstein, 2009), and, because punishment is a function of prior police contact, the marginal arrest leads to greater punishment down the line. This disadvantage can build if it is combined with such police practices as racial profiling when deciding whom to stop, question, and search (Ridgeway and MacDonald, 2010). Hispanics and African Americans are disproportionately confined in jails and prisons than would be predicted by their arrest rates, and Hispanic and African American juveniles are more likely to be referred to adult court rather than juvenile court relative to white juveniles (Harris et al., 2009).

Disadvantage can further compound inequities in other ways. Youth who live in stable two-parent, higher-income families are more likely to be released than youth living in single-parent, lower-income families, which has implications also for further sanctions and for educational disruptions. Moreover, minority youth are more likely to face harsh disciplinary action in schools by being suspended or referred to court (Mizel et al., 2016), and schools with stringent disciplinary policies that favor suspension can also contribute to greater arrests among youth (Cuellar and Markowitz, 2015).

The high budgetary and social costs of imprisonment have led federal and state policy makers to reconsider sentencing and sanctioning rules. At the federal level, although there are mandatory minimum laws, changes were instituted to lower punishments for low-level, nonviolent drug offenses by individuals with no ties to large-scale organizations or gangs and to reduce sentences for certain inmates (DOJ, 2013). Texas and Arkansas also have reduced their prison populations by identifying alternative sanctions for low-level drug offenders. Kentucky similarly has shifted resources from prison beds to treatment services for offenders with behavioral health problems and greater community supervision. Other state initiatives, such as drug courts, have been found to reduce disparities for Hispanics and, to some extent, for African Americans (Nicosia et al., 2013). At the juvenile level, states have also sought to promote treatment alternatives to incarceration for selected populations with behavioral health problems (Cuellar and Dave, 2016; Cuellar et al., 2006). Since 2007, the Justice Reinvestment Initiative—a public–private partnership that includes the DOJ Bureau of Justice Assistance—has also supported efforts in 33 states, all of which "aim to improve public safety and control taxpayer costs by prioritizing prison space for serious and repeat offenders and investing some of the savings in alternatives to incarceration for low-level offenders that are effective at reducing recidivism" (The Pew Charitable Trusts, 2016).

Recidivism is a large problem for the individuals who have been convicted. Recidivism has been linked in part to barriers faced by those with a criminal record. Federal, state, and local policies can exacerbate these barriers by stipulating legal sanctions and restrictions imposed on individuals with criminal records. The areas in which such challenges are faced include housing, employment, education, public benefits, and permission to travel. Some states "prohibit the employment of convicted felons in occupations ranging from child- and dependent-care service providers to barbers and hairdressers" (Bushway et al., 2007, p. 3). Some states also cut off their access to public employment, which has been an important source of work for inner-city minorities (Bushway et al., 2007). The American Bar Association has compiled the National Inventory of Collateral Consequences of Conviction, which catalogs the wide-ranging collateral consequences of criminal convictions contained in the numerous laws and regulations at the federal and state levels (ABA, 2016). As Bushway and colleagues suggest, policies like these can present formidable barriers to successful reintegration into society after release from prison (Bushway et al., 2007).

Recognizing the role that local policies play in marginalizing those with a criminal record, some communities have advocated for laws aimed at reducing the barriers to reentry for the formerly incarcerated. As of 2016 more than 150 cities and counties have adopted "ban the box" policies that prohibit employers from considering criminal records at the beginning of the application process. Ban-the-box policies instead require that employers first consider a job candidate's qualifications (Rodriguez and Avery, 2016). However, recent data reveal that ban-the-box policies may have a negative effect on work opportunities for young, low-skilled African American and Hispanic men (Doleac and Hansen, 2016). Reentry is also a difficult transition for juveniles. Many states have developed special programs for youth, including mentoring, mental health counseling, education supports, and family reunification supports, to facilitate successful reintegration and the transition to adulthood, and some have reformed their juvenile justice system (see, for example, The Pew Charitable Trusts, 2014).

While incarcerated, those confined to jail, prison, halfway houses, or juvenile facilities are reliant upon the justice system to provide for their health care needs. Many of these services are funded by criminal justice budgets. In addition, individuals may be eligible for Medicaid-funded services if they are not prisoners per se,[36] such as when they reside in transitional reentry institutions or if they are not committed (Gupta et al., 2005). State and federal Medicaid policies can affect the available funding for health care services for these groups. With the recent expansion of Medicaid under the ACA, states and the federal government are revisiting Medicaid regulations related to the adult criminal justice population and facilitating access to Medicaid for eligible individuals prior to and after a stay in a correctional institution (CMS, 2016).

Beyond the far-reaching effects of a criminal record, criminal justice policies can play a role in health equity by influencing the odds of victimization (e.g., through gun policies). Clearly, firearm violence remains an important public health concern for many communities across the country (Monuteaux et al., 2015). With more than 10,000 Americans killed by firearms in 2014 (Kochanek et al., 2016), the United States suffers from the highest rate of firearm homicides among industrialized nations (IOM and NRC, 2013), and the burden of gun violence is borne disproportionately by economically disadvantaged communities, particularly communities of color (Altheimer, 2008). Exceptional levels of gun violence coexist alongside deeply polarized views over gun rights and gun policy. On the one hand, repeated episodes of large-scale gun violence in the United States have provoked proponents of gun control to argue for stricter policies to regulate the availability of guns in communities. On the other hand, proponents of gun rights argue that gun availability deters crime and enhances personal defense. Recent research in the *American Journal of Preventive Medicine* (Monuteaux et al., 2015) finds household gun ownership rates associate positively with various forms of violence across states. Other research concludes that living in a city with high rates of household gun ownership leads to greater odds of gun assault or gun robbery victimization (Altheimer, 2008). This research suggests that policies aimed at curbing firearm availability might help reduce violence in communities. However, the overall state of research on the relationship between gun availability and violence is mixed and offers contrasting views about the importance of gun regulation for violence. Furthermore, research that focuses specifically on how gun control policies influence firearm violence is also inconclusive (IOM and NRC, 2013).

---

[36] Medicaid does not cover "inmates of a public institution."

The recommendations of a recent IOM and National Research Council report that calls for more research on the potential efficacy of gun control policies in preventing firearm violence in U.S. communities continue to resonate (IOM and NRC, 2013). Chapter 7 includes a discussion of actions in public safety that could be considered to begin to bring about change from the community level up.

CONCLUDING OBSERVATIONS

Chapter 4 discussed the importance of communities and the fact that they not only are the locus for change, they also possess agency and can draw on their own power and assets to help effect change. However, as acknowledged in that chapter, it can be difficult for communities to promote health equity on their own. The present chapter describes the effects that policies and laws can have on communities. To sustain change over the long term, the broader context of issues that influence community efforts and success needs to be addressed.

REFERENCES

ABA (American Bar Association). 2016. *National Inventory of Collateral Consequences of Conviction (NICCC).* http://www.abacollateralconsequences.org (accessed May 13, 2016).

Ackerman, B. A. 2014. *We the people, volume 3: The civil rights revolution, The civil rights revolution.* Cambridge, Massachusetts: Belknap Press of Harvard University Press.

Adler, N. E., and D. H. Rehkopf. 2008. US disparities in health: Descriptions, causes, and mechanisms. *Annual Review of Public Health* 29:235–252.

AHRQ (Agency for Healthcare Research and Quality). 2016a. *About the National Quality Strategy (NQS).* http://www.ahrq.gov/workingforquality/about.htm#priorities (accessed October 14, 2016).

AHRQ. 2016b. *Working for quality: National Quality Strategy (NQS).* http://www.ahrq.gov/workingforquality (accessed October 17, 2016).

Alley, D. E., C. N. Asomugha, P. H. Conway, and D. M. Sanghavi. 2016. Accountable health communities—addressing social needs through Medicare and Medicaid. *The New England Journal of Medicine* 374(1):8.

Altheimer, I. 2008. Do guns matter—a multi-level cross-national examination of gun availability on assault and robbery victimization. *Western Criminology Review* 9:9.

Andrews, N. O., D. J. Erickson, I. Galloway, and E. Seidman. 2012. Investing in what works for America's communities. *San Francisco: Federal Reserve Bank of San Francisco and Low Income Investment Fund.*

Autor, D. H., A. Manning, and C. L. Smith. 2016. The contribution of the minimum wage to U.S. wage inequality over three decades: A reassessment. *NBER Working Paper No. 16533.* http://www.nber.org/papers/w16533 (accessed October 24, 2016).

Baicker, K., S. L. Taubman, H. L. Allen, M. Bernstein, J. H. Gruber, J. P. Newhouse, E. C. Schneider, B. J. Wright, A. M. Zaslavsky, and A. N. Finkelstein. 2013. The Oregon experiment—effects of Medicaid on clinical outcomes. *New England Journal of Medicine* 368(18):1713–1722.

Bartilow, G. 2016. The safety net in Kentucky lifts 810,000 people out of poverty. *Kentucky Center for Economic Policy Policy Blog*. http://kypolicy.org/safety-net-kentucky-lifts-810000-people-poverty (accessed October 24, 2016).

Beatty, A., and D. Foster. 2015. *The determinants of equity: Identifying indicators to establish a baseline of equity in King County*. King County, WA.

Bell, J., and L. Cohen. 2009. *The transportation prescription: Bold new ideas for healthy, equitable transportation reform in America, 2009. Commissioned by the convergence partnership*. https://www.preventioninstitute.org/sites/default/files/publications/The%20 Transportation%20Prescription_0.pdf (accessed December 1, 2016).

Ben-Shalom, Y., R. A. Moffitt, and J. K. Scholz. 2011. *An assessment of the effectiveness of antipoverty programs in the United States*. Cambridge, MA: National Bureau of Economic Research.

Berwick, D. M., T. W. Nolan, and J. Whittington. 2008. The triple aim: Care, health, and cost. *Health Affairs* 27(3):759–769.

Bitler, M., and H. Hoynes. 2013. *The more things change, the more they stay the same? The safety net and poverty in the great recession*. Cambridge, MA: National Bureau of Economic Research.

Bitler, M., H. Hoynes, and E. Kuka. 2016. *Child poverty, the great recession, and the social safety net in the United States*. Cambridge, MA: National Bureau of Economic Research.

Blumstein, A. 2009. Race and the criminal justice system. *Race and Social Problems* 1(4):183–186.

Blumstein, A., and A. J. Beck. 1999. Population growth in U.S. prisons, 1980–1996. *Crime & Justice*. 26:17.

Branas, C. C., R. A. Cheney, J. M. MacDonald, V. W. Tam, T. D. Jackson, and T. R. Ten Have. 2011. A difference-in-differences analysis of health, safety, and greening vacant urban space. *American Journal of Epidemiology* 174(11):1296–1306.

Burke, M. P., E. A. Frongillo, S. J. Jones, B. B. Bell, and H. Harline-Grafton. 2016. Household food insecurity is associated with greater growth in body mass index among female children from kindergarten through eighth grade. *Journal of Hunger and Environmental Nutrition* 11(2):227–241.

Bushway, S., D. F. Weiman, and M. A. Stoll. 2007. *Barriers to reentry?: The labor market for released prisoners in post-industrial America*. New York, NY: Russell Sage Foundation.

CBO (Congressional Budget Office). 2016. *The distribution of household income and federal taxes, 2013*. https://www.cbo.gov/sites/default/files/114th-congress-2015-2016/reports/51361-HouseholdIncomeFedTaxes_OneCol.pdf (accessed October 24, 2016).

CDC (U.S. Centers for Disease Control and Prevention). 2009. *Health effects of gentrification*. http://www.cdc.gov/healthyplaces/healthtopics/gentrification.htm (accessed July 7, 2016).

ChangeLab Solutions. 2015. *Preserving, protecting, and expanding affordable housing: A policy toolkit for public health*. http://www.changelabsolutions.org/sites/default/files/Preserving_Affordable_Housing-POLICY-TOOLKIT_FINAL_20150401.pdf (accessed October 24, 2016).

ChangeLab Solutions. 2016. *Model comprehensive plan language on complete streets: A framework to embrace complete streets principle*. http://www.changelabsolutions.org/publications/comp-plan-language-cs (accessed October 24, 2016).

Chetty, R., M. Stepner, S. Abraham, S. Lin, B. Scuderi, N. Turner, A. Bergeron, and D. Cutler. 2016. The association between income and life expectancy in the United States, 2001–2014. *JAMA* 315(16):1750–1766.

CHOICES (Childhood Obesity Intervention Cost-Effectiveness Study). 2016. *Brief: Cost-effectiveness of a sugar-sweetened beverage excise tax in Philadelphia, PA*. http://choicesproject.org/brief-cost-effectiveness-of-a-sugar-sweetened-beverage-excise-tax-in-philadelphia-pa (accessed November 23, 2016).

Chow, J. C.-C., M. A. Johnson, and M. J. Austin. 2006. The status of low-income neighborhoods in the post-welfare reform environment. *Journal of Health & Social Policy* 21(1):1–32.

Christensen, J. 2016. *Environmental bonds should equitably benefit all communities: Looking forward based on an analysis of Prop 84.* Los Angeles: University of California, Los Angeles, Institute of the Environment and Sustainability.

CMS (Centers for Medicare & Medicaid Services). 2016. State health official letter re: to facilitate successful re-entry for individuals transitioning from incarceration to their communities. Baltimore, MD: U.S. Department of Health and Human Services.

Cohen, R. A., and M. E. Martinez. 2015. *Health insurance coverage: Early release of estimates from the National Health Interview Survey, January–March 2015.* Hyattsville, MD: National Center for Health Statistics.

Cohen, S., and N. Uberoi. 2013. Differentials in the concentration in the level of health expenditures across population subgroups in the US, 2010. *Statistical brief* 421.

Collinson, R., I. G. Ellen, and J. Ludwig. 2015. Low income housing policy. In *Economics of means-tested transfer programs in the United States, volume 2.* Chicago, IL: University of Chicago Press.

CSG (Council of State Governments). 2016. *States receiving technical assistance from the CSG Justice Center.* https://csgjusticecenter.org/jr (accessed October 24, 2016).

Cuellar, A., and D. M. Dave. 2016. Causal effects of mental health treatment on education outcomes for youth in the justice system. *Economics of Education Review* 54:321–339.

Cuellar, A. E., and S. Markowitz. 2015. School suspension and the school-to-prison pipeline. *International Review of Law and Economics* 43:98–106.

Cuellar, A. E., L. S. McReynolds, and G. A. Wasserman. 2006. A cure for crime: Can mental health treatment diversion reduce crime among youth? *Journal of Policy Analysis and Management* 25(1):197–214.

Cunningham, P. J. 2008. *Track report: Trade-offs getting tougher: Problems paying medical bills increase for U.S. families, 2003-2007.* Washington, DC: Center for Studying Health System Change.

Currie, J., and A. Yelowitz. 2000. Are public housing projects good for kids? *Journal of Public Economics* 75(1):99–124.

Cutler, D. M., and A. Lleras-Muney. 2006. *Education and health: Evaluating theories and evidence.* Working paper no. 12352. Cambridge, MA: National Bureau of Economic Research.

Dahl, G. B., and L. Lochner. 2005. *The impact of family income on child achievement.* Working paper no. 11279. Cambridge, MA: National Bureau of Economic Research.

Darcy, J. 2016. Memorandum for commander, U.S. Army Corps of Engineers. *Proposed Dakota Access Pipeline crossing at Lake Oahe, North Dakota.* https://www.army.mil/e2/c/downloads/459011.pdf (accessed December 5, 2016).

Ding, L., and J. Hwang. 2016. The consequences of gentrification: A focus on residents' financial health in Philadelphia: Working paper 16-22. *Research Department, Federal Reserve Bank of Philadelphia* 40.

Ding, L., J. Hwang, and E. Divringi. 2015. *Gentrification and residential mobility in Philadelphia.* Philadelphia, PA: Federal Reserve Bank of Philadelphia.

Dobkin, C., A. Finkelstein, R. Kluender, and M. J. Notowidigdo. 2016. *The economic consequences of hospital admissions.* Working paper no. 22288. Cambridge, MA: National Bureau of Economic Research.

DOJ (U.S. Department of Justice). 2013. Smart on crime: Reforming the criminal justice system for the 21st century. https://www.justice.gov/sites/default/files/ag/legacy/2013/08/12/smart-on-crime.pdf (accessed October 20, 2016).

Doleac, J. L., and B. Hansen. 2016. *Does "ban the box" help or hurt low-skilled workers? Statistical discrimination and employment outcomes when criminal histories are hidden.* Cambridge, MA: National Bureau of Economic Research.

DOT (U.S. Department of Transportation). 2012a. *Environmental justice policy guidance for Federal Transit Administration recipients (FTA c 4703.1).* U.S. government.

DOT. 2012b. *Title VI requirements and guidelines for Federal Transit Administration recipients (FTA C4702. 1B).* U.S. government.

Doty, M. M., S. R. Collins, S. D. Rustgi, and J. L. Kriss. 2008. Seeing red: The growing burden of medical bills and debt faced by U.S. families: Issue brief. *The Commonwealth Fund* 42(August).

ED (U.S. Department of Education). 2016a. *Healthy students, promising futures: State and local action steps and practices to improve school-based health toolkit.* http://www2.ed.gov/admins/lead/safety/healthy-students/index.html (accessed October 24, 2016).

ED. 2016b. *Racial and ethnic disparities in special education: A multi-year disproportionality analysis by state, analysis category, and race/ethnicity.* Washington, DC: U.S. Department of Education.

ED. 2016c. U.S. Department of Education takes action to deliver equity for students with disabilities. http://www.ed.gov/news/press-releases/us-department-education-takes-action-deliver-equity-students-disabilities (accessed November 23, 2016).

Ehlinger, E. P. 2015. We need a triple aim for health equity. *Minnesota Medicine:* 28–29.

Ellen, I. G., K. M. Horn, and A. E. Schwartz. 2016. Why don't housing choice voucher recipients live near better schools? Insights from big data. *Journal of Policy Analysis and Management* 35(4):884–905.

Environmental Justice Leadership Forum on Climate Change. 2016a. *Clean power plan tool kit.* http://www.ejleadershipforum.org/clean-power-plan-tool-kit (accessed October 24, 2016).

Environmental Justice Leadership Forum on Climate Change. 2016b. *Environmental justice state guidance: How to incorporate equity and justice into your state clean power planning approach.* http://www.eesi.org/files/EJ-State-Guidance-Final-v5-jan-15-2016.pdf (accessed October 24, 2016).

EPA (U.S. Environmental Protection Agency). 2016. EJScreen: Environmental justice screening and mapping tool (version 2016). https://ejscreen.epa.gov/mapper (accessed October 24, 2016).

Evans, W. N., and C. L. Garthwaite. 2014. Giving mom a break: The impact of higher EITC payments on maternal health. *American Economic Journal: Economic Policy* 6(2):258–290.

Executive Office of the President. 2015. *Long-term benefits of the Supplemental Nutrition Assistance Program.* https://www.whitehouse.gov/sites/whitehouse.gov/files/documents/SNAP_report_final_nonembargo.pdf (accessed November 23, 2016).

Finch, B. K., A. N. Beck, and H. Amaro. 2016. *Does gentrification contribute to segregation? A study of urban displacement.* Population Association of America Annual Meeting, Washington, DC. Poster presentation, March 18, 2016.

Finkelstein, A., S. Taubman, B. Wright, M. Bernstein, J. Gruber, J. P. Newhouse, H. Allen, K. Baicker, and Oregon Health Study Group. 2012. The Oregon health insurance experiment: Evidence from the first year. *The Quarterly Journal of Economics* 127(3):1057–1106.

Freeman, L. 2005. Displacement or succession? Residential mobility in gentrifying neighborhoods. *Urban Affairs Review* 40(4):463–491.

GAO (U.S. Government Accountability Office). 2015. *Federal low-income programs: Multiple programs target diverse populations and needs.* U.S. Government Accountability Office.

Garcia, R. 2013. The George Butler lecture, social justice and leisure: The usefulness and uselessness of research. *Journal of Leisure Research* 46:7–22.

Garcia, R., A. Collins, and C. De La Vega. 2016. Park funding for all! *Parks & Recreation* 32–33. http://www.cityprojectca.org/blog/archives/43709 (accessed October 24, 2016).

Garvin, E. C., C. C. Cannuscio, and C. C. Branas. 2013. Greening vacant lots to reduce violent crime: A randomised controlled trial. *Injury Prevention* 19(3):198–203.

Goldberg, D. 2016. Bay area and Boulder soda taxes would extend lives, avert millions in health care costs over 10 years, Harvard model projects. *Healthy Food America.* http://www.healthyfoodamerica.org/bay_area_and_boulder_soda_taxes_would_extend_lives_avert_millions_in_health_costs_over_10_years_harvard_model_projects (accessed November 23, 2016).

Goldman, D., and J. P. Smith. 2011. The increasing value of education to health. *Social Science & Medicine* 72(10):1728–1737.

Gross, T., and M. J. Notowidigdo. 2011. Health insurance and the consumer bankruptcy decision: Evidence from expansions of Medicaid. *Journal of Public Economics* 95(7-8):767–778.

Gupta, R. A., K. J. Kelleher, K. Pajer, J. Stevens, and A. Cuellar. 2005. Delinquent youth in corrections: Medicaid and reentry into the community. *Pediatrics* 115(4):1077–1083.

Hamad, R., and D. H. Rehkopf. 2015. Poverty, pregnancy, and birth outcomes: A study of the earned income tax credit. *Paediatric and Perinatal Epidemiology* 29(5):444–452.

Hamad, R., and D. H. Rehkopf. 2016. Poverty and child development: A longitudinal study of the impact of the earned income tax credit. *American Journal of Epidemiology* 183(9):775-784.

Harris, C. T., D. Steffensmeier, J. T. Ulmer, and N. Painter-Davis. 2009. Are blacks and Hispanics disproportionately incarcerated relative to their arrests? Racial and ethnic disproportionality between arrest and incarceration. *Race and Social Problems* 1(4):187–199.

Healthy Schools Campaign. 2016. A new national initiative highlights the link between health and education. *Healthy Schools Campaign.* https://healthyschoolscampaign.org/policy/a-new-national-initiative-highlights-the-link-between-health-and-education (accessed July 16, 2016).

HHS (U.S. Department of Health and Human Services). 2016. Summary: Final rule implementing Section 1557 of the Affordable Care Act.

Holahan, J., and L. Blumberg. 2006. Massachusetts health care reform: A look at the issues. *Health Affairs* 25(6):w432–w443.

Howard, T., and T. Norris. 2015. Can hospitals heal America's communities?: "All in for mission" is the emerging model for impact. Washington, DC: The Democracy Collaborative.

Hu, L., R. Kaestner, B. Mazumder, S. Miller, and A. Wong. 2016. *The effect of the Patient Protection and Affordable Care Act Medicaid expansions on financial wellbeing.* Working paper no. 22170. Cambridge, MA: National Bureau of Economic Research.

HUD (U.S. Department of Housing and Urban Development). 2016a. *Low-income housing tax credits (LIHTC) data sets* (May 15, 2016). https://www.huduser.gov/portal/datasets/lihtc.html (accessed December 16, 2016).

HUD. 2016b. *Picture of subsidized households datasets.* https://www.huduser.gov/portal/datasets/picture/yearlydata.html (accessed December 19, 2016).

Huynh, M., and A. R. Maroko. 2014. Gentrification and preterm birth in New York City, 2008-2010. *Journal of Urban Health* 91(1):211–220.

International Energy Agency. 2015. *Capturing the multiple benefits of energy efficiency.* http://www.iea.org/publications/freepublications/publication/capturing-the-multiple-benefits-of-energy-efficiency.html (accessed October 20, 2016).

IOM (Institute of Medicine). 2011. *For the public's health: Revitalizing law and policy to meet new challenges.* Washington, DC: The National Academies Press.

IOM and NRC (National Research Council). 2013. *Priorities for research to reduce the threat of firearm-related violence.* Washington, DC: The National Academies Press.

IRS (Internal Revenue Service). 2016. *Statistics for tax returns with EITC.* https://www.eitc.irs.gov/EITC-Central/eitcstats?_ga=1.80629535.982617637.1477348670 (accessed December 19, 2016).

Jacob, B. A., M. Kapustin, and J. Ludwig. 2015. The impact of housing assistance on child outcomes: Evidence from a randomized housing lottery. *The Quarterly Journal of Economics* 130(1):465–506.

Jacobs, L. R., and T. Callaghan. 2013. Why states expand Medicaid: Party, resources, and history. *Journal of Health Politics, Policy and Law* 38(5):1023–1050.

Jacobs, L. R., and J. Soss. 2010. The politics of inequality in America: A political economy framework. *Annual Review of Political Science* 13(1):341–364.

James, J. 2016. Health policy brief: Nonprofit hospitals' community benefit requirements. *Health Affairs* http://healthaffairs.org/healthpolicybriefs/brief_pdfs/healthpolicybrief_153.pdf (accessed August 8, 2016).

Kaiser Family Foundation. 2015. *Health insurance coverage of nonelderly 0-64.* http://kff.org/other/state-indicator/nonelderly-0-64/?currentTimeframe=0&sortModel=%7B%22colId%22:%22Location%2022,%22sort%22:%22asc%22%7D (accessed September 10, 2016).

Kaiser Family Foundation. 2016. *Current status of state action on the Medicaid expansion decision, KFF state health facts.* http://kff.org/health-reform/slide/current-status-of-the-medicaid-expansion-decision (accessed September 10, 2016).

Kessler, R. C., G. J. Duncan, L. A. Gennetian, L. F. Katz, J. R. Kling, N. A. Sampson, L. Sanbonmatsu, A. M. Zaslavsky, and J. Ludwig. 2014. Associations of housing mobility interventions for children in high-poverty neighborhoods with subsequent mental disorders during adolescence. *JAMA* 311(9):937–948.

Kochanek, K. D., S. L. Murphy, J. Q. Xu, and B. Tejada-Vera. 2016. Deaths: Final data for 2014. *National Vital Statistics Reports* 65(4).

Kochtitzky, C. S., H. Frumkin, R. Rodriguez, A. Dannenberg, J. Rayman, K. Rose, R. Gillig, and T. Kanter. 2006. Urban planning and public health at CDC. *Morbidity and Mortality Weekly Report Supplements* 55(2):34–38.

Kyureghian, G., R. M. Nayga, and S. Bhattacharya. 2013. The effect of food store access and income on household purchases of fruits and vegetables: A mixed effects analysis. *Applied Economic Perspectives and Policy* 35(1):69–88.

Mathur, C., D. J. Erickson, M. H. Stigler, J. L. Forster, and J. R. Finnegan. 2013. Individual and neighborhood socioeconomic status effects on adolescent smoking: A multilevel cohort-sequential latent growth analysis. *American Journal of Public Health* 103(3):543–548.

Mauer, M. 2001. The causes and consequences of prison growth in the United States. *Punishment & Society* 3(1):9–20.

Meltzer, D. O., and Z. Chen. 2011. The impact of minimum wage rates on body weight in the United States. In *Economic aspects of obesity*. Chicago, IL: University of Chicago Press. Pp. 17–34.

Miller, S. 2012. The impact of the Massachusetts health care reform on health care use among children. *American Economic Review* 102(3):502–507.

Mizel, M. L., J. N. Miles, E. R. Pedersen, J. S. Tucker, B. A. Ewing, and E. J. D'Amico. 2016. To educate or to incarcerate: Factors in disproportionality in school discipline. *Children and Youth Services Review* 70:102–111.

Mohai, P., P. M. Lantz, J. Morenoff, J. S. House, and R. P. Mero. 2009. Racial and socioeconomic disparities in residential proximity to polluting industrial facilities: Evidence from the Americans' changing lives study. *American Journal of Public Health* 99(Suppl 3):S649–S656.

Montez, J. K., and L. F. Berkman. 2014. Trends in the educational gradient of mortality among US adults aged 45 to 84 years: Bringing regional context into the explanation. *American Journal of Public Health* 104(1):e82–e90.

Monuteaux, M. C., L. K. Lee, D. Hemenway, R. Mannix, and E. W. Fleegler. 2015. Firearm ownership and violent crime in the US: An ecologic study. *American Journal of Preventive Medicine* 49(2):207–214.

Multnomah County. 2014a. *Foundational assumptions of the equity and empowerment lens logic model.* https://multco.us/file/31824/download (accessed October 28, 2016).
Multnomah County. 2014b. *Multnomah County Office of Diversity and Equity: Equity and empowerment lens.* https://multco.us/diversity-equity/equity-and-empowerment-lens (accessed October 24, 2016).
Multnomah County. n.d. *What is the equity and empowerment lens?* https://multco.us/diversity-equity/equity-and-empowerment-lens (accessed October 28, 2016).
NASEM (National Academies of Sciences, Engineering, and Medicine). 2015. *The growing gap in life expectancy by income: Implications for federal programs and policy responses.* Washington, DC: The National Academies Press.
NASEM. 2016a. *Accounting for social risk factors in Medicare payment: Identifying social risk factors.* Washington, DC: The National Academies Press.
NASEM. 2016b. *Accounting for social risk factors in Medicare payment: Criteria, factors, and methods.* Washington, DC: The National Academies Press.
NASEM. 2016c. *Accounting for social risk factors in Medicare payment: Data.* Washington, DC: The National Academies Press.
NASEM. 2016d. *The role of business in multisector obesity solutions: Working together for positive change: Workshop in brief.* Washington, DC: The National Academies Press.
NASEM. 2016e. *Systems practices for the care of socially at-risk populations.* Washington, DC: The National Academies Press.
Neumark, D., J. I. Salas, and W. Wascher. 2014. More on recent evidence on the effects of minimum wages in the United States. *IZA Journal of Labor Policy* 3(1):26.
Newman, K., and E. K. Wyly. 2006. The right to stay put, revisited: Gentrification and resistance to displacement in New York City. *Urban Studies* 43(1):23–57.
Nichols, A., and J. Rothstein. 2016. *The earned income tax credit from the economics of means-tested transfer programs in the United States, volume one.* Edited by R. A. Moffitt. Vol. 1, *Economics of means-tested transfer programs in the United States.* Chicago, IL: University of Chicago Press.
Nicosia, N., J. M. MacDonald, and J. Arkes. 2013. Disparities in criminal court referrals to drug treatment and prison for minority men. *American Journal of Public Health* 103(6):e77–e84.
NPS (National Park Service). 2013. *San Gabriel watershed and mountains special resource study.* https://parkplanning.nps.gov/document.cfm?documentID=43639 (accessed September 16, 2016).
NPS. 2014. Healthy parks healthy people community engagement e-guide: Edition 1.
NPS. 2015. *Rim of the valley corridor special resource study and environmental assessment.* https://parkplanning.nps.gov/document.cfm?documentID=65351 (accessed October 24, 2016).
NRC and IOM (National Research Council and Institute of Medicine). 2013. *U.S. health in international perspective: Shorter lives, poorer health.* Washington, DC: The National Academies Press.
Olshansky, S. J., T. Antonucci, L. Berkman, R. H. Binstock, A. Boersch-Supan, J. T. Cacioppo, B. A. Carnes, L. L. Carstensen, L. P. Fried, D. P. Goldman, J. Jackson, M. Kohli, J. Rother, Y. Zheng, and J. Rowe. 2012. Differences in life expectancy due to race and educational differences are widening, and many may not catch up. *Health Affairs* 31(8):1803–1813.
OMB (Office of Management and Budget). 2016. *Analytical perspectives, budget of the United States government, fiscal year 2017.* https://www.whitehouse.gov/omb/budget/Analytical_Perspectives (accessed October 24, 2016).
Palamar, J. J., S. Davies, D. C. Ompad, C. M. Cleland, and M. Weitzman. 2015. Powder cocaine and crack use in the United States: An examination of risk for arrest and socioeconomic disparities in use. *Drug and Alcohol Dependence* 149:108–116.
Pettit, B., and B. Western. 2004. Mass imprisonment and the life course: Race and class inequality in US incarceration. *American Sociological Review* 69(2):151–169.

PHAB (Public Health Accreditation Board). 2011. *Public Health Accreditation Board standards & measures, version 1.0*. http://www.phaboard.org/wp-content/uploads/PHAB-Standards-and-Measures-Version-1.01.pdf (accessed December 2, 2016).

Phillips, D., L. Flores Jr., and J. Henderson. 2014. *Development without displacement*. Oakland, CA: Causa Justa.

PolicyLink. 2016a. *Equity tools: Affordable housing*. http://www.policylink.org/equity-tools/equitable-development-toolkit/affordable-housing (accessed October 21, 2016).

PolicyLink. 2016b. *Equity tools: Economic opportunity*. http://www.policylink.org/equity-tools/equitable-development-toolkit/economic-opportunity (accessed October 21, 2016).

REACH Healthcare Foundation. 2016. *Mid-America Regional Council Community Services Corporation*. https://reachhealth.org/awarded-grants/mid-america-regional-council-community-services-corporation-9 (accessed October 14, 2016).

Ricklin, A., and N. Kushner. 2014. *Healthy plan making—integrating health into the comprehensive planning process: An analysis of seven case studies and recommendations for change*. Chicago, IL: American Planning Association.

Ridgeway, G., and J. MacDonald. 2010. Methods for assessing racially biased policing. *Race, ethnicity, and policing: New and essential readings*. Pp. 180–204.

Rodriguez, M. N., and B. Avery. 2016. *Ban the box: U.S. Cities, counties, and states adopt fair-chance policies to advance employment opportunities for people with past convictions*. National Employment Law Project. http://www.nelp.org/content/uploads/Ban-the-Box-Fair-Chance-State-and-Local-Guide.pdf (accessed December 17, 2016).

Rodriguez, M., M. Brenman, M. E. Lado, and R. Garcia. 2014. *Using civil rights tools to address health disparities*. Los Angeles, CA: The City Project.

Rosenbaum, S., and B. Choucair. 2016. Expanding the meaning of community health improvement under tax-exempt hospital policy. In *Health Affairs Blog*. http://healthaffairs.org/blog/2016/01/08/ expanding-the-meaning-of-community-health-improvement-under-tax-exempt-hospital-policy (accessed September 28, 2016).

Sanbonmatsu, L., J. Ludwig, L. F. Katz, L. A. Gennetian, G. J. Duncan, R. C. Kessler, E. Adam, T. W. McDade, and S. T. Lindau. 2011. Moving to opportunity for fair housing demonstration program--final impacts evaluation. Washington, DC: U.S. Department of Housing and Urban Development Office of Policy Development and Research.

Schill, M. H., and S. M. Wachter. 1995. The spatial bias of federal housing law and policy: Concentrated poverty in urban America. *University of Pennsylvania Law Review* 143(5):1285–1342.

Schwartz, A. F. 2014. *Housing policy in the United States*. New York: Routledge.

Sommers, B. D., K. Baicker, and A. Epstein. 2012. Mortality and access to care among adults after state Medicaid expansions. *New England Journal of Medicine* 367:1025–1034.

Strully, K. W., D. H. Rehkopf, and Z. Xuan. 2010. Effects of prenatal poverty on infant health: State earned income tax credits and birth weight. *American Sociological Review* 75(4):534–562.

Tax Policy Center. 2014. *State minimum wage rates, 1983–2014*. http://www.taxpolicycenter.org/sites/default/files/legacy/taxfacts/content/PDF/state_min_wage.pdf (accessed November 2, 2016).

The City Project. 2014a. Best practice HUD Los Angeles state historic park healthy green land use for all. In *The City Project Blog*. Los Angeles, CA: The City Project. http://www.cityprojectca.org/blog/archives/32984 (accessed June 3, 2016).

The City Project. 2014b. San Gabriel mountains best practice environmental justice framework for parks, health, and conservation values. In *The City Project Blog*. Los Angeles, CA: The City Project. http://www.cityprojectca.org/blog/ archives/32899 (accessed June 3, 2016).

The City Project. 2015. Environmental justice and civil rights frequently asked questions FTA best practices. In *The City Project Blog*. Los Angeles, CA: The City Project. http://www.cityprojectca.org/blog/ archives/38688 (accessed June 3, 2016).

The City Project. 2016a. National Park Service rim of the valley final study best practice environmental justice. In *The City Project Blog*. Los Angeles, CA: The City Project. http://www.cityprojectca.org/blog/archives/41777 (accessed June 3, 2016).

The City Project. 2016b. U.S. Civil rights commission civil rights and environmental justice and enforcement by EPA. In *The City Project Blog*. Los Angeles, CA: The City Project. http://www.cityprojectca.org/blog/archives/43798 (accessed June 3, 2016).

The City Project. 2016c. US Army Corps of Engineers best practice for revitalizing L.A. River for all. In *The City Project Blog*. Los Angeles, CA: The City Project. http://www.cityprojectca.org/blog/ archives/41580 (accessed June 3, 2016).

The City Project. 2016d. US EPA EJSCREEN park access and health disparities civil rights and environmental justice best practice. In *The City Project Blog*. Los Angeles, CA: The City Project. http://www.cityprojectca.org/blog/archives/43843 (accessed June 3, 2016).

The Pew Charitable Trusts. 2014. Judging for juvenile justice: 3 judges share lessons of juvenile justice reform: The Pew Charitable Trusts. http://www.pewtrusts.org/~/media/assets/2014/11/pspp_juvenilejudges_qa_brief_web.pdf (accessed October 24, 2016).

The Pew Charitable Trusts. 2016. *31 states reform criminal justice policies through justice reinvestment: Fact sheet*. http://www.pewtrusts.org/en/research-and-analysis/fact-sheets/2016/01/31-states-reform-criminal-justice-policies-through-justice-reinvestment (accessed October 24, 2016).

U.S. Army Corps of Engineers, LA District, and Tetra Tech Inc. 2015. *Los Angeles River ecosystem restoration integrated feasibility report: Final feasibility report and environmental impact statement/environment impact report: Volume 1: Integrated feasibility report: Los Angeles County, California*. Los Angeles, California.

U.S. Census Bureau. 2015. Latest local health insurance statistics available through Census Bureau's American Community Survey. Suitland, MD: U.S. Census Bureau.

USDA (U.S. Department of Agriculture). 2012. *Environmental justice strategic plan: 2012–2014*. Washington, DC: U.S. Department of Agriculture.

Van Der Wees, P., A. Zaslavsky, and J. Ayanian. 2013. Improvements in health status after Massachusetts health care reform. *The Millbank Quarterly* 91(4):663–689.

Waldron, H. 2007. Trends in mortality differentials and life expectancy for male social security-covered workers, by socieoeconomic status. *Social Security Bulletin* 67(3):1–28.

Wehby, G., D. Dave, and R. Kaestner. 2016. Effects of the minimum wage on infant health: Working paper no. 22373. Cambridge, MA: The National Bureau of Economic Research.

West, M. R. 2016. *From evidence-based programs to an evidence-based system: Opportunities under the Every Student Succeeds Act*. Washington, DC: The Brookings Institution.

Wherry, L. R., and S. Miller. 2016. Early coverage, access, utilization, and health effects associated with the Affordable Care Act Medicaid expansions: A quasi-experimental study. *Annals of Internal Medicine* 164(12):795–803.

Whittington, J. W., K. Nolan, N. Lewis, and T. Torres. 2015. Pursuing the triple aim: The first 7 years. *Milbank Quarterly* 93(2):263–300.

Wilson, S., M. Hutson, and M. Mujahid. 2008. How planning and zoning contribute to inequitable development, neighborhood health, and environmental injustice. *Environmental Justice* 1(4):211–216.

Woolf, S. H., R. E. Johnson, R. L. Phillips, and M. Philipsen. 2007. Giving everyone the health of the educated: An examination of whether social change would save more lives than medicine. *American Journal of Public Health* 2007(97):4.

Woolf, S. H., L. Aron, L. Dubay, S. M. Simon, E. Zimmerman, and K. X. Luk. 2015. *How are income and wealth linked to health and longevity?* Washington, DC: Urban Institute and Virginia Commonwealth University.

Wright, G. 2013. *Sharing the prize: The economics of the civil rights revolution in the American south.* Cambridge, MA: Belknap Press of Harvard University Press.

WXY and Hester Street Collaborative. 2016. *East Harlem neighborhood plan.* http://www.eastharlemplan.nyc/EHNP_FINAL_FINAL_LORES.pdf (accessed December 4, 2016).

Wyatt, R., M. Laderman, L. Botwinick, K. Mate, and J. Whittington. 2016. *Achieving health equity: A guide for health care organizations.* Cambridge, MA: Institute for Healthcare Improvement.

Wyly, E. K., and D. J. Hammel. 2004. Gentrification, segregation, and discrimination in the American urban system. *Environment and Planning* 36:1215–1241.

Yasaitis, L. C., W. Pajerowski, D. Polsky, and R. M. Werner. 2016. Physicians' participation in ACOs is lower in places with vulnerable populations than in more affluent communities. *Health Affairs* 35(8):1382–1390.

Zuk, M., A. H. Bierbaum, K. Chapple, K. Gorska, A. Loukaitou-Sideris, P. Ong, and T. Thomas. 2015 (unpublished). *Gentrification, displacement, and role of public investment: A literature review.* Federal Reserve Bank of San Francisco.

7

Partners in Promoting Health Equity in Communities

Effective partnerships are essential for community-based solutions for advancing health equity by making it a shared vision and value, increasing the community's capacity to shape outcomes, and fostering multi-sector collaboration. Many different stakeholders can lead or participate in championing and implementing such solutions. These include organizations with a health mission, such as public health agencies, hospitals, or federally qualified health centers. In some communities these traditional partners are joined by public- and private-sector partners, including community-based organizations, faith-based organizations, businesses (from Fortune 1,000 to small employers), the education sector and academia, philanthropy, housing, justice, planning and land use, public safety, and transportation agencies.

Partners are able to deploy unique skills and access resources to serve a variety of roles in community-based solutions for health equity. A partner, such as a public health agency or a congregation, may serve as the convener of coalitions as a source of data and analysis (e.g., the local hospital, university, or school district), as a funder (a foundation or community development financial institution), or all of the above. As philanthropy and other partners engage in actions and interventions that address the underlying or "upstream" causes of health inequity (Mitchell, 2016), innovative ideas from the private sector are being brought to bear in addressing health inequities.

The concepts of disruption, innovation, paradigm shift, and design thinking have become guiding principles for engaging in this emerging collaborative cross-sector work. Systems have functioned in silos for decades for good reason: efficiency, expertise, and logistics have all kept programs moving down the same course. However, the outcomes that result from those systems need to improve, and to get to the improved outcomes will require novel ways of both defining the challenges and thinking about how cross-sector partners can come together, leverage work from other fields, and work effectively as a team.

Human-centered design is an approach that places communities and individuals at the center of the solution. Particularly for health equity, community engagement plays a central role in finding solutions. Different models have used design thinking for place-based initiatives as well as solutions aimed at improving other social determinants of health. More of these partnerships with various cross-sector groups are likely to arise in the coming years (Active Living By Design, 2016).

In addition to new ways to bring cross-sector partners together across levels, new forums will likely emerge. These could include combining professional education, joint conferences, new educational tracks within professional schools, and new positions within institutions that span multiple skill sets—for example, a planner embedded in a health department and a health worker embedded in a planning department. In the following sections, different health equity actors are highlighted, with their unique roles in promoting health equity outcomes described and various examples offered of how they have been able to create partnerships to advance progress toward health equity. Innovative approaches to fostering multi-sector collaboration to achieve health equity will require participation from many different partners. Research on community engagement initiatives suggests that these partnerships generate benefits at both the individual and community levels (Attree et al., 2011). The remainder of this chapter is dedicated to describing these different stakeholders and the roles they may assume in supporting community interventions, ending with a discussion of cross-sector collaboration.

FINANCE

In recent years, the array of funding sources and financing structures for community-based efforts to address social, economic, and environmental factors that shape health has greatly expanded. In addition to federal government programs such as Promise Neighborhoods and the Sustainable Communities Partnership and foundations that support community work (e.g., the California Endowment's Building Healthy Communities, the multi-partner Build Health Challenge), the funding landscape now includes the community development sector, led by the Federal Reserve Bank of San Francisco and others, for-profit financial institutions, social investors, and others. Emerging financing structures include pay-for-success arrangements and private equity real estate funds (NASEM, 2016a; Super Church, 2015). The role of hospitals and health system as sources of financing—for example, through community benefit investments—is discussed in the section on anchor institutions.

Although the range of potential funders of efforts to advance community well-being and to address the roots of health inequity has expanded, the ongoing need to secure adequate and sustainable funding even in the face of constraints (e.g., both ongoing and acute, such as economic recession) is a fact of life. Partnerships need to be creative and cannot view their work in a silo; identifying leverage points and co-benefits is vital. Funding from the transportation, infrastructure improvement, development, climate resilience, and health sectors needs to be leveraged collaboratively to garner a synergistic effect. The Strong, Prosperous, and Resilient Communities Challenge (SPARCC) is an example that highlights this paradigm shift from silo to overlapping circles, from isolation to synergy. With a $20 million investment and additional capital, six regions will serve as pilot sites for learning about collaborative approaches at the regional level. The partners engaged will include "leaders from the for-profit, nonprofit, philanthropic, and government organizations working across diverse issue areas such as transportation, community development, racial equity, climate resiliency, and health," with a goal of promoting integrated outcomes and building capacity to effect systems change (SPARCC, n.d.). Existing funding programs can be leveraged with health and equity principles as a way to award and prioritize funding. For example, California has a cap-and-trade program as one of several strategies to reduce greenhouse gases, and a California legislative requirement allocates a certain amount of funding for disadvantaged communities (CalEPA, n.d.). This type of investment from a climate change program has the direct benefit of promoting health equity.

Role of Philanthropy

The philanthropy sector can use different tools to support communities as they design, implement, and evaluate interventions to achieve health equity. In broad categories, these tools include convening, leadership and capacity development, model testing, topic studies and reports, project and program funding, advocacy support, and social movement building.

Convening is a core strategy for foundations, which may serve the role of a trusted, neutral host in bringing together individuals and organizations from different sectors and disciplines. Most foundations aspire to achieve balance and inclusivity across the broad landscape of community members and other stakeholders and to support engaging across differences to achieve a common goal.

Leadership development and capacity building is another commonly used philanthropic tool that helps address gaps, especially within the nonprofit sector, though other private and public sectors can and do take advantage of these foundation programs. In the case of community interventions that are inclusive of multiple sectors and the affected community, funding both the capacity of all participants to fully engage and the development of new leaders within communities is essential to creating enduring change that will outlast the funding duration.

Model testing refers to smaller-scale, innovative interventions that, while based on robust theories and other inputs, may not have the evidence base to attract other funding sources such as local, state, and federal government agencies. Foundations can take risks with innovative programming, fund appropriate evaluation, and create the evidence that others require to address the issues of scale and sustainability. For most of the philanthropic sector, this is as close as philanthropy gets to funding empirical research.

Foundations do fund studies of specific topics: specifically, studies that review and synthesize existing knowledge, projects, or data and create reports, position papers, media, and other products that are intended to support and inspire other work. In fact, this report is an example of what foundations can do to promote community interventions.

Another core foundation strategy for community work involves grants made for explicit projects or programs. Such philanthropic grant making can be responsive (involving a cyclical review of unsolicited grants that advance the mission of the foundation) or directive (usually involving a request-for-proposals process where agencies such as community nonprofits apply to complete a scope of work created by the foundation). Some foundations are also using novel approaches involving community engagement to distribute decision making for program and project funding to the communities themselves.

Advocacy funding may present challenges for certain foundations for which funding issue-specific advocacy strategies, such as lobbying, is prohibited by federal tax law. Nevertheless, such foundations can support advocacy groups with general operating funds (as distinguished from program-specific funds) that can be used to lobby, as long as the foundation is not involved with decision making about what issues the advocacy group chooses to take on. Foundations can also support social movement building by providing support for organizations that use community organizing to address important social issues. However, many (if not most) foundations choose not to offer funding in the advocacy and policy arenas, despite the opportunities to create significant, sustainable change in health equity issues. This pattern may change over time, however, as foundations look for enduring upstream changes in areas that address their mission.

Another area for foundation support is civil rights law. A 2001 report to The Rockefeller Foundation on racial justice with findings and recommendations for funders that are relevant in considering community solutions to achieve health equity suggests that

- Foundation support is needed to expand civil rights and racial justice lawyering to take on injustice while deepening public understanding of the nature and causes of exclusion, including the complexities of race, ethnicity, and class.
- Civil rights and racial justice lawyering can be a powerful tool to strengthen philanthropic efforts across a range of programs. Creative approaches can help create broader constituencies in various foundation areas, including health, education, and community revitalization.
- Funding for organizational capacity is needed to permit the creation of broad networks and the development of sophisticated techniques.
- Strategic funding of national, regional, and local groups can have a substantial impact. Local groups can work for community solutions around the country while connecting with the broader national civil rights community. Support for problem-solving legal strategies can build trust, build partnerships, and empower community leaders speak for themselves. Lawyers can facilitate access to unresponsive institutions and provide legal leverage against unfair practices. Marginalized communities can use local democracy to challenge structures that isolate and impoverish them (Hair, 2001).

Through greater investments in communities of color and low-income communities, foundations can build on the civil rights movement and advance social justice through advocacy and organizing for structural change (Hansen, 2012; Skocpol, 2013). As an example, while strategic foundation support has enabled the success of the environmental justice movement, funding constraints have made it difficult to build organizational infrastructure, community organizing, leadership development, and effective participation in the policy and legal arenas. Reliable, predictable, and flexible multiyear core support for health, environmental justice, and racial equity organizations is necessary for them to carry out their mission, respond to new challenges and opportunities, and serve their communities (Bullard and Garcia, 2015; Joassart-Marcelli, 2010;

Joassart-Marcelli et al., 2011). For a community example of an environmental justice organization that successfully leverages foundation support to build healthier and more equitable communities, see the discussion of WE ACT for Environmental Justice in Chapter 5.

The California Endowment's Building Healthy Communities initiative offers a noteworthy example of a philanthropic multi-sector intervention to achieve health equity. This 10-year, 14-community strategy has, at its 5-year mark, achieved improved health coverage for the underserved, as grantees and partners fought for and supported the successful implementation of the Patient Protection and Affordable Care Act (ACA) and the expansion of Medicaid in California. There has been a stronger health coverage policy for undocumented residents as grantees and partners successfully crafted and led the #Health4All Campaign,[1] paving the way for state-supported health coverage for undocumented children. There have been school climate, wellness, and equity improvements as grantees, partners, and youth have led or supported efforts across the state to reform harsh school discipline and suspension policies, and they continue to work to successfully implement school equity funding formulas. Foundation grantees and partners have lent advocacy support for health- and prevention-oriented justice system reform; a key objective of justice reinvestment is to channel savings from a reduced need for prisons into prevention strategies. Grantees have joined with other coalitions supporting outcome improvement work in young men of color, bringing improved public policy and civic attention to the issue and resulting in the creation of a Select Committee on the Status of Boys and Men of Color in the state legislature. Finally, the Building Healthy Communities initiative has helped grantees in their efforts to enact more than 100 local policies and system changes, ultimately promoting a culture of health in local jurisdictions that emphasizes such community resources as more walkable neighborhoods, fresh food access, park space, and access to safe drinking water.

> **Recommendation 7-1: Foundations and other funders should support community interventions to promote health equity by:**
> - **Supporting community organizing around important social determinants of health;**
> - **Supporting community capacity building;**
> - **Supporting education, compliance, and enforcement related to civil rights laws; and**

---

[1] For more information, see http://www.calendow.org/prevention/health4all (accessed December 19, 2016).

- Prioritizing health equity and equity in the social determinants of health through investments in low-income and minority communities.

Reliable, predictable, and flexible multiyear core support for health, environmental justice, and racial equity organizations is necessary for them to carry out their missions, respond to new challenges and opportunities, and serve their communities. With available tools, philanthropy can play an important role in supporting community interventions to achieve health equity and should be considered as an important potential partner in this work.

Role of Business

The U.S. business community has a significant stake in correcting health inequities as a strategy for stabilizing and strengthening the U.S. economy. Business contributes positively (or negatively) to health and healthy conditions in several ways: as payers offering their employees health care benefits; as employers who have a role in ensuring workplace health and safety; as producers of goods and services that may have implications for health and well-being; as creators of externalities (e.g., causing environmental impacts through such things as the production of greenhouse gases) or promoters of sustainable technology; and through their philanthropic efforts, as funders of a range of activities that may contribute to improving public health. The various ways that businesses can affect health and well-being also illustrate the multiple pathways for business involvement in promoting health equity: through a focus on health care; through workplace wellness and safety; through corporate social responsibility (e.g., sustainability programs, impact investing of education, and other determinants of health); and through philanthropic endeavors.

Several major U.S. organizations that have addressed employee health for decades, including the U.S. Chamber of Commerce and the National Business Group on Health (NBGH), have in the past several years begun to consider the potential for a wider role for business, beyond workplace wellness and health care insurance, in addressing the social determinants of health and achieving health equity. Analogous to the gradual shift from focusing primarily on health care benefits and how their growing cost affects the corporate "bottom line," to achieving a better quality of care and better value—including by addressing inequities in health care— there has been an evolution in thinking about worker health and wellness to a greater consideration of the social determinants of health and ways for business to expand opportunity in communities.

Examples of the former include the NBGH Innovation in Advancing Health Equity Award (formerly called the Innovation in Reducing Health Care Disparities Award) and its development of a health disparities cost impact tool and an employer's guide to reducing racial and ethnic disparities in the workplace (Dan et al., 2011). In 2014 a U.S. Chamber of Commerce event entitled Innovations in Workplace and Community Wellness: Navigating the New Terrain included a session titled The Business Case for Equity of Care, in which Kenneth Thorpe spoke about how gaps in equity present "large human and economic costs" and how non-health factors, including community environments, affect health outcomes and the deep inequities among them.

Examples of the latter—the move toward considering what shapes health beyond the factory or office walls—include several high-profile efforts and reports published over the past 2 years. In a report making the business case for racial equity in Michigan, the author writes of the experience of America's Edge and ReadyNation, among other business-oriented efforts to expand opportunity, and concludes that "racially-based obstacles to the success of today's younger generation threaten our economy and security. Tackling these obstacles is not only the right thing to do; it can be a significant driver of our collective social and economic well-being" (Turner, 2015). One company that has taken on wellness outside of the office walls is the Rosen Hotels and Resorts, which has shifted its benefits for employees to include college tuition and the construction of a medical center for employees. Rosen has also contributed to funding for a local preschool in a community that was suffering from low graduation rates and high rates of violence.

In 2015 the Vitality Institute published a report that provided support for business leaders' interest in engaging with communities and others to improve health beyond the company walls. The report illuminated the links between an unhealthy workforce and conditions in their communities of residence. It echoed other research in asserting that the limited investment in disease prevention and social programs and services and heavy investment in treatment has contributed to disparities in outcomes. The authors concluded that "investments in community health have substantial potential to impact the health of the workforce in these sectors, to narrow occupation-related health disparities among working-age Americans, and to reduce the risk that non-communicable diseases pose to the economic vitality of the nation" (Oziransky et al., 2015). Notably, the report called for employer–community partnerships and recommended that employers "engage in strategic philanthropy and use market-driven solutions to create shared value and address health disparities" (Oziransky et al., 2015). Box 7-1 briefly describes a business–community partnership that seeks to improve community health.

> **BOX 7-1**
> **Campbell's Healthy Communities Initiative**
>
> In 2011 the Campbell's Soup Company made a commitment to measurably improve the health of the young people in its hometown, Camden, New Jersey, by reducing childhood obesity and hunger by 50 percent.[a] Along with this commitment, Campbell's Soup decided to keep its corporate headquarters housed in Camden, despite the city's social and economic challenges at the time. Since then, the company has been engaged in a collaborative effort to invest in the community by focusing on four strategic areas:
>
> - Ensuring access to affordable and fresh food;
> - Increasing physical activity in a safe environment;
> - Supporting healthy lifestyles through nutrition education; and
> - Partnering with the community to advance positive social change.
>
> ---
>
> [a] For more information, see https://www.campbellsoupcompany.com/newsroom/news/2015/03/23/campbells-healthy-communities-taking-shape-in-camden (accessed October 21, 2016).
> SOURCES: RWJF, 2015a; Campbell's, 2015.

Another development in the business sector that can be deployed to engage community-based partners on the topic of collaborative action to improve well being and economic vitality, if not explicitly health equity, is the notion of the triple bottom line (*The Economist*, 2009): profit, people, planet or achieving balance or harmony among financial, social, and environmental impacts. This notion is conceptually linked with the increasingly popular business sector definition of shared value (Porter and Kramer, 2011) as balancing profit with sustainability and social benefit and the evidence against viewing them as trade-offs (see Chapter 4).

In *Capitalism at Risk: Rethinking the Role of Business*, Harvard Business School professors highlighted chief executive officer remarks from a series of symposia on capitalism's greatest challenges (Bower et al., 2011). These include executives' concern about societal risks that tear the fabric of public trust, such as income and wealth inequality and its effects—exploitation and political and financial instability. Bower and colleagues observed that "health care costs affect the competitiveness of U.S. businesses but also constitute the leading cause of personal bankruptcy, contributing significantly to the burden of low income," and they added that, in light of these costs, "it is surprising that business has on the whole been so little engaged with the question" (Bower et al., 2011). Business leaders at all levels understand that poor health reduces business profits, and although they are not necessarily focused on health equity, they are thinking about health and its implications. Bower and colleagues point out that "it is not hard to imagine individual companies, industry associations, or international groups joining in some kind of program to drive widespread attention to these three aspects [smoking, obesity, and substance abuse] of improved health" (Bower et al., 2011). This attention is aligned with acknowledging that smoking, obesity, and drug abuse are the result of health inequities and that in addition to reducing profitability, these inequities widen economic and opportunity inequalities and political polarization that can lead to gridlock and prevent democracy from solving national problems.

To engage local, regional, and national business leaders in addressing health inequities, one effective approach is to discuss the challenges in terms that permit the leaders to participate as partners. This might involve talking about health inequity as weakening workforce productivity, increasing operating costs and hurting profits, and worsening inequality and political polarization. These approaches enable business people to become involved in matters that matter to most to them. Improving health equity enhances the reputations of those businesses involved. If such efforts are pursued constructively and systematically, business leaders will want to be publicly associated with these efforts because they are viewed as being "good for business." If community leaders and business leaders who are actually concerned about employee productivity, company profitability, and political stability work together effectively, the result will be meaningful improvements that help achieve health equity.

ANCHOR INSTITUTIONS

Many cities in the United States face significant challenges—such as high rates of poverty, high unemployment, and substandard schools—stemming from disinvestment, deindustrialization, globalization, and the related negative impacts on the manufacturing-based economies on which these cities previously relied. Over the past three decades, discussion has evolved on the role of institutions of higher education and medical centers in the economic, cultural, and social fabric of cities (Harkavy et al., 2014; Netter Center for Community Partnerships, 2008). These are only a few of what have been described as anchor institutions.[2] Anchor institutions were first described in 2001 (Harkavy et al., 2014) and sub-

---

[2] Key anchor institutions within a local community include educational, health care, and infrastructure. Additional anchor institutions include local government entities; faith-based organizations; and cultural institutions, such as museums, arts centers, or sports venues (Rubin and Rose, 2015).

sequently "emerged as [a] new paradigm for understanding the role that place-based institutions could play in building successful communities and local economies" (Taylor and Luter, 2013, p. 4). While there are many definitions of anchor institutions, Taylor and Luter note three agreed-upon features of anchor institutions: "anchors are large, spatially immobile, mostly nonprofit organizations that play an integral role in the local economy" (Taylor and Luter, 2013, p. 8). Because anchor institutions are "firmly rooted in their locales" (Norris and Howard, 2015, p. 8) and therefore are considered "sticky capital"—that is, they have "an economic self-interest in helping ensure that the communities in which they are based are safe, vibrant, and healthy" (Serang et al., 2013, p. 4).

Citing arguments by Hodges and Dubb (Hodges and Dubb, 2012), a report by Serang and colleagues defines an anchor mission as "a commitment to consciously apply their long-term, place-based economic power of the institution, in combination with its human and intellectual resources, to better the long-term welfare of the communities in which the institution is anchored" (Serang et al., 2013, p. 5).

Anchor institutions such as universities and hospitals have significant economic, social, and cultural impacts in their surrounding communities (ICIC, 2011). Their relevance for cities is particularly noteworthy: of the 100 largest city cores in the United States, 66 have an anchor institution as the largest employer, and 1 in 8 (about 925) U.S. colleges and universities and 1 in 15 (about 350) hospitals are based in such areas (ICIC, 2011).

Universities and hospitals are powerful local economic engines; they have significant holdings in real estate and expenditures related to procurement for goods and services, endowments, and employment (Norris and Howard, 2015). As shown in Figure 7-1, hospitals in the United States have annual expenditures of nearly $800 billion and nearly $350 billion in purchasing alone, and they employ 5.5 million individuals annually (Norris and Howard, 2015). Annually, the 4,100 universities in the United States educate 21 million students, employ 4 million people, and have more than $400 billion in endowments and $460 billion in economic activity (Harkavy et al., 2014; Snyder and Dillow, 2015). Together hospitals and universities employ 8 percent of the U.S. labor force and account for more than 7 percent of U.S. gross domestic product (Norris and Howard, 2015). Their economic, intellectual, and human capital places anchor institutions in a unique position to improve and enrich surrounding communities in partnership with other key place-based stakeholders from sectors such as government, business, faith, and community-based organizations and local residents. Yet, the economic and social impacts of universities, colleges, and hospitals in their local and surrounding communities can vary, are often undocumented, and contribute to the quality of relationships between such anchors and local residents. A number of scholars

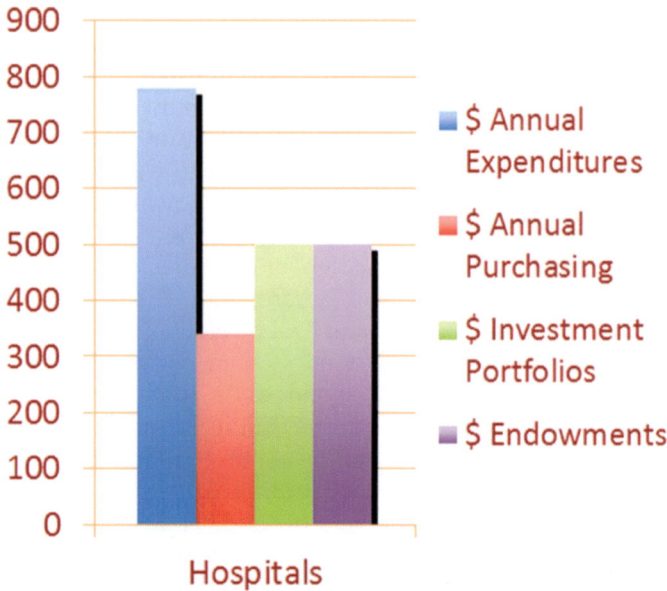

FIGURE 7-1 Annual hospital spending in the United States.
SOURCE: Norris and Howard, 2015.

have written about the often-conflicting relationships between such large organizations and local communities, particularly when local residents do not perceive their communities to be directly benefiting from the presence of such institutions (Martin et al., 2005; Miller and Rivera, n.d.; O'Mara, 2012). Rubin and Rose (2015) have noted that "[m]any anchors have a history of being distant from grassroots communities or of wielding their power and influence in ways that advance their immediate agenda but not that of nearby residents or the broader public" (Rubin and Rose, 2015, p. 2): for example, in terms of their human resources and procurement practices and real estate investments.

Consensus is growing regarding the benefits of such an anchor role. Harkavy and colleagues note that such institutions (1) are affected by their local environment and, as such, have a stake in the health of surrounding communities; (2) have a moral and ethical responsibility to contribute to the well-being of surrounding communities because they can make a difference; and (3) when involved in solving real-world local problems, they are more likely to advance learning, research, teaching, and service (Harkavy et al., 2014).

Becoming an "engaged anchor" (Rubin and Rose, 2015, p. 2) and adopting an anchor mission to implement and assess impacts on local communities requires a conscious and intentional approach in governance (Harkavy et al., 2014). For example, this includes the involvement of leadership from universities and hospitals, including the board of trustees, senior administration, and faculty in developing an operational strategy and new organizational structures in order to produce meaningful change.

Recent initiatives by the National Task Force on Anchor Institutions (NTFAI) (NTFAI, 2010) and the Democracy Collaborative (Democracy Collaborative, n.d.-a) have focused on leveraging the economic power of anchor institutions that reside within or next to low-income communities to improve community conditions and the health and well-being of local residents. While many universities and hospitals have community programs as part of their community engagement and community benefit efforts, the NFTAI-proposed anchor institution approach is different. It focuses on altering traditional anchor institution *business* practices in order to deploy anchor institutions' economic power locally to help improve the underlying conditions that shape health. The premise is that hospitals and universities have a unique responsibility and role, along with other anchor institutions (e.g., community foundations, local governments, and key infrastructure services), in helping solve local problems, including those affecting the health of local residents, and that they are uniquely positioned to use their vast economic knowledge and human resources to contribute to the improvement of the quality of life in their local communities. Furthermore, Birch and colleagues "suggest that the entire topic of the university as an engaged, anchor institution is a strategic element of the modern academy (Gaffikin and Perry, 2009) embedded in the practices of university leadership" (Birch et al., 2013).

Using the social determinants of health framework, the NTFAI and the Democracy Collaborative developed a framework, approach, and metrics that universities and hospitals can use to increase their economic investment in the local neighborhoods where they reside and to improve living conditions and quality of life (Dubb et al., 2013). Findings from interviews with anchor institution leaders, partnership directors, staff, and a broad range of representatives from national association and community development groups reveal the influential factors that led to the adoption of an anchor mission and strategy and the challenges related to this. Most importantly, the report outlines a set of equity and community benefits indicators and metrics with which anchor institutions can track their contributions and progress toward goals related to improving community well-being and wealth. A data dashboard was developed that allows anchors to use a shared metric for assessing such progress. The

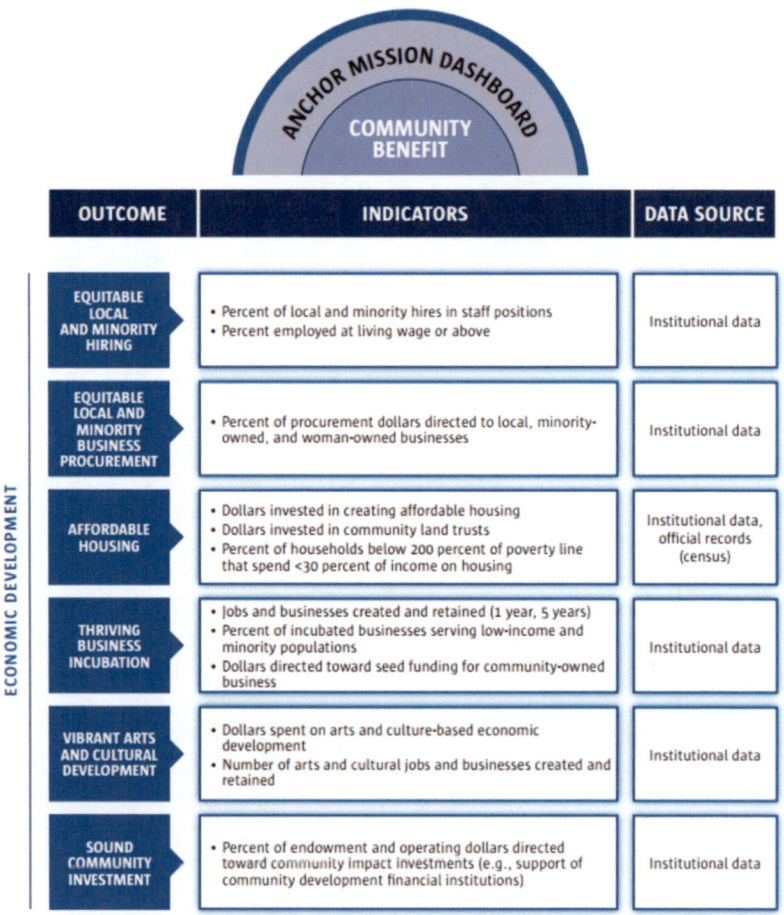

FIGURE 7-2 Anchor institution community benefit dashboard.
SOURCE: Democracy Collaborative, 2014.

dashboard identifies the desired outcome, indicators, and data sources for community benefits. As shown in Figure 7-2, these are couched in the social determinants of health framework and are highly consistent with the role of multi-sector collaboration and the critical role of community residents. Furthermore, the report highlights the importance of shared value and self-interest as motivating forces for anchor institutions to play an active and strategic role in improving conditions in their surrounding communities.

Six universities (Cleveland State University, Drexel University, the University of Memphis, the University of Missouri–St. Louis, Rutgers University–Newark, and SUNY Buffalo State) are participating in the Learning Cohort to pilot the Anchor Institution Mission and Metrics Dashboard (Democracy Collaborative, 2014). This effort is expected to lead to the identification of lessons learned and evidence-based strategies using a shared framework.

Examples of Anchor Institution Strategies

There are numerous examples of how universities and hospitals have implemented an anchor institution strategy to improve conditions in their local communities, particularly with a focus on the social determinants of health (Rooney and Gittleman, 2015; Rubin and Rose, 2015; Zuckerman, 2013). These new anchor institution approaches (Andrews and Erickson, 2012; Harkavy and Zuckerman, 1999) share a number of the features noted in the model discussed in this report (see Figure 1-3). For example, their focus is well aligned with upstream approaches relevant to the social determinants of health, such as the creation of workforce training and living-wage jobs with good benefits to increase employment among local residents; building wealth and reducing debt among community residents; creating and improving existing affordable housing; increasing community safety and access to safe green space and parks and affordable healthy food; enriching the presence of and participation in the arts; building advocacy and action capacity among community residents and community-based organizations; and engaging multiple private and public sectors in partnerships.

This new paradigm for anchor institution commitment to improve conditions in their local communities differs from past failed efforts. Such past efforts commonly relied only or primarily on government and foundation grants to universities to develop time-limited projects with their cities and communities without any real integration of the work into their institutional mission, culture, and organizational structure (Taylor and Luter, 2013). Treated as an add-on, these projects were not sustainable and are thought to have contributed little to improving local community conditions (Taylor and Luter, 2013).

For example, the Community–Campus Partnerships for Health (CCPH) is a nonprofit membership organization established in 1997 that promotes health equity and social justice through partnerships between communities and academic institutions (CCPH, n.d.). Members view health broadly as physical, mental, emotional, social, and spiritual well-being and emphasize partnership approaches to health that focus on changing the conditions and environments in which people live, work, study, pray, and play. By mobilizing knowledge, providing training and technical assistance, conducting research, building coalitions, and advocating for supportive policies, CCPH helps to ensure that the reality of community engagement and partnership matches the rhetoric (CCPH, 2007, 2012).

As noted in the examples below, anchor institutions can and are playing an important role in uplifting community conditions through a series of multilevel strategies and economic investment. However, an anchor institution approach is not a panacea, especially if it is not combined with an equitable approach to economic development that meaningfully uplifts the living conditions of long-term, poor residents. Without intentional attention paid to equitable benefits from economic development, such efforts risk contributing to gentrification and the displacement of existing poor residents. Thus, at the crux of anchor institution efforts is the challenge of how to improve community conditions without displacement but instead with observable and measureable indicators that living conditions have improved for the individuals and families living in these neighborhoods prior to reinvestment. The following are community examples of anchor institution approaches to improving community conditions and improving health outcomes. Box 7-2 highlights a few examples of institutions applying the anchor approach.

BOX 7-2
Anchor Institutions: Some Highlights

The Cleveland Model, Cleveland, Ohio

Within the new anchor institution paradigm, one of the most comprehensive and developed models is the Cleveland Greater University Circle Initiative, known as the Cleveland Model (ICIC, 2011; Serang et al., 2013; Wright et al., 2016). This effort involves multi-sectorial partnerships of more than 50 anchor institutions, including Case Western University, the Cleveland Orchestra, the Cleveland Museum of Art, the Cleveland Museum of Natural History, the Cleveland Public Library, University Hospitals of Cleveland, and several churches. Its approach is multipronged, synergistic, and coalesces around four high-level, shared, economic inclusion goals: (1) *buy locally*: increase opportunities for anchors to purchase goods and services locally, helping small businesses to grow and increase their capacity to meet these needs; (2) *hire locally*: increase the number of residents from the neighborhoods hired by the anchors, helping to improve the local workforce system; (3) *live locally*: support and improve employer-assisted housing for home purchase and renovations and apartment rental, and leverage these resources to help create more stable neighborhoods; and (4) *connect*: seek to eliminate silos

BOX 7-2 Continued

and create connections by reweaving community networks, fostering community engagement, and lifting residents' voices and connection to anchor institution resources (Wright et al., 2016).

The Cleveland Model stakeholders recognize that documenting impact is critical and thus have identified metrics and hired an evaluator to track changes, recognizing that accomplishing population-level changes will take time. Reports reflect impressive and significant financial investments by multiple anchor partners, the implementation of institutional changes aligned with the institutional goals noted above, and preliminary indicators that anchor institutions have pivoted in their approach through the implementation of major initiatives such as the establishment of three worker co-owned cooperatives, workforce training programs, local hiring practices, and housing assistance programs (ICIC, 2011; Serang et al., 2013; Wright et al., 2016).

Not surprisingly, among the areas of Cleveland with the greatest gentrification is University Circle, where the Cleveland Model's activities have been focused (Governing, n.d.). Cleveland's rank of 45th out of 50 metro areas in terms of upward mobility (Chetty and Hendren, 2015) underscores the need for equitable development approaches that benefit the poor.

Henry Ford Health System, Detroit, Michigan

Henry Ford Health System is Detroit's fifth largest employer and generates more than $1.7 billion per year (Henry Ford Health System, n.d.). In collaboration with other anchor institutions, its anchor strategy includes (1) neighborhood revitalization that includes campus expansion, transportation, and façade improvements in local neighborhood acquisition and the rehabilitation of properties with the state's housing development authority; (2) significant local and minority purchasing and a transparent sourcing policy to increase minority business opportunities; (3) land acquisition to attract large suppliers to Detroit; (4) contract opportunities for local small businesses; (5) employer-assisted housing programs; (6) a 5-year clinical degree program for high school students; (7) nonprofit technology business incubator services; and (8) health systems partnerships to reduce infant mortality (Wright et al., 2016).

Gentrification has not hit Detroit to the same degree as other major metro areas (Wright et al., 2016), likely because of the major economic challenges facing Detroit, including bankruptcy. Detroit is the most segregated city in the United States (Neavling, 2013). Detroit's economic challenges led some city leaders to call for gentrification with the hopes of increasing the city's tax base (Neavling, 2013). There is a concern that development and the resulting gentrification in some areas of the city do not address the needs of most residents, including the significant number living in poverty (Doucet, 2015; Woods, 2014).

Trinity Health, Headquarters: Livonia, Michigan

Trinity Health is one of the largest multi-institutional Catholic health care delivery systems in the nation (Trinity Health, n.d.). It serves individuals and communities in 22 states from coast to coast, with 93 hospitals and 120 continuing care

continued

> **BOX 7-2 Continued**
>
> locations, including home care, hospice, PACE (Program of All-inclusive Care for the Elderly), and senior living facilities. With annual operating revenues of $15.9 billion and assets of $23.4 billion,[a] the organization returns almost $1 billion to its communities annually in the form of charity care and other community benefit programs.
>
> Community health and well-being is central to Trinity Health's mission and to becoming a people-centered health system. An increased focus on policy, systems, and environmental change strategies across the organization through efforts such as Tobacco 21, launched in 2015, has yielded tremendous success. In partnership with the Campaign for Tobacco Free Kids, Trinity Health served as a catalyst to make Tobacco 21 a national priority with jurisdictions all over the country by starting the conversation, providing technical assistance, and helping pass legislation.
>
> In addition to leveraging its ability to affect policy, Trinity Health launched the Transforming Communities Initiative (TCI) in November 2015 to improve community health and well-being by providing up to $80 million in grants, loans, community match dollars, and services to address the root causes of poor health. Six community partnerships were announced as grant recipients to focus on the policy, systems, and environmental changes that directly affect areas of high local need. The programs focus on reducing tobacco use and obesity, both of which are leading drivers of preventable chronic disease and high health care costs in the United States. TCI also leverages Trinity Health's investment portfolio to enhance the built environment. The Reinvestment Fund and IFF, two community development financial institutions serving the geographic region, serve as capital partners. They will manage Trinity's loan capital and related technical assistance to ensure the implementation of capital projects that address gaps in the built environment. Specifically, Trinity Health will support affordable housing projects, healthy food access projects, and early childhood education projects.
>
> ---
>
> [a] As of March 22, 2016.

Role of Academic Research Centers

One federal strategy to promote the more rapid adoption of clinical research was the establishment of the Clinical and Translational Science Award (CTSA) program, which initially funded 12 institutions (NCATS, n.d.-a). The CTSA program, has grown and evolved over time to more than 60 organizations, but while funding support for community engagement efforts has decreased over the past few years, engaging patients and communities in every phase of the process of translating research into practice remains a program goal. Members of the CTSA consortium collaborated in the publication of community engagement principles (ATSDR, 2011) as well as other products that may be useful to communities, such as logic models (Eder et al., 2013) and suggested measures. A 2013 Institute of Medicine (IOM) report reinforced the critical role of community engagement in all phases of research, from basic research to clinical practice and community and public health research, and concluded that these partnerships with patients, family members, health care providers, and other community stakeholders need to be preserved, nurtured, and expanded (IOM, 2013).

Many CTSA program awardees make resources available to community-based organizations and community members through their community engagement activities. The Irving Institute, funded through Columbia University's CTSA, includes a freestanding community engagement center, the CCPH. From the perspective of university researchers, CCPH supports community-engaged research as well as recruitment and data collection at a convenient place in the primarily Latino community of Washington Heights/Inwood in New York City. However, CCPH also offers resources and services, including free blood pressure screening and meeting space for community-based organizations. (See the description of the community example WE ACT for Environmental Justice in Chapter 5 for information on other Columbia University programs that have fostered local engagement in community research in marginalized neighborhoods of northern Manhattan in New York City.)

Academic organizations funded through the CTSA program (NCATS, n.d.-b) have developed and made available resources that can be used to promote community-based solutions for health equity, such as a health literacy review service and computers for community members to use. The Partnership of Academicians and Communities for Translation (PACT) of the Colorado Clinical & Translational Science Institute includes the PACT Council, which comprises 18 members with equal representation from the university and community, with participants from more than 20 ethnic, geographic, and self-identified communities facing a range of health disparities (Westfall et al., 2013). Two activities are particularly relevant for community-based solutions to achieve health equity. First, more than $200,000 per year is awarded in pilot grants for innovative programs that address health disparities identified by the community. Second, there is a robust educational program aimed at graduate students, researchers, and community members. This includes a seminar series on community engagement as well as the Colorado Immersion Training program, which provides an intensive longitudinal experience for researchers to develop and sustain community-engaged research, including a placement in a local community.

As noted in Chapters 3 and 4, respectively, transdisciplinary research approaches are needed to produce more of the evidence necessary to inform work on health equity, and the knowledge base that communities can draw on today to design solutions to reduce health inequities is not well matched to the challenge (i.e., randomized controlled trials are not a good fit for generating evidence on approaches that address the social, economic, environmental, and structural factors that shape health). An increased knowledge base could inform and guide communities in applying the promising strategies needed to shed light on systems and how to change them, to increase the understanding of complex and interacting initiatives aimed at population-wide change, and to support the work of continuing adaptation to improve outcomes. Yet, longstanding traditions and institutional arrangements have favored a narrow swath of research—research using controlled experimental methods to identify circumscribed programs that have been found to be effective in controlled settings. Therefore, based on the committee's expertise and its examination of the available evidence, the committee recommends the following:

Recommendation 7-2: A number of actions to improve the knowledge base for informing and guiding communities should be taken, including
- **Public and private research funders should support communities and their academic partners in the collection, analysis, and application of evidence from the experience of practitioners, from leaders of community-based organizations, and from traditionally underrepresented participants who are typically left out of such partnerships.**
- **Universities, policy centers, and academic publications should modify current incentive[3] structures to encourage and reward more research on the social distribution of risks and resources and the systematic generation and dissemination of the evidence needed to guide the complex, multi-faceted interventions that are most likely to reduce inequities in health outcomes.[4]**

---

[3] Such incentives may include funding, publication standards, and rules governing tenure.

[4] SQUIRE (Standards for Quality Improvement Reporting Excellence) is an example of concerted efforts by leaders in one sector—health care—to change powerful incentives. The SQUIRE guidelines provide an explicit framework for reporting new knowledge about system-level work to improve the quality, safety, and value of health care in the hope of shifting the emphasis and rewards from a near-exclusive emphasis on experimental findings to examining interventions closely, carefully, and in detail; generating important new knowledge about systems of care; and learning about how best to change those systems (Davidoff and Batalden, 2005).

- Academic programs should promote the development of and dialogue on theory, methods, and the training of students to create a more useful knowledge base in the next generation of researchers on how to design, implement, and evaluate place-based initiatives to improve community health.

Regarding the final bullet in Recommendation 7-2, such programs would contribute to preparing population health researchers and practitioners to advance knowledge that leads to improved population health science. These future researchers will need to address several questions, such as

- Through which modifiable mechanisms do community-level factors affect health directly and indirectly? And for which populations and what health conditions?
- Which policy and community-level levers are the most powerful, feasible, and sustainable for improving health in varied community settings—and for what health conditions?
- What have been promising approaches for place-based interventions, and what methodological challenges have they faced in documenting change at the population level and scaling up?
- What is the role of social capital, collective efficacy, community organizing, and the empowerment of community residents as agents of change for improving community conditions in place-based interventions? And what effective or promising approaches have been used?
- How and under what circumstances can researchers and community-based organizers best partner with each other, and what are the most effective community organizing strategies to promote health equity?
- What is the role of anchor institution policies and practices, including for colleges and universities, within poor neighborhoods in contributing to improving community conditions and fostering health equity? What are the pros and cons of various campus-community partnership models? What evidence exists regarding the efficacy and impact of these partnerships on the factors that affect health and health outcomes among local poor communities? (Smedley and Amaro, 2016)

Hospitals and Health Systems

Hospitals and health care systems share in the responsibility to improve health equity. The American College of Healthcare Executives, the American Hospital Association (AHA), America's Essential Hospitals, the Association of American Medical Colleges, and the Catholic Health Association of the United States have urged all hospitals to "take the #123forEquity Pledge to Eliminate Health Care Disparities" (AHA, n.d.-a). The AHA provides a tool kit (AHA, 2015) and other resources (AHA, n.d.-b) for hospitals that pursue the #123forEquityPledge.

In a review of the literature and interviews with leaders of health care organizations, the Institute for Healthcare Improvement (IHI) outlines practical steps and a conceptual framework for guiding health care organizations that want to begin a journey to improved health equity. The IHI stresses the importance of "making health equity a strategic priority at every level of an organization, especially at the top" (IHI, 2016, p. 4) and outlines a number of concrete ways for health care systems to get started. The paper offers a framework for change and a self-assessment tool for health care organizations to assess their current state on each component of the IHI framework. In the IHI and AHA materials, hospitals are urged to start their health equity journey by looking at practices within their own institutions, with the stated goal of "dismantling the institutional racism and implicit biases that hold us back" (IHI, 2016). The AHA equity-of-care tool kit highlights the steps that hospitals can take—starting with leadership—including better collection and use of data on race and ethnicity, cultural competency training, and increasing diversity in governance and leadership (AHA, 2015). Key components of the IHI framework are outlined below:

- Begin quality improvement work by considering the needs and issues faced by populations experiencing worse health outcomes and the greatest disparities in the social determinants of health.
- Tailor quality improvement efforts to meet the needs of marginalized populations across the continuum of social determinants of health.
- Include traditionally disenfranchised people in health care transformation efforts and in advisory positions.
- Use the required community health needs assessment (CHNA) as an opportunity to pursue health equity issues in a more coordinated approach with other hospitals and diverse stakeholders committed to advancing health equity (see Box 7-3 for a brief overview of CHNA for charitable hospitals).
- Provide cultural competency education within the institution and in the community.
- Procure supplies and services from women- and minority-owned businesses and use hiring practices that promote diversity and

> **BOX 7-3**
> **Community Health Needs Assessment**
>
> The community health needs assessment (CHNA) is both the activity and product of identifying and prioritizing a community's health needs. Changes to the Internal Revenue Code with the passage of the Patient Protection and Affordable Care Act (ACA) in 2010 imposed new requirements on each charitable hospital beginning in the tax year 2 years after the passage of the ACA to conduct a CHNA and adopt an implementation strategy that addresses the identified needs. CHNAs can be used to address health equity in communities, and there are several examples of CHNAs that do (Providence Hospital, n.d.; Viveiros and Sturtevant, 2016). The ACA and the Internal Revenue Service (IRS) rules require a hospital's CHNA and implementation strategy be approved by an authorized body of the hospital, usually the hospital's board, which must represent the community. IRS rules implementing the CHNA provisions require hospitals to get input into their assessments from persons knowledgeable about disparities, specifically "medically underserved populations (including) populations experiencing health disparities or at risk of not receiving adequate medical care as a result of being uninsured or underinsured or due to geographic, language, financial, or other barriers."[a]
>
> ---
> [a] Affordable Care Act. Section 501(r)3(4)(b).

inclusion; increasing diversity in hospital leadership and governance is especially important.
- Increase access to health care and human services which includes, among other things, building health care facilities in underserved communities.

Hospitals also need to commit to looking beyond the walls of their institutions to address the root causes of poor health that are situated outside hospitals; the primary causes of growing health disparities in the United States do not begin in a doctor's office, and place heavily influences health (see Chapters 2 and 3). To truly advance health equity in the community, hospitals must also have a strong focus on improving the places where people live and work and where children learn and play.

Hospitals are well positioned to help lead multi-sector work aimed at advancing health equity. For example, hospitals are often trusted health leaders in the communities they serve. Nonprofit hospitals are already required to conduct CHNAs (see Chapter 6), a task that could be conducted with a health equity focus. For example

- Bon Secours in Baltimore and Virginia has partnered with community organizations to develop low-income housing.
- Catholic Health Initiatives, a health care system based in Denver, requires all of its hospitals to address one community-identified issue related to violence prevention.
- Our Lady of the Lake Hospital in Baton Rouge has a robust program of school health clinics that includes physical, dental, and mental health. The purpose of the program is to improve school attendance and to ensure that children are ready to learn.
- Presence Health in Chicago is partnering with Catholic Charities and others in the community to form an accountable health community and will be identifying and addressing issues related to social determinants.
- Innovations in the use and sharing of data are increasingly used to bring partners together across the social determinants of health to highlight connections, create a common language, and monitor progress across various sectors (e.g., see the Camden Coalition of Healthcare Providers[5]).

Moreover, as anchor institutions, hospitals are deeply rooted economic engines in the communities they serve, holding significant social capital and controlling vast amounts of real estate and other financial investments (see the section on the role of anchor institutions in this chapter). By leveraging their economic power, good will, and human resources, hospitals can make significant advancements in health equity. The role of hospitals is explored further in the discussion of anchor institutions below.

Community health centers and federally qualified health centers (FQHCs) have long played a role in providing primary care services to underserved populations, including uninsured and underinsured individuals and families (for a summary of the first rural FQHC, Delta Health Center, see Chapter 5). A 2010 report on FQHC partnerships with local health departments described "promoting health equity and eliminating health disparities" as one goal of such partnerships (Zakheim et al., 2010).

In 2015 the National Association of Community Health Centers (NACHC) implemented the Protocol for Responding to and Assessing Patients' Assets, Risks, and Experiences (PRAPARE), a national effort to help health centers and other providers collect the data needed to better understand and take action on their patients' social determinants

---

[5] For more information, see https://www.camdenhealth.org (accessed December 19, 2016).

of health.[6] The PRAPARE Core Measures include, in addition to race, ethnicity, and education, housing status and housing stability, migrant and seasonal farm worker status, material security, transportation, social integration and support, and stress. The PRAPARE tool is being used with different electronic health record systems and in different settings (NACHC, n.d.-b).

Anchor Institution Approaches

Anchor institutions, including universities, hospitals, and other entities discussed earlier in this chapter, that are located in low-income communities have an important role to play in improving local economies and the community conditions that affect health. The anchor institution approach of an articulated mission, strategies, and metrics to improve community conditions has gained increasing attention and buy-in in a number of major metropolitan areas. Such organizations have made significant investment, usually with a number of other anchor partners, including city government and, often, private investors. Data on how such efforts have improved the living conditions of long-term and poor residents are not yet available.

Yet, a number of the anchor investment areas have evidenced gentrification and displacement, and often local residents question whether long-term and poor residents have benefited compared to the benefits gained by anchor partners and wealthier residents who have moved into the areas. Thus, while anchor investment areas are promising, a major remaining challenge for anchor institutions is whether in fact they can improve the quality of life for low-income residents in their surrounding neighborhoods. This will require keeping a careful eye on the development of community initiatives that equitably benefit long-term and poor residents of their surrounding communities.

An alternative to the traditional approach to economic development described by the Democracy Collaborative focuses on community wealth building (Kelly and McKinley, 2015). Figure 7-3 shows the drivers of community wealth and the differences between traditional and community wealth-building approaches to economic development. Figure 7-4 shows six strategies for the wealth-building approach. The wealth-building approach does not assume that economic development will result in "trickle down" benefits to local residents and instead employs and builds

---

[6] "PRAPARE has been a multi-year effort between NACHC, the Association of Asian Pacific Community Health Organizations, the Oregon Primary Care Association, and the Institute for Alternative Futures, along with a group of pioneer health centers and health center networks in Hawaii, Iowa, New York, and Oregon" (NACHC, n.d.-a).

Drivers	Community Wealth Building	Traditional Approach
Place	Develops under-utilized local assets of many kinds, for benefit of local residents.	Aims to attract firms using incentives, which increases the tax burden on local residents.
Ownership	Promotes local, broad-based ownership as the foundation of a thriving local economy.	Supports absentee and elite ownership, often harming locally owned family firms.
Multipliers	Encourages institutional buy-local strategies to keep money circulating locally.	Pays less attention to whether money is leaking out of community.
Collaboration	Brings many players to the table: nonprofits, philanthropy, anchors, and cities.	Decision-making led primarily by government and private sector, excluding local residents.
Inclusion	Aims to create inclusive, living wage jobs that help all families enjoy economic security.	Key metric is number of jobs created, with little regard for wages or who is hired.
Workforce	Links training to employment and focuses on jobs for those with barriers to employment.	Relies on generalized training programs without focus on linkages to actual jobs.
System	Develops institutions and supportive ecosystems to create a new normal of economic activity.	Accepts status quo of wealth inequality, hoping benefits trickle down.

FIGURE 7-3 Approaches to and drivers of community wealth building to improve economic development.
SOURCE: Kelly and McKinley, 2015.

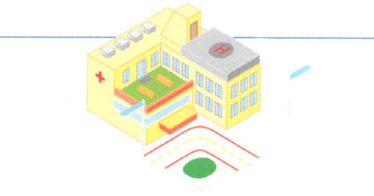

ANCHOR PROCUREMENT
Locally rooted nonprofit institutions (including hospitals, universities, community foundations, and governments) consciously direct resources to drive equitable development.

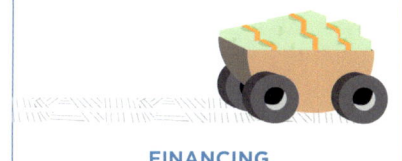

FINANCING
In partnership with CDFIs, foundations, banks, and impact investors, cities create loan funds, make equity investments, and introduce responsible banking ordinances.

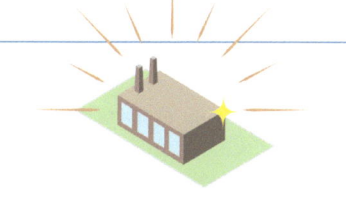

ENTERPRISE DEVELOPMENT
Cities build infrastructure for inclusive enterprises by supporting cooperative development, conversion to employee ownership, and incubator and accelerator creation.

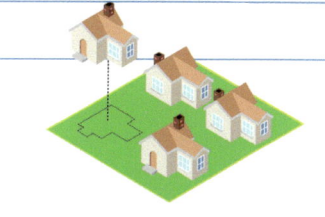

LAND USE & REAL ESTATE
Partnering with others, city governments support equitable land development through urban gardens, community land trusts, and land banks.

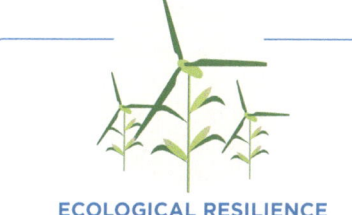

ECOLOGICAL RESILIENCE
Cities pair workforce and ecological goals as they promote energy efficiency, foster renewable energy, recycle materials, and create food hubs.

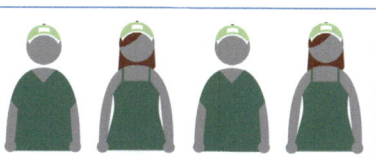

WORKFORCE
Cities consciously link workforce development efforts to employers, especially for residents with barriers to employment, creating pipelines for employment.

FIGURE 7-4 Strategies for building community wealth.
NOTE: CDFI = community development financial institution.
SOURCE: Kelly and McKinley, 2015.

on existing assets within the local community to build sustainable ecosystems that promote equity and provide direct benefit to local residents. This is the real distinction between wealth-building and more prevalent market-driven approaches that can be part of more traditional anchor approaches to development.

The concept of shared value discussed above also offers another approach to the traditional anchor approaches to community and/or economic development. Porter (2010) has described how anchor institutions should view community viability as a critical driver of an anchor's long-term success in workforce hiring, recruitment, and quality of life, and asserted that when anchors make progress working with communities with the greatest need, that can help create "the greatest shared value" (Porter, 2010).

> *Conclusion 7-1: Based on its judgment and its review of community-based efforts to promote health equity or address the determinants of health, the committee concludes that community-based innovations are often most effective when they build on efforts of various community entities (e.g., foundations, anchor institutions) with an existing foundation or body of work and a strong presence in the community.*

Recommendation 7-3: The committee recommends that anchor institutions (such as universities, hospitals, and businesses) make expanding opportunities to promote health equity in their community a strategic priority. This should be done by:
- **Deploying specific strategies to address the multiple determinants of health on which anchors can have a direct impact or through multi-sector collaboration; and**
- **Assessing the negative and positive impacts of anchor institutions in their communities and how negative impacts may be mitigated.[7]**

The literature on institutional racism and implicit bias and effects on health equity is generally focused on health care organizations and settings. Little or no evidence is available for other kinds of anchor institutions (aside from scholarship on racism and bias in academia, although not as anchor institutions or in the context of the production of health inequities). Based on the evidence and examples available from health care, however, and with the support of emerging tools on equity, diversity, and inclusion,[8] anchor institutions could develop a structure and

---

[7] See, for example, McNeely and Norris (2015).
[8] See examples outlined in NASEM, 2016b.

processes to identify and decrease institutional racism and implicit bias within their own institutions to enable them to evaluate their roles and engage with communities more effectively.

OTHER COMMUNITY-BASED PARTNERS

The Role of Faith Organizations

Faith organizations are often a key partner in advocating for and developing or providing health care services as well as in addressing the social determinants of health. Faith organizations are often the entities where issues are first identified at a point when they can be dealt with at a much earlier and resolvable stage. A community of caring and competent volunteers can be mobilized to address the community's needs and to advocate for appropriate legislation and the use of civic resources—including food, shelter, pregnancy care, child care, respite, elderly care, and addiction care—to address health equity (e.g., see a summary of work by ISAIAH, a faith-based community organization, in Box 7-4). Health care providers can be a partner and resource for the many faith communities in their service area. Whether for dental care, opioid addiction, advanced care planning, or domestic abuse, partnering with faith communities can be invaluable, as they often have the most confidence of and credibility with their communities (Schroepfer, 2016). Examples of faith organizations engaging in work to achieve health equity in their communities include the Health Ministries Association, Inc. (HMA, n.d.), the Maryland Faith Health Network (Health Care for All, n.d.), and the Methodist Healthcare Center of Excellence in Faith & Health (Methodist Healthcare, n.d.).

BOX 7-4
ISAIAH: Improving the Health and Wealth of Minnesotans through Grass Roots Organizing and Strategic Partnerships

As part of the PICO Network,[a] ISAIAH is a vehicle for congregations, clergy, and people of faith to act collectively and powerfully toward racial and economic equity in the state of Minnesota. ISAIAH believes that leadership development unites and allows people to take powerful steps to improve the quality of the community. ISAIAH's vision is a Minnesota

continued

> **BOX 7-4 Continued**
>
> - that ensures the conditions in which all Minnesotans can be healthy. ISAIAH is committed to eliminating place-based and race-based health inequities to ensure that all Minnesotans have an opportunity for good health.
> - where the benefits of public infrastructure—roads, bridges, transit, and residential and commercial development—are distributed equitably. This includes opportunities for economic growth, community health, and the increase in wealth that occurs with major transportation and housing or commercial developments.
> - that aligns public investments and applies collective resources to achieve equity in education and that opens access to opportunity to students of color across Minnesota.
> - that seeks fairness in all its dealings, eliminating financial discrimination against communities of color, supporting best practices in foreclosure prevention, and taking an aggressive approach to enforcing fair lending laws (ISAIAH, n.d.).
>
> ISAIAH's mechanisms of change include three components (IOM, 2015b). The first is grassroots leadership development. The second builds upon the first: democratic, accountable, sustainable, community-driven organizations, whose participants are "exercising democracy with each other." The third component of community organizing emphasizes the role of the power or the ability to act in change. In an IOM workshop, executive director Doran Schrantz explained that "differentials in power do not change because somebody else who has more power gives it to you. Differentials in power change because you take ownership

Almost all faith organizations are clear that in addition to preaching the doctrines of their faith, a critical call is to provide service for those in need and those most vulnerable. With their unique position in the community, they have the ability to be invaluable in achieving health equity.

Community Development Corporations

Community development corporations (CDCs) are nonprofit, community-based organizations focused on revitalizing the areas in which they are located, which are typically low-income, underserved neighborhoods that have experienced significant disinvestment (Democracy Collaborative. n.d.-b). The CDC movement is 45 years old, and the Democracy Collaborative reports that more than 4,000 CDCs across the United States engage in a variety of communities, including those with high proportions of racial and ethnic minorities (Democracy Collaborative, n.d.-b). Historically, the emphasis of CDCs has been housing, but today the functions and

and collective and community responsibility for negotiating for the power and the resources you need. When that power structure is in place, that is when change happens" (IOM, 2014, p. 50).

ISAIAH's multi-sectoral efforts target multiple determinants of health including education, employment, health systems and services, housing, income and wealth, the physical and social environments, and transportation. Several activities aimed at income and wealth are notable, including health impact assessments related to the impact of "pinklining" on the wealth and future of women (Bhaskaran, 2016) and the need for payday loan reforms (Purciel-Hill et al., 2016). Additionally, ISAIAH's recent work on paid family leave policy in partnership with the Minnesota Department of Health (MDH) has included

- legislation introduced and moved in 2015, with more than 1,500 faith leaders engaged;
- MDH reports written on income and health and paid leave and health;
- a fiscal and implementation study contracted and conducted from 2015 to 2016;
- state employees granted 6 weeks of paid leave in 2015, with other cities following suit;
- a small business coalition built for paid leave that is robust at the city and state levels;
- municipal campaigns launched for paid sick days in Minneapolis and Saint Paul; and
- paid family leave as the top election issue in 2016 (Schrantz, 2016).

---

[a] For more information, see http://www.piconetwork.org/about (accessed December 15, 2016).

services of CDCs vary widely, with some also offering direct health services. The work of the Thunder Valley CDC, for example, is summarized in Chapter 4. Additional examples below highlight the variety of CDC activities taking place.

Chicanos Por La Causa, Inc. (CPLC) is one of the largest Hispanic CDCs in the United States (CPLC, n.d.). For more than 40 years, CPLC has focused on building stronger, healthier communities by providing the political and economic empowerment that supports individuals to learn the skills and develop the resources necessary to become self-sufficient. Funded through a grant from the Helios Education Foundation, a new program in Arizona focuses on helping 2,000 Hispanic parents develop literacy and advocacy skills related to education and health services. Through the Northern New Mexico Food Hub, Siete Del Norte, a subsidiary of CPLC, is working with community partners to assist local farmers to access commercial markets and make local produce more readily available in rural New Mexico. Health services are provided through multiple CPLC components.

Since 1975 the East Bay Asian Local Development Corporation (EBALDC) has invested more than $200 million in assets in Oakland and the greater San Francisco East Bay area with a primary emphasis on *housing options, social supports,* and *income and wealth* (EBALDC, n.d.). Recently, EBALDC has developed and implemented a healthy neighborhood framework for assessing each potential project, program, and partnership for its potential to bring resources and opportunities that will enable the people who live there to make choices that lead to healthy and vibrant lives. This healthy neighborhood framework also informs assessments of the needs of particular communities as well as the particular approaches to be applied. While the primary emphasis areas remain consistent across activities, special attention is focused on other needs of the community, based on the assessment. EBALDC's work will be complemented by collaboration with local businesses on nearby commercial corridors to improve the business environment, create good jobs, and support business development in the neighborhood.

The Quitman County Development Organization (QCDO) was established in 1977 by a group of African American community activists with a history of engagement in the civil rights movement (QCDO, n.d.). Toward the overall goal of improving the quality of life in northwest Mississippi, QCDO has developed affordable housing, owns a community credit union, provides grants to churches for economic development projects, and engages in a variety of child care social services programs and microenterprise lending. A number of activities target early childhood. For example, the Raising a Reader program targets children 3 to 5 years of age to assist with early language development. In addition, the program equips parents with the skills and knowledge to successfully support their children's growth in reading and language through monthly parent meetings, monthly classroom readings, the provision of books for reading to the child, and parental tracking of books read to the child.

ROLE OF GOVERNMENT

Policy Makers and Elected Officials

Policy makers may be elected officials such as members of city councils or of municipal, county, or school boards; state legislators; mayors and governors; members of Congress; and the president of the United States. Policy makers also include policy and other staff at different jurisdictional levels and in different types of agencies and departments. Policy makers in a specific sector range from the local (e.g., zoning) to the national policy level (e.g., implementers of the Fair Housing Act).

Local policy decisions may have untoward effects that create conditions that contribute to health inequities. The IOM identified the role of policy as a determinant of health in its report *For the Public's Health: Revitalizing Law and Policy to Meet New Challenges* (IOM, 2011). The report provides examples of various policy decisions across sectors that can have impacts on health. For example, land use decisions can shape the physical environment (e.g., building freeways that divide neighborhoods) and agricultural policy can impact the food environment (e.g., corn subsidies contributing to poor diets) (IOM, 2011). There is also research that suggests that policy decisions can have a disproportionate impact on underserved populations. Fullilove and Wallace (2011) examine historical policies such as segregation, redlining, and urban renewal and their effects on minority populations. The displacement of these groups has been linked with violence, family disintegration, substance abuse, sexually transmitted diseases, and stress (Fullilove and Wallace, 2011). The committee finds that policy makers, discussed throughout the report, can play a significant leadership role to promote health equity.

> **Recommendation 7-4:** The committee recommends that local policy makers assess policies, programs, initiatives, and funding allocations for their potential to create or increase health inequities in their communities.

Policy makers and government executives can help spur innovations in connecting the dots for health equity, as in the case of geospatial data that can highlight associations. As an example, the city of Fresno, California, facilitates the collaborative Fresno Community Health Improvement Partnership to build a Health Priority Index, which looks at places that bear the highest burden of disease and serves as a starting point to think about policy, systems, and environmental change. This multi-sector network uses data as a point of conversation for shared priorities and decision making, bringing together city staff, the public health department, community members, planners, and community-based organizations.[9]

Centers for Medicare & Medicaid Services

Addressing unmet needs in the social determinants of health, such as food, housing, and social services, has gained momentum and interest among payers. For example, the Centers for Medicare & Medicaid

---

[9] For more information, see http://www.fchip.org (accessed December 21, 2016).

Services recently developed an innovation project, "accountable health communities," that required screening patient populations for unmet needs and referring them for services. Participating health care institutions were required to demonstrate linkages with local resources and joint planning. As part of the program, a common screening tool will be developed. A broad social-determinants-of-health lens would require comprehensive screening across many areas, including housing, food security, employment, transportation, and education. It would also elicit consumers' desire for assistance. Various tools along these lines have been developed in pediatrics.

Some evidence-based models exist that rely on screening and referral. In addition, there are pediatric models that embed intervention services related to social determinants of health (reading, early childhood education, and advocacy) within clinical settings. At times the referral is combined with dedicated staff, such as community health workers, patient navigators, or case managers, who refer and also facilitate linkage with available community programs (Shah et al., 2014). One challenge with broad screening programs is that they require maintaining up-to-date program and contact information for local private and public agencies. Another is the need to provide training at the screening site concerning sensitive screening, avoiding stigma, and broadening knowledge across the areas of need. Finally, screening programs can fail if resources in the community are not available to address identified needs, leading the screening to be both inefficient and ethically questionable.

Public Health Agencies

Public health agencies throughout the United States are focusing attention and resources on addressing health equity (e.g., the theme of the 2016 National Association of County and City Health Officials' [NACCHO's] annual meeting, "Cultivating a Culture of Health Equity," and the 2016 Association of State and Territorial Health Officials President's Challenge, "Advancing Health Equity and Achieving Optimal Health for All"). Addressing health equity will require the intentional investment of resources and support in the communities and populations with the greatest need. This approach is not new to state and local public health agencies accustomed to using infectious disease data to guide their investments in prevention and treatment measures to the highest risk individuals and communities. As an example, the number of newly diagnosed HIV infections decreased 19 percent from 2005 to 2014 (CDC, 2014), and reductions in the morbidity, mortality, and health care costs associated with vaccine-preventable diseases from 2000 to 2010 have been included among the top 10 public health achievements for the decade

(CDC, 2011). Public health agencies are working to adapt such approaches to address the non-health factors that shape health outcomes, including education, transportation, housing, and employment opportunities, and to exchange data with the traditional and nontraditional partners that are primarily responsible for addressing these social and economic factors. In addition, public health agencies will need to access other, nontraditional public health data sources on the social determinants of health as they continue to work in this area. Data on indicators such as high school graduation rates, poverty levels, affordable housing availability, median family income, unemployment rates, and limited English proficiency could be considered core public health data.

Public health agencies have the unique ability to use population-based health data to identify health priorities and health disparities; to inform and help mobilize the community and stakeholders to address health priorities; and to evaluate and monitor the health effects of new policies, programs, and changes to the built environment. Several public health agencies have prioritized addressing health equity in their community health plans (City of Chicago, 2016; OpenData KC, 2016). In March 2016, the Chicago Department of Public Health launched Healthy Chicago 2.0, a citywide plan that was developed and will be implemented in collaboration with representatives of more than 130 organizations across a broad range of sectors with the primary goal of achieving health equity (City of Chicago, 2016). NACCHO has developed a health equity and social justice program[10] to build the capacity of local health departments in confronting the root causes of health inequity, including resources such as a tool kit and a Web-based course for the public health workforce (NACCHO, 2016).

Because of existing relationships, public health agencies may be the natural conveners of certain health equity stakeholders, including health care systems, community organizations, and health insurance companies. They can also be partners with or conveners of community development organizations, faith-based organizations, businesses, and other governmental agencies (e.g., transportation, housing, education) because public health agencies have the data needed to link nontraditional partners' work and interests to health and to share with them evidence-based approaches. Box 7-5 highlights a few examples of public health agencies as conveners or partners. In recent years, due in to part to the evolution of public health accreditation standards (PHAB, 2013), many public health agencies have invested in the staff and training required to support community engagement for addressing acute or emerging health issues as

---

[10] For more information, see http://www.naccho.org/programs/public-health-infrastructure/health-equity (accessed October 21, 2016).

> **BOX 7-5**
> **Public Health Agencies as Conveners or Partners**
>
> **Seattle & King County Health Department**
>
> In early 2008, the Seattle & King County Health Department (SKCHD) (King County, n.d.-b) was a leader in launching the King County Equity and Social Justice Initiative, intended to eliminate longstanding and persistent inequities and social injustices. The initiative focused on working to provide access to livable wages, affordable housing, quality education and health care, and safe and vibrant neighborhoods. SKCHD participated in the creation of a strategic plan for equity and social justice, focusing on investments that address the root causes of inequities. One of the SKCHD activities is Communities Count, a public–private partnership that tracks social, economic, health, environmental, and cultural conditions important to King County residents. Nonprofit and philanthropic organizations, state and local government, service providers, and the public have Internet access to qualitative and quantitative data that they use to inform decisions in support of healthier King County communities.
>
> **Los Angeles County Department of Public Health**
>
> Public health agencies can play leadership or supportive roles in community-based solutions for addressing health equity. In 2015 the Los Angeles County Department of Public Health (LACDPH) received an Advancing Health Equity Award from the Office of Health Equity, California Department of Public Health (Gehlert, 2015). LACDPH plays a supportive role in the implementation of Parks after Dark (PAD), a place-based initiative that has improved access to health and social services, improved community safety, and increased physical activity among residents. This initiative was initially designed by the County Parks and Recreation Department, the Human Relations Commission, and the Sheriff's Department as a gang violence reduction initiative. PAD extended park hours and enhanced activities from 6 p.m. to 10 p.m. 3 days per week (Thursdays, Fridays, and Saturdays) during the summer. Shortly after the initiative began, the partner organizations recognized the potential for achieving improvements for a broader range of social and health outcomes. As a result, the LACDPH began providing health services,

well as ongoing public health priorities. Some innovative public health agencies have even invested in staff who can provide capacity building assistance to communities too.

As organizations initiate efforts to address health equity, public health agencies should be engaged in the early phases of plan development. Public health agencies can contribute data, epidemiologic expertise, partnerships, and community engagement capacity in addition to commitments to achieving health equity.

> including sexually transmitted infection screenings and health education about emergency preparedness and bike safety. In addition, the LACDPH established baseline health metrics in order to track progress toward meeting program objectives, including participation, and to monitor the impact of the program on violence.
>
> **Kansas City Health Department**
>
> Kansas City, Missouri, received a Robert Wood Johnson Foundation Culture of Health Award in 2015. The Kansas City Health Department (KCHD) played a leadership role in the city's efforts to achieve health equity (RWJF, 2015b). KCHD jump-started its activities with the release of its 2001 Community Health Improvement Plan, which highlighted the large disparity in life expectancy between whites and African Americans. This report catalyzed action from governmental agencies, community groups, nonprofit organizations, and businesses and helped them to focus efforts on addressing the social and economic factors that affect health. Health equity–focused efforts include violence-prevention initiatives, including trauma-informed school programs and community-based violence interrupter programs; a policy designed to encourage urban agriculture to improve food access; and a policy to increase the minimum wage. KCHD has played a leadership role in the development and implementation of these initiatives. KCHD's initial focus on data remains a priority as the progress and impact of policies and programs are continuously monitored and reported.
>
> **New York State Department of Health**
>
> Since 2013 the New York State Department of Health (NYSDOH) has played a leadership role in the Medicaid Redesign Team Affordable Housing Work Group which has allocated between $47 million and $388 million per year in funding to expand supportive housing units and to support home renovations for high-cost Medicaid populations who might otherwise require institutional care (NYSDOH, 2016). Initially, NYSDOH provided evidence to support the important role that housing plays in improving health. Currently, it funds research and evaluation to demonstrate the effectiveness of the program. Every Medicaid member using Medicaid housing is tracked to see if his or her health care use (avoidable hospitalization and emergency room visits) is decreasing and if primary care utilization is increasing.

Public health agencies can hire staff who have community development knowledge and experience. In addition, public health agencies and health care systems should tap into the expertise of community development organizations (e.g., community development organizations, community development financing institutions) when creating their community health plans.

As local jurisdictions start to come together to address the underlying social determinants of health, many of the legacy structures that continue to influence social issues will need to change, and change, although disruptive, can lead to greater effectiveness. In both Boulder, Colorado, and San Diego, California, housing and health departments have come together in recognition that health equity is difficult to achieve if homelessness or housing insecurity is a major issue (Quinn, 2016). Creating new ways to provide services is not only achievable through merging departments to create a more efficient system; it can also happen through how funding is allocated toward improving conditions related to the social determinants of health. Lead poisoning, poor housing conditions that exacerbate asthma, and physical risk from poor housing structures are physical environment factors that directly affect health and that disproportionately affect the health of vulnerable populations. The funding streams available to remediate such a problem can be complicated to apply for, and often there is a need to go through several funding sources and applications. Although there are co-benefits from retrofitting a house (e.g., energy efficiency, better health from addressing asthma triggers), funds are separated even if the retrofit achieves multiple benefits. The Green and Healthy Homes Initiative has been able to braid funding from federal, state, private, and philanthropic partners to address housing and health issues in a more holistic way (GHHI, n.d.). For a community example that addresses housing and health with a multi-sectoral approach, see the discussion of People for Sustainable Housing in Chapter 5.

In early 2016 the Governance Institute convened the first in a series of intensive trainings as part of Alignment of Governance & Leadership in Healthcare: Building Momentum for Transformation. The training, which will recur, was designed to orient health care delivery system executives to the potential of interfacing and partnering with the community development sector. Moreover, the Build Healthy Places Network, the Center on Social Disparities in Health, and the Robert Wood Johnson Foundation (RWJF) have put forward "Making the Case for Linking: Community Development and Health," a brief highlighting multiple models and examples of health and development sector partnerships from around the country (Edmonds et al., 2015).

> **Recommendation 7-5: The committee recommends that public health agencies and other health sector organizations build internal capacity to effectively engage community development partners and to coordinate activities that address the social and economic determinants of health. They should also play a convening or supporting role with local community coalitions to advance health equity.**

The Role of the Educational System

Schools and school systems have not typically thought of public health and health care professionals as potential partners in their efforts to confront the nonacademic aspects of low educational achievement, especially in the context of their required efforts to conduct needs assessments and develop school improvement plans. However, there are many potential stakeholders on which schools could rely for advice and support. Public health departments, managed care organizations, public health–focused community organizations, and others can serve as partners in assessing health needs and have an influence on educational success. Schools can go further by engaging both district-employed and contracted specialized instructional support personnel, union officials, and other community-based organizations as part of their efforts to assess and meet student needs, especially those related to health and wellness.

Community engagement and the partnerships that may emerge as a result are likely to affect educational outcomes as well. There are numerous examples of schools where well-conceived and well-coordinated partnerships appear to have affected both the physical and the mental health needs of student and academic achievement (Frankl, 2016). Although the strength of the evidence underlying these examples varies widely, as does the scale of these partnerships, there is reason to believe that the observed positive educational effects are related to the care with which these partnerships have been built (Freudenberg and Ruglis, 2007). High-quality community engagement is essential across all grade levels—early childhood, elementary grades, and high schools (ICF International, 2010; Legters and Balfanz, 2010; Sigler, 2016). Engaging low-income families is challenging for a variety of reasons, not the least of which is that all too often these are people who have had negative experiences with schools and school systems (Mitchell, 2008). Other factors range from logistical issues associated with the parents' or guardians' ability to get to schools, to social and cultural factors having to do with their ability to effectively navigate the organizational dynamics of schools, especially for schools that are not deliberately focused on family involvement (Hornby and Lafaele, 2011). See the description of the Eastside Promise Neighborhood in Chapter 5 for an example of a low-income community that seeks to improve both health and educational outcomes.

Another approach to the role of schools in health equity interventions is to address education and health disparities by focusing on health problems that are widely present in communities, for which there are strong linkages to academic success, and for which community-based intervention is possible. Basch suggests that it is important to think in terms of causal pathways, plausible explanations for why a particular health problem would cause a negative educational outcome (Basch, 2011). He identifies a variety of educationally relevant health factors, ranging from vision impairment, asthma, and dental disease to aggression and violence, nutrition and obesity, and sexual health issues, which taken together are likely to negatively affect educational opportunities and learning outcomes.

Collecting data on health determinants and health indicators as part of local needs assessments would help in the identification of health problems that affect student learning and achievement. The Every Student Succeeds Act[11] is a new federal mandate that requires school-level needs assessments, although access to quality data may persist as a barrier. A forthcoming health impact assessment conducted by the Health Impact Project (a joint initiative of the RWJF and The Pew Charitable Trusts) highlights the need to collect student-, household-, and community-level data on social determinants of health that influence student achievement (Morley, 2016). Unfortunately, not all schools have good data on chronic absenteeism, for example (Balfanz and Byrnes, 2012). Nor is information on school climate and neighborhood or on the community factors that affect learning widely available. The Health Impact Project's health impact assessment discusses that data on some community factors already being collected by local public health departments, hospitals, and other agencies and organizations can be examined as part of school-level needs assessments (Morley, 2016). Inclusion of such data in the development of school improvement plans can help to identify and build community partnerships beyond school settings to further improve student health and academic achievement as well as school performance (Morley, 2016). See Chapter 6 for a recommendation (Recommendation 6-2) on state department guidance for student health needs assessments.

Household and community factors figure prominently in educational outcomes and could be addressed through community-based education efforts. Neighborhood and household poverty have effects on the social, emotional, and physical resources available to children. Research indicates that violence gives rise to higher risks of posttraumatic stress and negative effects on school functioning (McGill et al., 2014). Housing instability creates attendance problems as well as affects the ability for sustained exposure to specific teachers and schools. Child welfare policies often exacerbate discontinuities in schooling. Other factors being equal, the more these neighborhood and household factors can be understood and addressed in concert with school efforts, the more likely it is that both health and educational outcomes will improve.

---

[11] S.1177—Every Student Succeeds Act. Public Law 114-95 (December 10, 2015), 114th Cong.

Mounting evidence suggests that focusing on measures of student engagement—especially those that have to do with sense of self, self-regulation, social awareness, and self-efficacy—both foster a sense of well-being in students and promote learning (see Dweck et al., 2014; Miyake et al., 2010). However, schools will need to broaden how they currently think about success for these measures to make sense. Schools might also have to adopt new data collection strategies, such as student and parent surveys, to generate this type of information. The CORE districts, a network of urban school districts in California, have developed such an instrument to collect data on factors they view as important indicators of student success (CORE, 2016).

Focusing on measures of school conditions may be another way to generate information about emotional well-being and learning. The research base about school climate and culture is substantial and suggests that in addition to leadership and instructional coherence, strong and trusting relationships among adults and between adults and students matter greatly to school and student success (Bryk et al., 2010). This, too, might require extra effort for school officials, but, given the evidence, it offers great potential in terms of improving the conditions for learning and student well-being. *A School Quality Review Guide for the New York City Public Schools* includes survey data on New York City schools' climate and culture (NYC Department of Education, 2016).

Measuring suspension and expulsion rates would give schools a sense of whether their disciplinary policies are excluding students from learning opportunities. Similarly, collecting and analyzing data on absenteeism is an important way to examine opportunities for students to learn. Given the emerging evidence, better data on absenteeism may be critical to addressing health and learning. Irregular attendance is often a function of underlying health factors and is correlated with credit accumulation in middle and high schools (Balfanz and Byrnes, 2012). Children who are chronically absent in the early grades are much less likely to read at grade level, and whether a young child reads at grade level in turn predicts academic performance at the middle and high school levels (Chang and Balfanz, 2016; Ginsburg et al., 2014). See Chapter 6 for more on the role of education at the federal and state levels.

> **Recommendation 7-6: Given the strong effects of educational attainment on health outcomes and their own focus on equity (ED, 2016), the U.S. Department of Education Institute for Educational Science and other divisions in the department should support states, localities, and their community partners with evidence and technical assistance on the impact of quality early childhood education programs, on interventions that reduce**

disparities in learning outcomes, and on the keys to success in school transitions (i.e., pre-K and K–12 or K–12 postsecondary).

Providing federal assistance to advance early childhood education programs is likely to provide many benefits for health equity because the evidence shows that disparities in development and achievement emerge early in the life course (Heckman, 2011), and thus this is a critical phase at which to intervene (Conti et al., 2011). Furthermore, this would leverage an already existing effort, as the U.S. Department of Education has committed to promoting the use of data to advance equity in the fiscal year 2017 (ED, 2016). There are potential limitations with the availability of evidence on reducing disparities in learning outcomes beyond early childhood and elementary levels. Additionally, the state of evidence on racial and ethnic minorities for whom English is not the first language needs to be taken into consideration. Otherwise, efforts to promote equity could unintentionally be hindered.

Role of Law Enforcement and the Justice System

It is increasingly clear that an important focus for community interventions should be building trust between law enforcement and local communities. The final report of The President's Task Force on 21st Century Policing highlights trust as the cornerstone for just and efficient law enforcement and community safety (The President's Task Force on 21st Century Policing, 2015). Yet, concerns about police brutality, bias, and a lack of accountability severely undermine trust in law enforcement, especially among racial and ethnic minority communities. Partnering with law enforcement agencies is essential to building trust between law enforcement and local communities.

One mechanism for building trust between law enforcement and local communities is community policing, which is based on the philosophy that police departments can join forces with the communities they serve to determine problems and identify solutions aimed at prevention and intervention (Skogan, 2006). In theory, proactive strategies that are implemented with a community policing approach address the proximal conditions that engender public safety issues such as crime, social disorder, and fear of crime (Bureau of Justice Statistics, 2016). Community policing can lead to greater permeability and interdependence between departments and communities (Gill et al., 2014). Building sufficient trust for effective community policing requires that police get to know residents, which can be achieved through police–resident social events, community gatherings, and public hearings.

The National Academies' Committee on Proactive Policing–Effects on Crime, Communities, and Civil Liberties in the United States[12] is conducting a study that reviews the evidence on the effects of various forms of proactive policing, including community policing. The review includes an assessment of proactive policing approaches and their effects on crime and disorder, discriminatory application, legality, and community receptiveness.

Specific strategies for community policing vary. One strategy to improve community oversight is the civilian review board, a mechanism by which community members can review police conduct (Finn, 2001). Although civilian review boards were a major focus of the civil rights movement, only some communities successfully convinced local governments to pass legislation establishing civilian review boards, which differ markedly from one another in form, structure, potency, and level of authority (Dunn, 2010; Harris, 2005).

Another approach to community policing is to achieve racially and ethnically representative police departments. Research suggests that communities have greater levels of trust in law enforcement when police demographics mirror the community (DOJ, 2015, 2016). This is rarely the case, however, as the proportion of sworn officers who are white is typically much higher than the proportion for the communities they serve (DOJ, 2015, 2016).

The predominant theory for why some communities have more violence than others centers on the differing capacity of communities to come together to control crime (Sampson, 2012). Communities experience different organizing against crime: some are able to come together and use their resources to control unwanted criminal elements, while others are less effective. Typically, able communities have greater financial resources and are relatively stable (i.e., residents have lived in the community for a long time and thus tend to know each other and have a vested stake in the community). These structural conditions—resources and stability—create conditions under which residents are more likely to agree on what constitutes a crime problem and under which they can work together to control crime via informal and formal means. Formally, residents will call the police when crimes are witnessed and otherwise work to develop positive relations with the police. Informally, they rely on healthy social capital and networks to transfer information and social control. For example, in a neighborhood where a resident knows his or her neighbors and feels a sense of belonging and attachment, he or she is more likely to recognize unwanted behavior as suspicious (e.g., a group of teenagers lurking in an

---

[12] Report forthcoming in 2017. For more information, see http://sites.nationalacademies.org/DBASSE/CLAJ/CurrentProjects/DBASSE_167718 (accessed December 2, 2016).

alleyway), notify other residents, or call the police. This is an example of collective efficacy: communities using their relationships, shared norms, trust, and social cohesion to come together to control crime.

Not all communities benefit from the same degree of collective efficacy (Sampson et al., 1997). In some communities, some neighbors may not know who is "suspicious," and different neighbors may not perceive the same individuals as "suspicious." Some neighbors may not alert other neighbors because they do not know or trust these neighbors. They may doubt that anything will be done about the issue and think it is a frequent occurrence. Witnesses may fear the police themselves and be reluctant to call. Such communities lack the collective efficacy to come together and address crime, and such places are often characterized by poverty and residential instability (where residents are not attached to neighborhoods).

One possible strategy to build and improve collective efficacy is to identify and obtain the resources necessary to improve the physical condition of neighborhoods. Various grant programs (such as the Seattle Department of Neighborhood's Neighborhood Matching Fund[13] and other Hope grants[14]) provide resources to communities that propose their own solutions (Ramey and Shrider, 2014). These community-driven approaches have been shown to increase attachment to place, reduce violence, and improve mental health (see work, for example, by Charles Branas at the University of Pennsylvania Urban Health Lab) (Culyba et al., 2016; University of Pennsylvania, 2013). Another approach to building collective efficacy involves improving the relationships between community and "external" actors who broker resources for the community, such as banks, politicians, and law enforcement (Vélez, 2001). Communities with stronger ties among these actors are more able to hold these actors accountable. Other potential strategies include creating community watch organizations and block groups, which can facilitate social cohesion; strengthening neighborhood institutions such as neighborhood associations, schools, churches, businesses, and community centers; and facilitating the ability of residents to own their homes, fostering a stronger attachment to their community. Community policing approaches are thus fundamentally multi-sectoral because they promote organizational strategies that facilitate collaborative relationships among various community stakeholders.

---

[13] For more information on the Neighborhood Matching Fund, see http://www.seattle.gov/neighborhoods/programs-and-services/neighborhood-matching-fund (accessed November 23, 2016).

[14] For more information on the HOPE VI Program, see http://portal.hud.gov/hudportal/HUD?src=/program_offices/public_indian_housing/programs/ph/hope6 (accessed November 23, 2016).

As noted earlier, the final report of The President's Task Force on 21st Century Policing highlights the importance of building and maintaining trust between law enforcement and local communities (The President's Task Force on 21st Century Policing, 2015). Recent events illustrate the crisis of trust and accountability that is taking place in many communities across the country. Concerns about police brutality, bias, and procedural injustice severely undermine the efficacy and legitimacy of law enforcement. This is especially acute among racial and ethnic minority communities. The committee supports the recommendations of The President's Task Force on 21st Century Policing that direct law enforcement agencies and communities toward the creation and maintenance of public safety

CROSS-SECTOR COLLABORATION—
HEALTH IN ALL POLCIES

The term "health in all policies" (HIAP) refers to the use of a social-determinants-of-health approach to solutions and structures that breaks down the siloed nature of government to advance collaboration. In 2006 Sihto and colleagues defined HIAP as "a horizontal, complementary policy-related strategy with a high potential to contributing to population health," at the core of which is the examination of "determinants of health, which can be influenced to improve health but are mainly controlled by policies of sectors other than health" (Sihto et al., 2006, p. 4). HIAP may be more accessibly described as the act of applying a health lens to decisions, policies, practices, and investments in other sectors, including in business (NASEM, 2016a).

Although the term has particular resonance for people working in the health field, it fits in a broader space of cross-sector collaboration which may include working across government agencies responsible for different aspects of the economy (e.g., the federal Sustainable Communities Partnership among the U.S. Department of Transportation [DOT], the U.S. Department of Housing and Urban Development [HUD], and the U.S. Environmental Protection Agency [EPA]) or at the intersection between the public and private sectors.

HIAP "engages diverse governmental partners and stakeholders to work together to promote health, equity, and sustainability, and simultaneously advance other goals such as promoting job creation and economic stability, transportation access and mobility, a strong agricultural system, and educational attainment" (Rudolph et al., 2013, p. 6). "There is no one 'right' way to implement a Health in All Policies approach, and there is substantial flexibility in process, structure, scope, and membership" (Rudolph et al., 2013, p. 17). *Health in All Policies: A Guide for State and Local Governments* outlines five key elements of HIAP, which are (1) promote health, equity, and sustainability; (2) support inter-sectoral collaboration; (3) benefit multiple partners (i.e., achieve "co-benefits"); (4) engage stakeholders; and (5) create structural or process change (Rudolph et al., 2013). HIAP approaches can prevent unintended negative consequences for health, potentially avoiding higher health care costs and other challenges.

There are numerous examples of unintended consequences that have surfaced when policy making did not consider the health implications of a policy (e.g., the use of antibiotics in agriculture or automobile-centered land use and planning). HIAP or cross-sector collaborative initiatives can use different tools to consider the health implications of new policies and programs. A health impact assessment (HIA) is sometimes used to systematically examine the likely effects of a policy decision, such as new infrastructure (see Chapter 8 for a more detailed discussion of the use of HIA to advance health equity). For example, transportation, planning, and health departments can collaborate to implement health impact assessments to ensure that new transportation projects are evaluated based on their health implications (such as walkability and safety) in addition to more traditional transportation metrics. The Minnesota Department of Health founded the Healthy Minnesota Partnership, a multi-sector coalition (specifically, transportation, education, and community organizations) to inform the development and implementation of a statewide health assessment and community health improvement plan. In 2014 the department released *Advancing Health Equity in Minnesota: Report to the Legislature* (MDH, 2014), a publication used as a resource by state and local coalitions in a range of policy initiatives, including the effort to advocate for an increase in the minimum wage (ASTHO, 2014).

The NACCHO website offers several HIAP resources, including success stories of local health departments working in cross-sector coalitions (NACHHO, n.d.). These include the county council in Prince George's County, Maryland, passing an ordinance in 2011 that requires the planning board to refer site, design, and master plan proposals to the Prince George's County Health Department for an HIA of the proposed development on the community and the distribution of potential effects within the population and to recommend design components that increase positive health outcomes and minimize adverse health outcomes for the community. In another example, the Mid-Ohio Regional Planning Commission passed a complete-streets policy mandating that all projects funded by the commission accommodate all users, including pedestrians, bicyclists, users of mass transit, people with disabilities, and older adults.

Governance for "Health in All Policies" or Cross-Sector Collaboration

State policies in such areas as education, development, and land use have clear parallels to federal policy and can significantly shape how communities respond to health disparities. There are several state-level examples of cross-sector collaboration intended to improve health and health equity. In 2010 the State of California created a Health in All Policies Task Force—representing 19 state agencies, departments, and offices—under the auspices of the state's Strategic Growth Council, aiming to build interagency partnerships across state government and to address issues of health, equity, and environmental sustainability. This is the first formal state-level body of its kind. Its goals describe a broad definition of health which includes air and water quality, natural resources and agricultural lands, the availability of affordable housing, infrastructure systems, public health, sustainable communities, and climate change. Such HIAP approaches and governance structures have also been adopted at the community level.

Several regions, including Seattle–King County (Washington state), Nashville, and Atlanta, have implemented cross-sector public sector and public–private partnership approaches to addressing challenges to the well-being of local communities by including a social justice and equity lens in all policies and collaborating to change the local conditions for health (King County, n.d.-a; Minyard et al., 2016; T4A, n.d.). The Nashville Metropolitan Planning Organization, for example, increased the percentage of projects that incorporate safe walking and biking elements from 2 percent in 2005 to 70 percent in its 2010 plan (Nashville Area Metropolitan Planning Organization, 2010). Although the plan does not use the term "health equity," its monitoring of performance and impacts is framed by Title VI of the Civil Rights Act of 1964 and by the 1994 Executive Order on Environmental Justice, and the overall planning process is informed by transportation equity principles. Specifically, the project evaluation factors described in the plan include questions on health and environment, such as: "Does the project aid/harm the advancement of social justice and equity opportunity to destinations throughout the region?" and "How can the project be scoped to mitigate any negative impacts to predominantly low-income or minority communities or persons with a disability?" (Nashville Area Metropolitan Planning Organization, 2010).

National Initiatives

Several national initiatives have served to further cross-sector partnerships to improve health, livability, and economic development. In 2015, NACCHO funded three HIAP demonstration sites (Houston,

Baltimore city, and San Diego) with funding from the National Center for Environmental Health and the Agency for Toxic Substances and Disease Registry, both of the U.S. Centers for Disease Control and Prevention (CDC). In September 2014, the CDC provided support for the 3-year Plan4Health initiative, jointly led by the American Public Health Association (APHA) and the American Planning Association (APA) and implemented through 18 local coalitions, which include APHA and APA local affiliates. Plan4Health coalitions "incorporate equity into many aspects of their work to increase opportunities for active living and access to health foods" (Norcross, 2016). However, "getting to the root issues of why inequities exist can be complex, time consuming, and takes the buy-in and contributions of traditional and non-traditional cross-sector partners" (Makara, 2016). Plan4Health has assembled a collection of resources to support coalitions in this vital work, including *A Refresher on Health Equity* and the *Transportation and Health Tool* developed by the DOT and the CDC (Hartig, 2015; Makara, 2016). In 2016 the Association of Collegiate Schools of Architecture and the Association of Schools and Programs of Public Health (ASPPH) held their first-ever joint conference, titled Building for Health and Well-being: Structures, Cities, Systems. One conference track focused on what it called Acupunctural Urbanism: Advocacy, Equity, and Community Based Initiatives. In 2014 the American Institute of Architects held a summit on health and design, keynoted by the acting U.S. Surgeon General, and launched the Design and Health Research Consortium in 2015 (of which ASPPH has become a member). The consortium's inaugural proceedings included a session on resilience and equity which concluded that ethnic and racial minorities are disproportionately exposed to harmful environmental factors and that "resilience in the context of health and environment must engage questions of race, ethnicity, income, and institutionalized prejudice" (AIA and ACSAAF, 2015). Such efforts—interprofessional, interdisciplinary, and cross-sectoral—enhance opportunities for fruitful collaboration to promote health equity in the practice of public health, architecture, and planning.

Financing and other support for a range of built environment and economic development projects comes from community development organizations. Community development corporations and community development financial institutions manage "billions in housing, real estate and small business assets and investments" and build community wealth and expand opportunities by increasing affordable housing access and building "green" affordable housing (Phillips, 2006).

Federal Government Initiatives on Health Equity

Over the past decade, there has been significant federal effort to coordinate actions aimed at advancing health equity. Below, the committee describes the considerable infrastructure for health equity that has been constructed within the federal government. As discussed earlier in this chapter, similar efforts to create a public-sector infrastructure for equity more generally or health equity specifically exist in some states and even some local jurisdictions.

The National Partnership for Action to End Health Disparities (NPA) has been a key driver. Its stakeholders are the Federal Interagency Health Equity Team (FIHET), the offices of minority health at the U.S. Department of Health and Human Services (HHS), regional health equity councils, and health equity champions. Federal leadership for NPA is provided by FIHET, whose mission is to convene federal leaders to end health inequities by building capacity for equitable policies and programs, cultivating strategic partnerships, and sharing relevant models for action (FIHET, 2016). The partnership includes leaders from the Consumer Product Safety Commission and the departments of agriculture, commerce, defense, education, housing and urban development, justice, labor, transportation, veterans affairs, and health and human services. The ACA mandated the establishment of offices of minority health within six agencies of HHS: the Agency for Healthcare Research and Quality, the CDC, the Centers for Medicare & Medicaid Services (CMS), Health Resources and Services Administration, Substance Abuse and Mental Health Services Administration, and the U.S. Food and Drug Administration. The 10 regional health equity councils are independent, nongovernmental organizations comprising leaders and stakeholders from both nonfederal public (e.g., state government) and private sectors (e.g., academia, community-based organizations, health systems, health insurers) from within that region. The health equity champions program further extends the NPA's reach through pledges of support from organizations, advocacy groups, foundations, academic institutions, technical or subject matter experts, and community members.

The NPA has produced two major products to date. The National Stakeholder Strategy (NSS) for Achieving Health Equity laid out five goals and associated strategies in the areas of awareness, leadership, health system and life experience, cultural and linguistic competency, and data, research, and evaluation (NPA, 2016b). Within the NSS, the priorities for action and associated progress are to

- Educate and facilitate outreach on the Patient Protection and Affordable Care Act of 2010 (ACA): The Office of Minority Health is supporting implementation of the ACA by helping connect

minority consumers and communities of color with information about affordable health insurance options and partnering with CMS and other federal agencies and private-sector organizations to support to outreach efforts.
- Support the implementation of the National Standards for Culturally and Linguistically Appropriate Services in Health and Health Care: The Think Cultural Health website (HHS, n.d.) includes resources as well as an interactive map for monitoring activities by state.
- Educate youth and emerging leaders about health inequities and the social determinants of health so that they become champions for health equity: The youth National Partnership for Action to End Health Disparities priority area was developed in response to this need and is preparing young people to become future leaders and practitioners by educating them about health inequities and the social determinants of health and engaging youth in health equity work (NPA, 2016a).
- Strengthen the nation's network of community health workers, who play a key role in disease prevention and health promotion: NPA activities primarily focus on supporting the integration of community health workers into clinical and preventive care workforces through the regional health equity councils (RHECs) (NPA, n.d.).
- Promote the integration of health equity into policies and programs: Activities include a "health equity mapping" pilot to work collaboratively with volunteer FIHET organizations to map the relationship between their priorities and core functions and the attainment of health equity; FIHET has partnered with the Democracy Collaborative to convene federal and nonfederal leaders from health, community economic development, and other sectors to identify key conditions needed to drive strategic cross-sector collaboration to promote health equity; RHECs have published regional blueprints and health equity report cards; and NPA has collaborated with nongovernmental partners who are key conveners of decision makers at the local and state levels (e.g., the National Indian Health Board and the Association of State and Territorial Health Officials) (NPA, 2016c).

The complementary HHS Action Plan to Reduce Racial and Ethnic Health Disparities includes an HHS commitment to an ongoing assessment of the effectiveness of policies and programs related to reducing racial and ethnic health inequities and accountability for increasing health insurance coverage, improving quality, building data capacity, preventing disease, and strengthening cultural competency to create a nation free

> **BOX 7-6**
> **Office of Minority Health Report on Health Equity in the Federal Government**
>
> To further support the work of FIHET within the NPA, the Office of Minority Health funded a report by the Democracy Collaborative that reflects a synthesis of information collected via interviews of leaders in the federal and non-federal sectors on cross-sector collaboration for health equity. The interviewees identified ways to strengthen and sustain collaboration and resource alignment to achieve health equity goals.
>
> - Establish partnerships between federal and private sectors for the funding of technical assistance, data analysis, and other items that the federal government is challenged to support, such as marketing, launching pilots, or meeting-related expenses such as travel and facilitation.
> - Use a backbone organization or facilitator for control of day-to-day and meeting logistics.
> - Invest resources in building the capacity of mid- and senior-level career civil servants to ensure the continuity of initiatives, particularly those started by political appointees.
> - Demonstrate leadership engagement to communicate institutional investment to collaborators and other stakeholders.
> - Co-create cohesive messaging and branding.
> - Develop shared data and metrics of success for sustained collaboration.
> - Provide technical assistance to grantees to enhance grantee capacity to effectively apply for resource-aligned funds and manage resource streams allocated to their communities.
> - Focus on a deliberate effort to educate existing and potential partners about the relationships among their program missions, priorities, and goals and the issue for which their participation is needed, achieving health equity.
>
> The study also identified six actionable opportunities for stakeholders focused on advancing a health equity agenda at the federal level:
>
> 1. Develop a "health equity learning community" of federal mid- and senior-level civil servants in partnership with philanthropy;
> 2. Develop a federal "Healthy Communities" designation, employing Promise Zone design principles;
> 3. Collaborate with the National Institute on Minority Health and Health Disparities to expand research linked to place-based initiatives around how social and economic conditions are linked to health outcomes;
> 4. Facilitate increased coordination at the local level around community health needs assessments through federal funder encouragement and information sharing;
> 5. Increase collaboration between the National Prevention Strategy, the FIHET, and the Convergence Partnership, a collaborative of national funders and health care organizations working to foster healthier and more equitable environments for all children and families; and
> 6. Embed equity as a value in Executive Core Qualifications for Senior Executive Service.
>
> SOURCE: Zuckerman et al., 2015.

of inequities in health and health care (HHS, 2011). Box 7-6 summarizes an Office of Minority Health report on the federal government's role in health equity.

Finally, CMS is implementing several activities that will provide opportunities for partnering across sectors in the community. Its quality strategy details agency priorities for health care quality improvement and identifies the elimination of disparities as a foundational principle along with enabling local innovations, strengthening infrastructure and data systems, and fostering learning organizations (CMS, 2016). The CMS Equity Plan for Medicare will affect change through several unique CMS levers (CMS, 2015). These include quality improvement networks and quality improvement organizations, CMS programs, policy, data, access to stakeholders, and communication tools. The plan focuses on Medicare populations that experience disproportionately high burdens of disease, worse quality of care, and barriers to accessing care.

Guided by a framework that includes three interconnected domains—better understanding and awareness of inequities, identifying and creating solutions based on that understanding, and accelerating the implementation of measurable actions to achieve health equity—the CMS Equity Plan for Medicare has six priority areas. Three focus on meeting the needs of diverse populations through enhanced language access, physical access, and community health worker training. The other three center on data collection, reporting, and analysis; evaluating impact and integrating solutions across CMS programs; and the development and dissemination of promising approaches to reduce health disparities.

The current state of health disparities is both deeply troubling and a call to action to stem the high human and economic cost of health inequity. Clearly, considerable support for addressing health equity has been established in HHS and across the executive branch through the Federal Interagency Health Equity Taskforce. Sustaining and elevating this cross-government effort will be important in helping to galvanize a national effort toward promoting health equity and encouraging ongoing efforts around the country.

In November 2016, the president signed an executive order establishing a community solutions council charged with fostering "collaboration across agencies, policy councils, and offices to coordinate actions, identify working solutions to share broadly, and develop and implement policy recommendations that put the community-driven, locally led vision at the center of policymaking" (The White House, 2016).

The council builds on the foundation of earlier efforts, including a 2010 executive order, and it seems to signal attention at the highest level of government to the notion of helping all communities to successfully confront their challenges "including crime, access to care, opportunities to pursue quality education, lack of housing options, unemployment, and deteriorating infrastructure" (The White House, 2016).

> **Recommendation 7-7: The committee recommends that key federal government efforts, such as the Community Solutions Council, that are intended to support communities in addressing major challenges, consider integrating health equity as a focus.**

A health equity focus could mean undertaking such efforts as

- Determining how government decisions in health and non-health sectors could affect low-income and minority populations, including unintended negative consequences.
- Convening key stakeholders to explore financing structures through which companies, philanthropy, and government can together fund key health equity initiatives, including efforts to generate better, timelier, and more locally relevant data.

The importance of considering the unintended consequences of government policies is evident. For example, Chapter 3 outlines several examples of historical government policies that shaped government investment, land use, transportation planning, and other features of communities with disproportionately negative effects on access to housing, safety, social cohesion, family stability, and health outcomes in low-income and minority populations (Freeman and Braconi, 2002; IOM, 2003; Levy et al., 2006; Prevention Institute, 2011; Vélez, 2001; Zuk et al., 2015). Weighing the consequences on health outcomes, however, will require access to more varied and meaningful sources of data and may demand resources for analysis and assessment. The unique circumstances and context of each community (e.g., defined by census tract or zip code) may make it difficult to undertake such an assessment of potential consequences in a way that considers their full scope.

Public–private partnerships offer opportunities for innovation and alignment of resources that can achieve greater efficiency and effectiveness. Examples include pay-for-success financing models to support early childhood development and other programs, the Sustainable Communities federal partnership that brought together public- and private-sector actors to align their efforts, and clean energy financing arrangements (IOM, 2015a; PolicyLink, n.d.; Probst, 2014).

The language of the Executive Order (excerpted in Box 7-7) demonstrates recognition of the importance of equity (not explicitly health equity) and the determinants of health and well-being: for example,

> **BOX 7-7**
> **Excerpt from Executive Order Establishing**
> **a Community Solutions Council**
>
> "Specific challenges in communities—including crime, access to care, opportunities to pursue quality education, lack of housing options, unemployment, and deteriorating infrastructure—can be met by leveraging Federal assistance and resources. While the Federal Government provides rural, suburban, urban, and tribal communities with significant investments in aid annually, coordinating these investments, as appropriate, across agencies based on locally led visions can more effectively reach communities of greatest need to maximize impact. In recent years, the Federal Government has deepened its engagement with communities, recognizing the critical role of these partnerships in enabling Americans to live healthier and more prosperous lives. Since 2015, the Community Solutions Task Force, comprising executive departments, offices, and agencies across the Federal Government, has served as the primary interagency coordinator of agency work to engage with communities to deliver improved outcomes. This order builds on recent work to facilitate inter-agency and community-level collaboration to meet the unique needs of communities in a way that reflects these communities' local assets, economies, geography, size, history, strengths, talent networks, and visions for the future" (The White House, 2016).

"Place is a strong determinant of opportunity and well-being. Research shows that the neighborhood in which a child grows up impacts his or her odds of going to college, enjoying good health, and obtaining a lifetime of economic opportunities" (The White House, 2016). This executive order builds on and revokes Executive Order 13560 of December 14, 2010, which had previously established a "community solutions council" within the Corporation for National and Community Service, a federal agency, and was intended to be comprised solely of 30 members from outside the federal government and charged "to support the social innovation and civic participation agenda of the Domestic Policy Council" (The White House, 2010). The new executive order also references the Community Solutions Task Force, created in 2015 and which the new Council is intended to replace. Since 2015, the Community Solutions Task Force, comprising executive departments, offices, and agencies across the federal government, has served as the primary interagency coordinator of agency work to engage with communities to deliver improved outcomes. This order builds on recent work to facilitate interagency and community-level collaboration to meet the unique needs of communities in a way that reflects these communities' local assets, economies, geography, size, history, strengths, talent networks, and visions for the future. The distinguishing feature of the new council is that it is to be located in the White House and be cochaired by an Assistant to the President or the

Director of the Office of Management and Budget, as designated by the President and by one of several cabinet secretaries identified in the order (e.g., DOJ, HHS, HUD).

The Executive Order also calls on the council to conduct outreach to "representatives of nonprofit organizations, civil rights organizations, businesses, labor and professional organizations, start-up and entrepreneurial communities, State, local, and tribal government agencies, school districts, youth, elected officials, seniors, faith and other community-based organizations, philanthropies, technologists, other institutions of local importance, and other interested or affected persons with relevant expertise in the expansion and improvement of efforts to build local capacity, ensure equity, and address economic, social, environmental, and other issues in communities or regions" (The White House, 2016).

The committee hopes that the council could build on the foundations of health equity work presented in this report and elsewhere and take action toward solutions, including cross-sector, community-driven, and public–private partnerships. It needs to be more than merely a symbol to avoid a disempowering effect on communities. Furthermore, there is a large power differential between a group of such high profile actors and communities and community members. The committee hopes that council engagement of community members will be conducted in the spirit of respect and authentic partnership. As outlined in this report, communities are where change takes place, and the members of communities are best equipped to know what is needed to effect change in their community.

CONCLUDING OBSERVATIONS

There are many potential multi-sector partners that can come together in creating community interventions to promote health equity, and multiple examples of effective approaches exist. Regardless of the sectors and organizations that make up these partnerships, a key element of success is the authentic engagement of members of the affected community. Partners will vary based on the target of the intervention, from the education sector (schools) and criminal justice (law enforcement) to the private sector (businesses, health care systems, and payers) and local, state, and federal government agencies (including public health). Anchor institutions can play key partner and leadership roles by virtue of their stable presence and economic resource power. Regardless of the participants, effective and enduring interventions depend on collaboration across multiple sectors. Cross-sector collaborations, as modeled by approaches aiming to achieve co-benefits (e.g., expanded employment and improved health status; increased energy efficiency and decreased asthma rates), bring together the partners discussed in this chapter to address the social determinants of health and achieve health equity.

REFERENCES

Active Living By Design. 2016. *Finding common ground with human-centered design.* http://activelivingbydesign.org/finding-common-ground-with-human-centered-design (accessed October 19, 2016).

AHA (American Hospital Association). 2015. Equity of care: A toolkit for eliminating health care disparities. http://www.hpoe.org/Reports-HPOE/equity-of-care-toolkit.pdf (accessed October 20, 2016).

AHA. n.d.-a. *#123forequity pledge to eliminate health care disparities.* http://www.equityofcare.org/pledge/index.shtml (accessed October 20, 2016).

AHA. n.d.-b. *Equity of care: Resources.* http://www.equityofcare.org/resources/index.shtml (accessed October 20, 2016).

AIA and ACSAAF (American Institute of Architects and the Association of Collegiate Schools of Architecture and Architects Foundation). 2015. *Pulse on progress: Proceedings of the inaugural meeting of the aia design & health research consortium.* Princeton, NJ: The American Institute of Architects and the Association of Collegiate Schools of Architecture and Architects Foundation.

Andrews, N. O., and D. J. Erickson. 2012. *Investing in what works for America's communities: Essays on people, place & purpose.* Federal Reserve Bank of San Francisco and Low Income Investment Fund.

ASTHO (Association of State and Terriorial Health Officials). 2014. *Minnesota Department of Health changes the narrative on health with the healthy Minnesota partnership.* http://www.astho.org/Health-Equity/MN-Health-Equity-in-All-Policies-Story (accessed October 20, 2016).

ATSDR (Agency for Toxic Substances and Disease Registry). 2011. Principles of community engagement (second edition). *NIH Publication No. 11-7782.* http://www.atsdr.cdc.gov/communityengagement (accessed October 19, 2016).

Attree, P., B. French, B. Milton, S. Povall, M. Whitehead, and J. Popay. 2011. The experience of community engagement for individuals: A rapid review of evidence. *Health & Social Care in the Community* 19(3):250–260.

Balfanz, R., and V. Byrnes. 2012. *Chronic absenteeism: Summarizing what we know from nationally available data.* Baltimore, MD: Johns Hopkins University Center for Social Organization of Schools.

Basch, C. E. 2011. Healthier students are better learners: A missing link in school reforms to close the achievement gap. *Journal of School Health* 81(10):593–598.

Bhaskaran, S. 2016. Pinklining: How Wall Street's predatory products pillage women's wealth, opportunities, & futures. http://isaiahmn.org/newsite/wp-content/uploads/2016/06/Pinkling-June-2016.pdf (accessed October 19, 2016).

Birch, E., D. C. Perry, and H. L. Taylor. 2013. Universities as anchor institutions. *Journal of Higher Education Outreach and Engagement* 17(3):7–15.

Bower, J. L., H. B. Leonard, and L. S. Paine. 2011. *Capitalism at risk: Rethinking the role of business.* Boston, MA: Harvard Business Review Press.

Bryk, A. S., P. B. Sebring, E. Allensworth, S. Luppescu, and J. Q. Easton. 2010. *Organizing schools for improvement: Lessons from Chicago.* Chicago, IL: University of Chicago Press.

Bullard, R. D., and R. Garcia. 2015. Diversifying mainstream environmental groups is not enough. *Parks & Recreation.* http://www.parksandrecreation.org/2015/July/Diversifying-Mainstream-Environmental-Groups-Is-Not-Enough (accessed October 19, 2016).

Bureau of Justice Statistics. 2016. *Community policing.* http://www.bjs.gov/index.cfm?ty=tp&tid=81 (accessed December 1, 2016).

CalEPA (California Environmental Protection Agency). n.d. *Greenhouse gas-reduction investments to benefit disadvantaged communities.* http://www.calepa.ca.gov/EnvJustice/GHGInvest (accessed October 19, 2016).

Campbell's Soup Company. 2015. *Campbell's healthy communities taking shape in Camden.* https://www.campbellsoupcompany.com/newsroom/news/2015/03/23/campbells-healthy-communities-taking-shape-in-camden (accessed October 21, 2016).

CCPH (Community–Campus Partnerships for Health). 2007. *Community-campus partnerships for health: Celebrating a decade of impact.* Community-Campus Partnerships for Health. https://ccph.memberclicks.net/assets/Documents/ 10annivreportfinal.pdf (accessed November 16, 2016).

CCPH. 2012. *Creating the space to ask "why?" Community-campus partnerships as a strategy for social justice.* https://ccph.memberclicks.net/assets/Documents/conf12-draftpaper.pdf (accessed October 20, 2016).

CCPH. n.d. *Community-campus partnerships for health.* https://ccph.memberclicks.net (accessed October 20, 2016).

CDC (U.S. Centers for Disease Control and Prevention). 2011. Ten great public health achievements—United States, 2001-2010. *Morbidity and Mortality Weekly Report* 60(19):619–623.

CDC. 2014. Diagnoses of HIV infection in the United States and dependent areas, 2014. *HIV Surveillance Report* (26). https://www.cdc.gov/hiv/pdf/library/reports/surveillance/cdc-hiv-surveillance-report-us.pdf (accessed September 12, 2016).

Chang, H., and R. Balfanz. 2016. Preventing missed opportunity: Taking collective action to confront chronic absence. *Attendance Works and Everyone Graduates Center.* http://www.attendanceworks.org/research/preventing-missed-opportunity (accessed October 19, 2016).

Chetty, R., and N. Hendren. 2015. The impacts of neighborhoods on intergenerational mobility: Childhood exposure effects and county-level estimates. http://www.equality-of-opportunity.org/images/nbhds_paper.pdf (accessed October 20, 2016).

City of Chicago. 2016. *Healthy Chicago 2.0: Partnering to improve health equity 2016–2020.* Chicago, IL: Chicago Department of Public Health.

CMS (Centers for Medicare & Medicaid Services). 2015. *The CMS equity plan for improving quality in Medicare.* Baltimore, MD: Centers for Medicare & Medicaid Services, Office of Minority Health.

CMS. 2016. *CMS quality strategy.* Baltimore, MD: Centers for Medicare & Medicaid Services.

Conti, G., J. Heckman, and S. Urzua. 2011 (unpublished). *Early endowments, education, and health.* Chicago, IL: University of Chicago.

CORE. 2016. *Student, staff, parent culture-climate survey.* Sacramento, CA: John W. Gardner Center for Youth and their Communities.

CPLC (Chicanos Por La Causa). n.d. *Chicanos por la causa.* http://www.cplc.org (accessed October 20, 2016).

Culyba, A. J., S. F. Jacoby, T. S. Richmond, J. A. Fein, B. C. Hohl, and C. C. Branas. 2016. Modifiable neighborhood features associated with adolescent homicide. *JAMA Pediatrics* 170(5):473–480.

Dan, D., R. Finch, D. Harrison, and D. Kendall. 2011. *An employer's guide to reducing racial & ethnic health disparities in the workplace.* Washington, DC: National Business Group on Health.

Davidoff, F., and P. Batalden. 2005. Toward stronger evidence on quality improvement. Draft publication guidelines: The beginning of a consensus project. *Quality & safety in health care* 14(5):319–325.

Democracy Collaborative. 2014. *Press release: Six universities partner with the democracy collaborative to develop and share best practices for measuring community impact.* http://democracycollaborative.org/content/press-release-six-universities-partner-democracy-collaborative-develop-best-practices (accessed October 20, 2016).

Democracy Collaborative. n.d.-a. *Anchor institutions.* http://democracycollaborative.org/democracycollaborative/anchorinstitutions/Anchor%20Institutions (accessed October 20, 2016).

Democracy Collaborative. n.d.-b. *Community development corporations (CDCs).* http://community-wealth.org/strategies/panel/cdcs/index.html (accessed November 1, 2016).

DOJ (U.S. Department of Justice). 2015. *Diversity in law enforcement: A literature review.* http://www.cops.usdoj.gov/pdf/taskforce/Diversity_in_Law_Enforcement_Literature_Review.pdf (accessed October 19, 2016).

DOJ. 2016. *Advancing diversity in law enforcement.* https://www.justice.gov/crt/case-document/file/900761/download (accessed October 18, 2016).

Doucet, B. 2015. Detroit's gentrification doesn't address poverty. *Portside.* http://portside.org/2015-02-18/detroits-gentrification-doesnt-address-poverty (accessed October 20, 2016).

Dubb, S., S. McKinley, and T. Howard. 2013. *Achieving the anchor promise: Improving outcomes for low-income children, families and communities.* Democracy Collaborative.

Dunn, R. A. 2010. Race and the relevance of citizen complaints against the police. *Administrative Theory And Praxis* 32(4):557–577.

Dweck, C. S., G. M. Walton, and G. L. Cohen. 2014. *Academic tenacity: Mindsets and skills that promote long-term learning.* Bill and Melinda Gates Foundation.

EBALDC (East Bay Asian Local Development Corporation). n.d. *East Bay Asian Local Development Corporation.* http://www.ebaldc.org (accessed October 19, 2016).

ED (U.S. Department of Education). 2016. The fiscal year 2017 budget: Promoting greater use of evidence and data as a lever for advancing equity. In *Homeroom: The Official Blog of the U.S. Department of Education.* Washington, DC: U.S. Department of Education.

Eder, M. M., L. Carter-Edwards, T. C. Hurd, B. B. Rumala, and N. Wallerstein. 2013. A logic model for community engagement within the clinical and translational science awards consortium: Can we measure what we model? *Academic Medicine* 88(10):1430–1436.

Edmonds, A., P. Braveman, E. Arkin, and D. Jutte. 2015. *Making the case for linking community development and health: A resource for those working to improve low-income communities and the lives of the people living in them.* http://www.buildhealthyplaces.org/resources/making-the-case-for-linking-community-development-and-health (accessed October 24, 2016).

FIHET (Federal Interagency Health Equity Team). 2016. *Federal interagency health equity team.* http://minorityhealth.hhs.gov/npa/templates/browse.aspx?lvl=1&lvlid=36 (accessed December 1, 2016).

Finn, P. 2001. *Citizen review of police: Approaches & implementation.* https://www.ncjrs.gov/pdffiles1/nij/184430.pdf (accessed October 19, 2016).

Frankl, E. 2016. *Community schools: Transforming struggling schools into thriving schools.* https://populardemocracy.org/news/publications/community-schools-transforming-struggling-schools-thriving-schools (accessed October 19, 2016).

Freeman, L., and F. Braconi. 2002. Gentrification and displacement. *The Urban Prospect* 8(1).

Freudenberg, N., and J. Ruglis. 2007. Reframing school dropout as a public health issue. *Preventing Chronic Disease* 4(4).

Fullilove, M. T., and R. Wallace. 2011. Serial forced displacement in American cities, 1916–2010. *Journal of Urban Health* 88(3):381–389.

Gaffikin, F., and D. C. Perry. 2009. Discourses and strategic visions: The U.S. research university as an institutional manifestation of neoliberalism in a global era. *American Educational Research Journal* 46(1):115–144.

Gehlert, H. 2015. *Advancing health equity: Case studies of health equity practice in four award-winning California Health Departments.* Berkeley, CA: Berkeley Media Studies Group.

GHHI (Green and Healthy Homes Initiative). n.d. *What is GHHI?* http://www.greenandhealthyhomes.org/about-us/what-ghhi (accessed October 19, 2016).

Gill, C., D. Weisburd, C. W. Telep, Z. Vitter, and T. Bennett. 2014. Community-oriented policing to reduce crime, disorder and fear and increase satisfaction and legitimacy among citizens: A systematic review. *Journal of Experimental Criminology* 10:399–428.

Ginsburg, A., P. Jordan, and H. Chang. 2014. Absences add up: How school attendance influences student success. *Attendance Works*. http://www.attendanceworks.org/research/absences-add (accessed October 19, 2016).

Governing. n.d. *Cleveland gentrification maps and data*. http://www.governing.com/gov-data/cleveland-gentrification-maps-demographic-data.html (accessed October 20, 2016).

Hair, P. D. 2001. *Louder than words: Lawyers, communities and the struggle for justice*. http://www.racialequitytools.org/resourcefiles/hair.pdf (accessed October 19, 2016).

Hansen, S. 2012. Cultivating the grassroots: A winning approach for environment and climate funders. https://www.ncrp.org/files/publications/Cultivating_the_grassroots_final_lowres.pdf (accessed October 19, 2016).

Harkavy, I., and H. Zuckerman. 1999. *Eds and meds: Cities' hidden assets*. Washington, DC: The Brookings Institution Center on Urban and Metropolitan Policy.

Harkavy, I., M. Hartley, R. A. Hodges, A. Sorrentino, and J. Weeks. 2014. Effective governance of a university as an anchor institution: University of Pennsylvania as a case study. *Leadership and Governance in Higher Education* 2.

Harris, D. A. 2005. *Good cops: The case for preventive policing*. New York: New Press.

Hartig, E. 2015. *Explore the transportation and health tool*. http://plan4health.us/explore-the-transportation-and-health-tool (accessed October 20, 2016).

Health Care for All. n.d. *Maryland faith health network*. http://healthcareforall.com/get-involved/maryland-faith-community-health-network (accessed October 20, 2016).

Heckman, J. 2011. The economics of inequality: The value of early childhood education. *American Educator* 31–47.

Henry Ford Health System. n.d. *About Henry Ford Health System*. https://henryford.referrals.selectminds.com/info/page1 (accessed October 20, 2016).

HHS (U.S. Department of Health and Human Services). 2011. *HHS action plan to reduce racial and ethnic health disparities*. Washington, DC: U.S. Department of Health and Human Services.

HHS. n.d. *Think cultural health*. https://www.thinkculturalhealth.hhs.gov (accessed October 20, 2016).

HMA (Health Ministries Association). n.d. *Health Ministries Association, Inc*. http://hmassoc.org/about-us/what-we-do (accessed October 20, 2016).

Hodges, R. A., and S. Dubb. 2012. *The road half traveled: University engagement at a crossroads*.

Hornby, G., and R. Lafaele. 2011. Barriers to parental involvement in education: An explanatory model. *Educational Review* 63(1):37–52.

ICF (Inner City Fund) International. 2010. *Communities in schools national evaluation: Five year summary report*. Fairfax, VA: ICF International.

ICIC (Initiative for a Competitive Inner City). 2011. Inner city, anchor institutions and urban economic development: From community benefit to shared value. *Inner City Highlights* 1(2). http://community-wealth.org/content/inner-city-anchor-institutions-and-urban-economic-development-community-benefit-shared-value (accessed October 20, 2016).

IHI (Institute for Healthcare Improvement). 2016. *Achieving health equity: A guide for health care organizations*. Cambridge, MA: Institute for Healthcare Improvement.

IOM (Institute of Medicine). 2003. *Unequal treatment: Confronting racial and ethnic disparities in health care*. Washington, DC: The National Academies Press.

IOM. 2011. *For the public's health: Revitalizing law and policy to meet new challenges*. Washington, DC: The National Academies Press.

IOM. 2013. *The CTSA program at NIH: Opportunities for advancing clinical and translational research*. Washington, DC: The National Academies Press.

IOM. 2014. *Supporting a movement for health and health equity: Workshop summary.* Washington, DC: The National Academies Press.

IOM. 2015a. *Financing population health improvement: Workshop summary.* Washington, DC: The National Academies Press.

IOM. 2015b. *The role and potential of communities in population health improvement: Workshop summary.* Washington, DC: The National Academies Press.

ISAIAH. n.d. *Vision.* http://isaiahmn.org/vision-3 (accessed October 19, 2016).

Joassart-Marcelli, P. 2010. Leveling the playing field? Urban disparities in funding for local parks and recreation in the Los Angeles region. *Environment and Planning A* 42(5):1174–1192.

Joassart-Marcelli, P., J. Wolch, and Z. Salim. 2011. Building the healthy city: The role of nonprofits in creating active urban parks. *Urban Geography* 32(5):682–711.

Kelly, M., and S. McKinley. 2015. *Cities building community wealth.* Democracy Collaborative.

King County. n.d.-a. *Equity and social justice.* http://www.kingcounty.gov/elected/executive/equity-social-justice.aspx (accessed October 20, 2016).

King County. n.d.-b. *Public health—Seattle & King County.* http://www.kingcounty.gov/healthservices/health.aspx (accessed October 20, 2016).

Legters, N., and R. Balfanz. 2010. Do we have what it takes to put all students on the graduation path? *New directions for youth development* 2010(127):11–24.

Levy, D. K., J. Comey, and S. Padilla. 2006. *In the face of gentrification: Case studies of local efforts to mitigate displacement.* Washington, DC: Urban Institute.

Makara, M. 2016. *A refresher on health equity.* http://plan4health.us/a-refresher-on-health-equity (accessed October 20, 2016).

Martin, L. L., H. Smith, and W. Phillips. 2005. Bridging 'town & gown' through innovative university-community partnerships. *The Innovation Journal: The Public Sector Innovation Journal* 10(2). http://www.innovation.cc/volumes-issues/martin-u-partner4final.pdf (accessed October 20, 2016).

McGill, T. M., S. R. Self-Brown, B. S. Lai, M. Cowart-Osborne, A. Tiwari, M. Leblanc, and M. L. Kelley. 2014. Effects of exposure to community violence and family violence on school functioning problems among urban youth: The potential mediating role of post-traumatic stress symptoms. *Front Public Health* 2:8.

McNeely, E., and G. Norris. 2015. *Shine summit 2015: Innovating for netpositive impact: Summary report.* Boston, MA: Sustainability and Healthy Initiative for NetPositive Enterprise.

MDH (Minnesota Department of Health). 2014. *Advancing health equity in Minnesota: Report to the legislature.* St. Paul: Minnesota Department of Health.

Methodist Healthcare. n.d. *Community.* http://www.methodisthealth.org/about-us/faith-and-health/community/ (accessed October 20, 2016).

Miller, D. S., and J. D. Rivera. n.d. Town and gown: Understanding the past to improve the future. *International Journal of the Humanities* 3(8):215–224.

Minyard, K., K. Lawler, E. Fuller, M. Wilson, and E. Henry. 2016. Reducing health disparities in Atlanta. *Stanford Social Innovation Review.* https://ssir.org/articles/entry/reducing_health_disparities_in_atlanta (accessed October 20, 2016).

Mitchell, C. 2008. Parental involvement in public education: A literature review. *Research for Action.* http://www.researchforaction.org/wp-content/uploads/2016/02/Mitchell_C_Parent_Involvement_in_Public_Education.pdf (accessed October 19, 2016).

Mitchell, F. 2016. Innovations in health equity and health philanthropy. *Stanford Social Innovation Review.* https://ssir.org/articles/entry/innovations_in_health_equity_and_health_philanthropy (accessed October 19, 2016).

Miyake, A., L. E. Kost-Smith, N. D. Finkelstein, S. J. Pollock, G. L. Cohen, and T. A. Ito. 2010. Reducing the gender achievement gap in college science: A classroom study of values affirmation. *Science* 330:1234–1237.

Morley, R. 2016. *Re: Comments on title i, § 200.21(c) school-level needs assessment; proposed rule. Docket ID: Ed-2016-oese-0032 title i, § 200.21(c).* http://www.pewtrusts.org/~/media/assets/2016/10/health-impact-project-comments-20021c/hip-comments-20021c.pdf (accessed November 18, 2016).

NACCHO (National Association of County and City Health Officials). 2016. *Health equity and social justice.* http://www.naccho.org/programs/public-health-infrastructure/health-equity (accessed October 19, 2016).

NACCHO. n.d. *Resources.* http://archived.naccho.org/topics/environmental/HiAP/resources (accessed October 20, 2016).

NACHC (National Association of Community Health Centers). n.d.-a. *Prapare.* http://nachc.org/research-and-data/prapare (accessed October 20, 2016).

NACHC. n.d.-b. *Research and data.* http://nachc.org/research-and-data (accessed October 20, 2016).

NASEM (National Academies of Sciences, Engineering, and Medicine). 2016a. *Applying a health lens to business practices, policies, and investments: Workshop summary.* Washington, DC: The National Academies Press.

NASEM. 2016b. *Framing the dialogue on race and ethnicity to advance health equity: Proceedings of a workshop.* Washington, DC: The National Academies Press.

Nashville Area Metropolitan Planning Organization. 2010. *2035 Nashville area regional transportation plan.* http://www.nashvillempo.org/docs/lrtp/2035rtp/Docs/2035_Doc/2035Plan_Complete.pdf (accessed March 8, 2016).

NCATS (National Center for Advancing Translational Sciences). n.d.-a. *Clinical and translational science awards (ctsa) program.* http://www.ncats.nih.gov/ctsa (accessed October 19, 2016).

NCATS. n.d.-b. *CTSA program hubs.* http://www.ncats.nih.gov/ctsa/about/hubs (accessed October 19, 2016).

Neavling, S. 2013. 'Bring on more gentrification,' declares Detroit's economic development czar. *Motor City Muckraker.* http://motorcitymuckraker.com/2013/05/16/bring-on-more-gentrification-declares-detroits-economic-development-czar-george-jackson (accessed December 2, 2016).

Netter Center for Community Partnerships. 2008. *Anchor institutions toolkit: A guide for neighborhood revitalization.* Philadelphia: University of Pennsylvania.

Norcross, A. 2016. *Health equity and planning.* http://plan4health.us/health-equity-and-planning (accessed October 20, 2016).

Norris, T., and T. Howard. 2015. Can hospitals heal America's communities? "All in for mission" is the emerging model for impact. *Democracy Collaborative.* http://democracycollaborative.org/content/can-hospitals-heal-americas-communities-0 (accessed October 20, 2016).

NPA (National Partnership for Action to End Health Disparities). 2016a. *Education youth and emerging leaders about the social determinants of health and health disparties through the youth national partnership to action to end health disparities (YNPA).* http://minorityhealth.hhs.gov/npa/templates/content.aspx?lvl=1&lvlid=38&ID=356 (accessed October 20, 2016).

NPA. 2016b. *National stakeholder strategy for achieving health equity.* Rockville, MD: National Partnership for Action to End Health Disparities, U.S. Department of Health and Human Services, Office of Minority Health.

NPA. 2016c. *Promoting the integration of equity in all policies & programs.* http://minorityhealth.hhs.gov/npa/templates/content.aspx?lvl=1&lvlid=38&ID=355 (accessed December 1, 2016).

NPA. n.d. *Regional health equity councils.* http://minorityhealth.hhs.gov/npa/templates/browse.aspx?lvl=1&lvlid=42 (accessed December 1, 2016).

NTFAI (National Task Force on Anchor Institutions). 2010. *Anchor institutions task force.* http://www.margainc.com/files_images/general/anchor_task_force_statement.pdf (accessed October 20, 2016).

NYC (New York City) Department of Education. 2016. *Quality review.* http://schools.nyc.gov/Accountability/tools/review/default.htm (accessed December 19, 2016).

NYSDOH (New York State Department of Health). 2016. *Supportive housing initiatives.* https://www.health.ny.gov/health_care/medicaid/redesign/supportive_housing_initiatives.htm (accessed October 20, 2016).

O'Mara, M. P. 2012. Beyond town and gown: University economic engagement and the legacy of the urban crisis. *Journal of Technology Transfer* 37(2):234–250.

OpenData KC. 2016. *Kansas City, MO., community health improvement plan 2011 through 2016.* https://data.kcmo.org/Health/KCMO-CHIP-2011-2016/gunq-ki6v (accessed October 20, 2016).

Oziransky, V., D. Yach, T. Tsu-Yu, A. Luterek, and D. Stevens. 2015. *Beyond the four walls: Why community is critical to workforce health.* New York: Vitality Institute.

PHAB (Public Health Accreditation Board). 2013. *Public health accreditation board standards & measures.* Alexandria, VA: Public Health Accreditation Board.

Phillips, R. 2006. Interview of Ron Phillips, CEO of Coastal Enterprises, Inc. (CEI) of Maine, edited by S. Dubb. Washington, DC: Democracy Collaborative.

PolicyLink. n.d. *Center for infrastructure equity: Sustainable communities.* http://www.policylink.org/focus-areas/infrastructure-equity/sustainable-communities (accessed December 1, 2016).

Porter, M. E. 2010. Anchor institutions and urban economic development: From community benefit to shared value. Presented at Inner City Economic Forum Summit San Francisco, CA.

Porter, M. E., and M. R. Kramer. 2011. Creating shared value. *Harvard Business Review* 89(1-2):62–77.

Prevention Institute. 2011. *Fact sheet: Links between violence and health equity.* Oakland, CA: Prevention Institute.

Probst, C. S. 2014. *Private sector financing and public-private partnerships for financing clean energy.* Research Program on Sustainability Policy and Management, Earth Institute, Columbia University.

Providence Hospital. n.d. *Community health assessment.* http://www.provhosp.org/about-us/community-health-assessment (accessed December 1, 2016).

Purciel-Hill, M., F. Santiago, L. Farhang, A. Tesfai, K. Ito, and K. H. Pace. 2016. Drowning in debt: A health impact assessment of how payday loan reforms improve the health of Minnesota's most vulnerable. http://isaiahmn.org/newsite/wp-content/uploads/2016/03/PaydayLendingHIA-FinalReport41616.pdf (accessed October 19, 2016).

QCDO (Quitman County Development Organization). n.d. *Quitman County Development Organization.* http://www.qcdo.org (accessed October 20, 2016).

Quinn, M. 2016. Boulder County, CO.: Blueprint for merging health and housing under one roof. *Governing.* http://www.governing.com/topics/health-human-services/gov-housing-health-mergers-boulder.html (accessed October 19, 2016).

Ramey, D. M., and E. A. Shrider. 2014. New parochialism, sources of community investment, and the control of street crime. *Criminology & Public Policy* 13(2):193–216.

Rooney, J. D., and J. Gittleman. 2005. *A new era of higher education-community partnerships: The role and impact of colleges and universities in greater Boston today.* The Boston Foundation and the University College of Citizenship and Public Service at Tufts University.

Rubin, V., and K. Rose. 2015. *Strategies for strengthening anchor institutions' community impact.* Oakland, CA: PolicyLink.

Rudolph, L., J. Caplan, K. Ben-Moshe, and L. Dillon. 2013. *Health in all policies: A guide for state and local governments*. Washington, DC, and Oakland, CA: American Public Health Association and Public Health Institute.

RWJF (Robert Wood Johnson Foundation). 2015a. *From vision to action: A framework and measures to mobilize a culture of health*. Princeton, NJ: Robert Wood Johnson Foundation.

RWJF. 2015b. *Kansas City, MO: 2015 culture of health prize winner*. http://www.rwjf.org/en/library/articles-and-news/2015/10/coh-prize-kansas-city-mo.html (accessed October 20, 2016).

Sampson, R. J. 2012. *Great American city: Chicago and the enduring neighborhood effect*. Chicago; London: The University of Chicago Press.

Sampson, R. J., S. W. Raudenbush, and F. Earls. 1997. Neighborhoods and violent crime: A multilevel study of collective efficacy. *Science* 277(5328):918–924.

Schrantz, D. 2016. PowerPoint presentation to the Committee on Community-Based Solutions to Promote Health Equity in the United States in Washington, DC, April 27, 2016. http://www.nationalacademies.org/hmd/~/media/Files/Activity%20Files/PublicHealth/COH_Community%20Based%20Solutions/April%20Meeting/Schrantz%20D.pdf (accessed October 18, 2016).

Schroepfer, E. 2016. A renewed look at faith community nursing. *MEDSURG Nursing* 25(1):61–66.

Serang, F., J. P. Thompson, and T. Howard. 2013. *The anchor mission: Leveraging the power of anchor institutions to build community wealth*. Takoma Park, MD: The Democracy Collaborative.

Shah, M. K., M. Heisler, and M. M. Davis. 2014. Community health workers and the Patient Protection and Affordable Care Act: An opportunity for a research, advocacy, and policy agenda. *Journal of health care for the poor and underserved* 25(1):17–24.

Sigler, M. K. 2016. Expanding transition: Redefining school readiness in response to toxic stress. *Voices in Urban Education (Annenberg Institute for School Reform)*(43):37–45.

Sihto, M., E. Ollila, and M. Koivusalo. 2006. Principles and challenges of health in all policies. In *Health in all policies: Prospects and potentials*, edited by T. Ståhl, M. Wismar, E. Ollila, L. E. and K. Leppo. Helsinki, Finland: Finland Ministry of Social Affairs and Health and the European Observatory on Health Systems and Policies.

Skocpol, T. 2013. Naming the problem: What it will take to counter extremism and engage Americans in the fight against global warming. http://www.scholarsstrategynetwork.org/sites/default/files/skocpol_captrade_report_january_2013_0.pdf (accessed October 19, 2016).

Skogan, W. G. 2006. *Police and community in Chicago: A tale of three cities*. Oxford; New York: Oxford University Press.

Smedley, B., and H. Amaro. 2016. Advancing the science and practice of place-based intervention. *American Journal of Public Health* 106(2):197.

Snyder, T. D., and S. A. Dillow. 2015. *Digest of educational statistics 2013*. Washington, DC: U.S. Department of Education, National Center for Education Statistics, Institute of Education Sciences.

SPARCC (Strong, Prosperous, and Resilient Communities Challenge). n.d. *Strong, prosperous, and resilient communities challenge*. http://sparccub.org (accessed October 19, 2016).

Super Church, M. 2015. *Using data to address health disparities and drive investment in healthy neighborhoods*. Washington, DC: National Academy of Medicine. https://nam.edu/wp-content/uploads/2015/12/SuperChurch.pdf (accessed July 16, 2016).

T4A (Transportation for America). n.d. *Transportation for America*. http://t4america.org (accessed October 20, 2016).

Taylor, H. L., and G. Luter. 2013. *Anchor institutions: An interpretative review essay*. New York: Anchor Institutions Task Force.

The Economist. 2009. *Triple bottom line: It consists of three ps: Profit, people and planet.* http://www.economist.com/node/14301663 (accessed December 1, 2016).
The President's Task Force on 21st Century Policing. 2015. *Final report of the president's task force on 21st century policing.* Washington, DC: Office of Community Oriented Policing Services.
The White House. 2010. *Executive order 13560—White House council for community solutions.* https://www.whitehouse.gov/the-press-office/2010/12/14/executive-order-13560-white-house-council-community-solutions (accessed December 1, 2016).
The White House. 2016. *Executive order—establishing a community solutions council.* https://www.whitehouse.gov/the-press-office/2016/11/16/executive-order-establishing-community-solutions-council (accessed December 1, 2016).
Trinity Health. n.d. *Trinity health.* http://www.trinity-health.org (accessed October 20, 2016).
Turner, A. 2015. *The business case for racial equity in Michigan.* Washington, DC: Altarum Institute.
University of Pennsylvania. 2013. *Urban health lab.* http://www.urbanhealthlab.org (accessed December 2, 2016).
Vélez, M. B. 2001. Role of public social control in urban neighborhoods: A multi-level analysis of victimization risk. *Criminology* 39(4):837–864.
Viveiros, J., and L. Sturtevant. 2016. *The role of anchor institutions in restoring neighborhoods: Health institutions as a catalyst for affordable housing and community development.* Washington, DC: National Housing Conference.
Westfall, J. M., K. Nearing, M. Felzien, L. Green, N. Calonge, F. Pineda-Reyes, G. Jones, M. Tamez, S. Miller, and A. Kramer. 2013. Researching together: A CTSA partnership of academicians and communities for translation. *Clinical and Translational Science* 6(5):356–362.
Woods, A. 2014. Detroit doesn't need hipsters to survive, it needs black people. *The Huffington Post.* http://www.huffingtonpost.com/2014/03/10/saving-detroit-thomas-sugrue-hipsters_n_4905125.html (accessed October 20, 2016).
Wright, W., K. W. Hexter, and N. Downer. 2016. *Cleveland University's circle initiative: An anchor-based strategy for change.* Takoma Park, MD: Democracy Collaborative.
Zakheim, M., K. McNamara, and J. Joseph. 2010. *Partnerships between federally qualified health centers and local health departments for engaging in the development of a community-based system of care.* Bethesda, MD: National Association of Community Health Centers.
Zuckerman, D. 2013. *Hospitals building healthier communities: Embracing the anchor mission.* College Park: The Democracy Collaborative at the University of Maryland.
Zuckerman, D., D. V., and K. Parker. 2015. *Cross-sector collaboration and resource alignment strategies to achieve health equity.* Washington, DC: Democracy Collaborative.
Zuk, M., A. H. Bierbaum, K. Chapple, K. Gorska, A. Loukaitou-Sideris, P. Ong, and T. Thomas. 2015 (unpublished). *Gentrification, displacement, and role of public investment: A literature review.* San Francisco, CA: Federal Reserve Bank of San Francisco.

8

Community Tools to Promote Health Equity

TOOLS FOR COMMUNITY SUCCESS

There are many tools available to communities to help them design, implement, and evaluate community-based solutions that advance health equity. These tools can be organized by the three elements identified in the committee's conceptual model (see Figure 8-1): (1) creating a shared vision and value of health equity, (2) increasing community capacity to shape health outcomes, and (3) fostering multi-sector collaboration. The tools described here encompass approaches, methods, measures, and necessary infrastructure. The committee identified these tools based on the lessons learned from communities that have implemented solutions (see Chapter 5), a review of the literature, input from information-gathering meetings (see Appendix C for agendas), and committee expertise. This chapter first describes tools that support community-based solutions in a manner that applies across the three elements of this report's conceptual model. Second, tools are organized according to the three elements in the report's conceptual model. Third, widely available community toolboxes are summarized. Some of the tools shared in this chapter are explicitly designed to address social determinants of health, while others address the consequences of poor health outcomes, and some do both. The tools also vary in the time frame for implementation; some can be employed within a relatively short time, while others will take more time to plan and implement.

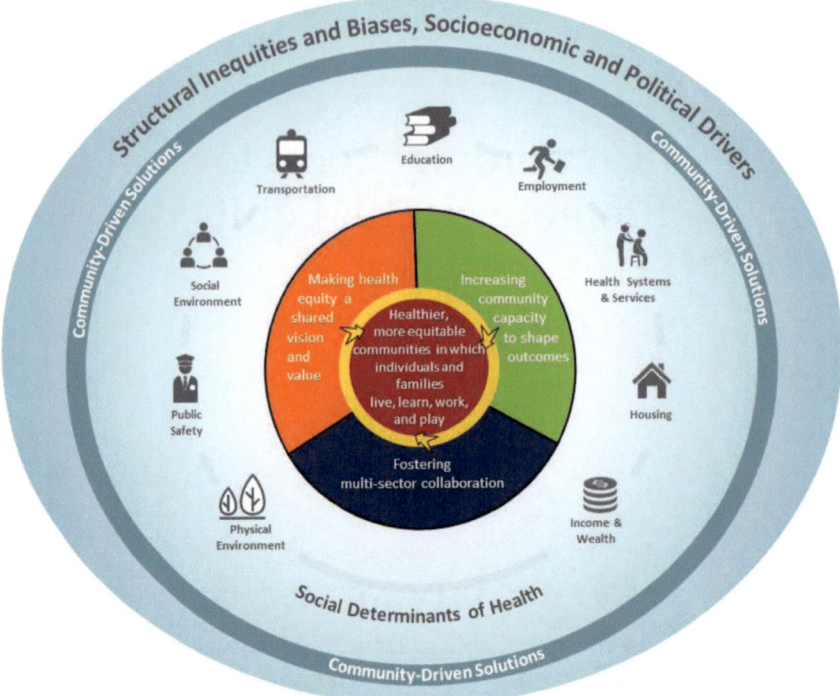

FIGURE 8-1 Report conceptual model for community solutions to promote health equity.

CROSSCUTTING TOOLS AND PROCESSES

A number of crosscutting tools provide a foundation for developing community-based solutions. Because each community is unique, the tools different communities need will vary. The tools described below are organized according to the types of actions that communities may need to take to address health equity, such as (1) making the case for health equity; (2) meeting information needs; (3) adopting or developing logic models or theories of change; (4) using civil rights law to promote health equity; (5) medical–legal partnerships; (6) using health impact assessments to understand policy implications; and (7) securing funding to support community action.

Making the Case for Health Equity

The Cost of Health Inequity

The cost of health inequity is usually calculated as a difference in cost, specifically, the excess burden that arises from certain groups experiencing disparate levels of health. Health-related economic costs are higher among minority racial and ethnic groups than among whites both because they have more chronic conditions and because they have lower average education, which is correlated with poorer health and earlier death. By some calculations, the lower levels of self-reported health and higher levels of chronic disease among African Americans, Hispanics, and non-Hispanic whites relative to whites cost public and private insurers an estimated $24 billion in 2009 (Waidmann, 2009). But the costs are more widespread, affecting not just insurers but also families and employers (Dan et al., 2011; Gaskin et al., 2012). Combining the cost of lower health with the cost of lower productivity pushes the estimated 2009 economic burden to $82 billion (Gaskin et al., 2012). Factoring in early death raises the estimates even more. The economic burden for 2050, when the representation of minorities in the population will have increased substantially, is predicted to be more than twice as large as it is now (Gaskin et al., 2012; Waidmann, 2009).

Strategies for Investment

Recognizing that health inequities arise from many factors, decision makers face a challenge in weighing different strategies to improve health equity and health outcomes and decrease the cost of inequity. One model that informs health care cost reduction allows the user to simulate outcomes across geographic areas across a host of factors, such as changes to health care delivery, health care payment (e.g., global payments with reinvested savings), factors that influence healthier behaviors, some social determinants, and some socioeconomic factors. This approach, taken by the ReThink Health Dynamics Model, was used to simulate outcomes for typical midsize U.S. cities (Homer et al., 2016). In that work, a combination of approaches—expanding global payment, enabling healthier behaviors, and expanding socioeconomic opportunities—was estimated to lower health care costs by 14 percent and to improve productivity by 9 percent over 24 years. The most costly intervention component addressed socioeconomic opportunities, and the simulation assumed that the more costly investments occurred after savings from changes in health care delivery and payments. However, this was also the component that resulted in the greatest estimated improvements in the disadvantaged fraction of the population.

Participating in health equity improvement is a voluntary activity on the part of actors in the community. As such it is most likely to be maintained if there is a "business case," meaning that benefits will accrue to the decision maker's bottom line. What are the advantages of investments in improved health equity and raising awareness among individuals, employers, and communities as a whole? While much of the health equity discussion rests on a moral argument, there are several economic arguments to support health equity promotion and improving the social determinants of health. One example of a social determinant of health for which there are large disparities among communities is education. By some estimates the annual economic value of better health from education is very high: if less educated populations improved their health and longevity to the level of college-educated Americans, the economic gain would be on the order of $1.02 trillion in 2006[1] (Schoeni et al., 2011).

Starting with education as an illustration, achieving health equity by reaching the poorest and most marginalized groups of people will require strong community ownership of the value and purpose of education, whether it be primary education, job training, or adult literacy. Disparities in education perpetuate disparities in income and health. What is the incentive—the business case—to improve education and training at individual, employer, and community levels? To individuals, education confers significant wage advantages; therefore, in theory, individuals have a strong incentive to pursue education (Blundell et al., 1999). Educational achievement is also shaped by ability; early childhood education; family background, including family income and parent education; and the local environment, including the quality of schools. The same amount of schooling could lead to very different skills, college experience, and earnings if one person goes to a much better school, with better teachers, instruction, and resources (Deming et al., 2014). Individuals can also achieve higher job earnings through employer training programs, but those most likely to receive additional training have greater skills and more education to begin with (Cappelli, 2004). This reinforcing nature of skills and education highlights how disparities can widen and create a "vicious circle" for those who do not have a strong start with initial qualifications.

Part of the reason a community's commitment to education is important is that any one employer in the community is likely to invest in education, whether by supporting secondary education or general training. Using a standard model a typical firm's calculus would be that education and training could improve worker productivity, making the firm more competitive and profitable (Becker, 1993). However, the more skilled workers could leave and work for a competing firm. Even if the firm were willing to pay a higher wage to retain the now higher-skilled worker, it would have "lost" its investment in training. In the real world, firms do

---

[1] "[This estimate does] not capture the causal effects of education on health. Instead, [it estimates] the foregone benefits if indeed the less-educated individuals experienced the same health and mortality as the college graduates" (Schoeni et al., 2011, p. S70).

support education and training, and this appears to be driven by contextual factors such as minimum wages, unionization, and employer competition in local areas (Acemoglu and Pischke, 1999; Autor, 2001). Firms also engage in particular or firm-specific training rather than general training. In contrast to general training, local employers may be more willing to invest in firm-specific training because the skills do not transfer to competitors as readily. Thus, the immediate business case for individual firms to act on behalf of general education and training in the community is somewhat narrow.

Mobilizing the Private Sector

While there is strong motivation at the individual level to pursue improvement, such as education, because of the prospect of higher incomes in the future, there is also a societal component at play. The spillover benefits of a more educated community accrue to everyone. Communities benefit from having an educated and literate population with greater civic engagement, lower crime, greater social cohesion, and economic growth. Firms can adapt their use of technology and equipment to the skills of a more educated, local work force, and more educated workers may exchange new ideas, furthering innovation. These spillover benefits mean that the community together, not just any one actor, should play an important role in supporting education. The challenge is that education benefits accrue over the long run and are thus investments that politically may be difficult to sustain. Private–public partnerships, such as Made in Durham, which works through a multi-sector collaborative to increase high school graduation rates and employment (NASEM, 2016; Stratton et al., 2012), have appeared to overcome some of the disincentives faced by any one actor operating in isolation.

Community momentum for changes in education, employment, or housing, whether through a school reform movement or a housing revitalization effort, may in part be understood as an attempt to mobilize the private sector on behalf of a public effort. The Aspen Institute describes such efforts as integrating social purposes with business methods (Sabeti, 2009). Such programs are often structured with public funding—for example, vouchers, grants, or tax credits—and private or shared public–private delivery of services and with public accountability structures. The impetus is often to introduce private-sector competition or innovation and to improve efficiency and performance. Frequently these mobilization efforts draw the attention of foundations, individual philanthropy, or private investors who provide additional resources and bolster further improvements. If these efforts around the social determinants of health can lead to resources being more effectively and more equitably distributed, this could make inroads in health equity as well.

Other health drivers can be viewed through a similar lens. Often individuals have an incentive to improve their own situations, but this is shaped by local circumstances. Businesses have an interest in reducing the cost of health care; lowering the cost of employer-provided benefits, including workers compensation costs; lowering turnover; improving worker productivity; and reducing the number of sick days. A healthy workforce is less costly to employers. Yet, firms left to themselves may underinvest in health activities for workers. Thus, communities have a strong case for coming together and devising joint solutions.

Several investors have become involved in "social impact bonds," also called "pay for success" programs (NASEM, 2016). Generally the programs are well-defined, are focused on "human capital" improvements over a 5- to 7-year span, and are limited in scope. For example, some such programs have addressed early childhood education, home visiting, prison avoidance, chronic homelessness, and foster care avoidance for children born to homeless mothers. They commonly involve private investors and foundations along with public payers. When early intervention programs yield desired outcomes—which means savings to the public down the line—the programs pay their investors from public or foundation funds. These solutions are appealing in part as a mechanism for community-building, for reinvigorating local dialogue on the social determinants of health, and for leveraging private institution participation and promoting transparency and efficiency. At the moment, however, because few such programs have run their course, there is relatively little empirical evidence concerning their effectiveness.

Another form of business-driven venture is the employment social enterprise. In this case, various entities, typically nonprofits, invest in disadvantaged groups, including those with low job skills and experience. They provide employment, training, and social services along with wages and experiential learning, working closely with local businesses (Maxwell et al., 2013; NASEM, 2016; Rotz et al., 2015). Social enterprises may also receive technical support and capital funding from entities such as REDF in California, which is itself grant-, foundation-, and donor-supported, as well as funding through tax credits. Social enterprises represent another form of public–private partnership and arise from a shared sense of purpose and common incentives.

Framing Outcomes and Success in Community Solutions

The major outcome of interest for community solutions is impact on health. Life expectancy can be a useful measure of impact on health because it is straightforward and easy to interpret, compare, and value.

However, it is less likely that community solutions will have data or measured impact on mortality indicators in the short term, as it takes considerable time to see changes in these long-term outcomes. In addition, the quantity of life is only one metric of health and does not capture quality, satisfaction, well-being, happiness, and opportunity. Instead, the committee sought out community-based solutions that target the social determinants of health with strong links to health outcomes as evidenced by the literature. However, community-level outcomes cannot be measured without community-level data. The section below outlines what is currently available to communities as well as the gaps in data and data tools.

Meeting Information Needs to Drive Community-Based Solutions

In 2011 the Institute of Medicine (IOM) Committee on Public Health Strategies to Improve Health highlighted the lack of accurate local data on the social, environmental, and behavioral determinants of health and recommended that the U.S. Department of Health and Human Services (HHS) support and implement: (1) a core, standardized set of indicators that can be used to assess the health of communities, including social determinants of health; (2) a core, standardized set of health outcome indicators for national, state, and local use; and (3) a summary measure of population health that can be used to estimate and track health-adjusted life expectancy (IOM, 2012). Since the publication of that report, there has been an increased emphasis on the use of common data elements (CDEs) in some parts of HHS, and a CDE resource portal is hosted by the National Library of Medicine (NIH, 2016). However, with a few exceptions (e.g., the National Health and Nutrition Evaluation Survey and the Patient Reported Outcomes Measurement Information System), CDE initiatives are disease-focused, and most are not linked to localities such as neighborhoods or census tracts. To address the issue of measurement heterogeneity, an IOM committee generated a framework, a core measure set, and an initial set of indicators (IOM, 2015b). Beyond addressing the challenges of what should be measured and how it should be measured, communities need data and interactive tools to easily access data as well as metrics that are specific to their situations and needs. Such data are critical to raising awareness to make health equity a shared vision and value, increasing a community's capacity to design community-based solutions and shape outcomes, and fostering multi-sector collaboration and evaluation of solutions.

Data Sources

Increasingly, there are sources of electronic data that are publicly available and can be used to examine issues related to health and health equity and to inform the development of community-based solutions. Some data sets are specific to health and others are from sectors relevant to health and health equity.

Thousands of data sets are accessible for public use through the U.S. government's Health Data Initiative and the open data portal (HHS, n.d.-a). These include data sets from federal agencies, including U.S. Department of Health and Human Services agencies such as the U.S. Centers for Disease Control and Prevention (CDC), the Centers for Medicare & Medicaid Services, the Health Resources and Services Administration, the National Institutes of Health, and the U.S. Food and Drug Administration, as well as from states (e.g., Hawaii, Michigan, New York) and cities (e.g., Boston, Fort Collins). For instance, Boston's open data portal includes data sets from many sectors that are relevant to health and health equity. These include hospital locations, healthy corner stores, farmers markets, community culinary and nutrition programs, crime incident reports, building code violations, and economic indicators (City of Boston Data Portal, 2013). Such data are sometimes organized into community dashboards that display key indicators. In Fort Collins, Colorado, for example, the dashboard includes quarterly summaries of factors that are related to a culture of health that advances health equity: neighborhood livability and social health, environment, transportation, economic health, environmental health, and safe community. The community dashboard for Travis County, Texas, presents data according to goals (CAN, 2016). For example, the municipality's goal of "Being safe, just, and engaged" includes data related to crime, the proportions of jail bookings by race and ethnicity, and voting. The goal of "Realizing full potential" uses indicators related to kindergarten readiness, high school graduation, college success, and unemployment.

Some nongovernmental organizations also offer public access to various data sources relevant to community-based solutions that advance health equity. These include data sets from surveys such as the Robert Wood Johnson Foundation (RWJF) National Survey of Health Attitudes, which includes data on such values as health interdependence, sense of community, and social support; the University of Michigan's Monitoring the Future series of youth surveys; and the Corporate Giving in Numbers survey. In other instances, data are available as files (e.g., the National Association of County and City Health Officials [NACCHO] National Profile of Local Health Departments) or reports (e.g., Best Complete Street Policies of 2015). Such resources (see Box 8-1) are currently more valuable for national-, state- or city-level assessments, as most of the data sets lack data at the neighborhood or community level. Moreover, many of these data sources are more suitable for use by researchers than by communities.

BOX 8-1
Examples of Governmental and Nongovernmental Data Sources

The Agency for Healthcare Research and Quality's Area Health Resources Files is a family of health data resource products that draws from an extensive county-level database assembled annually from more than 50 sources. Available at http://ahrf.hrsa.gov (accessed June 15, 2016).

American Community Survey (ACS). ACS 2013 is available at https://www.census.gov/programs-surveys/acs/data.html (accessed June 18, 2016). A product of the U.S. Census Bureau, the ACS is an ongoing survey that provides information on a yearly basis about the United States and its people.

Basic Economic Security Tables (BEST) Index. The BEST Index is available at http://www.basiceconomicsecurity.org/best (accessed June 15, 2016). A collaboration of the Institute for Women's Policy Research, the National Council on Aging, and the University of Massachusetts at Boston, the BEST Index measures the income that a working adult requires to meet his or her basic needs at the city, state, and national levels.

Best Complete Streets Policies report. Data tables are available at http://www.smartgrowthamerica.org/best-complete-streets-policies-of-2015 (accessed June 15, 2016). A product of Smart Growth America, the focus of a Complete Streets approach is an integrated transportation system that supports safe travel for people of all ages and abilities.

Bureau of Justice Statistics Census of State and Local Law Enforcement Agencies (CSLLEA). A public file is available at http://www.icpsr.umich.edu/icpsrweb/NACJD/studies/27681 (accessed June 19, 2016). CSLLEA is conducted every 4 years to enumerate agencies and their employees.

Center for Climate and Energy Solutions (C2ES). A publicly available table is available at http://www.c2es.org/us-states-regions/policy-maps/climate-action-plans (accessed June 15, 2016). Data are available at the state level.

Community Diversity Data creates customized reports describing more than 100 measures of diversity, opportunity, and quality of life for 362 metropolitan areas. Available at www.diversitydata.org (accessed July 1, 2016).

Current Population Survey (CPS) March Annual Social and Economic Supplement. A public use data set for the CPS March Annual Social and Economic Supplement is available at https://www.census.gov/cps/data (accessed June 14, 2016). A product of the U.S. Census Bureau and the U.S. Bureau of Labor Statistics, CPS is the primary source of labor force statistics for the United States and also includes data on income and health insurance coverage.

continued

BOX 8-1 Continued

Current Population Survey's Volunteer and Civic Engagement Supplement. A public use data set is available at http://www.nationalservice.gov/about/open-government-initiative/opengovernment-gallery (accessed June 18, 2016). A service of the Corporation for National and Community Service, data on volunteering are available at the state, city, and geographic region levels.

The Equality of Opportunity Project. Raj Chetty and Nathaniel Hendren, principal investigators, Harvard University. Available at http://www.equal-opportunity.org (accessed June 15, 2016).

Giving in Numbers survey. Reports presenting the data are available at http://cecp.co/measurement/tools.html (accessed September 1, 2016). The reports present a profile of corporate philanthropy and detail corporate investments.

The Harvard Public Health Disparities Geocoding Project Monograph provides an introduction to geocoding and to using area-based socioeconomic measures with public health surveillance data, based on the work of the Public Health Disparities Geocoding Project at the Harvard School of Public Health, Department of Society, Human Development, and Health. Available at https://www.hsph.harvard.edu/thegeocodingproject (accessed June 20, 2016).

HealthData.gov provides access to almost 3,000 data sets. Data files are accessible at http://www.healthdata.gov (accessed June 15, 2016). More than 65 data sets are tagged as community level, and many of these are also tagged as health.

Monitoring the Future. A public use data set is available at http://www.icpsr.umich.edu/icpsrweb/ICPSR/series/35 (accessed July 1, 2016). The Continuing Study of the Lifestyles and Values of Youth surveys gathers data on important values, behaviors, and lifestyle orientations of contemporary American youth.

The National Association of County and City Health Officials (NACCHO) National Profile of Local Health Departments. Data can be requested from http://nacchoprofilestudy.org/data-requests (accessed June 15, 2016). There is a fee to access the analytic file. The files include data on local health department infrastructure and practice, including partnerships, programs and services, and public health policy.

The National Center for Education Statistics provides fiscal and non-fiscal data for public schools through data tables and searchable tools. Available at https://nces.ed.gov/ccd (accessed June 13, 2016).

National Survey on Drug Use and Health (NSDUH). A public use data set can be downloaded for free at http://www.samhsa.gov/data/population-data-nsduh/reports (accessed June 18, 2016). Data on drug use and health are available at national, state, and sub-state/metro levels.

Office of Management and Budget (OMB) budget historical tables can be downloaded at https://www.whitehouse.gov/omb/budget/Historicals (accessed September 3, 2016). OMB files provide data on budget receipts, outlays, surpluses or deficits, federal debt, and federal employment over an extended time period, generally from 1940 or earlier to 2017.

The Robert Wood Johnson Foundation (RWJF) National Survey of Health Attitudes is accessible through RWJF's Health and Medical Care Archive (HMCA) through the Inter-University Consortium for Political and Social Research at the University of Michigan at http://www.icpsr.umich.edu/icpsrweb/ICPSR/studies?searchSource=find-analyze-home&sortBy=&q=rwjf (accessed June 15, 2016). Developed by RWJF and RAND, the survey primarily addresses the culture of health action area of making health a shared value.

The Uniform Crime Report (UCR) is available through the Federal Bureau of Investigation at https://ucr.fbi.gov (accessed June 20, 2016). The UCR Program collects statistics on violent crime (murder and nonnegligent manslaughter, forcible rape, robbery, and aggravated assault) and property crime (burglary, larceny/theft, and motor vehicle theft). Using the table-building tool, users can specify offenses, locality (city, county, state), and year(s).

U.S. Centers for Disease Control and Prevention's Behavioral Risk Factor Surveillance System (BRFSS). The BRFSS undertakes health-related telephone surveys (more than 400,000 adult interviews each year) that collect state data about U.S. residents regarding their health-related risk behaviors, chronic health conditions, and use of preventive services. Available at http://www.cdc.gov/brfss (accessed June 18, 2016).

U.S. Department of Education data include data on enrollment demographics, preschool, discipline, school expenditures, teacher experience, among others; 2013–2014 data were collected for the first time on chronic student absenteeism, the availability of free or partial-payment preschool, educational access in justice facilities, civil rights coordinators, and other data points. Data from 2004, 2006, and 2009–2010 are based on a rolling stratified sample of approximately 7,000 districts and 70,000 schools, whereas 2000, 2011–2012, and 2013–2014 were based on data collected from all of the nation's school districts and schools, making them more useful for communities addressing education disparities. Available at http://ocrdata.ed.gov (accessed June 18, 2016).

U.S. Department of Interior Office of Budget fund receipts can be downloaded at https://www.doi.gov/budget/budget-data (accessed June 14, 2016). Data include Land and Water Conservation Fund receipts and federal funding for Native American programs.

Indicators

For the purpose of this report, the committee uses the definition of *indicator* from the 2011 IOM report: a statistic or measure that is widely acknowledged to be useful for measuring something of concern to policy makers or the public (IOM, 2012). In the following section, indicators are summarized according to the components of the conceptual model for the report: (1) social determinants of health, (2) making health equity a shared vision and value, (3) increasing community capacity to shape outcomes, and (4) healthier, more equitable communities in which individuals and families live, learn, work, and play. The indicators selected for inclusion were based on a recent environmental scan on social-determinants-of-health indicators (Koo et al., 2016), an IOM report (IOM, 2012) that summarized national indicator sets for public health action, and a targeted literature search. The intent was to provide examples pertinent to community-based solutions rather than to provide an exhaustive summary. Further details of selected indicators by data set or index are provided in Appendix B.

Social determinants of health There are many data sources that contain indicators related to various social determinants of health. These include America's Health Rankings, County Health Rankings, Community Health Status Indicators, and the National Equity Atlas. Indicators are most frequently available at the state or county level. Some cities have local equity atlases; Denver (Mile High Connects, 2016; Sadler et al., 2012) and Los Angeles (Reconnecting America, 2013) have noninteractive local equity atlases with a strong emphasis on transit. The Metro Atlanta Equity Analysis examines eight dimensions of community well-being (demographics, economic development, education, environment, health, housing, public safety, and transportation) through online tools.[2] In some cases, such as the AARP Livability Index;[3] the Brandeis University Diversity Data Kids dataset;[4] the University of California, Davis, Regional Opportunity Index;[5] and the Virginia Health Opportunity Index,[6] data are available for smaller areas such as school districts or neighborhoods. Some indicators occur in the majority of the data sets reviewed. For example, high school

---

[2] For more information, see http://atlantaequityatlas.com/about-maea (accessed December 19, 2016).

[3] For more information, see https://livabilityindex.aarp.org (accessed December 19, 2016).

[4] For more information, see http://www.diversitydatakids.org (accessed December 19, 2016).

[5] For more information, see http://interact.regionalchange.ucdavis.edu/roi (accessed December 19, 2016).

[6] For more information, see http://www.vdh.virginia.gov/health-equity/virginia-health-opportunity-index-hoi (accessed December 19, 2016).

graduation 4 years after starting 9th grade, health insurance, and air pollution are common indicators for education, health systems and services, and physical environment, respectively. There are also summarizing projects, such as Community Commons, that make these data available to a broader range of users (IP3, n.d.).

Making health equity a shared vision and value Although they were not conceptualized as explicit measures to demonstrate the extent to which health equity is a shared vision and value, some existing indicators are likely relevant. For instance, the Virginia Health Opportunity index includes a measure of segregation that includes community diversity and distances between communities with different racial or ethnic profiles. The JustSouth Index[7] also includes a measure related to public school segregation along with measures of wage and employment equity. The National Equity Atlas[8] characterizes diversity through the inclusion of a Diversity Index and a Culture of Health measure set that uses residential segregation.

None of these indicators explicitly measure attitudes or beliefs related to health equity, which are central to making health equity a shared vision and value. There is certainly the potential to construct indicators through standard techniques for survey development. However, attitudes and beliefs are sentiments or opinions that can be monitored through newer analytic techniques applied to social media. Sentiment analysis—the application of natural language processing, text mining, or computational linguistic tools to determine positive or negative effect—is widely used to assess opinions in written texts, including tweets. For example, it has been used to assess emotions associated with global warming and climate change (Lineman et al., 2015) and the moods of patients in online cancer communities (Rodrigues et al., 2016), and it has been used in the "Geography of Happiness" in combination with demographics and objective characteristics of place (Mitchell et al., 2013). Sentiment analysis tools are increasingly available as open sources or built into quantitative (e.g., R) or qualitative (e.g., NVivo) analysis programs.

In the short term, there will be a need to determine which existing indicators are most relevant for measuring and monitoring progress toward making health equity a shared vision and value. Moreover, new indicators are needed. The sentiment analysis of texts such as tweets and other social media communication represents a promising approach to capturing changes in popular opinions over time.

---

[7] For more information, see http://www.loyno.edu/news/documents/just-south-index-2016.pdf (accessed December 19, 2016).

[8] For more information, see http://nationalequityatlas.org (accessed December 19, 2016).

Increasing community capacity to shape outcomes As part of its culture of health agenda, RWJF developed measures organized by its action framework (Chandra et al., 2016). Four of those indicators relate to this report's focus on increasing community capacity to shape outcomes: (1) a sense of community, (2) social support, (3) voter participation, and (4) volunteer engagement. The latter two are also present in several other data sources. Other aspects of community capacity building are leadership development, community organizing, organizational development, and fostering collaborative relations among organizations. These may be relevant areas for future measure development.

Fostering multi-sector collaboration RWJF's culture of health metrics (Chandra et al., 2016) include nine indicators related to fostering multi-sector collaboration: local health department collaboration; opportunities to improve health for youth in schools; business support for workplace health promotion and culture of health; U.S. corporate giving; federal allocations for health investments related to nutrition and indoor and outdoor physical activity; community relations and policing; youth exposure to advertising for healthy and unhealthy food and beverage products; climate adaptation and mitigation; and health in all policies. In addition to the RWJF National Attitudes survey, the indicators reflect several novel data sources, including the Nielsen ratings for measuring youth exposure to advertising for health and unhealthy food and beverage products and community climate action plans for measuring climate adaptation and mitigation.

Healthier more equitable communities in which individuals and families live, learn, work, and play The measurement of progress toward "healthier more equitable communities in which members and families live, learn, work, and play" requires health indicators as well as equity indicators, including those related to the social determinants of health. National health indicator data sets contain a large variety of indicators for which health disparities exist (see Table B-1 in Appendix B for examples of indicators relevant to health equity in public data sources). These include indicators related to health behaviors (e.g., smoking, binge drinking), health status (e.g., poor mental health days, overall health status), morbidity (e.g., high blood pressure, diabetes), and mortality (e.g., premature death, addiction-related death). In addition, a report that RWJF commissioned from the Health Enhancement Research Organization proposed five indicators related to costs that could be used by collaborations wishing to engage nontraditional partners such as business entities: (1) annual end-of-life care expenditures, (2) family health care cost, (3) per capita expenditures on health care, (4) potentially preventable hospitalization rates, and (5) social spending relative to health expenditure (May et al., 2016).

Interactive Tools

Although lists of indicators are useful in determining what to measure and how it should be measured, Web-based interactive tools make data sets more accessible to communities. Box 8-2 lists a collection of selected interactive tools, and their contents are summarized in Appendix B. Moreover, many of the interactive tools allow queries by geographic location, making it easy for communities to target their state, county, or neighborhood. In some instances, comparisons are made with other similar locations. For example, the CDC's Community Health Status Indicators presents a target county's data in comparison with "peer" counties and lists the indicators in three categories according to quartiles: better, moderate (middle two quartiles), and worse than the comparators (CDC, 2015). Other interactive tools display a composite index. The AARP Livability Index integrates multiple indicators in areas that are relevant to advancing health equity (housing, neighborhood, transportation, environment, health, engagement, and opportunity) to create an overall score (AARP Public Policy Institute, n.d.).

Some interactive tools are designed explicitly with health equity in mind. For example, the National Equity Access provides detailed demographic data as well as indicators in three key areas: economic vitality, readiness, and connectedness. In addition, it includes metrics related to the economic benefits of racial equity (gross domestic product gains with racial equity and income gains with racial equity) (PolicyLink and USC Program for Environmental and Regional Equity, 2016). Tools such as EJSCREEN (EPA, 2016) and the Food Access Research Atlas (U.S. Department of Agriculture Economic Research Service, 2016) focus on other important social determinants of health. While education level is found in many indexes, the Children's Health and Education Mapping Tool explicitly links school population and resources, including school-based clinics, with health (School-Based Health Alliance, n.d.). The Diversity Data Kids interactive tool includes early childhood education and provides rankings and child opportunities by race and ethnicity for states, counties, large cities, and large school districts (Brandeis University, n.d.).

Another area of emphasis for interactive tools that is relevant to advancing health equity is opportunity indexes. Some indexes are at the state or county level. In contrast, the Virginia Health Opportunity Index has dashboards for counties, legislative districts, and health districts, thus providing a more local view of indicators to drive or evaluate community action (Virginia Department of Health, 2016).

> **BOX 8-2**
> **Examples of Interactive Tools**
>
> AARP Livability Index: https://livabilityindex.aarp.org/categories/neighborhood (accessed June 30, 2016)
>
> Children's Health and Education Mapping Tool: http://www.sbh4all.org/resources/mapping-tool (accessed June 30, 2016)
>
> Community Health Status Indicators: http://wwwn.cdc.gov/CommunityHealth/info/AboutProject (accessed June 30, 2016)
>
> Diversity Data Kids data set: http://www.diversitydatakids.org (accessed June 30, 2016)
>
> Environmental Justice Screening and Mapping Tool (EJSCREEN): https://www.epa.gov/ejscreen (accessed June 30, 2016)
>
> Food Access Research Atlas: http://www.ers.usda.gov/data-products/food-access-research-atlas.aspx (accessed June 30, 2016)
>
> Health Equity Index: http://www.cadh.org/health-equity/health-equity-index.html (accessed June 30, 2016)
>
> JustSouth Index: http://www.loyno.edu/jsri/news/inaugural-justsouth-index-2016
>
> National Equity Atlas: http://nationalequityatlas.org (accessed June 30, 2016)
>
> Opportunity Index: http://opportunityindex.org/#4.00/40.00/-97.00 (accessed June 30, 2016)
>
> The Housing and Transportation (H+T®) Affordability Index: http://www.htaindex.org (accessed June 30, 2016)
>
> Virginia Health Opportunity Index: https://www.vdh.virginia.gov/OMHHE/policyanalysis/virginiahoi.htm (accessed June 30, 2016)

The good news is there are many existing data sources, indicators, and interactive tools that can inform community-based solutions. Challenges include the facts that many communities may be unaware that such tools exist or may not be well positioned to use them effectively; that there is a need for indicators that can ascertain the extent to which health equity is a shared vision and value; that there is a persistent dearth of indicators and interactive tools based on neighborhood- or community-level data; and that although some interactive tools allow queries by racial or ethnic group, gender, or age, they may not be informative for other groups for which health disparities exist, such as incarcerated, formerly incarcerated, and lesbian, gay, bisexual, and transgender (LGBT) populations.

> *Conclusion 8-1: Accessible and community-friendly interactive tools with data and metrics specific to individual communities are needed. Such data are critical to raising awareness to make health equity a shared vision and value, increasing community capacity to design community-based solutions and shape outcomes, and fostering multi-sector collaboration and the evaluation of solutions.*
> - *In the short term there is a need to determine which existing indicators are most relevant for measuring and monitoring progress toward making health equity a shared vision and value, developing community capacity to shape outcomes, and encouraging multi-sector collaboration.*
> - *Other aspects of community capacity building, including leadership development, community organizing, organizational development, and fostering collaborative relations among organizations are additional areas for potential indicator development.*
>
> *Conclusion 8-2: There are many existing data sources, indicators, and interactive tools that are relevant to meeting the information needs that drive community-based solutions; however,*
> - *Many communities may be unaware that such tools exist or lack some of the prerequisite skills for their effective use. Furthermore, these tools need to be made more user-friendly to facilitate use by community members.*
> - *Many of the indicators and interactive tools provide data at the national, state, or county level. More tools are needed that provide interactive access to data at the neighborhood or community level.*

Adopting or Developing Logic Models or Theories of Change

Engaging communities, developing community interventions, and developing projects addressing health equity all deal with very complex issues. To maximize the likelihood of success as well as of the potential for learning, those individuals, groups, and organizations pursuing such work must create and follow some sort of framework to guide strategies and activities. This framework might be as simple as project management, which involves identifying activities, specifying timelines, and measuring progress, or can involve more structured approaches such as logic models and theories of change.

Logic models are popular tools in the public health, nonprofit, and other fields. These models are frameworks that describe the different components of a program with the intent that the activities that make up a program are matched to the desired outcomes. Logic models graphically illustrate program components and usually include inputs, or what resources are used by the program; activities, or what the program does in terms of tasks, actions, etc.; outputs, or what the activities produce; outcomes, or the changes and benefits of the program in the short, medium, and long term; and impact, or the long-term intended change in organization, communities, or systems resulting from the program. These frameworks are outcomes-focused and assume causal links between activities and outcome. Using logic models helps stakeholders clearly identify a program's components and intended results.

Another popular framework for complex interventions is the theory of change, which is specifically ideal for developing interventions to address complex social issues, such as health equity. In contrast to the logic model, which progresses from resources to outcomes, a theory of change starts by identifying a long-term goal and works backward to identify the preconditions that must be met in order to achieve the goal. Interventions to create the preconditions, as well as indicators of the performance of the interventions, are developed. Planners explicitly explain why the preconditions are necessary in order to achieved short-term objectives and why these are necessary to meet the long-term goal; in essence, the narrative concludes that the goal cannot be achieved unless the preconditions are met. Theories of change link outcomes and activities to explain how and why the desired change is expected to come about. Theories of change are dynamic and can be refined based on ongoing evaluation and strategic learning information; they provide guidance for stakeholders, support resource planning, and can help determine why an intervention worked—or did not. Done correctly, the process depends on the inclusion of different perspectives and participants in developing and implementing successful interventions. Additional details about specific approaches for change within organizations are provided later in this chapter. Box 8-3 highlights the development and application of theories of change in the community examples discussed in Chapter 5.

Using Civil Rights Law to Promote Health Equity

Civil rights laws can support community-based solutions to promote health equity and are an integral part of the culture of health in the United States. Chapter 6 contains a discussion on the broader context of using civil rights law to promote health equity, including background, the relationship to federal and state laws, and implementation of the

> **BOX 8-3**
> **Examples of Developing and Applying Theories of Change from Community Examples in Chapter 5**
>
> In New York City, WE ACT's theory of change is logic model-based and details short-term, intermediate, and long-term outcomes as well as the ultimate societal change of transforming northern Manhattan into a healthy community (see Figure 5-21).
>
> In San Antonio, Texas, the Eastside Promise Neighborhood's theory of change is supported by 21 neighborhood goals, which include targets set by community members and stakeholders to address 10 promises: (1) Children enter kindergarten ready to succeed in school; (2) students improve academic performance and are proficient in core subjects; (3) students successfully transition from elementary to middle to high school; (4) students graduate from high school; (5) students earn a college degree or a job training certification; (6) students are healthy and their educational performance improves by accessing aligned learning and enrichment activities; (7) students feel safe at school and in their community; (8) students live in stable communities; (9) families and community members support learning in Promise Neighborhood schools; and (10) students have access to 21st-century learning tools.
>
> In Los Angeles, California, the Magnolia Community Initiative, along with the Children's Council of Los Angeles and First 5 LA, developed a Community Level Change Model (see Figure 5-15) in which the foundation for achieving family and community-level change is relationship-based resident groups.

law—including many examples. As noted in Chapter 6, the Civil Rights Act of 1964 is an essential tool for addressing health disparities. (See below for a few civil rights law examples at the community level, and Box 8-4 provides an example from Baldwin Hills in Los Angeles County, California, of using the Clean Water Act for a civil rights, environmental justice, and health victory.) Civil rights laws offer tools that stakeholders working with public interest attorneys, public health professionals, community groups, government agencies, and recipients of federal, state, and local funds can use to promote health equity. As noted in Chapter 6, it is important to emphasize that these legal tools are not by any means limited to a litigation strategy. Voluntary compliance with civil rights laws can be preferable to litigation as a way of achieving equal justice goals. The civil rights movement uses many strategies to promote human dignity, equal justice, and just democracy and to overcome discrimination.[9]

---

[9] DOJ Title VI Legal Manual at page II-3 (supporters of Title VI considered it an efficient alternative to ponderous, time-consuming, and uncertain litigation) (2016). Available at https://www.justice.gov/crt/fcs/T6manual (accessed July 15, 2016); Rodriguez et al. (2014).

> **BOX 8-4**
> **Baldwin Hills in Los Angeles County, California**
>
> The battle for clean water justice in the historic African American part of Los Angeles shows how attorneys working with the community can be more effective than the community acting alone.
> The Baldwin Hills area in Los Angeles County is a center of excellence for African Americans in the United States. For decades the black community complained without success of noxious sewer odors permeating their neighborhoods and homes, making people nauseated and contributing to stress and other health disorders. "The odors smell like rotten eggs and are caused by naturally occurring hydrogen sulfide escaping from the sewers" (Garcia and Sivasubramanian, 2012). Finally, in 2001 the U.S. Environmental Protection Agency (EPA) partnered in court with community leaders, including Concerned Citizens of Southcentral Los Angeles and the Baldwin Hills Home Owners' Association—represented by civil rights attorneys—and a mainstream environmental organization. Together they sued the City of Los Angeles to repair the sewer system city-wide and to eliminate the persistent and offensive odors concentrated in the African American parts of town. After the city admitted liability for 3,500 sewer spills, the parties reached a $2 billion settlement agreement, and the city and the community continued to work together even after the suit ended. Because the Los Angeles sewer system is one of the largest, this work is significant to the nation. It was the first time the Clean Water Act was used to address sewage odors, which are separate from overflows. The case is one of the largest sewage cases in U.S. history, according to the EPA.
>
> SOURCE: Garcia and Sivasubramanian, 2012.

Related Examples of Policies and Actions to Promote Health Equity

Agencies can also promote health equity through broad-based, more equitable community engagement. The National Park Service's (NPS's) Healthy Parks Healthy People U.S. program was established in 2011 to reframe the role of parks and public lands in terms of an emerging health and prevention strategy. The program seeks to work with national, state, and local parks as well as businesses, new health partners, funding resources, stakeholders, and advocacy organizations to foster and build upon the role that parks play in the health of our society (NPS, 2014). The NPS views civic engagement as an important part of its work and has created a number of tools, guides, and handbooks to promote engagement across diverse communities.[10]

---

[10] See https://www.nps.gov/civic for tools such as *Beyond Outreach Handbook: A Guide to Designing Effective Programs to Engage Diverse Communities; Learning to Make Choices for*

Civil rights and health equity can also be promoted through programmatic priorities. For example, NPS recognizes that transportation is a significant barrier for many low-income communities and communities of color in reaching existing parks and open space. Many families do not have cars and do not live near efficient and reliable public transit that provides access to regional parks (NPS, 2015). Similarly, the NPS Every Kid in a Park provides every 4th grader in the nation and their families with a free pass to the national parks. NPS is providing transportation grants to schools with a high proportion of low-income students who qualify for free or reduced-price meals. In Los Angeles, 1 of 11 target cities in the nation, NPS and the U.S. Forest Service are working with the Los Angeles Unified School District, the second largest in the nation. Similarly, the Transit to Trails programs in the Los Angeles region provides transit and education materials for free, fun, healthy, and educational trips to mountains, beaches, rivers, and deserts (The City Project, n.d.-b).

Physical Education in Public Schools

A successful community-based effort to promote health equity through wellness and prevention is physical education in public schools. The IOM recommends monitoring physical education minutes, addressing disparities, improving teacher education, making physical education a core subject, and addressing physical activity in the whole school environment (IOM, 2013). Failure to provide physical education may adversely impact health outcomes as well as academic achievement. According to studies, physical education can have a neutral or positive effect on testing (Basch, 2011a; Diamant et al., 2011; HHS, 2002); cognitive function may be linked positively with physical activity among low-income and minority students in elementary and middle school (Efrat, 2011); physical education may be associated with reduced overweight or obesity, lower blood pressure, and improved bone health (Basch, 2011b); and physical education is an important component in the fight against obesity and other related chronic conditions (Diamant et al., 2011; Springer et al., 2009) The Los Angeles County Department of Public Health publishes a physical education model action plan (MAP) and a tool kit to support community action for compliance with physical education and civil rights requirements in public schools (LA County Department of Public Health, 2015). The Los Angeles Unified School District adopted a plan to comply with physical education and civil rights requirements in 2008 (Lafleur et al., 2013).

---

the Future: Strategies for National Parks and Other Special Places; and Leading in a Collaborative Environment: Six Case Studies Involving Collaboration and Civic Engagement.

A 2016 University of Southern California study analyzed physical education and physical fitness in almost 900 California public school districts. According to the report, there are significant racial and ethnic, economic, and achievement indicators that affect student fitness across all districts. The California Education Code mandates that all public schools both provide physical education for students and assess students' physical fitness annually through the Fitnessgram standardized test. Yet many schools fail to meet physical education requirements, and less than half of all assessed students demonstrate full physical health. The major findings of the study include

- Fitnessgram passing rates differed significantly based on race and ethnicity.
- Non-Hispanic white students had the highest average passing rate, at 34 percent, followed by Asian students, at 31 percent. Students identifying as "Other" had an average passing rate of 29 percent. Hispanic students had a Fitnessgram passing rate of 26 percent. African American students had the lowest passing rate at 22 percent. Additionally, African American students had the highest percentage of poor scores, with nearly 400 districts reporting an overall passing rate of 10 percent or less among this racial group.
- School districts with more low-income students (eligible for free or reduced-price meals) tended to have lower Fitnessgram passing rates.
- Districts with higher API (academic performance index) scores tended to have higher Fitnessgram passing rates (Green et al., 2015).

According to the California Courts of Appeal, the state Education Code requires an average of 20 minutes of physical education per day in elementary schools, and parents and students have the right to sue a school district for not complying with that law. Half the public school districts audited in California from 2005 to 2009 did not comply with the minute requirements (Lafleur et al., 2013). According to a 2013 study, 83 percent of elementary schools in San Francisco reported that they met the minute requirements, but when the schools were monitored on-site only 5 percent met the requirements (Thompson, 2013). Districts that did not comply had a higher percentage of African American and Latino students than districts that did, according to a separate study (Rodriguez et al., 2014; Sanchez-Vaznaugh et al., 2012).

The shared use of parks, schools, and pools can help address the lack of places for healthy active living in underserved communities. In recent years the Los Angeles Unified School District has raised $27 billion for new school construction and modernization. The school district has built more than 130 new schools, modernized hundreds more, cleaned up acres of polluted brownfields, and made the future brighter for generations of students (The City Project, n.d.-a).

Schools and parks can combine education materials on ethnic studies on places and people with studies of STEM (science, technology, engineering, and mathematics) subjects to make health and environmental quality and justice personal to students. According to a recent study from Stanford University, ethnic studies programs improve grade point averages across all subjects, increase school attendance, and increase courses taken (Dee and Penner, 2016).

There are national and community resources available for communities seeking help with civil rights issues. Community organizations are discussed throughout this report. National resources include the NAACP Legal Defense & Educational Fund, Inc., which works on racial and ethnic justice (NAACP LDF, n.d.). The American Bar Association lists many pro bono programs (ABA, 2009). The University of California, Los Angeles (UCLA), Civil Rights Project website houses many resources, including community tools for education, transportation, and housing (UCLA, 2016). The Human Rights Campaign is the largest civil rights organization with the goal of achieving LGBT equality (Human Rights Campaign, 2016). NOW, the National Organization for Women, is dedicated to women's rights (NOW, 2016).

Medical–Legal Partnerships

In contrast to civil legal aid organizations that provide assistance to community members on issues that affect health through a justice-driven framework, medical–legal partnerships operate through a public health framework that includes the social determinants of health and values population outcomes as well as individual outcomes. Formally established in the early 1990s, medical–legal partnership is defined as "an approach to health that integrates the expertise of health care, public health and legal professionals, and staff to address and prevent health-harming social and legal needs for patients, clinics, and populations. By partnering together, health care, public health, and legal institutions transform the health care system's response to social determinants of health" (National Center for Medical–Legal Partnership, 2014b, p. 2). The National Center for Medical–Legal Partnership reports the participants in U.S. medical–legal partnerships to be 155 hospitals, 139 health centers, 34 health schools, 52 law schools, 126 legal aid agencies, and 64 pro bono partners (National Center for Medical–Legal Partnership, 2016). The legal care provided by medical–legal partnerships focuses on social, financial, or environmental problems that have a deleterious impact on a person's health and can be addressed through civil legal aid. It is distinctive from that of civil legal aid organizations in five key ways (National Center for Medical–Legal Partnership, 2014b).

First, medical–legal partnerships train health care team members and often health professional students to recognize health-harming civil legal needs. The training can take the form of specialized training for medical champions (Pettignano et al., 2014), social workers (University of Colorado Law School, n.d.), family specialists (Sege et al., 2015), or broader training for a group of physicians and nurse practitioners in a particular clinical setting (Taylor et al., 2015). Sometimes, the medical–partnership includes a law school as well as community-based legal aid services, thus affording the opportunity for collaborative interprofessional training of law, medical, nursing, social work, and other types of students. For example, through a service learning project, law and medical students at Florida International University partnered with community members and Florida Legal Services to collect patient narratives, disseminate information on Medicaid expansion to community members, and present patient stories to state lawmakers (Martinez et al., 2016).

Second, medical–legal partnerships support screening patients for health-harming civil legal needs. Increasingly, this is done through formal checklists that screen for the breadth of civil legal needs rather than a single high-priority need (Pettignano et al., 2013; Taylor et al., 2015). In some instances, computer-based clinical decision support has been used to screen for health-harming legal and social needs as well as to improve the delivery of appropriate physician counseling and to streamline access to legal and social service professionals when nonmedical remedies are required (Gilbert and Downs, 2015).

Third, legal professionals and others with specialized training provide triage, consultation, and legal representation services for patients—most typically on-site. The Atlanta-based Health Law Partnership, comprised of three community partners—Children's Healthcare of Atlanta, the Atlanta Legal Aid Society, and the Georgia State University College of Law—has attorneys in hospitals and clinics, and weekly interprofessional case conferences support triage of potential cases into those that require legal representation versus other types of services (Pettignano et al., 2014). Through the Colorado Health Equity Project, case management teams (physician, attorney, and social worker or behavior health specialist) provide on-site services to the Salud Family Health Center in Commerce City and the Colorado Center for Refugee Health (University of Colorado Law School, n.d.).

Fourth, changes to clinical or health care institution policy are made jointly by health care or legal professionals or both to treat and prevent health-harming legal needs. The Medical–Legal Partnership at Legal Aid of Western Missouri reported on the role of advocacy in occasioning community and organizational change in a medical–legal partnership (National Center for Medical–Legal Partnership, 2014a). Partners included a pediatric hospital, a federally qualified health center (FQHC), and a nonprofit social service organization focused on youth living in poverty. During a 3-year period, 158 advocacy efforts targeted 11 community sectors (e.g., civic groups, government, housing, education), resulting in multiple changes, including a community advisory board at the pediatric hospital and the establishment of a medical–legal partnership at a federally funded health care organization.

Fifth, health care or legal professionals or both jointly advance changes to local, state, and federal policies and regulations to improve population health. For example, to decrease injuries in motor vehicle accidents for children after they are too big for baby car seats, the Atlanta-based Health Law Partnership[11] drafted state legislation to mandate that booster seats be used with seat belts for children under 8 years old. The key partners were Georgia State University students in a health legislation and advocacy course, who identified and researched the problem, assessed political will, and drafted the legislation, and government affairs staff of Children's Healthcare of Atlanta, who found sponsors. The bill was subsequently signed into law.

Given the vulnerability of children, especially those with chronic diseases and who live in environments with inadequate heat, cooling, and light, children's health has been a particularly fertile area for the implementation of medical–legal partnerships. Consequently, a number of medical–legal partnerships have targeted energy insecurity and demonstrated positive effects in preventing utility shut-offs. For example, the PhilaKids medical–legal partnership implemented a multifaceted intervention that included the training of health care staff, the implementation of a needs screener, and the development of consensus criteria for certification of medical need approvals for stable utilities (Taylor et al., 2015). During a 1-year period, this process increased the certification of medical need approvals by 65 percent, preventing utility shut-offs for 396 families with vulnerable children. Another study focused on children with asthma in Atlanta and demonstrated both financial and nonfinancial outcomes. Over 7 years, half of the nonfinancial outcomes achieved were in the area of housing (e.g., protection from foreclosure, improved housing,

---

[11] For more information, see https://healthlawpartnership.org (accessed December 20, 2016).

and obtained or retained housing) and utilities (Pettignano et al., 2013). Recently, some authors have advocated for better integration of palliative medicine and medical–legal partnerships to address issues across the life course (Hallarman et al., 2014).

Medical–legal partnerships are growing and are currently present in all 50 states and the District of Columbia (National Center for Medical–Legal Partnership, 2016). Evidence, including the examples provided here, suggest that medical–legal partnerships play an important role in addressing the social determinants of health and are a relevant community-based solution for advancing health equity.

Using Health Impact Assessments to Understand Policy Implications

Health impact assessment (HIA) is a tool for analyzing the health effects of proposed programs, policies, and projects. The assessment process uses data and input from local stakeholders to understand the often overlooked benefits and consequences of a given proposal. HIA relies on the premise that most policy and programs will inevitably affect population health in some way and that it is better to understand those outcomes before final decisions are made. Recommendations to change a proposal based on HIA results can help improve health outcomes. To date, public health practitioners have conducted HIAs in a variety of policy areas—including, but not limited to, transportation, housing, land use, criminal justice, and development (NACCHO, 2016; The Pew Charitable Trusts, 2016).

Since the early 2000s when HIA was first used, the practice has become increasingly prominent as a method to apply a health context to policy decisions. At a 2002 meeting hosted by the CDC focused on the built environment's effect on health, workshop participants identified HIA as a promising approach (Kemm, 2013). To date, more than 240 HIAs have been conducted within the United States, and there is movement to make the practice more widespread (Ross et al., 2014). The White House Task Force on Childhood Obesity, Health and Human Services's Healthy People 2020 Policy, and the CDC's Transportation and Healthy Policy all advocate for the use of HIA (Kemm, 2013).

HIA remains an optional tool for policy analysis, unlike environmental impact assessments, which can be required on federally funded or licensed projects (Ross et al., 2014). The Massachusetts legislature emerged as one of the few bodies mandating HIAs when it passed the Healthy Transportation Compact in 2009, which requires state agencies to "institute a health impact assessment for use by planners, transportation administrators, public health administrators, and developers."[12] Due to HIA's noncompulsory status, regulations guiding the practice do not exist. Practitioners are awarded much flexibility, and the resultant reports vary in content, methodology, messaging, and audience.

In 2007, a group of business and community leaders from North Omaha, Nebraska, formed a coalition to return the neighborhood to its former glory (CDC, 2013). The plan included improving Adams Park, a 68-acre green space next to the Malcolm X birthplace. The Douglas County Health Department led the HIA with its partners, the African American Empowerment Network and the North Omaha Neighborhood Alliance. They collected and analyzed data on health, demographics, food access, crime, traffic crashes, and land use; interviewed experts; and reviewed scientific research to understand how changes in Adams Park could impact health. The HIA showed that the Adams Park plan could greatly improve health in North Omaha in multiple ways: (1) provide greater access to affordable fruits and vegetables; (2) create space for social interaction and exercise; (3) increase physical activity levels; and (4) raise property values and reduce crime within a quarter-mile span. See Box 8-5 for an example of a community-driven health impact assessment of a rezoning proposal.

To make conducting an HIA more accessible and to increase the number of practitioners, members of the HIA community have begun to publish guidelines. A methodology that includes six main stages—screening, scoping, recommendations, assessment, reporting, and monitoring and evaluation—is often considered common practice and a useful way for approaching the HIA process. Recently, 12 equity metrics related to four HIA outcomes have been proposed (Heller et al., 2014):

1. The HIA process and product focused on equity: (1) the proposal analyzed in the HIA was identified by or relevant to communities facing inequities; (2) the HIA scope—including goals, research questions, and methods—clearly addresses equity; (3) the distribution of health and equity impacts across the population was analyzed (e.g., existing conditions, impacts on specific populations predicted to address inequities; the HIA utilized community knowledge and experience as evidence); (4) the recommendations focus on impacts to communities facing inequities and are responsive to community concerns; (5) the findings and recommendations are disseminated in and by communities facing inequities using a range of culturally and linguistically appropriate media

---

[12] The 189th General Court of the Commonwealth of Massachusetts. 2009. Chapter 25. An Act Modernizing the Transportation Systems of the Commonwealth.

and other platforms; and (6) the monitoring and evaluation plan included clear goals to monitor equity impacts over time and an accountability mechanism (i.e., accountability triggers, actions, and responsible parties) to address adverse impacts that may arise.
2. The HIA process built the capacity and ability of communities facing health inequities to engage in future HIA and in decision making more generally: (1) communities facing inequities lead or are meaningfully involved in each step of the HIA; and (2) as a result of the HIA, communities facing inequities have increased knowledge and awareness of decision-making processes and have attained greater capacity to influence decision-making processes, including the ability to plan, organize, fundraise, and take action within the decision-making context.

BOX 8-5
Health Impact Assessment of the Housing Component of the East Harlem Neighborhood Plan

Gentrification and decreased amounts of affordable housing are a concern in East Harlem, and the East Harlem Neighborhood Plan (EHNP) was created to mitigate the potential effects of a rezoning proposal (see Box 6-1). The New York Academy of Medicine conducted a health impact assessment (HIA) of the housing component of the EHNP to inform future decisions made by Community Board 11, the EHNP Steering Committee, the Department of City Planning, and the City Council as specific proposals for zoning changes and new development emerge in East Harlem.

Key findings of the HIA highlight social determinants of health and include

- Health: higher rates of chronic disease than other Manhattan residents; the major health concerns identified by the community include hypertension, diabetes, asthma, infant mortality, mental health, and violence
- Housing affordability and displacement: more than half of East Harlem residents are rent-burdened or severely rent-burdened; East Harlem is losing nearly 300 rent-controlled or rent-stabilized units each year
- Mixed-income development and increased density: mixed-income development could address health disparities through the provision of new, well-maintained housing which could offset the potential effects of increased density
- Increased commercial activity or manufacturing in the neighborhood: the great need for increased economic opportunity that would come from increased commercial activity is expected to counterbalance negative health outcomes; it could potentially have a positive effect through increase in job opportunities and increased social cohesion

3. The HIA resulted in a shift in power benefiting communities facing inequities: (1) communities that face inequities have increased influence over decisions, policies, partnerships, institutions, and systems that affect their lives; and (2) government and institutions are more transparent, inclusive, responsive, and collaborative.
4. The HIA contributed to changes that reduced health inequities and inequities in the social and environmental determinants of health: (1) the HIA influenced the societal and environmental determinants of health within the community and a decreased differential in these determinants between communities facing inequities and other communities; and (2) the HIA influenced physical, mental, and social health issues within the community and a decreased differential in these outcomes between communities facing inequities and other communities.

- New development on New York City Housing Authority (NYCHA) property: it could provide revenue to maintain existing housing as well as create the opportunity for more affordable housing

Conclusion: Creating more affordable housing, increased neighborhood amenities, and better maintenance of NYCHA housing could result in improved health outcomes.

Selected strategies to maximize health-promoting potential and reduce the potential health risks of the EHNP zoning and affordable housing recommendations include, among others:

- Reduce the risk of displacement and provide new, affordable housing options for existing East Harlem residents by striving to include the 25 percent affordable housing set-aside at 60 percent Area Median Income (AMI) with 20 percent required at 40 percent AMI and the additional option of 20 percent units at 40 percent AMI in all developments.
- Focus efforts and available funding on improving the indoor environmental conditions of existing housing stock.
- Mitigate potential negative health outcomes of commercial development: provide technical assistance programs for small employers on health benefits, develop a business improvement district, or provide capacity-building support to existing merchant associations and neighborhood chambers of commerce.
- Monitoring and evaluation: augment regular monitoring of health outcomes with measures such as residential mobility, population density, ethnic diversity, changes in rent-stabilized housing, and investments in neighborhood improvements (Realmuto et al., 2016).

Funding Mechanisms for Communities

Regardless of the intended impact and the process of development and implementation of any community intervention to promote health equity, a key element is identifying the necessary fiscal resources for the project or program. Funding for community interventions can be described in terms of sources and mechanisms or strategies. Potential sources include federal, state, and local governmental agencies; business and other private-sector sources; and foundations or individual (or group) philanthropy. Mechanisms and strategies include grants, endowments and trusts, braided funding, leveraging or shared funding, investments (including social impact bonds and program-related investments or other low-interest loan programs or sub-market investments), and public–private partnerships. Community collaboratives working on health equity benefit from knowing the potential sources of funding and from using different strategies to diversify their revenue mix in order to bring more resources to bear and to increase the likelihood of success and sustainability.

Government funding sources are particularly attractive because, in general, they tend to be available for longer durations and can be quite substantial and even entirely sufficient for the development, implementation, and long-term sustainability of a program. Agencies have a broad set of potential funding mechanisms: including direct program or project funding, such as Medicaid and the U.S. Department of Housing and Urban Development (HUD) project grants; specific grant programs, such as community development block grants; low or below-market interest loan programs, such as the Federal Student Aid program; credit assistance, such as that provided by the Transportation Infrastructure Finance and Innovation Act; use fees, such as tolls; directly allocated taxes, such as the federal gasoline tax; and subsidies, such as HUD tenant and project-based assistance programs and public housing operating subsidies. Agencies can also pursue public–private partnerships where community services are financed by the government and provided by private agencies.

Many of the examples in Chapter 5 illustrate government as a source of funding for their initiatives. Both the Dudley Street Neighborhood Initiative and the Eastside Promise Neighborhood received Promise Neighborhood funding from the U.S. Department of Education through planning and implementation grants. In addition, Dudley Neighbors, Inc., as a certified state community development corporation, secured $100,000 in community tax investment credits. As an FQHC, Delta Health Center receives funding from the Health Resources and Services Administration Health Center Program through the Health Center Program Statute of the Public Health Service Act. Mandela MarketPlace has received essential funding support from the U.S. Department of Agriculture, specifically from its Agricultural Marketing Service agency, the Food Insecurity Nutrition Incentive program, the Risk Management Agency, and the Healthy Food Financing Initiative.[13] The Sustainable Neighborhoods Program of People United for Sustainable Housing (PUSH) was awarded a state grant to develop affordable housing units. In one example of city-level funding, during the first year of the Blueprint for Action, the city budget adopted by the Minneapolis mayor included $175,000 to support implementation.

The private sector is another potential funding source. Traditional mechanisms include corporate philanthropy, either voluntary or in response to regulated community benefit spending in support of a business's nonprofit status, such as that required of nonprofit hospitals under the ACA. In order to sustain its work, the Indianapolis Congregation Action Network (IndyCAN) raises funds from corporations as well as others. The Dudley Street Neighborhood Initiative's membership includes local businesses. Among Mandela MarketPlace's partners is Mercury LLC, an advertising and marketing firm. A new and innovative mechanism is the social impact bond, with which private-sector investments pay for improved social outcomes that result in private-sector savings; these bonds are repaid contingent on attaining certain social outcomes. An example is the Denver Permanent Supportive Housing Social Impact Bond Initiative, which would decrease the cost associated with acute services for heavy-utilizing homeless persons by providing housing and on-site support services.

Philanthropy, often called the "third sector," is another important source of funding for community interventions. Foundations have an advantage in terms of having greater flexibility to be more innovative and take greater risks than government agencies. Depending on the foundation, funding can be quite flexible, including providing "general operating support" which gives the grantee decision making concerning how best to bring resources to bear in addressing an issue. Foundation funding also presents challenges: compared to government sources, the total amount of dollars available is less. Projects much be aligned with the unique mission and vision of the foundation. Foundations are unlikely to be a source of sustainable funding over time, as foundation boards tend to be interested in moving on to new, innovative projects that promote their mission. And, despite the ability to be flexible and innovative, foundations can be as risk-averse and as proscriptive as any public agency—sometimes even more so. There are many types of foundations, with different sources of funding and different regulatory requirements, including

---

[13] The Healthy Food Financing Initiative is operated jointly by the U.S. Department of Agriculture, the U.S. Department of Health and Human Services, and the U.S. Department of the Treasury.

private foundations, family foundations, community foundations, and corporate foundations, and each has myriad approaches to grant making. A relatively new foundation mechanism that has been used to support community health equity interventions is program-related investment, whereby a foundation makes a below-market loan or investment, such as in an affordable housing project, and any return on investment becomes a source for future grant making.

Foundations have been a prominent source of funding for the community examples in Chapter 5. For example, the Dudley Street Neighborhood Initiative was founded with assistance from the Boston-based Mabel Louise Riley Foundation. The Delta Health Care's state and federal funding has been supplemented by the W.K. Kellogg Foundation. WE ACT's development of the Northern Manhattan Climate Action Plan was supported through a $100,000 grant from The Kresge Foundation. The Magnolia Community Initiative recently received a $2 million collaborative gift from the Doris Duke Charitable Foundation and the Tikun Olam Foundation. Thunder Valley Community Development Corporation has secured funding from multiple foundations, including the Northwest Area Foundation, Doris Duke Charitable Foundation, Surdna Foundation, Novo Foundation, and W.K. Kellogg Foundation.

Community collaborations that are developing funding for a program or project will benefit from being aware of all potential funding sources. An affordable housing project might rely on more than half a dozen different sources, including private sources (such as traditional loans), government sources (such as community development funds), and philanthropic loans from foundations and individuals. All of the community examples in Chapter 5 relied on a diversity of funding sources to develop, implement, and maintain their activities. In many instances there was substantial governmental as well as philanthropic funding. There are financing strategies available to community organizations themselves, such as school districts and local public health agencies, as well as "braided" or "blended" funding, which refers to pooling funding from separate funding streams, usually created with different priorities but with enough flexibility and overlap to permit supporting a single intervention (Clary and Riley, 2016). A common strategy in attracting philanthropic funding is "leveraging," whereby the investment from one foundation is used to attract additional grants from others. This also has the advantage of creating additional stakeholders and may translate to better chances of program sustainability as the ongoing costs are shared among a group of interested organizations.

In summary, an awareness of potential sources and creativity in financing are important in developing the resources required for community interventions. While sustainability is most often the intent of projects and programs, communities should also be aware of the value of other enduring products that can come from interventions. Policy changes, for example, can endure and affect the health of a community for a long time. Leadership and collaborative relationships endure and can be repurposed to address new community issues. New knowledge of what works and what does not work is a key enduring product from any intervention. And, of course, the direct benefit to individuals affected by the intervention can be lifelong.

The following sections discuss the tools available to communities based on the three elements in the committee's conceptual model: (1) making health equity a shared vision and value, (2) building community capacity to act, and (3) fostering multi-sector collaboration. The chapter then ends with examples of community tool kits that are readily available to communities and incorporate many of the tools outlined in this chapter.

MAKING HEALTH EQUITY A SHARED VISION AND VALUE

General Principles

Multiple approaches to making health equity a shared vision and value through community-based solutions share three characteristics:

1. A shared sense of urgency about the issue to be addressed, and the need for a community-based solution (Hanleybrown et al., 2012).
2. Clearly stated shared purpose and values. This may include a commitment to collective impact, which is described later in this chapter (Public Health Agency of Canada, 2016).
3. A champion. An effective champion is trusted, respected, non-partisan, and works effectively with political leaders; is strongly committed to the determinants of health philosophy; and welcomes, encourages, and successfully brokers multiple and varying perspectives to shape a health equity agenda (Public Health Agency of Canada, 2016).

A shared vision, aligned with a clearly stated purpose and values and fueled by a sense of urgency, is highlighted in the community examples in Chapter 5. Community-level data regarding the social determinants of health were essential in establishing a sense of purpose to facilitate a shared vision among all partners. In some instances, the shared vision targeted youth and families. For example, a shared vision of improved outcomes among children and families binds the Magnolia Community Initiative network of more than 70 government and private-sector partner organizations. Driven by public safety concerns, Blueprint for Action was motivated by a shared vision of a unified city in which all youth are safe and able to thrive (Blueprint for Action, 2013). The Dudley Street Neighborhood Initiative has cultivated a shared vision among residents, families, local organizations, and local businesses regarding their power to achieve a healthier and more vibrant community. IndyCAN's main platform, Opportunity for All, is based on a shared vision that every person should have equal opportunity to access the conditions and resources to achieve racial and economic equity. WE ACT has nurtured a shared vision of improved health in northern Manhattan through its environmental justice and climate activities.

The role of a champion or a group of champions is illustrated throughout the community examples. A prominent example of an individual champion was Jack Geiger's role at both the policy level, to advocate to the Office of Equal Opportunity for the concept of neighborhood health centers, and later as project director of the Delta Health Center, the first FQHC. In contrast, the leaders who convened to develop the Blueprint for Action represented multiple champions from law enforcement, juvenile supervision, public health, youth programs, education, social services, faith communities, neighborhoods, and city and county government.

Public Will Building

Public will building differs in a number of ways from other approaches to making health equity a shared vision and value in that it is an explicit communication approach that "builds public support for social change by integrating grassroots outreach methods with traditional mass media tools in a process that connects an issue to the existing, closely held values of individuals and groups" (Metropolitan Group, 2009). In contrast to public opinion-based campaigns, which often target a short-term goal, public will-based approaches focus on long-term change building over time using four principles: (1) connecting through closely held core values rather than trying to change values; (2) respecting cultural context, including the dynamics of power, language, relationships, values, traditions, worldview, and decision making; (3) including target audiences in development and testing of key strategies and methods to ensure authenticity, clarity of message, and credibility of messengers; and (4) integrating grassroots and traditional communication methods. While not explicitly reflected in the Chapter 5 community examples, public will-based approaches have been applied to multiple topics, including the arts, behaviors that influence the outcomes of children and families (Leiderman et al., 2000), and out-of-school programs (Padgette et al., 2010). An example of the last topic is summarized in Box 8-6.

> **BOX 8-6**
> **Strengthening Partnerships and Building Public Will for Out-of-School Time Programs: A Municipal Leadership Example**
>
> With funding from the Wallace Foundation, the National League of Cities Institute for Youth, Education, and Families developed a strategy guide for municipalities to promote out-of-school time programs. Such programs aim to keep children and youth engaged and safe during the hours between the end of school and the end of parental workdays. Public will building is often used in conjunction with other approaches, and the guide integrates strategies in three areas:
>
> 1. Engage and involve a broad set of partners to take full advantage of all community resources
> 2. Keep out-of-school time on the public agenda
> 3. Lead efforts by city, school, and community leaders to establish a common set of outcomes and a shared vision for out-of-school time
>
> Specific strategies for building public will for municipal leadership include
>
> - Using their "bully pulpit" to highlight needs and increase public awareness
> - Aligning efforts with other important priorities
> - Developing a coordinated approach and communications plan
> - Using high-profile events (e.g., state of the city) to sustain public attention
> - Seeking authentic community input on a regular basis (Padgette et al., 2010)

INCREASING COMMUNITY CAPACITY TO SHAPE HEALTH OUTCOMES

Successful and sustainable community interventions require the engagement of individuals and leaders from multiple sectors, not the least of which are the affected individuals in the community and the organizations that are perhaps closest to the affected population. In many instances, these individuals and grassroots organizations have less power, experience, and capacity to represent the unique goals and needs of the population that health equity interventions are meant to address. Community capacity refers to the ability of community members to make a difference over time and across different issues (Work Group for Community Health and Development, 2016b).

Capacity building enables an organization to be more effective in pursuing its mission, vision, and goals; to be sustainable; and to grow as needs require. Skill building includes such areas as basic business planning and practices, communication tools and strategies, strategic planning, grant writing, and fundraising. Capacity building is a key element of sustainability. Strengthening community capacity to develop, implement, and sustain successful interventions depends on specific strategies, which include leadership development, community organizing, supporting the relationships between organizations necessary for collaboration, and organizational development (Chaskin, 1999).

Capacity Building for Leadership Development

Capacity building in regards to leadership development at the individual level includes building the skill sets that committed participants need to take a key role in representing the interests of their community and enhancing their effectiveness in helping shape intervention elements that respond to the specific community member needs. Leadership development, which usually includes specific skill building around communication and presentation skills as well as specific knowledge transfer and often project development, also creates lasting change for those individuals who engage in training.

Leadership development has different components within organizations. ISAIAH, located in Minneapolis, is a vehicle for congregations, clergy, and people of faith to act collectively and powerfully toward racial and economic equity in the state of Minnesota. ISAIAH's mechanisms of change include three components (IOM, 2015a). The first component is grassroots leadership development. The second component builds upon the first: democratic, accountable, sustainable, and community-driven organizations, whose participants are "exercising democracy with each other" (IOM, 2014). The third component of community organizing emphasizes that the power or the ability to act drives change. In an IOM workshop, ISAIAH's executive director Doran Schrantz explained, "Differentials in power do not change because somebody else who has more power gives it to you. Differentials in power change because you take ownership and collective and community responsibility for negotiating for the power and the resources you need. When that power structure is in place, that is when change happens" (IOM, 2014, p. 50).

Leadership development is an essential strategy emphasized in the community examples in Chapter 5. The Dudley Street Neighborhood Initiative offers internship programs to develop leadership capacity and provide career opportunities for talented youth in order to create the next generation of community leaders. Mandela Foods Cooperative, a venture of Mandela MarketPlace, has supported youth leadership development through the West Oakland Youth Standing Empowered program and also enabled employee leadership development through pathways from employment to ownership. WE ACT offers an 11-week environmental

> **BOX 8-7**
> **Multistep Leadership Development Plan:**
> **An Organizational Perspective**
>
> One tool for leadership development is a multistep leadership development plan. From the perspective of an existing leader wishing to develop others, these include
>
> - Envisioning your leadership team (e.g., the number, skills, being representative of the community, having a commitment to the organization's goals)
> - Assessing current personnel (e.g., staff, members, volunteers) as compared to an ideal leadership team and set goals with actions and timelines to address areas of need for the group (e.g., working as a team, awareness of diversity)
> - Selecting methods for developing leaders, including things that existing leaders can do personally (e.g., model good leadership, teach as you lead, expect individuals to act like leaders, invest in each person, provide mentoring) or structures that can be put in place (e.g., exchange programs with other organizations, orientations, workshops and training sessions, retreats, leadership groups)
> - Setting leadership development goals for individuals in the context of what leadership skills are needed in the organization and the individuals best suited to learn those skills and write individual leadership development plans with each
> - Recruiting new members and volunteers to lead, bring new ideas, and challenge existing assumptions and ideas
> - Continuing to develop as a leader through an individual development plan (Work Group for Community Health and Development, 2016c)

health and justice leadership training program to educate community members about the environmental health issues confronting their northern Manhattan neighborhoods. WE ACT recently adapted its leadership training model for high school students in collaboration with academic partners and offers the Climate Change and Health Fellows program aimed at fostering climate literacy. Another example is Magnolia Community Initiative's Belong Campaign,[14] which is building social connections and creating leaders ("neighborhood ambassadors") who can help connect residents to the resources available in the community. Box 8-7 outlines a multistep leadership development plan.

---

[14] For more information, see https://www.youtube.com/watch?v=CUEtCD_I9iU (accessed October 21, 2016).

Capacity Building for Community Organizing

Community organizing through local outreach brings together individuals with shared interests and gives voice and power to individuals who traditionally are excluded and marginalized. Organizing can use grassroots approaches, often recruiting through one-on-one outreach interactions; faith- or congregation-based organizing, which works more at building networks of groups and institutions; and broad-based organizing, which may include secular, faith-based, or individual groups. Community organizing gives planners access to specific insights into what interventions are critical (and which are not) and increases the power and voice of community members in decision-making settings.

Community organizing may take different forms. In a seminal publication, Rothman characterized three models of practice: social planning, social action, and locality development (Rothman, 1996). Importantly for sustainability, the relationships created by community organizing often last longer than the lifespan of a program or project.

Social planning uses information and analysis to address substantive community issues and helps build agreement on common results. HIAs are one approach to social planning. Another strategy is the use of the variety of data sources described earlier in this chapter to characterize a particular issue.

Social action involves efforts to increase the power and resources of low-income, relatively powerless, or marginalized people. This may include the use of political action or disruptive events such as lawsuits, sit-ins, or boycotts to draw attention and focus to their concerns from those in power. IndyCAN's Ticket to Opportunity field program mobilizes marginalized voters of color through large-scale voter engagement to build sustained capacity for transit equity. Community residents are also taught to use the tools of democracy to improve their communities.

Locality development is the process of reaching group consensus about common concerns and collaborating in problem solving. Promise Neighborhoods are an example of community organizing with an emphasis on locality development. The Dudley Street Neighborhood Initiative and Eastside Promise Neighborhood have received Promise Neighborhood funding, and their activities, which are described in Chapter 5, are exemplars of locality development. Another example of locality development is the Northside Achievement Zone (NAZ), which strives to permanently close the achievement gap and end generational poverty in North Minneapolis, a neighborhood with approximately 5,500 children with major educational achievement gaps at baseline. Only 29 percent of entering kindergartners living in North Minneapolis are ready to learn, 37 percent of African American youth graduate on time from Minneapolis Public Schools, 16 percent of African American youth graduate ready for college, and 13 percent of those who attend a public university graduate in four years (Northside Achievement Zone, n.d.). This low achievement occurs in the context of other important social determinants of health: 73 percent of NAZ families earn $19,000 or less per year, single-parent families represent 51 percent of NAZ households, 25 percent of North Minneapolis students are homeless or highly mobile, and this small area is responsible for the majority of violent crime in Minneapolis. Consequently, the program's community-based solutions are multi-sectoral and not solely focused on education:

- Education: early childhood, K–12, expanded learning, and mentoring
- Economic development: Emerge Community Development, Twin Cities RISE!
- Housing: Minneapolis Public Housing Authority, Project for Pride in Living, Urban Homeworks
- Health care: Visiting Nurse Agency, The Family Partnership, Northpoint Health & Wellness Center, Washburn Center for Children

In reality, community organizing often integrates aspects of multiple models, as reflected in several of the community examples in Chapter 5 (e.g., the Magnolia Community Initiative) and by Aim4Peace. Based in Kansas City, Missouri, Aim4Peace focuses on the neighborhood factors that most often contribute to violence, helping those who are considered at highest risk of committing offenses due to their living or employment situation. Aim4Peace includes locality development through its Life Skills Learning Program that works to prevent school delinquency and dropouts; supporting community actions to keep students in school; its Job Readiness Program that helps participants prepare for obstacles that can happen when they enter the workforce; and its Job Fair Initiative that links trainees and local employers. Through Aims4Peace's Hospital Prevention Program, hospital workers respond to gunshot and violence-related trauma situations, intervene in conflicts, and aim to prevent further violence. Aim4Peace also engages in advocacy, a mechanism for social action.

Capacity Building for Organizational Development

In the United States, fairness is obtained by efforts that begin at the community level. Historically, in fact, advances in voting, education, and civil rights all followed from the efforts of people working first in specific communities. Some communities are issue-linked. Some are geographic.

It was the dedicated communities of women across the nation who won women's right to vote. It was the efforts of teenagers in specific counties that set education equity in motion.[15] Communities can be defined in many ways, including by geography, ethnicity, faith, race, need, age, and even aspiration.

Though communities vary greatly, successful change efforts are the same in key respects. They all involve people working together with a shared vision and commitment to improve some aspect of life. Importantly, the actions required to organize a community effort that has lasting effects are similar to those needed to restructure a company or an institution and to bring a group of people together to successfully achieve long-lasting desired change. Thinking and talking about systematic approaches to achieving health equity has several advantages. First, systematic efforts are more likely to be successful, and second, pursuing change in focused, orderly ways is more likely to attract the support of essential businesses, faith-based organizations, and the media.

Achieving change is a process. One well-documented process was developed at the Harvard Business School by Professor John Kotter. His "eight steps" for leading change have been used over the past 30 years to restructure and build successful private companies, public institutions, and nonprofit organizations. These steps, described from the perspective of errors that led to transformation failures in 1995 (Kotter, 1995), were further delineated in 1996 in the book *Leading Change* (Kotter, 1996). The eight steps provide a process for achieving desired changes and a foundation for community, business, faith, media, and other sectors to communicate effectively with each other to increase health equity in concrete ways.

Leading Change is the result of studying many thousands of companies and institutions and describes the steps required to change the culture of an organization. The steps are universal in that they are not about a single business or institution, but rather they are about human behavior and motivation. They apply to corporate, institutional, and even national restructuring efforts. The wording of the steps sometimes changes depending on the application, but the essential components are constant.

According to Kotter (1996), successful change requires close attention to these eight steps:

---

[15] The April 1951 Farmville, Virginia, high school strike led by teenager Barbara Johns was followed by others in the south. Lawsuits were filed, the cases worked their way up the court system, and in May 1954, just 36 months after the Farmville walk-out, the Supreme Court handed down its landmark *Brown v. Board of Education* decision declaring that the principle of "separate but equal" is unconstitutional.

1. Identify the urgency: Leaders need to describe health inequities and the high personal, social, political, and economic costs associated with them in ways that appeal to people's heads and hearts and use this statement to raise a large army of volunteers.
2. Build a guiding coalition: A volunteer army needs a coalition of effective people—coming from its own ranks—to guide it, coordinate it, and communicate its activities.
3. Form a strategic vision and initiatives: Strategic initiatives are targeted and coordinated activities that, if designed and executed fast and well enough, will make the vision a reality.
4. Enlist a volunteer army: Large-scale change can only occur when significant numbers of local, regional, or national citizens amass under a common opportunity and drive action in the same direction.
5. Enable action by removing barriers: By removing barriers such as inefficient processes or hierarchies, leaders provide the freedom necessary for volunteers to work across boundaries and create real impact.
6. Generate short-term wins: Wins are the molecules of results. They must be collected, categorized, and communicated—early and often—to track progress and energize volunteers to drive change.
7. Sustain acceleration: Change leaders must adapt quickly in order to maintain their speed. Whether it is a new way of finding talent or removing misaligned processes, the leaders must determine what can be done—every day—to stay the course toward the vision.
8. Institute change: To ensure that new behaviors are repeated over the long term, it is important to define and communicate the connections between these behaviors and society's political and economic success (Kotter, 1996).

Other theories of organizational change (such as Lewin's Change Management Model, *Harvard Business Review*'s Seven Steps to Change, and *Managing Organizational Change in the Public Sector: Theory to Practice* by Fernandez and Rainy) have many of the same elements and are relevant to communities as they consider their paths forward (Fernandez and Rainey, 2006; *Harvard Business Review*, 2002; Levasseur, 2001).

Building community capacity to shape health outcomes is an essential component of advancing health equity. Multiple groups have developed integrated resources for strengthening community capacity in leadership development, community organizing, supporting the relationships between organizations necessary for collaboration, and organizational development. One such multilingual resource is the Community Tool

Box at the University of Kansas (Work Group for Community Health and Development, 2016a). This resource and others are summarized in Table 8-2 later in this chapter.

FOSTERING MULTI-SECTOR COLLABORATION

Collaboration skills represent a specific area for capacity building and are key to bringing together the different sectors necessary to create, implement, and sustain a successful community intervention to achieve health equity. Convening strategies involve meetings that bring together representatives from different sectors to explore shared values, visions, and interventions; to identify roles and collaborative activities; and to braid different sources of funding to create greater impact than a single sector or organization can achieve alone. Collaboration is not always easy, given the disparate missions, goals, organizational cultures, and languages of the key participants, yet creating a shared and compelling vision can be successful in bringing individuals and organizations together to address critical health equity issues. As with all of the elements of community capacity building, the relationships created through collaboration can endure after specific projects or programs end.

Collaboration requires coalition building. A community coalition is a group of individuals or organizations with a common interest who agree to work together toward a common goal aimed at bettering their community (Community Health Innovation, n.d.; Community Tool Box, n.d.). The primary motivation for coalition building is to create a shared response to a community concern (e.g., an urgent issue, policy change, or release of new information) or opportunity (e.g., the availability of new funding) because the existing community response is either nonexistent or insufficient to meet the community's need. Community coalitions vary in their scope and structure, but most often include the elements of influencing public policy, changing health behavior, and building healthy communities. They may be multi-issue or topic-specific.

Supported by the Greater Nashua Public Health Advisory Council, Plan4Health Nashua is a coalition of planning and public health professionals, including the Nashua Regional Planning Commission, the City of Nashua, the New Hampshire Public Health Association, and Healthy Eating Active Living (HEAL NH) (Plan4Health, n.d.). The Plan4Health Nashua goal is to advance street planning and design that support safer and easier ways to get around for pedestrians and bicyclists. During its 15-month grant period, the Plan4Health Nashua coalition conducted a street study to assess the bikeability and walkability of Nashua streets, developed a Complete Streets guidebook and policy recommendations, and provided training to city staff, planners, elected officials, and other community members.

The DC Tobacco Free Coalition focuses on a single health issue, tobacco use and exposure (DC Tobacco Free Coalition, n.d.). Partners of the initiative include faith- and community-based organizations in Washington, DC, and individuals who employ multiple strategies spanning education, public policy, and advocacy using culturally and linguistically competent approaches.

The Prevention Institute describes eight steps to building an effective coalition among organizations within the same sector or across sectors (Cohen et al., 2002):

1. Analyze the program's objectives and determine whether or not to form a coalition.
2 Recruit the right people.
3. Devise a set of preliminary objectives and activities.
4. Convene the coalition.
5. Anticipate the necessary resources.
6. Define elements of a successful coalition structure.
7. Maintain coalition vitality.
8. Make improvements through evolution.

The community examples in Chapter 5 highlight the important role of partnership building in the success of their organizations and the importance of investing in partnerships. Multi-sector collaboration was a criterion in the selection of the community examples. As part of community-based solutions, multi-sectoral collaborations can benefit from the following general principles that have been delineated by a number of authors:

- The ability of partners to commit resources: Multi-sectoral collaboration requires a human resource plan that is documented and agreed to by all partners, the identification of skill requirements and opportunities for training and development, the sharing of examples of innovative working methodologies, and consensus on a cost-sharing plan (Public Health Agency of Canada, 2016). Investment in partnership includes financial obligations such as time, personnel, and money and may also include forgoing other opportunities and taking on risks (Public Health Agency of Canada, 2016).
- The health sector as a leader or facilitator: Depending on the focus of the multi-sectoral community-based solution, the health sector may assume a leadership role when the solution is tied

to its primary interests and capacities or a facilitation or participant role when the necessary capacities belong to another sector such as education, transportation, or public safety (Public Health Agency of Canada, 2016).
- Political support and a public policy environment that supports collective action: A direct link to the political level facilitates visible political support, sustained partner participation, and access to necessary resources (Public Health Agency of Canada, 2016).
- Successful working relationships: Relationships are characterized by trust and mutual respect; being inclusive of all participants; reflecting clear and unambiguous communication; being transparent, clear, timely, and fair in the handling of issues; being supported by a clearly articulated vision; being enabled by effective leadership that ensures the various partners participate on an equitable footing; and having clarity around roles and responsibilities (Danaher, 2011).
- Ability to share leadership, accountability, and rewards among partners: Sharing should be supported through careful planning, mechanisms for monitoring progress and accountability, and plans for sharing anticipated gains (Public Health Agency of Canada, 2016).

These principles are illustrated in multiple community examples. PUSH has collaborated with multiple sectors, such as housing, energy, and parks departments, as well as more than 20 nongovernmental organizations ranging from national organizations and foundations to local nonprofits. The important aspects of Blueprint for Action's partnerships have been communication to decrease redundancy in efforts across partners and the coordination of data collection from various sectors both to inform the Blueprint's objectives and priorities and to systematically track progress. As with other case studies, the Dudley Street Neighborhood Initiative has multi-sector collaboration as a core organizational strength. The diversity of partnerships goes beyond nonprofits and governmental organizations to include businesses through the Dudley Workforce Collaborative as well as arts and cultural institutions through the Fairmont Cultural Corridor.

Different approaches may be used in developing community-based collaboration. One is the Framework for Collaborative Community Action on Health. This framework includes assess, prioritize, plan; implement targeted action; change community conditions and systems; achieve widespread change in behaviors and risk factors; and improve population health (IOM, 2003; Roussos and Fawcett, 2000). Collective impact is another approach for facilitating multi-sector collaboration through a focus on shared benefits that accrue to the participating organizations.

Beyond these general principles for fostering multi-sector collaboration, collective impact initiatives are long-term commitments by a group of important actors from different sectors to a common agenda for solving a specific social problem. Collective impact approaches are not needed for all social problems; they are best suited for adaptive problems (i.e., problems with a complex, unknown solution, for which no single entity has the resources nor authority to solve the problem alone) (Kania and Kramer, 2011).

Collective impact initiatives have three preconditions: (1) an influential champion or small group of champions, (2) financial resources to last for at least 2 to 3 years, and (3) a sense of urgency for change around a problem. These preconditions create the opportunity and motivation necessary to convene and maintain multi-sector collaborations. Collective impact initiatives are also characterized by five conditions relevant to advancing community-based solutions for health equity: a common agenda, shared measurement, mutually reinforcing activities, continuous communication, and backbone support.

The phases of collective impact and related activities are summarized in Table 8-1 according to the four components for success (Hanleybrown et al., 2012). The phases include activities that have been discussed elsewhere in this chapter, such as community engagement, public will building, and the data to meet community information needs. With Phases I

TABLE 8-1 Phases of Collective Impact

Components for Success	Phase I Initiate Action	Phase II Organize for Impact	Phase III Sustain Action and Impact
Governance and infrastructure	Identify champions and form cross-sector group	Create infrastructure (backbone and processes)	Facilitate and refine
Strategic planning	Map the landscape and use data to make the case	Create a common agenda (goals and strategy)	Support implementation (align with goals and strategies)
Community involvement	Facilitate community outreach	Engage the community and build public will	Continue engagement and conduct advocacy
Evaluation and improvement	Analyze baseline data to identify key issues and gaps	Establish shared metrics (indicators, measurement, and approach)	Collect, track, and report progress (process to learn and improve)

SOURCE: Hanleybrown et al., 2012.

and II taking up to 2 years for completion and Phase III lasting a decade or more, Hanleybrown et al. emphasize that collective impact is a "marathon, not a sprint" (Hanleybrown et al., 2012).

The Community Tool Box at the University of Kansas includes several assessments related to collective impact. The Collective Impact Readiness Impact assesses the extent to which preconditions are met or will require further investment. The Collective Impact Progress Assessment details progress on the five collective impact conditions (Work Group for Community Health and Development, 2016c).

The Magnolia Community Initiative exemplifies a collective impact approach, and a description of its efforts is also included in the Community Tool Box. Communication is facilitated through a shared website that offers access to discussion forums, group blogs, e-mail blasts, a shared calendar, and shared files and documents. Shared measurement is informed by a shared theory of change. Backbone support is provided by the network partners.

COMMUNITY TOOL KITS

In addition to individual strategies and tools, a number of tool kits have been developed. Koo et al. conducted an environmental scan and identified six tool kits that met their definition of a comprehensive resource for community health. Their criteria for inclusion were: (1) a conceptual model or theory of change for improving the community's health, (2) a suggested set of actions or steps to improve community health, (3) resources to support collaboration with other sectors, and (4) examples of successful collaborative partnerships to improve health. In addition, they required that the tools targeted more than one sector and were freely available on the Internet. The six tool kits and their contents are summarized in Table 8-2 (Koo et al., 2016).

Other tool kits also provide guidance on various specific aspects of community-based solutions. For example, the National Partnership for Action to End Health Disparities Toolkit for Community Action was developed to help individuals, organizations, and policy makers: (1) raise awareness about health disparities by providing descriptions of health disparities and their causes; (2) engage others in conversations about the problem and solutions with tools to guide efforts to promote programs and policies for change; and (3) take action for change by providing information and tools to help individuals and organizations to address health in their communities (HHS, n.d.-b). The Health Equity and Social Justice Toolkit from NACCHO is targeted to local health departments and includes journal articles, video clips, reports, PowerPoint

TABLE 8-2 Comprehensive Tool Kits Supporting Community Health, United States, June 2014–December 2015

Name	Lead Organization	Primary Audience	Features Unique to Tool Kit
Build Healthy Places Network[a]	Build Healthy Places Network	Health and community development sectors	Logic models for various health conditions; MeasureUp (mapping and measurement tools); community close-ups that highlight the role of community development
Community Commons[b]	IP3 and CARES–University of Missouri	Broad	Access to and ability to visualize social determinants data in graphs, maps, and other formats; content from the field organized in "channels," including economy, education, environment, equity, food, and health; houses ("hubs") where organizations, initiatives, and collaboratives can share content, data, and resources
Community Health Improvement Navigator[c]	U.S. Centers for Disease Control and Prevention	Hospitals, public health sector, community partners	Community health improvement infographic; key quotes from Internal Revenue Service final rule on community health needs assessments for charitable hospitals; search engine for evidence-based community interventions
Community Tool Box[d]	University of Kansas	Broad	Online training, curriculum, community workstations; materials in multiple languages; troubleshooting guide; guestbook to describe use of toolbox

continued

TABLE 8-2 Continued

Name	Lead Organization	Primary Audience	Features Unique to Tool Kit
County Health Rankings and Roadmaps Action Center	University of Wisconsin Population Health Institute	Broad, community partners	County Health Rankings; What Works for Health database; model of population health; partner guides (including for public health)
Practical Playbook[e]	Duke University School of Medicine, Department of Community and Family Medicine	Public health sector, primary care providers	Similar content also published as a textbook: J. L. Michener, D. Koo, B. C. Castrucci, and J. B. Sprague (eds.), *The Practical Playbook: Public Health and Primary Care Together*, New York: Oxford University Press, 2016; first national meeting May 2016.

[a] For more information, see http://buildhealthyplaces.org (accessed November 17, 2016).
[b] For more information, see http://www.communitycommons.org (accessed November 17, 2016).
[c] For more information, see http://www.cdc.gov/chinav (accessed November 17, 2016).
[d] For more information, see http://ctb.ku.edu/en (accessed November 17, 2016).
[e] For more information, see http://practicalplaybook.org (accessed November 17, 2016).

presentations, book references, action guides, and websites.[16] Another example that is particularly relevant to fostering multi-sector collaboration is the Prevention Institute's coalition and collaboration tools, including (1) Developing Effective Coalitions: An Eight Step Guide,[17] (2) Collaboration Multiplier,[18] (3) Collaboration Assessment Tool,[19] and (4) The

---

[16] For more information, see http://archived.naccho.org/topics/justice/hesj-tools.cfm (accessed November 17, 2016).
[17] For more information, see https://www.preventioninstitute.org/publications/developing-effective-coalitions-an-eight-step-guide (accessed November 17, 2016).
[18] For more information, see https://www.preventioninstitute.org/tools/collaboration-multiplier (accessed November 17, 2016).
[19] For more information, see https://www.preventioninstitute.org/publications/collaboration-assessment-tool (accessed November 17, 2016).

Tension of Turf: Making it Work for the Coalition[20] (Prevention Institute, 2016a). There are also specific guides that demonstrate the application of the tools in a specific domain: for example, multi-sector partnerships for preventing violence (Tsao and Davis, 2014). The Guide to Community Preventive Services is a collection of evidence-based findings from the Community Preventive Services Taskforce, a panel appointed by the CDC director. The resource is designed to help select interventions to improve health and prevent disease at the community level as well as at other levels. The Community Guide contains reviews designed to answer three questions of key relevance to those wishing to implement community-based solutions: (1) What has worked for others, and how well? (2) What might this intervention cost, and what am I likely to achieve through my investment? and (3) What are the evidence gaps?

In addition, another type of tool kit—collections of community exemplars—are useful to inform community-based solutions by highlighting successful practices at the local level through narrative. For example, the Prevention Institute offers a searchable database of more than 100 community profiles that address a variety of social determinants of health (Prevention Institute, 2016b). The Community Guide also provides stories featuring those who have used the Community Guide to make people safer and healthier.

CONCLUSION

Chapters 4 and 5 described why communities matter and highlighted nine examples of community-based solutions to promote health equity in the United States. This chapter outlines specific tools that communities can use to move toward health equity organized by: (1) those tools that apply across all three elements of health equity as a shared vision, cross-sector collaboration, and community capacity to shape outcomes; (2) those that apply specifically to one of the elements; and (3) prominent tool kits that can inform community-based efforts to promote health equity.

REFERENCES

AARP (American Association of Retired Persons) Public Policy Institute. n.d. *Livability index.* https://livabilityindex.aarp.org/categories/neighborhood (accessed October 18, 2016).

ABA (American Bar Association). 2009. *Standing committee: Pro bono and public service.* http://apps.americanbar.org/legalservices/probono/directory/programlinks.html (accessed November 21, 2016).

---

[20] For more information, see https://www.preventioninstitute.org/publications/the-tension-of-turf-making-it-work-for-the-coalition (accessed November 17, 2016).

Acemoglu, D., and J. S. Pischke. 1999. Beyond Becker: Training in imperfect labour markets. *Economic Journal* 109(453):112–142.

Autor, D. H. 2001. Why do temporary help firms provide free general skills training? *Quarterly Journal of Economics* 116(4):1409–1448.

Basch, C. E. 2011a. Healthier students are better learners: A missing link in school reforms to close the achievement gap. *Journal of School Health* 81(10):593–598.

Basch, C. E. 2011b. Physical activity and the achievement gap among urban minority youth. *Journal of School Health* 81(10):626–634.

Becker, G. S. 1993 [1964]. *Human capital: A theoretical and empirical analysis, with special reference to education.* 3rd ed. Chicago, IL: The University of Chicago Press.

Blueprint for Action. 2013. *Minneapolis Blueprint for Action to Prevent Youth Violence.* Minneapolis, MN: City of Minneapolis Health Department.

Blundell, R., L. Dearden, C. Meghir, and B. Sianesi. 1999. Human capital investment: The returns from education and training to the individual, the firm and the economy. *Fiscal Studies* 20(1):1–23.

Brandeis University. n.d. *Diversity data kids.* http://www.diversitydatakids.org (accessed October 21, 2016).

CAN (Community Advancement Network). 2016. *CAN dashboard.* http://www.can communitydashboard.org (accessed December 20, 2016).

Cappelli, P. 2004. Why do employers pay for college? *Journal of Econometrics* 121(1):213–241.

CDC (U.S. Centers for Disease Control and Prevention). 2013. *HIA stories from the field: Douglass County Health Department.* https://www.cdc.gov/healthyplaces/stories/omaha.htm (accessed November 21, 2016).

CDC. 2015. *The Community Health Status Indicators (CHSI).* http://wwwn.cdc.gov/CommunityHealth/ info/AboutProject (accessed October 18, 2016).

Chandra, A., J. Acosta, K. G. Carman, T. Dubowitz, L. Leviton, L. T. Martin, C. Miller, C. Nelson, T. Orleans, and M. Tait. 2016. *Building a national culture of health.* Santa Monica, CA: RAND Corporation.

Chaskin, R. J. 1999. *Defining community capacity: A framework and implications from a comprehensive community initiative.* Chicago, IL: Chapin Hall Center for Children at the University of Chicago.

City of Boston Data Portal. 2013. *City of Boston data portal.* https://data.cityofboston.gov (accessed October 18, 2016).

Clary, A., and T. Riley. 2016. *Braiding and blending funding streams to meet health-related social needs of low-income persons: Considerations for state health policymakers.* Washington, DC: National Academy for State Health Policy.

Cohen, L., N. Baer, and P. Satterwhite. 2002. *Developing effective coalitions: An eight step guide.* https://www.preventioninstitute.org/sites/default/files/uploads/8steps_040511_WEB.pdf (accessed October 21, 2016).

Community Health Innovation. n.d. *Fundamentals of community coalition building.* http://chsolutions.typepad.com/elevation/2010/04/community-coalition-building-part-1-fundamentals.html (accessed October 19, 2016).

Community Tool Box. n.d. *Coalition building I: Starting a coalition.* http://ctb.ku.edu/en/table-of-contents/assessment/promotion-strategies/start-a-coaltion/main (accessed October 19, 2016).

Dan, D., R. Finch, D. Harrison, and D. Kendall. 2011. *An employer's guide to reducing racial & ethnic health disparities in the workplace.* Washington, DC: National Business Group on Health.

Danaher, A. 2011. *Reducing health inequities: Enablers and barriers to inter-sectoral collaboration.* Toronto, ON: Wellesley Institute.

DC Tobacco Free Coalition. n.d. *DC Tobacco Free Coalition.* http://www.dctfc.org (accessed October 19, 2016).

Dee, T., and E. Penner. 2016. *The causal effects of cultural relevance: Evidence from an ethnic studies curriculum.* National Bureau of Economic Research working paper no. 21865.

Deming, D. J., J. S. Hastings, T. J. Kane, and D. O. Staiger. 2014. School choice, school quality, and postsecondary attainment. *The American Economic Review* 104(3):991–1013.

Diamant, A. L., S. H. Babey, and J. Wolstein. 2011. Adolescent physical education and physical activity in California. Healthy policy brief, May. Los Angeles: University of California, Los Angeles, Center for Health Policy Research.

Efrat, M. 2011. The relationship between low-income and minority children's physical activity and academic-related outcomes: A review of the literature. *Health Education & Behavior* 20(10):1–11.

EPA (U.S. Environmental Protection Agency). 2016. *EJS: Environmental justice screening and mapping tool.* https://www.epa.gov/ejscreen (accessed October 18, 2016).

Fernandez, S., and H. G. Rainey. 2006. Managing successful organizational change in the public sector. *Public Administration Review* 66(2):168–176.

Garcia, R., and R. Sivasubramanian. 2012. Environmental justice for all: Struggle in Baldwin Hills and south central Los Angeles. *Clearinghouse Review: Journal of Poverty Law and Policy* 46(7–8):374–378.

Gaskin, D. J., T. A. LaVeist, and P. Richard. 2012. *The state of urban health: Eliminating health disparities to save lives and cut costs.* New York: National Urban League Policy Institute.

Gilbert, A. L., and S. M. Downs. 2015. Medical–legal partnership and health informatics impacting child health: Interprofessional innovations. *Journal of Interprofessional Care* 29(6):564–569.

Green, G., J. Henry, and J. Power. 2015. Physical fitness disparities in California school districts: A practicum issue briefer for The City Project. *University of Southern California: Price School of Public Policy.* http://www.cityprojectca.org/blog/wp-content/uploads/2015/06/FINAL-Physical-Education-Briefer-20150601.pdf (accessed July 20, 2016).

Hallarman, L., D. Snow, M. Kapoor, C. Brown, K. Rodabaugh, and E. Lawton. 2014. Blueprint for success: Translating innovations from the field of palliative medicine to the medical–legal partnership. *Journal of Legal Medicine* 35(1):179–194.

Hanleybrown, F., J. Kania, and M. Kramer. 2012. Channeling change: Making collective impact work. *Stanford Social Innovation Review.* http://jcisd.org/cms/lib/MI01928326/Centricity/Domain/ 218/Making%20Collective%20Impact%20Work%20Stanford%20 2012.pdf (accessed October 31, 2016).

Harvard Business Review. 2002. *Seven steps to change: A systematic approach.* Cambridge, MA: Harvard Business School Press.

Heller, J., M. L. Givens, T. K. Yuen, S. Gould, M. B. Jandu, E. Bourcier, and T. Choi. 2014. Advancing efforts to achieve health equity: Equity metrics for health impact assessment practice. *International Journal of Environmental Research and Public Health* 11(11):11054–11064.

HHS (U.S. Department of Health and Human Services). 2002. *Physical activity is fundamental to preventing disease.* Washington, DC: Office of the Assistant Secretary for Planning and Evaluation, U.S. Department of Health and Human Services.

HHS. n.d.-a. *Healthdata.gov.* https://www.healthdata.gov (accessed October 18, 2016).

HHS. n.d.-b. *National partnership for action to end health disparities: Toolkit for community action.* http://minorityhealth.hhs.gov/npa/files/Plans/Toolkit/NPA_Toolkit.pdf (accessed October 31, 2016).

Homer, J., B. Milstein, G. B. Hirsch, and E. S. Fisher. 2016. Combined regional investments could sustainably enhance health system performance and be financially affordable. *Health Affairs* 35(8):1435–1443.

Human Rights Campaign. 2016. *Human Rights Campaign.* http://www.hrc.org (accessed October 21, 2016).

IOM (Institute of Medicine). 2003. *The future of the public's health in the 21st century.* Washington, DC: The National Academies Press.
IOM. 2012. *For the public's health: The role of measurement in action and accountability.* Washington, DC: The National Academies Press.
IOM. 2013. *Educating the student body: Taking physical activity and physical education to school.* Washington, DC: The National Academies Press.
IOM. 2014. *Supporting a movement for health and health equity: Lessons from social movements: Workshop summary.* Washington, DC: The National Academies Press.
IOM. 2015a. *The role and potential of communities in population health improvement: Workshop summary.* Washington, DC: The National Academies Press.
IOM. 2015b. *Vital signs: Core metrics for health and health care progress.* Washington, DC: The National Academies Press.
IP3. n.d. *Community commons.* http://www.communitycommons.org (accessed October 18, 2016).
Kania, J., and M. Kramer. 2011. Collective impact. *Stanford Social Innovation Review* Winter. https://ssir.org/images/articles/2011_WI_Feature_Kania.pdf (accessed October 24, 2016).
Kemm, J. R. 2013. *Health impact assessment: Past achievement, current understanding, and future progress.* Oxford, UK: Oxford University Press.
Koo, D., P. W. O'Carroll, A. Harris, and K. B. DeSalvo. 2016. An environmental scan of recent initiatives incorporating social determinants in public health. *Preventing Chronic Disease* 13:E86.
Kotter, J. P. 1995. Leading change: Why transformation efforts fail. *Harvard Business Review* March–April.
Kotter, J. P. 1996. *Leading change.* Cambridge, MA: Harvard Business Press.
LA (Los Angeles) County Department of Public Health. 2015. *School district physical education model action plan (PE MAP) toolkit.* http://publichealth.lacounty.gov/cardio (accessed October 7, 2016).
Lafleur, M., S. Strongin, B. L. Cole, S. L. Bullock, R. Banthia, L. Craypo, R. Sivasubramanian, S. Samuels, and R. García. 2013. Physical education and student activity: Evaluating implementation of a new policy in Los Angeles public schools. *Annals of Behavioral Medicine* 45(1):122–130.
Leiderman, S. A., W. C. Wolf, and P. York. 2000. *Some thoughts about public will.* Center for Assessment and Policy Development. http://www.racialequitytools.org/resourcefiles/leiderman.pdf (accessed August 15, 2016).
Levasseur, R. E. 2001. People skills: Change management tools—Lewin's change model. *Interfaces* 31(4):71–73.
Lineman, M., Y. Do, J. Y. Kim, and G.-J. Joo. 2015. Talking about climate change and global warming. *PLOS One* 10(9):e0138996.
Martinez, I. L., N. Castellanos, C. Carr, C. J. Plescia, A. L. Rodriguez, S. Thommi, L. Zaremski, D. Weithorn, P. Maisel, and A. L. Wells. 2016. Increasing awareness in health care access in Florida: A community-based medical–legal practicum project. *Progress in Community Health Partnerships: Research, Education, and Action* 10(1):141–147.
Maxwell, N., D. Rotz, A. Dunn, L. Rosenberg, and J. Berman. 2013. *The structure and operations of social enterprises in redf's social innovation fund portfolio: Interim report.* Oakland, CA: Mathematica Policy Research.
May, J., K. Moseley, and P. Terry. 2016. *Developing culture of health metrics that really matter to companies and communities.* Health Enhancement Research Organization.
Metropolitan Group. 2009. *Building public will: Five-phase communication approach to sustainable change.* http://www.metgroup.com/assets/Public-Will.pdf (accessed October 30, 2016).

Mile High Connects. 2016. *Denver regional equity atlas.* http://www.denverregionalequity atlas.org (accessed October 18, 2016).
Mitchell, L., M. R. Frank, K. D. Harris, P. S. Dodds, and C. M. Danforth. 2013. The geography of happiness: Connecting twitter sentiment and expression, demographics, and objective characteristics of place. *PLOS One* 8(5):e64417.
NAACP LDF (National Association for the Advancement of Colored People Legal Defense Fund). n.d. *Home.* http://www.naacpldf.org (accessed October 21, 2016).
NACCHO (National Association of County and City Health Officials). 2016. *Health impact assessment.* http://archived.naccho.org/topics/environmental/health-impact-assessment (accessed October 24, 2016).
NASEM (National Academies of Sciences, Engineering, and Medicine). 2016. *Applying a health lens to business practices, policies, and investments: Workshop summary.* Washington, DC: The National Academies Press.
National Center for Medical–Legal Partnership. 2014a. *Medical–legal partnership at legal aid of Western Missouri.* http://medical-legalpartnership.org/wp-content/uploads/2014/02/MLP-at-LAWMO-2013-Kansas-City-MO.pdf (accessed November 21, 2016).
National Center for Medical–Legal Partnership. 2014b. *Medical–legal partnership toolkit.* http://medical-legalpartnership.org/mlptoolkit (accessed October 21, 2016).
National Center for Medical–Legal Partnership. 2016. *Partnerships across the U.S.* http://medical-legalpartnership.org/partnerships (accessed October 21, 2016).
NIH (National Institutes of Health). 2016. *U.S. National Library of Medicine: Common data element (CDE) resource portal.* https://www.nlm.nih.gov/cde/summaries.html (accessed October 18, 2016).
Northside Achievement Zone. n.d. *Northside Achievement Zone (NAZ).* http://northside achievement.org (accessed October 21, 2016).
NOW (National Organization for Women). 2016. National Organization for Women. http://now.org (accessed October 21, 2016).
NPS (National Park Service). 2014. *Healthy parks healthy people community engagement eguide: Edition 1.* https://www.nps.gov/public_health/hp/hphp/press/HealthyParks HealthyPeople_eGuide.pdf (accessed October 23, 2016).
NPS. 2015. *Rim of the valley corridor special resource study and environmental assessment.* https://parkplanning.nps.gov/document.cfm?documentID=65351 (accessed October 24, 2016).
Padgette, H., S. Deich, and L. Russell. 2010. *Strengthening partnerships and building public will for out-of-school time programs.* Washington, DC: National League of Cities' Institute for Youth, Education, and Families.
Pettignano, R., L. R. Bliss, S. B. Caley, and S. McLaren. 2013. Can access to a medical–legal partnership benefit patients with asthma who live in an urban community? *Journal of Health Care for the Poor and Underserved* 24(2):706–717.
Pettignano, R., L. Bliss, and S. Caley. 2014. The health law partnership: A medical–legal partnership strategically designed to provide a coordinated approach to public health legal services, education, advocacy, evaluation, research, and scholarship. *Journal of Legal Medicine* 35(1):57–79.
Plan4Health. n.d. *Plan4health Nashua: A collaborative project integrating planning and public health where we live, learn, work, and play.* http://plan4health.us/plan4health-coalitions/nashua-nh-plan4health-nashua-an-initiative-of-the-greater-nashua-public-health-network (accessed November 21, 2016).
PolicyLink and USC (University of Southern California) Program for Environmental and Regional Equity. 2016. *National equity atlas.* http://nationalequityatlas.org (accessed October 18, 2016).
Prevention Institute. 2016a. *Tools.* https://www.preventioninstitute.org/tools (accessed October 21, 2016).

Prevention Institute. 2016b. *Tools: Communities taking action: Profiles of health equity.* https://www.preventioninstitute.org/tools/communities-taking-action-profiles-health-equity (accessed October 21, 2016).

Public Health Agency of Canada. 2016. *Canadian best practices portal: Key element 6.* http://cbpp-pcpe.phac-aspc.gc.ca/population-health-approach-organizing-framework/key-element-6-collaborate-sectors-levels (accessed October 21, 2016).

Realmuto, L., S. Owusu, and K. Libman. 2016. *East Harlem neighborhood plan health impact assessment: Connecting housing affordability and health.* New York: The New York Academy of Medicine.

Reconnecting America. 2013. *Los Angeles equity atlas.* http://reconnectingamerica.org/laequityatlas/index.php (accessed October 18, 2016).

Rodrigues, R. G., R. M. das Dores, C. G. Camilo-Junior, and T. C. Rosa. 2016. Sentihealth-cancer: A sentiment analysis tool to help detecting mood of patients in online social networks. *International Journal of Medical Informatics* 85(1):80–95.

Rodriguez, M., M. Brenman, M. E. Lado, and R. Garcia. 2014. *Using civil rights tools to address health disparities.* Los Angeles, CA: The City Project.

Ross, C. L., M. Orenstein, and N. Botchwey. 2014. *Health impact assessment in the United States.* New York: Springer.

Rothman, J. 1996. The interweaving of community intervention approaches. *Journal of Community Practice* 3(3–4):69–99.

Rotz, D., N. Maxwell, and A. Dunn. 2015. *Economic self-sufficiency and life stability one year after starting a social enterprise job.* Oakland, CA: Mathematica Policy Research.

Roussos, S. T., and S. B. Fawcett. 2000. A review of collaborative partnerships as a strategy for improving community health. *Annual Review of Public Health* 21:369–402.

Sabeti, H. 2009. *The emerging fourth sector: Executive summary.* Washington, DC: The Aspen Institute.

Sadler, B., E. Wampler, J. Wood, M. Barry, and J. Wirfs-Brock. 2012. *The Denver regional equity atlas: Mapping access to opportunity at a regional scale.* Denver, CO: Mile High Connects, Reconnecting America, and The Piton Foundation.

Sanchez-Vaznaugh, E. V., B. N. Sánchez, L. G. Rosas, J. Baek, and S. Egerter. 2012. Physical education policy compliance and children's physical fitness. *American Journal of Preventive Medicine* 42(5):452–459.

Schoeni, R. F., W. H. Dow, W. D. Miller, and E. R. Pamuk. 2011. The economic value of improving the health of disadvantaged Americans. *American Journal of Preventive Medicine* 40(1):S67–S72.

School-Based Health Alliance. n.d. *The children's health and education mapping tool.* http://www.sbh4all.org/resources/mapping-tool (accessed October 21, 2016).

Sege, R., G. Preer, S. J. Morton, H. Cabral, O. Morakinyo, V. Lee, C. Abreu, E. De Vos, and M. Kaplan-Sanoff. 2015. Medical–legal strategies to improve infant health care: A randomized trial. *Pediatrics* 136(1):97–106.

Springer, A. E., D. M. Hoelscher, B. Castrucci, A. Perez, and S. H. Kelder. 2009. Prevalence of physical activity and sedentary behaviors by metropolitan status in 4th-, 8th-, and 11th-grade students in Texas, 2004–2005. *Preventing Chronic Disease* 6(1):1–16.

Stratton, C., M. Rose, A. Parcell, and J. Mooney. 2012. *Made in Durham: Building an education-to-career system.* Durham, NC: MDC, Inc.

Taylor, D. R., B. A. Bernstein, E. Carroll, E. Oquendo, L. Peyton, and L. M. Pachter. 2015. Keeping the heat on for children's health: A successful medical–legal partnership initiative to prevent utility shutoffs in vulnerable children. *Journal of Health Care for the Poor and Underserved* 26(3):676–685.

The City Project. n.d.-a. *Quality education, physical education, and schools of hope.* http://www.cityprojectca.org/quality-education-physical-education-and-shared-use#summary (accessed July 8, 2016).

The City Project. n.d.-b. *Transit to trails.* http://www.cityprojectca.org/transit-to-trails (accessed October 21, 2016).

The Pew Charitable Trusts. 2016. Issue brief: Is health impact assessment effective in bringing community perspectives to public decision-making? Lessons from 4 case studies in California. *The Pew Charitable Trusts.* http://www.pewtrusts.org/en/research-and-analysis/issue-briefs/2016/10/is-health-impact-assessment-effective-in-bringing-community-perspectives-to-public-decision-making (accessed October 24, 2016).

Thompson, H. R. 2013. Are physical education policies working?: A snapshot from San Francisco, 2011. *Preventing Chronic Disease* 10.

Tsao, B., and R. Davis. 2014. *Multi-sector partnerships for preventing violence: A guide for using collaboration multiplier to improve safety outcomes for young people, communities, and cities.* Oakland, CA: Prevention Institute.

UCLA (University of California, Los Angeles). 2016. *The Civil Rights Project.* https://www.civilrightsproject.ucla.edu (accessed October 21, 2016).

University of Colorado Law School. n.d. *Colorado Health Equity Project (CHEP).* http://chep.colorado.edu (accessed October 21, 2016).

USDA (U.S. Department of Agriculture) Economic Research Service. 2016. *The food access research atlas.* http://www.ers.usda.gov/data-products/food-access-research-atlas.aspx (accessed October 21, 2016).

Virginia Department of Health. 2016. *Virginia health opportunity index (HOI).* https://www.vdh.virginia.gov/OMHHE/policyanalysis/virginiahoi.htm (accessed October 21, 2016).

Waidmann, T. 2009. *Estimating the cost of racial and ethnic health disparities.* Washington, DC: Urban Institute.

Work Group for Community Health and Development. 2016a. *The community tool box.* http://ctb.ku.edu/en (accessed October 21, 2016).

Work Group for Community Health and Development. 2016b. *The community tool box: Chapter 1, section 3. Our model of practice: Building capacity for community and system change.* http://ctb.ku.edu/en/table-of-contents/overview/model-for-community-change-and-improvement/building-capacity/main (accessed October 21, 2016).

Work Group for Community Health and Development. 2016c. *The community tool box: Chapter 13, section 1. Developing a plan for building leadership.* http://ctb.ku.edu/en/table-of-contents/leadership/leadership-ideas/plan-for-building-leadership/main (accessed October 21, 2016).

9

Conclusion

"Of all the forms of inequality, injustice in health care is the most shocking and inhumane." —Dr. Martin Luther King, Jr.

"Poverty is not an accident. Like slavery and apartheid, it is man-made and can be removed by the actions of human beings." —Nelson Mandela

For many years researchers, public health practitioners, and others have known that health status in this country and around the world is determined as much by socioeconomic as biologic or behavioral factors. Despite that recognition, approaches to improving health status and health outcomes have narrowly centered on improving medical interventions, technologies, systems, and access. Beyond clinical approaches, some health promotion strategies have focused on changing behavior, despite the robust evidence indicating that they are ineffective in addressing health inequities (Baum and Fisher, 2014). Although these strategies play a role in improving population health, it has become amply clear that they are necessary but not sufficient. Health is the result of much more than health care; the social, economic, environmental, and structural factors—for example, education, poverty, housing, and structural racism—that shape health outcomes also create health inequities. Addressing and putting an end to health inequities will only be possible if society and decision makers broaden their view of health to fully grasp how steep and unjust disparities in social and other conditions limit, thwart, and even destroy some people's ability to live healthy and full lives.

This report spotlights community interventions to address health inequity because communities are the unit in which individuals and families live, learn, work, and play. Thriving communities provide opportunities for people to live healthy lives. The opposite is also true. Communities that are unsafe, provide poor educational and economic opportunities, and offer weak infrastructure and surroundings also have poor health status. However, such realities are not destiny, and communities across the country have shown their resilience and ability to be agents of social change, as described throughout this report and especially in the community examples highlighted in Chapter 5. This ability to catalyze change can not only affect social and economic status but can also have a powerful impact on reducing health inequity.

This report highlights what is known about health inequity and its root causes: social, economic, environmental, and structural inequities. Because of their historically entrenched nature, such structural inequities as structural racism are highlighted as a major root cause of health inequity. Other root causes include inequities in education—which is highlighted as a key social determinant of health because of the well-documented impact it has on health and income—and income, which affects health status along with housing, transportation, and access to health care services. The committee concluded that health inequities are the result of much more than individual choice; they are the result of the historic and ongoing interplay of inequitable structures, policies, norms, and demographic and geographic patterns that shape lives and play out in the social, economic, environmental, and structural determinants of health (Braveman and Gottlieb, 2014; Krieger et al., 1997; Marmot et al., 2010; Williams and Collins, 2001).

Community solutions, such as those described in the report, have the best chance of being effective in addressing health inequities when implemented in the context of an enabling environment with supportive laws and policies (described in Chapter 6) and with a range of collaborators from a variety of relevant sectors (described in Chapter 7). The community-based solutions that the committee highlights as promising are characterized by (1) having a shared vision and values regarding what was needed in their community—whether or not health equity was explicitly acknowledged in that vision—and on how to move forward to address those needs; (2) enhancing community capacity by harnessing the power of communities; and (3) embracing and building on cross-sector collaboration. The committee also found that (see Chapters 4 and 5 for more details)

- Advances in health equity involve local community action, but always in collaboration with a range of partners.

CONCLUSION

- Community initiatives create positive change and improve results through many different pathways, and no one solution can serve as an exact template to be scaled or generalized.
- Robust initiatives demonstrate a focus on developing the next generation of leaders as well as flexibility, creativity, and resilience.
- Community collaboration can help create lasting change when all stakeholders agree on a shared commitment to results and to systematic learning from their experience and evolving research.
- Effective community solutions involve collaboration across professional, organizational, and bureaucratic boundaries; draw on the experience of practitioners and residents; and are informed by evidence.
- A mutual commitment to realizing co-benefits can facilitate the creation and sustainability of partnerships across sectors.
- Effective community solutions create a capacity for residents to identify key issues and to participate in devising strategies to meet their needs and build on their strengths while recognizing the power of systems and other forces outside the community to enhance or undermine the effectiveness of their efforts.
- Communities recognize the importance of sustainability in their approach to multiple and diverse sources of funding, to maintaining accountability, and to nurturing leadership.

In addition to providing a rationale for the community as the locus for confronting health inequities (see Chapter 4) and exploring community examples (see Chapter 5), the report highlights some of the helpful tools available to communities (see Chapter 8); describes the evidence on root causes and outlines some research and data needs (see Chapter 3); reviews the state of health disparities (see Chapter 2); discusses the national policy terrain (see Chapter 6); and explores the actions and engagement of different sectors and potential community partners (see Chapter 7).

As discussed in the report, communities have agency, voice, and power, and multi-actor, multi-sectoral community partnerships can drive the identification, development, and implementation of solutions to promote health equity. However, a supportive policy and resource environment is needed to facilitate community efforts. The report provides evidence of both the critical need and the opportunity to address health inequity and of the key role that community-based solutions can play. It also outlines a path toward using a health focus as a lever in building a more equal, just, and fair society and to approaching the goal depicted at the center of the report conceptual model (see Figure 9-1): healthier, more equitable communities in which individuals and families live, learn, work, and play.

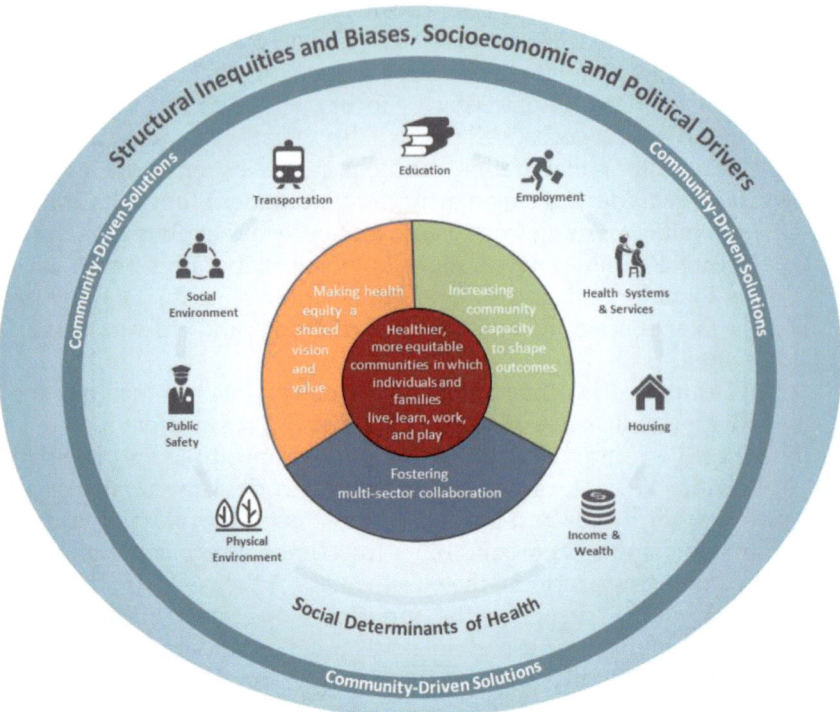

FIGURE 9-1 Report conceptual model for community solutions to promote health equity.

REFERENCES

Baum, F., and M. Fisher. 2014. Why behavioural health promotion endures despite its failure to reduce health inequities. *Sociology of Health & Illness* 36(2):213–225.
Braveman, P., and L. Gottlieb. 2014. The social determinants of health: It's time to consider the causes of the causes. *Public Health Reports* 129(Suppl 2):19–31.
Krieger, N., D. R. Williams, and N. E. Moss. 1997. Measuring social class in U.S. public health research: Concepts, methodologies, and guidelines. *Annual Review of Public Health* 18(1):341–378.
Marmot, M., J. Allen, P. Goldblatt, T. Boyce, D. McNeish, M. Grady, and I. Geddes. 2010. *Fair society, healthy lives: Strategic review of health inequalities in England post-2010.* London: The Marmot Review.
Williams, D. R., and C. Collins. 2001. Racial residential segregation: A fundamental cause of racial disparities in health. *Public Health Reports* 116(5):404–416.

Appendix A

Native American Health: Historical and Legal Context

FEDERAL TRUST RELATIONSHIP

To sufficiently examine and ultimately address health disparities affecting Native Americans, it is essential to understand the unique historical and legal context of Native American communities in the United States. Native American tribes have a legal relationship with the federal government that can be traced back to the 18th century, which has shaped the conditions that impact the health of this population. According to a report transmitted by the U.S. Commission on Civil Rights (2004), the special relationship between the federal government and Native Americans, referred to as a "trust" relationship, requires the government to protect tribal lands, assets, resources, treaty rights, and health care, in addition to other responsibilities (United States Commission on Civil Rights, 2004). The original basis for the federal–tribe relationship is rooted in Article I, Section 8 of the U.S. Constitution, which grants Congress the power "to regulate commerce . . . with the Indian tribes."[1]

While there is no single legal source of the federal government's trust obligation to Native American tribes, there is an extensive history of treaties, laws, and judicial decisions that collectively form the legal basis of this obligation. The American Indian Policy Review Commission Report commissioned by Congress (1977) cites treaties in which the United States acquired land in exchange for its commitment to protect the people and

---

[1] U.S. CONST. art. I, § 8, cl. 3.

property of tribes from encroachment by U.S. citizens (American Indian Policy Review Commission, 1977). Among the most noteworthy court cases is *Cherokee Nation v. Georgia*,[2] in which the Supreme Court concluded that the relationship of states to Indian nations is analogous to "that of a ward to his guardian." The following year, in *Worcester v. Georgia*, the Supreme Court held that Indian tribes are guaranteed protection against interference from the states, as they are domestic sovereigns of the United States.[3] These two cases established that only the federal government has jurisdiction over Indian nations and that, as a trustee, the federal government must ensure that states do not interfere with tribes' self-governance or intrude on their land (U.S. Commission on Civil Rights, 2004). The aforementioned cases and legislation, in addition to other policies and treaties, have shaped the unique "trust" relationship between Native American tribes and the federal government.

Role of Policies Over Time

It is important to highlight the role of assimilation policies that began in the late 1800s because these policies have had sustained effects on Native American communities and, ultimately, their health conditions. As the United States expanded westward, Native Americans were forced to move to reservations, and the federal government made efforts to assimilate Native Americans into mainstream society. As tribes resettled, they continued to suffer from the infectious diseases that plagued the population during the prior decades of warfare. Assimilation policies took on many forms, including the General Allotment Act of 1887,[4] legislation that abolished the group title of a tribe to land and replaced it with individual plots. In addition, the Bureau of Indian Affairs implemented a boarding school system, which prohibited traditional Native American practices, including religion, medicine, language, and other traditional cultural expressions (e.g., dress, hairstyle, etc.) (Shelton, 2004). This boarding school system, coupled with the prohibition of traditional health care activities, exacerbated the already dismal health and living conditions of Native American communities at the time. The results included rampant infectious diseases, poor sanitation, malnutrition, poverty, overcrowding and inadequate ventilation in homes, poor education practices, and isolation. The harsh conditions that Native Americans had to endure on reservations were extensively documented in *The Meriam Report*, a study

---

[2] *Cherokee Nation v. Georgia*, 30 U.S. (5 Pet.) 17 (1831).
[3] *Worcester v. Georgia*, 31 U.S. (6 Pet.) 515, 557 (1832).
[4] The General Allotment Act of 1887, Ch. 119, 24 Stat. 388-91 (1887) (also known as the "Dawes Act").

commissioned to assess the status of tribes across the country at the time (Meriam, 1928).

After the assimilation era, there was a series of policies and legislation that formed the periods of Native American policy known as reorganization and, subsequently, termination. In his report on the legal and historical roots of health care for Native Americans, Shelton detailed the chronology and impact of these policies, including the Indian Reorganization Act of 1934 (IRA).[5] The IRA was designed to stimulate economic development and self-determination, while also promoting the adoption of modern business-like practices for governing tribes (Shelton, 2004). This positive shift in power was short-lived, as it was followed by termination policies in the 1950s, which had enduring effects on Native American communities regarding mental health, identity, and social and family networks (Walls and Whitbeck, 2012). Congress passed legislation discontinuing the special federal–tribe "trust" relationship with 109 tribes and bands (Shelton, 2004). The termination policies resulted in the removal of tribes' federal recognition, the elimination of their reservations, and the forced relocation of Native Americans from their tribal lands to major urban areas.

Following the termination-era policies, the federal government made the official transition to tribal self-determination and passed laws to restore tribal sovereignty. In 1975 Congress recognized the importance of tribal decision making in tribal affairs and the significance of the nation-to-nation relationship between the United States and tribes through the passage of the Indian Self-Determination and Education Assistance Act (ISDEAA).[6] The ISDEAA directs the Secretary of the U.S. Department of Interior and the Secretary of the U.S. Department of Health and Human Services to enter self-determination contracts or compacts with tribal organizations, upon the request of any Native American tribe (Bauman and Floyd, 1999). Subsequent amendments to the ISDEAA strengthened the federal policies supporting tribal self-determination and self-governance.

Health Care Services

Unlike other racial and ethnic minority groups in the United States, Native Americans have legal rights to federal health care services. Federal responsibility for Native American health care was codified in the Snyder

---

[5] Ch. 576, 48 Stat. 984 (codified as amended at 25 U.S.C. §§ 461, 462, 463, 464, 465, 466–470, 471–473, 474, 475, 476–478, 479) (1934).

[6] The Indian Self-Determination and Education Assistance Act of 1975, Public Law 93-638.

Act of 1921[7] and the Indian Health Care Improvement Act[8] (IHCIA) of 1976, which together form the legislative authority for the federal agency known today as the Indian Health Service (IHS) (U.S. Commission on Civil Rights, 2004). The Snyder Act authorized funding for health care services to federally recognized tribes, and the IHCIA defined the structure for the delivery of health services and authorized the construction and maintenance of health care and sanitation facilities on reservations (U.S. Commission on Civil Rights, 2004). Although these pieces of legislation marked significant progress, the Snyder Act has been criticized for its use of broad and vague language, which does not facilitate long-term planning or provide resources based on need. This is considered to have influenced the piecemeal approach that has shaped the funding and distribution of health care resources for Native Americans (IOM, 2003).

The IHS is the federal agency responsible for fulfilling the trust obligation to provide health services to Native Americans. When the federal responsibility for health care services was transferred from the U.S. Department of the Interior to the U.S. Department of Health, Education, and Welfare in 1955, the IHS was established under the Public Health Service. This transfer resulted in the doubling of appropriations for the IHS. Currently, the IHS operates within the U.S. Department of Health and Human Services. IHS is only required to provide federal health care services to federally recognized tribes. Individual eligibility for services is determined by a number of criteria, including, but not limited to, the requirement that the individual is of Native American descent, is regarded as a tribal member, has some legal evidence of tribal enrollment or certificate of origin, and resides on or near a federal reservation (IOM, 2003). The IHS consists of a network of hospitals, clinics, field stations, and other programs that collectively serve approximately 2.2 million Native Americans (IHS, 2015). The IHS system is divided into three major branches: the federally operated direct health care services, tribally operated health care services, and urban Native American health care services and resource centers. For those who are eligible, health care services can be received at any IHS facility; however, there are complex rules that restrict the delivery of contract medical care that is not available in IHS facilities (Jim et al., 2014).

Since the passage and amendments of the ISDEAA, there has been an increasing trend toward tribal self-governance with respect to all domains of life, including health care. As a result, tribes have the option to receive direct services from the IHS, to assume responsibility for health care with

---

[7] The Snyder Act of 1921, Ch. 115, 42 Stat. 208 (1921) (codified as amended at 25 U.S.C. § 13 [2004]).

[8] The Indian Health Care Improvement Act of 1976, Public Law 94-437. The IHCIA was permanently reauthorized in 2010 as part of the Patient Protection and Affordable Care Act.

the option to contract with IHS, or to fund the establishment of their own programs or supplementation of ISDEAA programs (IHS, 2016). The option of self-governance allows tribes to tailor health care services to the needs of their communities. The IHS operates from the understanding that tribal leaders are in the best position to assess and address the needs of their communities. More than half of the IHS appropriation is currently administered by tribes, through self-determination contracts or self-governance compacts (IHS, 2015).

There are a number of barriers that preclude the IHS from reaching its full potential of providing quality, efficient health care services to its target population to reduce disparities (U.S. Commission on Civil Rights, 2004). The persistent lack of adequate funding is often cited as a barrier to reducing the pervasive health disparities that affect Native Americans (Sequist et al., 2011; Warne and Frizzell, 2014). Every year, Congress appropriates funds to IHS to fulfill the trust responsibility to provide health care services. According to the National Congress of American Indians, in 2014 the IHS per capita expenditures for patient health services were only $3,107, compared to $8,097 per person for health care spending nationally, and when examining medical spending only, IHS per capita was approximately $1,904 (National Congress of American Indians, 2016).

A physician survey conducted in 2007 explored barriers to quality improvement within the IHS. The findings revealed that access to high-quality specialists within geographic proximity, nonemergency hospital admission, high-quality imaging services, and high-quality outpatient mental health services were high-priority barriers for physicians (Sequist et al., 2011). Furthermore, a majority of the physicians felt that a lack of IHS funding to support provision of care through subspecialists was a crucial barrier to quality improvement (Sequist et al., 2011).

SOCIAL DETERMINANTS OF HEALTH

As is the case with all other populations, Native Americans' opportunities to achieve optimal health are affected by the social determinants of health in their communities, which in turn have been shaped by social and political processes, both historical and contemporary. A keen understanding of the root causes and determinants of health will help inform the most effective and just solutions to address health inequities among Native Americans.

Income and Wealth

Native Americans are one of the most economically impoverished populations in the United States. The median household income for this group is $37,227, as compared with $53,657 in the nation as a whole (U.S. Census Bureau, 2015). Given that income is a strong predictor of health outcomes and life expectancy (Chetty et al., 2016; Woolf et al., 2015), this disparity in income has severe consequences for the health and well-being of Native Americans. This particular population also has a higher proportion of people living in poverty than the rest of the country, with 28.3 percent of Native Americans living in poverty, compared with 15.5 percent of the total population (U.S. Census Bureau, 2015). Income and poverty are inextricably tied to employment opportunities, of which there are too few for Native Americans. Native Americans have the highest unemployment rate (9.9 percent in 2015) of any racial or ethnic group in the United States (U.S. Bureau of Labor Statistics, 2016).

In terms of recent trends in economic well-being, it is important to recognize the lasting effects of the economic recession of 2008. Native Americans saw declines in employment and income that were similar to other racial and ethnic groups; however, this population on average was in a more vulnerable financial condition than other groups at the beginning of the period. The unemployment rate for Native Americans spiked from 11 percent in 2008 to 18 percent in 2010 (Pettit et al., 2014). In that same time period, Native Americans also experienced almost double the percentage increase in the poverty rate as other racial and ethnic groups did, with the largest increase observed in the West (Pettit et al., 2014). By 2013 the overall Native American unemployment rate had dropped to 11.3 percent, but rates were still high in the Midwest (16.9 percent), Northern Plains (15 percent), and Southwest (15 percent) regions of the country (Austin, 2013).

Education

Education is a significant determinant of health for Native Americans, as the U.S. educational system has historically been a source of discrimination and, in many cases, trauma for this population. One of the most overt examples of this is the implementation of the boarding school system, which was designed with the purpose of eliminating students' tribal identity and facilitating assimilation into mainstream American culture (Executive Office of the President, 2014; Shelton, 2004). Today, educational progress for Native Americans is far behind that of other racial and ethnic groups. A report from the National Center for Education Statistics reveals that Native Americans have the highest high school dropout rate in the country, which was at 14.6 percent in 2012, compared with a low of 3.3 percent among Asians/Pacific Islanders (Stark and Noel, 2015). In addition, Native Americans had the lowest high school completion rate in 2012, which was at 79.0 percent compared with a high of 94.9 percent among Asians/Pacific Islanders (Stark and Noel, 2015). This disparity has serious implications for health inequities among Native Americans because the evidence demonstrates that there is a strong link between high school completion and health (Cutler and Lleras-Muney, 2006).

Since the civil rights movement in the 1960s, there has been an emergence of grassroots educational institutions that seek to support tribal identity, address academic deficiencies, and resolve the lack of quality education experiences and sense of displacement among tribal students (Crazy Bull, 2015). Research suggests that culturally relevant education increases the likelihood that a young Native American stays in school. Currently, approximately 20,000 students attend tribal colleges and universities full time in the United States (Crazy Bull, 2015).

Housing

Housing conditions for Native Americans are a major consideration for health disparities, on and off of reservations. Housing affordability is a community-level factor that affects Native Americans' access to shelter. According to a recent U.S. Department of Housing and Urban Development report, from 2006 to 2010 roughly 4 out of 10 Native American households had excessive cost burdens, paying more than 30 percent of their income on housing (Pettit et al., 2014). This was comparable to households among other racial and ethnic groups; however, Native American households were more likely to be severely cost-burdened (i.e., paying more than 50 percent of their income on housing) than households of other racial and ethnic groups (Pettit et al., 2014). While home ownership rates in tribal areas were relatively high (67 percent) in 2010, the overall homeownership rate for Native Americans lagged behind that of other racial and ethnic groups, at 54 percent and 65 percent, respectively (Pettit et al., 2014).

Safe and healthy housing is a determinant of health to which many Native Americans do not have access. For example, the U.S. Environmental Protection Agency reports that as of 2011, there were more than 120,000 tribal homes lacking access to basic water sanitation (EPA, 2012), and the IHS reports that almost 1 in 10 Native American homes are without safe and reliable water (Indian Health Service, 2011). It should also be noted that there are certain Native American communities that are particularly affected by the lack of quality housing (i.e., not having complete plumbing and kitchen facilities) in the Alaska, Arizona, and New Mexico regions (Pettit et al., 2014). Those living in extreme climate conditions, such as Alaska, are especially vulnerable to potential damages to their poor-quality housing caused by extreme weather.

Overcrowding in homes is an issue for Native Americans that research suggests is linked to the onset or exacerbation of many health problems. These health issues include respiratory conditions, the transmission of infectious diseases, child well-being (i.e., academic achievement, behavior problems, physical health), depression, and sleep deprivation (Angel and Bittschi, 2014; Solari and Mare, 2012; Webster, 2015). From 2006 to 2010, Native American households were much more likely to be overcrowded than all households in general, with 8.1 percent of Native American households being overcrowded and about one-third of these being severely overcrowded (Pettit et al., 2014). The highest incidence of overcrowding in Native American homes was in larger tribal areas, where 11 percent of households were overcrowded, compared with 3.1 percent of all U.S. households (Pettit et al., 2014). When examining overcrowding and its effects, it is important to recognize the cultural values and customs that shape household traditions in Native American communities.

Living in Urban and Rural Places

Whether Native Americans live in urban or rural areas has implications for the types of barriers and health disparities they face. The 2010 U.S. Census reported that 71 percent of Native Americans live in urban areas (UIHI, 2013). Racial misclassification is more of an issue for collecting mortality data on Native Americans in urban areas than those in rural areas because there is less awareness of Native American status off of reservations (Jacobs-Wingo et al., 2016). This population reportedly has less access to hospitals, health clinics, or contract health services that are managed by the IHS and tribal health programs, but they may have greater access to other health care resources that reduce mortality (HHS, 2016; Jacobs-Wingo et al., 2016). This group of Native Americans must also face the lasting effects of the termination policies from the 1950s, which lead to the coerced migration of many individuals and, in some cases, the breakdown of familial ties and social structures. Although the leading causes of death are similar between urban and rural Native Americans, death rates are generally higher among rural Native Americans (Jacobs-Wingo et al., 2016). Furthermore, rural residence has been associated with later cancer stage diagnosis, inadequate cancer treatment, and increased cancer mortality (Campbell et al., 2001; Monroe et al., 1992; Singh and Siahpush, 2014).

Public Safety

Similar to the case for other racial and ethnic minority groups, Native Americans experience systematic differences in exposure to violence and interactions with the criminal justice system as compared to whites. The findings from the 2010 National Intimate Partner and Sexual Violence survey showed that relative to white women, Native American women are 1.2 times more likely to have experienced violence in their lifetime and that relative to white men, Native American men are 1.3 times more likely to have experienced violence in their lifetime (Rosay, 2016). In particular, violence against Native American women is being addressed as a major public health and public safety issue (Crossland et al., 2013). In terms of the criminal justice system, Native Americans are arrested at 1.5 times the rate that whites are, with a larger disparity for specific violent and public order offenses (Hartney and Vuong, 2009). Furthermore, Native Americans are incarcerated and on parole at twice the rate that whites are (Hartney and Vuong, 2009). Research suggests that, when convicted, Native Americans are often sentenced more harshly than white, African-American, and Hispanic offenders (Franklin, 2013).

Native American youth, specifically, are at an elevated risk for delinquency and incarceration. The risk factors for delinquency can be directly linked to the social determinants of health. For example, Native American youth are more likely to live in poverty, drop out of school, and be exposed to violence than youth in the general population (Rolnick, 2016). A 2014 report from the University of Wisconsin Population Health Institute on the Wisconsin juvenile justice system revealed that Native American youth were twice as likely to be arrested and almost twice as likely to be detained following arrest as white youth, with little change from 2006–2012 (Lecoanet et al., 2014). This disparity was found to be much higher in certain counties in Milwaukee (Rolnick, 2016). The Indian Law and Order Commission reports that the federal and state juvenile justice systems incarcerate Native American youth and remove them from their families, reducing opportunities for positive contact with their communities and often contributing to trauma in this population (Rolnick, 2016).

REFERENCES

American Indian Policy Review Commission. 1977. *American Indian Policy Review Commission final report, submitted to Congress May 17, 1977.* Washington, DC: Congress of the United States.

Angel, S., and B. Bittschi. 2014. *Housing and health.* Mannheim, Germany: Centre for European Economic Research.

Austin, A. 2013. *High unemployment means Native Americans are still waiting for an economic recovery.* Washington, DC: Economic Policy Institute.

Bauman, D., and J. Floyd. 1999. *Indian tribal health systems governance and development: Issues and approaches.* Menlo Park, CA: Kaiser Family Foundation.

Campbell, N. C., A. M. Elliott, L. Sharp, L. D. Ritchie, J. Cassidy, and J. Little. 2001. Rural and urban differences in stage at diagnosis of colorectal and lung cancers. *British Journal of Cancer* 84(7):910–914.

Chetty, R., M. Stepner, S. Abraham, S. Lin, B. Scuderi, N. Turner, A. Bergeron, and D. Cutler. 2016. The association between income and life expectancy in the United States, 2001–2014. *JAMA* 315(16):1750–1766.
Crazy Bull, C. 2015. Helping native youth succeed with culturally responsive education. *The Aspen Journal of Ideas*, July/August. http://aspen.us/journal/editions/julyaugust-2015/helping-native-youth-succeed-culturally-responsive-education (accessed November 5, 2016).
Crossland, C., J. Palmer, and A. Brooks. 2013. NIJ's program of research on violence against American Indian and Alaska native women. *Violence Against Women* 19(6):771–790.
Cutler, D. M., and A. Lleras-Muney. 2006. *Education and health: Evaluating theories and evidence.* National Bureau of Economic Research working paper no. 12352. http://www.nber.org/papers/w12352 (accessed November 5, 2016).
EPA (U.S. Environmental Protection Agency). 2012. The Clean Water Indian Set Aside Grant Program. https://www.epa.gov/sites/production/files/2015-01/documents/epa-cwisa-report-final-2012-11-29-12_508cmpl.pdf (accessed October 24, 2016).
Executive Office of the President. 2014. *2014 native youth report.* Washington, DC.
Franklin, T. W. 2013. Sentencing Native Americans in U.S. federal courts: An examination of disparity. *Justice Quarterly* 30(2):310–339.
Hartney, C., and L. Vuong. 2009. *Created equal: Racial and ethnic disparities in the U.S. criminal justice system.* Oakland, CA: National Council on Crime and Delinquency.
HHS (U.S. Department of Health and Human Services). 2016. Profile: American Indian/Alaska native. http://minorityhealth.hhs.gov/omh/browse.aspx?lvl=3&lvlid=62 (accessed August 25, 2016).
IHS (Indian Health Service). 2011. *Public Law 86-121 annual report for 2011.* Rockville, MD: U.S. Department of Health and Human Services.
IHS. 2015. IHS year 2015 profile. https://www.ihs.gov/newsroom/factsheets/ihsyear2015profile (accessed October 24, 2016).
IHS. 2016. IHS year 2016 profile. https://www.ihs.gov/newsroom/index.cfm/factsheets/ihsprofile (accessed November 5, 2016).
IOM (Institute of Medicine). 2003. *Unequal treatment: Confronting racial and ethnic disparities in health care.* Washington, DC: The National Academies Press.
Jacobs-Wingo, J. L., D. K. Espey, A. V. Groom, L. E. Phillips, D. S. Haverkamp, and S. L. Stanley. 2016. Causes and disparities in death rates among urban American Indian and Alaska native populations, 1999–2009. *American Journal of Public Health* 106(5):906–914.
Jim, M. A., E. Arias, D. S. Seneca, M. J. Hoopes, C. C. Jim, N. J. Johnson, and C. L. Wiggins. 2014. Racial misclassification of American Indians and Alaska natives by Indian Health Service contract health service delivery area. *American Journal of Public Health* 104(Suppl 3):S295–S302.
Lecoanet, R., D. Kuo, S. Lindsley, and S. Seibold. 2014. *Disproportionate minority contact in Wisconsin's juvenile justice system.* Madison, WI: University of Wisconsin Population Health Institute.
Meriam, L. 1928. *Meriam report: The problem of Indian administration.* Washington, DC: The Institute for Government Research.
Monroe, A. C., T. C. Ricketts, and L. A. Savitz. 1992. Cancer in rural versus urban populations: A review. *Journal of Rural Health* 8(3):212–220.
National Congress of American Indians. 2016. *Fiscal year 2017 Indian country budget request: Upholding the promises, respecting tribal governance: For the good of the people.* Washington, DC: National Congress of American Indians.
Pettit, K. L. S., G. T. Kingsley, J. Biess, K. Bertumen, N. Pindus, C. Narducci, and A. Budde. 2014. *Continuity and change: Demographic, socioeconomic, and housing conditions of American Indians and Alaska natives.* Washington, DC: U.S. Department of Housing and Urban Development.

Rolnick, A. C. 2016. Locked up: Fear, racism, prison economics, and the incarceration of native youth. *American Indian Culture and Research Journal* 40(1):55–92.

Rosay, A. B. 2016. *Violence against American Indian and Alaska native women and men: 2010 findings from the National Intimate Partner and Sexual Violence Survey.* Washington, DC: National Institute of Justice.

Sequist, T. D., T. Cullen, K. Bernard, S. Shaykevich, E. J. Orav, and J. Z. Ayanian. 2011. Trends in quality of care and barriers to improvement in the Indian Health Service. *Journal of General and Internal Medicine* 26(5):480–486.

Shelton, B. L. 2004. *The legal and historical roots of health care for American Indians and Alaska natives in the United States.* Menlo Park, CA: The Henry J. Kaiser Family Foundation.

Singh, G. K., and M. Siahpush. 2014. Widening rural–urban disparities in life expectancy, U.S., 1969–2009. *American Journal of Preventive Medicine* 46(2):e19–e29.

Solari, C. D., and R. D. Mare. 2012. Housing crowding effects on children's wellbeing. *Social Science Research* 41(2):464–476.

Stark, P., and A. M. Noel. 2015. *Trends in high school dropout and completion rates in the United States: 1972–2012 (NCES 2015-015).* Washington, DC: National Center for Education Statistics.

UIHI (Urban Indian Health Institute). 2013. U.S. Census marks increase in urban American Indians and Alaska natives. http://www.uihi.org/wp-content/uploads/2013/09/Broadcast_Census-Number_FINAL_v2.pdf (accessed October 24, 2016).

U.S. Bureau of Labor Statistics. 2016. *Labor force characteristics by race and ethnicity, 2015. Report 1062.* Washington, DC: U.S. Bureau of Labor Statistics.

U.S. Census Bureau. 2015. *FFF: American Indian and Alaska Native Heritage Month: November 2015.* http://www.census.gov/newsroom/facts-for-features/2015/cb15-ff22.html (accessed October 24, 2016,).

U.S. Commission on Civil Rights. 2004. *Broken promises: Evaluating the Native American health care system.* Washington, DC: U.S. Commission on Civil Rights.

Walls, M. L., and L. B. Whitbeck. 2012. The intergenerational effects of relocation policies on indigenous families. *Journal of Family Issues* 33(9):1272–1293.

Warne, D., and L. B. Frizzell. 2014. American Indian health policy: Historical trends and contemporary issues. *American Journal of Public Health* 104(Suppl 3):S263–S267.

Webster, P. C. 2015. Housing triggers health problems for Canada's first nations. *The Lancet* 385(9967):495–496.

Woolf, S. H., L. Aron, L. Dubay, S. M. Simon, E. Zimmerman, and K. X. Luk. 2015. *How are income and wealth linked to health and longevity?* Washington, DC: Urban Institute and Virginia Commonwealth University.

Appendix B

Community-Level Indicators and Interactive Tools for Health Equity

Chapter 8 summarizes the current state of indicators and interactive tools available to communities. This appendix contains two resources relevant to that discussion. Table B-1 contains publicly accessible indicators related to health equity. This includes measures of demographics, the social determinants of health, and four aspects of the conceptual model for this report: (1) making health equity a shared vision and value, (2) building community capacity to shape outcomes, (3) fostering multi-sector collaboration, and (4) creating healthier more equitable communities in which members and families live, learn, work, and play. Table B-2 describes interactive tools that communities can use to examine health equity indicators by geographic region as the foundation for community-based solutions and to monitor progress over time.

TABLE B-1 Examples of Indicators Relevant to Health Equity in Publicly Available Data Sources

	HP2020[a]	CoH[b]	AHR[c]	CHR[d]	CHSI[e]	NEA[f]	VHOI[g]	DDK[h]	AARP[i]
Demographics									
Age			•	•	•	•		•	
Race	•		•	•	•	•	•	•	
Ethnicity	•		•	•	•	•	•	•	
Immigrant status						•			
Social Determinants of Health									
Education									
Early childhood education		•							
Education levels and job requirements								•	
Grade school achievement						•			
High school graduation			•	•					•
High school graduation 4 years after starting 9th grade	•		•	•	•			•	
Public school enrollment and racial/ethnic composition								•	
School poverty						•	•		
Years of schooling of adults						•	•	•	
Employment									
Annual unemployment rate				•	•	•	•	•	

	HP2020[a]	CoH[b]	AHR[c]	CHR[d]	CHSI[e]	NEA[f]	VHOI[g]	DDK[h]	AARP[i]
Social Determinants of Health									
Eligibility for Family Medical Leave Act									
Job quality								•	
Jobs per worker									•
Underemployment rate			•						
Working poor						•			
Health Systems and Services									
Access to care							•		
Access to mental health services		•							
Access to stable health insurance	•	•							
Cost barrier to care				•	•				
Hospice use				•					
Primary care physicians			•	•	•				
Primary care provider rate	•			•					
Preventable hospitalizations			•		•				
Preventable hospitalizations: Older adults			•						
Public health funding									
Unmet care need									

continued

TABLE B-1 Continued

	HP2020[a]	CoH[b]	AHR[c]	CHR[d]	CHSI[e]	NEA[f]	VHOI[g]	DDK[h]	AARP[i]
Social Determinants of Health									
Housing									
Home ownership									
Housing affordability		•							
Income spent on housing and transportation (i.e., Affordability Index)								•	
Renters									
Income and Wealth									
Children in poverty			•	•					
Gross domestic product (GDP) gains with racial equity						•			
Income disparity/inequality			•	•		•	•	•	
Income disparity ratio			•						
Income gains with racial equity						•			
Income growth						•			
Job and GDP growth						•			
Job and wage growth						•			
Median household income					•				
Median wage						•			
Minimum wage								•	

	HP2020[a]	CoH[b]	AHR[c]	CHR[d]	CHSI[e]	NEA[f]	VHOI[g]	DDK[h]	AARP[i]
Social Determinants of Health									
Per capita personal income			•						
Poverty								•	
Wages $15/hour						•			
Physical Environment									
Access to healthy food			•		•		•		•
Access to jobs via auto						•			•
Access to jobs via transit									•
Access to libraries		•							•
Access to parks		•			•	•			•
Air pollution	•		•	•	•		•		
Children exposed to secondhand smoke	•								
Housing accessibility									•
Housing burden						•			
Housing costs									•
Housing options									•
Housing stress					•				
Liquor-store density			•						
Living near highways					•				

continued

TABLE B-1 Continued

Social Determinants of Health	HP2020[a]	CoH[b]	AHR[c]	CHR[d]	CHSI[e]	NEA[f]	VHOI[g]	DDK[h]	AARP[i]
Neighborhood: Activity density									•
Neighborhood: Mixed use									•
Neighborhood: Poverty						•			•
Neighborhood: Vacancy rate									
Population churning/turnover							•		
Population density						•	•		•
Population growth rates							•		
Walkability									
Public Safety									
Crime rate									
Homicides	•								
Violent crime				•	•				
Youth safety		•							
Social Environment									
Disconnected youth						•			
Home language								•	
Inadequate social support				•	•				
Linguistic isolation								•	

	HP2020[a]	CoH[b]	AHR[c]	CHR[d]	CHSI[e]	NEA[f]	VHOI[g]	DDK[h]	AARP[i]
Social Determinants of Health									
Residential segregation		•							
Single-parent households				•					
Transportation									
Car/vehicle access						•	•		
Commute time						•			
Safe and convenient options									•
Making Health Equity a Shared Vision and Value									
Community diversity/Diversity index						•	•		
Distances between communities with different racial or ethnic profiles							•		
Public school racial/ethnic composition								•	
Racial generation gap						•			
Increasing Community Capacity to Shape Outcomes									
Sense of community		•							
Social support		•							

continued

TABLE B-1 Continued

	HP2020[a]	CoH[b]	AHR[c]	CHR[d]	CHSI[e]	NEA[f]	VHOI[g]	DDK[h]	AARP[i]
Increasing Community Capacity to Shape Outcomes									
Volunteer engagement		●							●
Voter participation		●							●
Fostering Multi-Sector Collaboration									
Business support for workplace health promotion and culture of health	●								
Climate adaptation and mitigation	●								
Community relations and policing	●								
Health in all policies	●								
Local health department collaboration	●								
Opportunities to improve health for youth at schools	●								
Youth exposure to advertising for health and unhealthy food and beverage products	●								
Healthier More Equitable Communities in Which Members and Families Live, Learn, Work, and Play									
Caregiving									
Caregiving burden		●							

526

	HP2020[a]	CoH[b]	AHR[c]	CHR[d]	CHSI[e]	NEA[f]	VHOI[g]	DDK[h]	AARP[i]
Healthier More Equitable Communities in Which Members and Families Live, Learn, Work, and Play									
Consumer/Patient Satisfaction									
Consumer experience		●							
Patient–clinician communication satisfaction		●							
Costs									
Annual end-of-life care expenditures		●							
Family health care cost		●							
Potentially preventable hospitalization rates		●							
Social spending relative to health expenditure		●							
Health Status: Self-rated									
Poor physical health days			●	●					
Self-rated overall health status			●	●	●				
Unhealthy days					●				
Well-being rating		●							

continued

TABLE B-1 Continued

Healthier More Equitable Communities in Which Members and Families Live, Learn, Work, and Play	HP2020[a]	CoH[b]	AHR[c]	CHR[d]	CHSI[e]	NEA[f]	VHOI[g]	DDK[h]	AARP[i]
Injury and Violence									
Fatal injuries	•		•						
Motor vehicle crash deaths				•	•				
Occupational fatalities			•						
Unintentional injury (including motor vehicle)					•				
Maternal, Infant, and Child Health									
Adolescent health issues								•	
Adverse child experiences (ACEs)		•							
Birth rate								•	
Infant mortality	•		•						
Low birth weight			•	•					
Teen birth rates			•	•	•				
Total preterm live births	•				•				
Mental Health									
Depression: Adolescents	•								
Depression: Older adults					•				

	HP2020[a]	CoH[b]	AHR[c]	CHR[d]	CHSI[e]	NEA[f]	VHOI[g]	DDK[h]	AARP[i]
Healthier More Equitable Communities in Which Members and Families Live, Learn, Work, and Play									
Poor mental health days	•								
Suicides	•		•						
Morbidity									
Alzheimer's diseases/dementia						•			
Asthma					•	•			
Cancer									
Diabetes			•		•	•			
Diabetes: Adult					•				
Disability associated with chronic conditions		•							
Heart attack			•						
Heart disease			•						
High blood pressure			•						
High cholesterol			•						

continued

TABLE B-1 Continued

	HP2020[a]	CoH[b]	AHR[c]	CHR[d]	CHSI[e]	NEA[f]	VHOI[g]	DDK[h]	AARP[i]
Healthier More Equitable Communities in Which Members and Families Live, Learn, Work, and Play									
Infectious disease			•						
Stroke			•						
Mortality									
Deaths: All causes			•		•				
Deaths: Alzheimer's disease					•				
Deaths: Cancer			•		•				
Deaths: Cardiovascular disease			•						
Deaths: Chronic kidney disease					•				
Deaths: Chronic lower respiratory disease					•				
Deaths: Coronary heart disease					•				
Deaths: Diabetes			•		•				
Deaths: Premature				•					
Deaths: Stroke					•				
Life expectancy						•			

	HP2020[a]	CoH[b]	AHR[c]	CHR[d]	CHSI[e]	NEA[f]	VHOI[g]	DDK[h]	AARP[i]
Healthier More Equitable Communities in Which Members and Families Live, Learn, Work, and Play									
Nutrition, Physical Activity, and Obesity									
Adult obesity	●		●						
Body mass index						●			
Child and adolescent obesity	●		●						
Fruit consumption			●						
Physical activity			●	●					
Physical inactivity	●		●						
Vegetable consumption	●		●						
Oral Health									
Annual dental visit	●								
Dental care		●							
Teeth extractions			●						
Reproductive and Sexual Health									
Adult female routine Pap test					●				

continued

TABLE B-1 Continued

	HP2020[a]	CoH[b]	AHR[c]	CHR[d]	CHSI[e]	NEA[f]	VHOI[g]	DDK[h]	AARP[i]
Healthier More Equitable Communities in Which Members and Families Live, Learn, Work, and Play									
Chlamydia screening			•						
Gonorrhea				•					
HIV					•				
Knowledge of serostatus among HIV-positive persons	•				•				
Sexually active females ages 15 to 44 years who received reproductive health services in the past 12 months	•								
Syphilis					•				
Sleep									
Insufficient sleep			•						
Substance Abuse									
Addiction death rate						•			
Adolescents using alcohol or any illicit drugs during the past 30 days	•		•	•	•				
Binge drinking	•			•					

	HP2020[a]	CoH[b]	AHR[c]	CHR[d]	CHSI[e]	NEA[f]	VHOI[g]	DDK[h]	AARP[i]
Healthier More Equitable Communities in Which Members and Families Live, Learn, Work, and Play									
Chronic drinking			•						
Drug deaths			•	•					
Excessive drinking				•					
Tobacco Use									
Adolescent smoking		•		•					
Adult smoking		•		•					

[a] Healthy People 2020, https://www.healthypeople.gov/2020/leading-health-indicators/2020-lhi-topics (accessed December 22, 2016).
[b] Culture of Health Metrics, http://hero-health.org/wp-content/uploads/2016/04/HERO-Final-Report-Developing-Culture-of-Health-Metrics-That-Really-Matter-to-Companies-and-Communities.pdf (accessed December 22, 2016).
[c] America's Health Rankings, http://www.americashealthrankings.org (accessed December 22, 2016).
[d] County Health Rankings, http://www.countyhealthrankings.org/our-approach (accessed December 22, 2016).
[e] Community Health Status Indicators, http://wwwn.cdc.gov/CommunityHealth/info/AboutProject (accessed December 22, 2016).
[f] National Equity Atlas, http://nationalequityatlas.org (accessed December 22, 2016).
[g] Virginia Health Opportunity Index, https://www.vdh.virginia.gov/OMHHE/policyanalysis/virginiahoi.htm (accessed December 22, 2016).
[h] Diversity Data Kids Data Set, http://www.diversitydatakids.org (accessed December 22, 2016).
[i] AARP Livability Index, https://livabilityindex.aarp.org/categories/neighborhood (accessed December 22, 2016).

TABLE B-2 Interactive Tools for Examining Health Equity Indicators by Geographical Region

Name/How to Access	Components
AARP Livability Index https://livabilityindex. aarp.org/categories/ neighborhood (accessed December 22, 2016). City, zip code, address	*Housing* (affordability and access), *Neighborhood* (access to life, work, and play), *Transportation* (safe and convenient options); *Environment* (clean air and water); *Health* (prevention, access, quality); *Engagement* (civil and social involvement); *Opportunity* (inclusion and possibilities)
Children's Health and Education Mapping Tool http://www.sbh4all.org/ resources/mapping-tool (accessed December 22, 2016).	*Health Insurance and Coverage* (under 18 percent on Medicaid or CHIP, under 18 percent uninsured), *Health* (teen birth rate, percent adult obesity, percent food insecure, chlamydia rate), *Education* (percent adults over 25 without high school diploma), *Demographic and Socioeconomic Indicators* (percent free lunch, percent kids in poverty, percent kids in single-parent households, percent households with severe housing problems, violent crime rate)
	School and School-Based Health Center (SBHC) Characteristics (Title I eligibility, lowest grade offered, highest grade offered, total school enrollment, free and reduced lunch eligibility; SBHC location, sponsor, staffing models [primary care only, primary care and mental health, primary care and mental health plus], hours of operation, populations served)
Community Health Status Indicators http://wwwn.cdc.gov/ CommunityHealth/info/ AboutProject (accessed December 22, 2016). County level	*Physical* (access to parks, annual average particulate matter concentration, housing stress, limited access to healthy food, living near highways), *Social Factors* (children in single-parent households, high housing costs, inadequate social support, on-time high school graduation, poverty, unemployment, violent crime), *Health Behaviors* (adult binge drinking, adult female routine pap tests, adult physical inactivity, adult smoking, teen births), *Health Care Access and Quality* (cost barrier to care, older adult preventable hospitalizations, primary care provider access, uninsured), *Morbidity* (adult diabetes, adult obesity, adult overall health status, Alzheimer's disease/dementia, cancer, gonorrhea, HIV, older adult asthma, older adult depression, preterm births, syphilis), *Mortality* (Alzheimer's disease deaths, cancer deaths, chronic kidney disease deaths, chronic lower respiratory disease deaths, coronary heart disease deaths, diabetes deaths, female life expectancy, male life expectancy, motor vehicle deaths, stroke deaths, unintentional injury, including motor vehicle)

TABLE B-2 Continued

Name/How to Access	Components
Diversity Data Kids dataset http://www.diversitydatakids.org (accessed December 22, 2016).	Rankings and child opportunities by race and ethnicity by states, counties, large cities, large school districts including *Population Demographics and Diversity* (population and racial/ethnic composition), *Household Composition and Family Structure* (home language and linguistic isolation); *Early Childhood Care and Education* (Head Start); *Education* (public school enrollment and racial/ethnic composition, student achievement [Grade 4 reading, Grade 8 reading, Grade 4 math, Grade 8 math, graduation rates]); *Health* (infant mortality, natality, adolescent health issues); *Parental Employment* (employment and labor force participation, employment characteristics, job quality, eligibility for Family Medical Leave Act [FMLA]); *Policy* (Head Start, FMLA); *Income and Poverty* (minimum wage, child poverty, parental poverty)
EJSCREEN: Environmental Justice Screening and Mapping Tool https://www.epa.gov/ejscreen (accessed December 22, 2016).	*Environmental Indexes* (National-Scale Air Toxics Assessment [NATA] Air Toxics Cancer Risk, NATA Respiratory Hazard Index, NATA Diesel Particulate Matter, particulate matter 2.5, ozone, traffic proximity and volume; lead paint, proximity to risk management plan sites, proximity to treatment, storage, and disposal facilities, proximity to National Priorities List sites, proximity to major direct water dischargers; *Demographic Indexes* (Demographic Index [average of percent low-income and percent minority] and Supplemental Demographic Index [average of percent low-income, percent minority, percent less than high school education, percent linguistic isolation, percent under 5, percent over 64])
Food Access Research Atlas http://www.ers.usda.gov/data-products/food-access-research-atlas.aspx (accessed December 22, 2016).	*General Census Tract Characteristics* (population, low-income tract, urban/rural status, housing units), *Low-Access and Distance Measures* (1 and 10 mile access), *Low-Income and Low-Access* (0.5, 1, 10, 20, or more mile access), *Vehicle Availability* (no vehicle and 0.5, 1, 10, 20, or more mile access), *Group Quarters* (census tract with 67 percent or more living in group quarters), *Low Access by Population Subgroups* (measures above by seniors and children)
Health Equity Index Connecticut	*Community-Specific Scores on Seven Social Determinants of Health* (civic involvement, community safety, economic security, education, employment, environmental quality, housing) *and 13 Health Outcomes* (accidents/violence, cancer, cardiovascular, childhood illness, diabetes, health care access, infectious disease, life expectancy, liver disease, mental health, perinatal care, renal disease, respiratory illness)

continued

TABLE B-2 Continued

Name/How to Access	Components
JustSouth Index http://www.loyno.edu/jsri/news/inaugural-justsouth-index-2016 (accessed December 22, 2016)	*Demographics*, nine social justice indicators in three categories: *Poverty* (average income per household, health insurance coverage for the poor white-minority, housing affordability white-minority), *Racial Disparity* (public school segregation, wage equity, employment equity); *Immigrant Exclusion* (immigrant youth outcomes, immigrant English proficiency, health insurance coverage for immigrants)
National Equity Atlas http://nationalequityatlas.org (accessed December 22, 2016).	*Demographics* (detailed race/ethnicity, people of color, race/ethnicity, population growth rates, contribution to growth: immigrants, contribution to growth: people of color, racial generation gap, diversity index, median age); *Economic Vitality* (poverty, working poor, unemployment, wages: median, wages: $15/hour, income growth, job and wage growth, job and gross domestic product growth, income inequality: Gini, income inequality: 95/20 ratio, homeownership); *Readiness* (school poverty, air pollution: exposure index, air pollution: unequal burden, education levels and job requirements, disconnected youth, overweight and obese, asthma, diabetes); *Connectedness* (neighborhood poverty, housing burden, car access, commute time); *Economic Benefits* (GDP gains with racial equity, income gains with racial equity)
Opportunity Index http://opportunityindex.org/#4.00/40.00/-97.00 (accessed December 22, 2016).	*Jobs and Local Economy* (jobs, wages, poverty, inequality, access to banking, affordable housing, Internet access); *Education* (preschool enrollment, high school graduating, postsecondary completion); and *Community Health and Civic Life* (group membership, volunteerism, youth economic and academic inclusion, community safety, access to health care, access to healthy food)
The Housing and Transportation (H+T®) Affordability Index http://www.htaindex.org (accessed December 22, 2016).	Provides a comprehensive view of affordability that includes both the cost of housing and the cost of transportation at the neighborhood level for more than 200,000 neighborhoods. *Neighborhood Characteristics* (gross density, regional household intensity, fraction of single-family detached housing, block density, Employment Access Index, Employment Mix Index, Transit Connectivity Index, transit access shed, transit access shed jobs, average available transit trips per week; *Household Characteristics* (median household income, average commuters per household, average household size), *Transit* (auto ownership, auto usage, public transit usage)

TABLE B-2 Continued

Name/How to Access	Components
Virginia Health Opportunity Index https://www.vdh.virginia.gov/OMHHE/policyanalysis/virginiahoi.htm (December 22, 2016).	Index consists of 13 indicators organized into 4 profiles: *Community Environmental* (air quality, population churning, population density, walkability); *Consumer Opportunity* (affordability, education, food accessibility, material deprivation); *Economic Opportunity* (employment accessibility, income inequality, job participation); *Wellness Disparity* (access to care, segregation [community diversity and distances between communities with different racial or ethnic profiles])

Appendix C

Public Meeting Agendas

MEETING ONE

January 6, 2016
Keck Center of the National Academies of Sciences,
Engineering, and Medicine
500 Fifth Street NW, Washington, DC

1:00–1:10 p.m.	Welcome and Opening Remarks Victor Dzau President, National Academy of Medicine
1:10–1:15 p.m.	Meeting Overview and Introductions James Weinstein Committee Chair
1:15–1:45 p.m.	Presentation of the Statement of Task and Discussion James S. Marks Executive Vice President, Robert Wood Johnson Foundation

PANEL 1

1:45–2:15 p.m.	What Shapes Health (and Health Inequities)? Steven H. Woolf Director, Virginia Commonwealth University Center on Society and Health
2:15–2:45 p.m.	State of Health Disparities in the United States: Challenges and Opportunities J. Nadine Gracia Deputy Assistant Secretary for Minority Health and the Director of the Office of Minority Health, U.S. Department of Health and Human Services
2:45–3:15 p.m.	Achieving Health Equity: Naming and Addressing the Impacts of Racism on Health Camara Jones President, American Public Health Association Senior Fellow, Satcher Health Leadership Institute and Cardiovascular Research Institute, Morehouse School of Medicine
3:15–3:35 p.m.	Discussion with Panel 1 Speakers
3:35–3:45 p.m.	BREAK

PANEL 2

3:45–4:10 p.m.	Countering the Production of Inequities to Achieve Health Equity: A Systems Approach Rachel Davis Managing Director, Prevention Institute
4:10–4:35 p.m.	The Politics of Health Inequity: Getting to the Roots Richard Hofrichter Senior Director, Health Equity, National Association of County and City Health Officials

APPENDIX C 541

4:35–5:00 p.m.	Advancing Health Equity and Optimal Health for All Edward Ehlinger President, Association of State and Territorial Health Officials Commissioner, Minnesota Department of Health
5:00–5:20 p.m.	Discussion with Panel 2 Speakers
5:20–5:30 p.m.	Public Comment
5:30 p.m.	Adjourn

MEETING TWO

March 7, 2016
National Academy of Sciences Building
2101 Constitution Avenue, NW, Washington, DC

8:30–9:00 a.m.	Arrival and Registration (coffee and tea will be provided)
9:00–9:05 a.m.	Welcoming Remarks James Weinstein Committee Chair
9:05–10:15 a.m.	Cuyahoga County Community Health Improvement Plan Presentation and Q&A Martha Halko Deputy Director, Prevention and Wellness, Cuyahoga County Board of Health Gregory Brown Executive Director, PolicyBridge President, Brown & Associates Consulting Services
10:15–10:30 a.m.	BREAK

10:30–11:00 a.m.	Planning and Health Anna Ricklin Manager, Planning and Community Health Center, American Planning Association
11:00–11:30 a.m.	Transportation and Health Sam Zimbabwe Associate Director, Policy, Planning & Sustainability Administration, District Department of Transportation
11:30 a.m.–12:00 p.m.	Q&A
12:00–12:45 p.m.	LUNCH
12:45–1:15 p.m.	Environmental Justice and Health Robert Bullard Dean, School of Public Affairs Texas Southern University
1:15–1:45 p.m.	Civil Rights Law and Health Marianne Engelman Lado Senior Staff Attorney, EarthJustice
1:45–2:15 p.m.	Q&A
2:15–2:45 p.m.	Overview of Health Disparities Tom LaVeist Chair, Professor, Health Policy and Management Department, George Washington University, Milken Institute of Public Health
2:45–3:05 p.m.	Q&A
3:05–3:35 p.m.	Building Community Wealth and Anchor Institutions David Zuckerman Manager, Healthcare Engagement, Anchor Institution Initiative, Democracy Collaborative
3:35–3:55 p.m.	Q&A

APPENDIX C

3:55–4:20 p.m.	Private Sector and Health
	Michelle Chuk Zamperetti
	Manager, Community Health Programs
	Healthymagination, GE

4:20–4:45 p.m.	Katie Loovis
	Director, Corporate Responsibility
	Communications and Government Affairs
	GlaxoSmithKline

4:45–5:05 p.m.	Q&A

5:05–5:30 p.m.	Public Comment

MEETING THREE

April 27, 2016
Arnold and Mabel Beckman Center
National Academies of Sciences, Engineering, and Medicine
100 Academy Drive, Irvine, CA

9:30–10:00 a.m.	Arrival and Registration

10:00–10:10 a.m.	Welcoming Remarks
	James Weinstein
	Committee Chair

PANEL 1

10:10–10:40 a.m.	Faith-Based Community Organizing for Health Equity
	Doran Schrantz
	Executive Director, ISAIAH

10:40–11:10 a.m.	Community-Based Participatory Research and Health Equity
	Nina Wallerstein
	Director, Center for Participatory Research
	University of New Mexico, Health Sciences Center

11:10–11:40 a.m.	Q&A

11:40 a.m.–12:30 p.m.   LUNCH

                          PANEL 2
12:30–1:00 p.m.   Place Based Factors and Policy at the
                              Community Level
                          Manal Aboelata
                          Managing Director, Prevention Institute

1:00–1:30 p.m.   Building Healthy Communities
                          Beatriz Solís
                          Director, Healthy Communities, South Region
                              The California Endowment

1:30–2:00 p.m.   Q&A

2:00–2:15 p.m.   BREAK

2:15–2:50 p.m.   Economics and Community Development
                          David Erickson
                          Director, Center for Community Development
                              Investments
                          Federal Reserve Bank of San Francisco

2:50–3:15 p.m.   Q&A

3:15–3:30 p.m.   Public Comment

Appendix D

Committee Biographical Sketches

James N. Weinstein, D.O., M.S. (*Chair*), is the chief executive officer and president of Dartmouth-Hitchcock and is also the Peggy Y. Thomson Professor in the Evaluative Clinical Sciences at Darmouth-Hitchcock Medical Center. He leads a health system that includes New Hampshire's only academic medical center and a network of clinics across two states, serving a patient population of 1.4 million. Dr. Weinstein also chairs the executive committee of the High Value Healthcare Collaborative, which he founded along with leaders of Denver Health, Intermountain Healthcare, and Mayo Clinic. Prior to being named as Dartmouth-Hitchcock's first system-wide chief executive officer in 2011, Dr. Weinstein served as the president of Dartmouth-Hitchcock Clinic and the director of the Dartmouth Institute for Health Policy and Clinical Practice (TDI), home of the Dartmouth Atlas. He is also the founding chairman of the Departments of Orthopedics at Dartmouth-Hitchcock and Dartmouth Medical School (now the Geisel School of Medicine), and the co-founder of the Dartmouth Center for Health Care Delivery Science, a collaborative effort between the Tuck School of Business and TDI. He is a principal investigator for the 13-center, 11-state National Institutes of Health (NIH)-funded SPORT (Spine Patient Outcomes Research Trial) study, in its 15th year of funding, the first large-scale trial to look at the effectiveness of the three most common surgical procedures for back pain, as compared to non-operative treatment. As a leader in advancing "informed choice" to ensure that patients receive evidence-based, safe, effective, efficient, and appropriate care, he established the first-in-the-nation Center for

Shared Decision-Making at Dartmouth-Hitchcock in 1999, where patient preferences and values are an integral part of diagnostic and treatment decisions.

Dr. Weinsten has a D.O. in osteopathic medicine from the Chicago College of Osteopathic Medicine (1977) and an M.S. in health services research from Dartmouth Medical School (1995). An internationally renowned spine surgeon, he is known as one of the foremost experts on spine tumors and developed the first-ever spine tumor classification system, which continues to be used around the world. In 1998 Dr. Weinstein founded the multidisciplinary spine center at Dartmouth-Hitchcock, which has become an international model for patient-centered health care delivery, incorporating shared decision making and patient self-reported outcomes into clinical practice. He is the winner of the Wiltse Lifetime Achievement Award from the International Society for the Study of the Lumbar Spine. He is the editor in chief of the journal *Spine* and author of more than 290 papers and articles, including the *Musculoskeletal Dartmouth Atlas of Health Care*. He is a member of the National Academy of Medicine (2011) and currently serves on the National Academies of Sciences, Engineering, and Medicine's Board on Population Health and Public Health Practice.

Hortensia de los Angeles Amaro, Ph.D., is Dean's Professor of Social Work and Preventive Medicine and the associate vice provost of community research initiatives at the University of Southern California (USC). She has dramatically advanced the understanding of substance abuse disorder treatment, HIV prevention, and other urgent public health challenges through a distinguished career that has spanned scholarly research, translation of science to practice, top-level policy consultation, and service on four Institute of Medicine committees. Before joining USC in 2012, Dr. Amaro was with Northeastern University for 10 years, serving as an associate dean and a distinguished professor of health sciences and counseling psychology of the Bouvé College of Health Sciences and also as the founder and director of the university's Institute on Urban Health Research. For 18 years before that, she was a professor in the Boston University School of Public Health and in the Department of Pediatrics at the Boston University School of Medicine. Dr. Amaro received her doctorate in psychology from the University of California, Los Angeles, in 1982 and was awarded honorary doctoral degrees in humane letters by Simmons College in 1994 and the Massachusetts School of Professional Psychology in 2012. She has received numerous awards, most recently the American Public Health Association's Elizabeth Beckman Professors Who Inspire Award (2014) and the Sedgwick Memorial Medal for Public Health

Service (2015). She has authored more than 140 scholarly publications, many of them widely cited, and she has made landmark contributions to improving behavioral health care in community-based organizations by launching addiction treatment programs that have helped thousands of families and by informing practice in agencies around the world. Dr. Amaro is a member of the National Academy of Medicine (2010) and currently serves on the Board on Population Health and Public Health Practice; the Standing Committee on Integrating New Behavioral Health Measures in the Substance Abuse and Mental Health Services Administration's Data Collection Programs; and the Workshop Steering Committee on Integrating New Measures of Trauma and Recovery (chair) into the Substance Abuse and Mental Health Services Administration's Data Collection Programs.

Elizabeth Baca, M.D., M.P.A., is passionate about innovations to foster total health and well-being. She currently serves as the senior health advisor in the State of California Governor's Office of Planning and Research (OPR). She is engaged in innovation in the public sector to foster health through multiple projects, including healthy planning, big data, and public–private partnerships. For healthy planning she works across sectors to foster collaboration and elevate the connection between health and the built environment, and she leads the effort to incorporate health considerations into the planning process to build healthy, resilient communities. A significant part of her work is aligning win-wins for projects that offer co-benefits, particularly with respect to climate mitigation and adaptation efforts. For big data, she is working on projects to link data sets to the planning process. Additionally, she serves as a lead for the Governor's Initiative to Advance Precision Medicine. Through her role in OPR, she is an advisor for the U.S. Green Building Council's Building Health Initiative and FS6, a new Food System Accelerator.

Previously, she served on the general pediatric faculty at Stanford Medical School and directed the community pediatric and child advocacy rotation. In addition to teaching medical students and residents about the social, economic, and environmental factors that affect health, Dr. Baca was the lead faculty mentor on several projects to increase access to healthy foods, reduce environmental triggers of asthma, increase physical activity opportunities, and improve the built environment.

Dr. Baca studied health policy at Universidad Simon Bolivar in Venezuela. She completed her master's in public administration at the Harvard Kennedy School of Government and her doctorate of medicine at Harvard Medical School. Dr. Baca completed her pediatric residency in the Pediatric Leadership for the Underserved (PLUS) program at the University of California, San Francisco.

B. Ned Calonge, M.D., M.P.H., is the president and chief executive officer of The Colorado Trust, a private grant-making foundation dedicated to achieving health equity for all Coloradans. Dr. Calonge is an associate professor of family medicine at the Colorado School of Medicine at the University of Colorado, Denver, and an associate professor of epidemiology at the Colorado School of Public Health. Nationally, he chairs the Evaluating Genomic Applications for Practice and Prevention (EGAPP) Working Group of the U.S. Centers for Disease Control and Prevention (CDC); chairs the Agency for Healthcare Research and Quality's Electronic Data Methods Forum Advisory Committee; and is a member of the CDC's Task Force on Community Preventive Services and of the CDC's Breast and Cervical Cancer Early Detection and Control Advisory Committee. Dr. Calonge received his B.A. in chemistry from The Colorado College, his M.D. from the University of Colorado, and his M.P.H. from the University of Washington, where he also completed his preventive medicine residency. He completed his family medicine residency at the Oregon Health and Science University. He is a past chair of the U.S. Preventive Services Task Force and is a past member of the Secretary's Advisory Committee on Heritable Disorders in Newborns and Children. Prior to coming to The Trust, Dr. Calonge was the chief medical officer of the Colorado Department of Public Health and Environment. He is a National Academy of Medicine member (elected in 2011). Dr. Calonge serves on the National Academies of Sciences, Engineering, and Medicine's Board on Population Health and Public Health Practice as well as on the Roundtable on the Promotion of Health Equity and the Elimination of Health Disparities.

Bechara Choucair, M.D., M.S., is the senior vice president of Community Health and Benefit, and chief community health officer for Kaiser Permanente. Prior to his role at Kaiser, Dr. Choucair was senior vice president of safety net transformation and community health at Trinity Health. Dr. Choucair was responsible for working directly with Trinity Health Regional Health Ministries to improve the health of populations and affect the community-based social determinants of health. He was responsible for the development of new care delivery models and new relationships with payers, public health agencies, and community organizations. He and his team were also responsible for leading community benefits throughout the ministry. For 5 years prior to joining Trinity Health, Dr. Choucair was the commissioner of the Chicago Department of Public Health (CDPH). There he and his team launched Healthy Chicago, the city's first comprehensive public health agenda. Since its launch, CDPH has reported historic lows in childhood obesity rates and both teen and adult smoking rates, as well as significant increases in overall life expectancy. Under his leadership, CDPH became the first big city public health agency to be awarded national accreditation. Prior to his appointment as CDPH commissioner, he served as the executive director of Heartland Health Centers in Chicago and as the medical director of Crusader Community Health in Rockford, Illinois. Dr. Choucair serves on numerous boards and has a faculty appointment at the Feinberg School of Medicine, Northwestern University. Dr. Choucair, a family physician by training, holds an M.D. from the American University of Beirut and a master's degree in health care management from The University of Texas at Dallas. In addition to earning a number of local and national awards, he was named one of Chicago's 40 under 40 by Crain's Chicago Business in 2012.

Alison Evans Cuellar, Ph.D., M.B.A., is an associate professor of health administration and policy at George Mason University and has extensive research experience in health care systems, Medicaid, mental health, and justice-involved populations. Her contributions include work on identifying and evaluating new organizational forms, such as hospital systems and physician alliances, and their effects on quality, efficiency, costs, prices, and technology adoption. In work supported by the National Institute of Mental Health, she has examined the intersection of behavioral health and the juvenile justice systems; Medicaid policies and their impact on justice-involved youth and youth with behavioral health problems; mental health courts as an innovative alternative for juvenile delinquents; and health care services for incarcerated youth and adults returning to the community. She was a member of a national collaborative Mental Health Policy network supported by the MacArthur Foundation. She also was co-investigator on a pediatric health needs assessment in Washington, DC, with a special focus on vulnerable and minority populations. In addition, she spent the 2005–2006 academic year as a visiting economist to the U.S. Department of Justice. She is co-editor of the Economic Grand Rounds column in the journal *Psychiatric Services*. Her work has been published in several journals, including *Journal of Policy Analysis and Management, Journal of Health Economics, American Journal of Public Health, Health Affairs, Archives of Pediatric and Adolescent Medicine,* and *American Journal of Psychiatry and Psychiatric Services,* among others. Previously, Dr. Cuellar was an assistant professor in the Department of Health Policy and Management at Columbia University.

Robert H. Dugger, Ph.D., is a co-founder of ReadyNation and the chairman of its advisory board. ReadyNation is the preeminent business leader organization working to strengthen business through better policies for children and youth. Dr. Dugger's main interest is early child development and organizing strong business coalitions in states to support high-return investment spending in children, prenatal to 5 years old.

Dr. Dugger began his career at the Federal Reserve Board in 1972, and in the 1980s he served on the staffs of the House and Senate banking committees and with the American Bankers Association. From 1992 to 2008 he was a partner in Tudor Investment Corporation. Together with Dr. James Heckman, the University of Chicago professor and Nobel Prize winner, and Dr. Steven Durlauf of the University of Wisconsin–Madison, Dr. Dugger heads the Global Working Group on Human Capital and Economic Opportunity at the Becker-Friedman Institute at the University of Chicago. Dr. Dugger is also the former board chairman of Singita-Grumeti Reserves, a Tanzanian wildlife conservation and tourism project regularly ranked number one in the world. Dr. Dugger received his Ph.D. in economics from the University of North Carolina at Chapel Hill on a Federal Reserve Dissertation Fellowship. He has received numerous awards and recognitions, including the McCormick Foundation's Center for Early Childhood Leadership's Corporate Champion for Change award in 2014, ZERO TO THREE's Reiner Award for Outstanding Advocacy on Behalf of Very Young Children in 2013, the Committee for Economic Development's Trustee Leadership Award in 2008, and, most recently, ReadyNation's 2015 Business Leader Champion for Children award.

Chandra Ford, Ph.D., M.P.H., M.S., is an associate professor in the Department of Community Health Sciences at the University of California, Los Angeles. Her areas of expertise include HIV/AIDS prevention and care; HIV testing among older adults; the social determinants of health/social epidemiology; conceptualizing and measuring racism, race, and ethnicity; public health critical race praxis (PHCRP)/critical race theory; and lesbian, gay, bisexual, and transgender (LGBT) health disparities. Dr. Ford earned her Ph.D. from the Gillings School of Public Health at the University of North Carolina and received her M.P.H. and M.L.I.S. from the University of Pittsburgh. She completed postdoctoral fellowships in the Department of Social Medicine at the University of North Carolina and the Department of Epidemiology at Columbia University, where she was a W.K. Kellogg Foundation Kellogg Health Scholar. Dr. Ford has received several competitive awards. She currently is a Kaiser Permanente Chris Burch Leadership Awardee.

Robert García, J.D., is a civil rights and human rights advocate who engages, educates, and empowers communities to fight for equal justice, human dignity, and equal access to public resources. He is the founding director and counsel of The City Project, a nonprofit legal and policy advocacy team in Los Angeles, California. He is an assistant professor at Charles Drew University of Medicine and Science. The City Project works with diverse allies on equal access to (1) healthy green land use through community planning, (2) climate justice, (3) quality education, including physical education, (4) health equity, and (5) economic vitality for all, including creating jobs and avoiding displacement. Mr. García has extensive experience in legal advocacy, public policy, mediation, and litigation involving complex social justice, civil rights, human health, environmental, education, and criminal justice matters. He has influenced the investment of more than $43 billion in underserved communities, working at the intersection of equal justice, public health, and the built environment. Previously he served as the chairman of the Citizens' School Bond Oversight Committee for 5 years, helping raise more than $27 billion to build new and modernize existing public schools as centers of their communities in Los Angeles. Mr. García served as an assistant United States attorney for the Southern District of New York and an attorney with the NAACP Legal Defense and Education Fund. Mr. García graduated from Stanford University and Stanford Law School, where he served on the board of editors of the *Stanford Law Review*. He received the President's Award from the California Attorneys for Criminal Justice for helping release Geronimo Pratt, the former Black Panther leader, from prison after 27 years for a crime he did not commit. He represented people on death row in Florida, Georgia, and Mississippi. Stanford Law School called him a "civil rights giant" and Stanford Magazine "an inspiration." Mr. García received the President's Award from the American Public Health Association. *Hispanic Business* magazine named him as one of the 100 most influential Latinos in the United States, and *PODER* magazine one of the Top 100 Latino Green Leaders. Green 2.0 celebrates his work as a leader of color in the environmental field. He serves on the boards of NEEF (National Environmental & Education Foundation), a nonprofit chartered by Congress; National Recreation and Parks Association (NRPA); and GreenLatinos. Mr. García is an immigrant who came to the United States with his family from Guatemala when he was 4.

Helene D. Gayle, M.D., M.P.H., is the chief executive officer of the McKinsey Social Initiative. She was formerly the president and chief executive officer of CARE USA. She also has served as the director of the Bill & Melinda Gates Foundation's HIV, TB, and Reproductive Health Program and directed HIV, STD, and TB prevention activities at the U.S. Centers for Disease Control and Prevention (CDC). During her nearly two decades at the CDC, Dr. Gayle also studied malnutrition in children in the United States and internationally, evaluated and implemented child survival programs in Africa, and worked on HIV/AIDS research, programs, and policy. Dr. Gayle received her M.D. from the University of Pennsylvania and a master's in public health from Johns Hopkins University. She has published numerous articles on public health and has received many awards for her scientific and public health contributions. She is a National Academy of Medicine member (1998) and has served on the Council of the National Academy of Medicine; the Committee on the U.S. Commitment to Global Health; and the Keck Futures Initiative Genomics Steering Committee.

Andrew Grant-Thomas, Ph.D., is the co-director at EmbraceRace, an online community of parents, grandparents, aunts and uncles, teachers and guidance counselors, day care providers, young people, and caring adults. He is also a race and social justice consultant, currently serving or having served in that capacity with the Haas Institute, the Democracy Fund, Open Society Foundations, Kellogg Foundation, Tufts Public Health Programs, and the Fetzer Institute, among others. Previously he was the director of programs at the Proteus Fund, a national foundation committed to advancing justice through democracy, human rights, and peace. At Proteus, Dr. Grant-Thomas worked on issues that include race and redistricting; money in politics; civil liberties, human rights, and national security policy; death penalty abolition; and social equity in philanthropy. Dr. Grant-Thomas was previously the deputy director of the Kirwan Institute for the Study of Race and Ethnicity at the Ohio State University, where he oversaw much of the institute's U.S.-based and global justice programming, directed its biannual Transforming Race conference, and served as the editor in chief of its journal, *Race/Ethnicity: Multidisciplinary Global Contexts*. Dr. Grant-Thomas came to Kirwan Institute from the Civil Rights Project at Harvard University, where he oversaw preparations for the 2003 Color Lines Conference and managed a range of policy-oriented racial justice projects. He earned his bachelor's in literature from Yale University, his master's in international relations from the University of Chicago, and his Ph.D. in political science from the University of Chicago.

Sister Carol Keehan, R.N., M.S., is the ninth president and chief executive officer of the Catholic Health Association of the United States (CHA). She assumed her duties in October 2005. She is responsible for all association operations and leads CHA's staff at offices in Washington, DC, where she is based, and in St. Louis. Sr. Carol worked in administrative and governance positions at hospitals sponsored by the Daughters of Charity for more than 35 years. Prior to joining CHA, she was the board chair of Ascension Health's Sacred Heart Health System in Pensacola, Florida. Previously, she served for 15 years as president and chief executive officer of Providence Hospital, which includes the Carroll Manor Nursing and Rehabilitation Center in Washington, DC. Currently Sr. Carol serves on the boards of St. John's University, Queens, New York, and Georgetown

University, Washington, DC. She has served on the boards of the District of Columbia Hospital Association, of which she is a past chair; Care First/Blue Cross of Maryland and the National Capital Area, Owings Mills, Maryland; and its affiliate, Group Hospitalization and Medical Services, Inc. In addition, she previously served on the nominating committee of the American Hospital Association and the finance committee of the Maryland Hospital Association and is a past chair of the Florida State Human Rights Advocacy Commission. Sr. Carol earned a B.S. in nursing from St. Joseph's College, Emmitsburg, Maryland, where she graduated magna cum laude, and an M.B.A. from the University of South Carolina, from which she received the School of Business Distinguished Alumna Award in 2000 and was honored in 2009 as "an outstanding alumna who has served others in a manner that goes beyond what is required by the individual's job or profession." She is the recipient of numerous awards and honors, including the American Hospital Association's Trustee Award; the Pro Ecclesia et Pontifice (Cross for the Church and Pontiff), bestowed by Pope Benedict XVI; the American Cardinals' Encouragement Award; and the Medal of Honor and the Monsignor George C. Higgins Labor Advocacy Award from the Archdiocese of Washington. Sr. Carol was named in 2010 one of *Time* magazine's 100 Most Influential People in the World and has been on Modern Healthcare's list of 100 Most Influential People in Healthcare several years, having topped the list as number one in 2007. Sr. Carol received honorary doctorates from Niagara University, New York.; the College of the Holy Cross, Worcester, Massachusetts; St. John's University, Queens, New York; The Catholic University of America, Washington, DC; Marymount University, Arlington, Virginia; and DePaul University, Chicago. Sr. Carol is a National Academy of Medicine member.

Christopher J. Lyons, Ph.D., an associate professor of sociology at the University of New Mexico (UNM), studies violence and social control as a window into the sources and consequences of social inequality. His research has developed around two principal areas: (1) race/ethnicity and socio-legal control, and (2) the spatial distribution of violence across communities. Work within these two areas explores themes relevant to urban and political sociology, stratification, and intergroup relations. He has sought to advance theoretical and empirical inquiries into the social construction and etiology of hate crime and racially motivated crime, race/ethnicity and crime clearance, the stratification consequences of incarceration and criminal justice intervention, perceptions of racial discrimination, the political foundations of neighborhood inequality and violence, and domestic violence. Along with colleagues Maria Velez (UNM) and Laurie Krivo (Rutgers), he is currently working on a National Science Foundation–funded project to collect a second wave of the National

Neighborhoods and Crime Study (NNCS-2) which will provide unique two-panel crime and demographic data for neighborhoods across 91 large cities in the United States.

Kent McGuire, Ph.D., is the president and chief executive officer of the Southern Education Foundation (SEF). Dr. McGuire is responsible for SEF's mission to advance equity and excellence in education in the American South. Prior to joining SEF, Dr. McGuire served as the dean of the College of Education at Temple University and was a tenured professor in the Department of Educational Leadership and Policy Studies. Previously, Dr. McGuire was a senior vice president at MDRC, Inc. Before that he served in the Clinton administration as an assistant secretary of the U.S. Department of Education. His previous nonprofit work included being the education program officer for the Philadelphia-based Pew Charitable Trusts and serving as the education program director for the Lilly Endowment. He received his Ph.D. in public administration from the University of Colorado Boulder and his M.A. in education administration and policy from Columbia University Teacher's College. He has written and co-authored various policy reports, book chapters, and papers in professional journals. He currently serves on many boards, including Cornerstone Literacy, the Institute for Education Leadership, The New Teacher Project, and Alliance for Excellent Education. He is currently serving on the National Research Council's Committee for the Five-Year (2009–2013) Summative Evaluation of the District of Columbia Public Schools (2012–2015), and he previously served on the Committee on Defining Deeper Learning and 21st Century Skills and the Committee on Independent Evaluation of DC Public Schools.

Julie Morita, M.D., is the commissioner for the Chicago Department of Public Health (CDPH). She was appointed to this position following 15 years of service to the department. As medical director for the immunization program, Dr. Morita fostered partnerships with health systems and the private sector, achieving recognition for both the improvements in coverage and the overall coverage rates. In 2009 Dr. Morita led the city's response to the pandemic influenza outbreak, developing a system to distribute more than 1 million doses of vaccine to clinics and residents across the city. In 2014, as chief medical officer, Dr. Morita led the city's efforts to prevent the introduction and spread of the Ebola virus, including developing and launching the Chicago Ebola Resource Network, the first local network of medical centers working jointly to prepare and respond to a possible Ebola case. Dr. Morita has represented local public health as a member of the Advisory Committee on Immunization Practices, the National Vaccine Advisory Committee, the Illinois Immunization

Advisory Committee, the Chicago Area Immunization Campaign, and the Illinois Chapter of American Academy of Pediatrics. Prior to her time with CDPH, Dr. Morita served as an epidemic intelligence service officer with the U.S. Centers for Disease Control and Prevention and worked in private practice. Dr. Morita is a graduate of the University of Illinois at Chicago Medical School.

Patricia (Tia) Powell, M.D., is the director of the Montefiore Einstein Center for Bioethics and of the Einstein Cardozo Master of Science in Bioethics program at the Albert Einstein College of Medicine and Montefiore Health System. She is also a professor of clinical epidemiology in the Division of Bioethics, and of clinical psychiatry. Dr. Powell has bioethics expertise in public policy, dementia, consultation, end-of-life care, decision-making capacity, bioethics education, and the ethics of public health disasters. Prior to her positions at Einstein and Montefiore, she served 4 years as the executive director of the New York State Task Force on Life and the Law, which functions as New York State's bioethics commission. Dr. Powell graduated magna cum laude from Harvard-Radcliffe College. At Yale Medical School (from which she earned her M.D. in 1987) she earned the Parker Prize, Yale's highest award for a graduating medical student. She completed her internship, psychiatric residency, and Consultation-Liaison fellowship at Columbia. She is a board-certified psychiatrist and a fellow of the New York Academy of Medicine, the American Psychiatric Association, and The Hastings Center. She has worked with the National Academies of Sciences, Engineering, and Medicine on many projects related to public health and ethics and most recently served on the Committee on the Public Health Dimensions of Cognitive Aging.

Lisbeth (Lee) Schorr is a senior fellow of the Center for the Study of Social Policy. Her work is currently focused on efforts to broaden the conventional understanding of evidence as applied to the design, improvement, and evaluation of complex initiatives and on promoting a results orientation to the reform of social policies and programs. With a group of colleagues, she recently founded The Friends of Evidence, which works to strengthen the role of evidence in efforts (public and philanthropic, local, regional, and national) to ensure the wise allocation of scarce resources and to improve outcomes among the children and families who are not faring well in today's society. Ms. Schorr has extensive experience in social policy, community building, education, health, and human service programs—which has helped her to become a national authority on how to improve the future of disadvantaged children and their families and neighborhoods. She serves on the board of the SEED Foundation, was the founding co-chair of the Aspen Institute's Roundtable on Community

Change, and has held leadership positions in many of the major national efforts on behalf of children and youth, including the National Center for Children in Poverty, City Year, and the Foundation for Child Development. From 1998 to 2007 she was a member of the National Selection Committee of the Ford Foundation/Kennedy School Awards for Innovations in American Government. From 1965 to 1967, she headed the health division of the Community Action Program at the federal Office of Economic Opportunity.

Ms. Schorr has published two books regarding social problems and children and families. Her 1988 book, *Within Our Reach: Breaking the Cycle of Disadvantage*, analyzed programs and strategies that succeeded in effectively combating serious social problems. In *Common Purpose: Strengthening Families and Neighborhoods to Rebuild America*, published in September 1997, she laid out the evidence that by acting strategically and focusing on the systems contexts in which programs are implemented, it is possible to strengthen children and families and to rebuild communities. She has been awarded honorary doctorate degrees from Whittier College, Lewis and Clark College, Wheelock College, the University of Maryland, Bank Street College of Education, and Wilkes University. She is a member of the National Academy of Medicine and has served on numerous committees, forums, and boards, including the Committee for Increasing High School Students' Engagement and Motivation to Learn; the Board on Children, Youth, and Families; the steering group of the National Forum on the Future of Children and Their Families; and the Forum on Global Violence Prevention.

Nick Tilsen is a member of the Oglala Sioux Tribe and the founding executive director of the Thunder Valley Community Development Corporation. He has more than 11 years of experience in working with nonprofit organizations and tribal nations on projects that have a social mission. Mr. Tilsen's goal is to shift the narrative on Indian reservations from victimhood and negativity to empowerment and possibility, with a youth movement as the primary catalyst. His strategy is three-fold: first, reconnect youth with their cultural and spiritual identities as a foundation for responsibility and ownership; second, engage youth as both the drivers and the beneficiaries of a new wave of citizen-led activity on the reservation; and third, facilitate (by demonstrating success and through advocacy) a new framework through which governments, philanthropy, and tribes themselves address the social and economic conditions that persist on Indian land. Mr. Tilsen is also currently the project director for Oyate Omnicye, a process funded by the U.S. Department of Housing and Urban Development's Office of Sustainable Housing and Communities to create a reservation-wide plan for sustainable development for the Oglala

Lakota Nation. In 2012 Mr. Tilsen was recognized by President Barack Obama at the White House Tribal Nations Conference, who said, "day by day, family by family, community by community, Nick and his nonprofit have helped inspire a new beginning for Pine Ridge."

William W. Wyman, M.B.A., began his career at the management consulting firm Booz Allen Hamilton. After working for the firm in New York; Düsseldorf, Germany; Athens, Greece; and Dallas, Texas, he returned to New York to become the president of the Management Consulting Group, a member of the executive committee, and a member of the board of directors. In 1984 Mr. Wyman co-founded Oliver Wyman & Co, a general management consulting firm focused on the financial industries. The firm grew rapidly, and in 2004 it became part of Marsh & McLennan. Today, the firm is one of the world's leading management consulting firms, employing nearly 4,000 professionals in 26 countries. More recently, Mr. Wyman has served as a director or an advisor to nearly two dozen public and private companies in the finance and technology industries. He also has served as an advisor to several private equity partnerships.

Mr. Wyman has been a member of the board of the Dartmouth Hitchcock Medical Center, Mary Hitchcock Hospital, and the Dartmouth Hitchcock clinic. Some years ago, he and his wife founded an organization in Rwanda that has developed a model for the delivery of primary health care in rural Africa. Mr. Wyman received his B.A. from Colgate University and his M.B.A. from the Harvard Business School. He served in the U.S. Navy before starting his career. He resides in Hanover, New Hampshire.